Hx
Dsm
compare/contrast

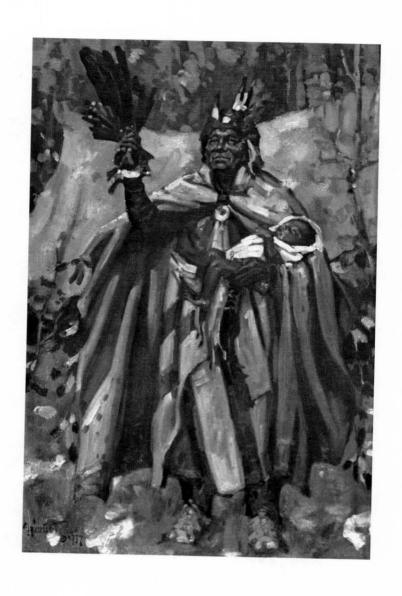

Children's Surgery

A Worldwide History

JOHN G. RAFFENSPERGER, M.D.

With Contributing Specialists

McFarland & Company, Inc., Publishers
Jefferson, North Carolina, and London

Frontispiece: *Blessing the Children* (1997), from the Blackfeet Sundance
Series of paintings by Gary Schildt at the C.M. Russell Museum in
Great Falls, Montana. The oil on canvas painting depicting a Blackfoot
medicine man holding an infant is similar to the logo of the American
Pediatric Surgical Association, a surgeon in cap and gown holding a
baby (courtesy Gary Schildt; Darrell Beauchamp, executive director;
and Lori Thompson, executive assistant of the C.M. Russell Museum).

LIBRARY OF CONGRESS CATALOGUING-IN-PUBLICATION DATA

Raffensperger, John G., 1928–
Children's surgery : a worldwide history / John G. Raffensperger ;
with contributing specialists.
p.   cm.
Includes bibliographical references and index.

ISBN 978-0-7864-6825-6
softcover : acid free paper ∞

I. Title.
[DNLM: 1. Child.   2. General Surgery—history.   3. Surgical Procedures, Operative—methods. WO 11.1]
617.9'8009 — dc23   2011053324

BRITISH LIBRARY CATALOGUING DATA ARE AVAILABLE

On the cover: *center: Blessing the Children* (1997), oil on canvas painting (courtesy
Gary Schildt, artist; Darrell Beauchamp, executive director; and Lori Thompson, executive
assistant of C. M. Russell Museum); *top left:* portrait of Percival Pott by George Romney, 1788
(courtesy Hunterian Museum at the Royal College of Surgeons); *top right:* surgeon © 2012
Shutterstock; *bottom left:* child © 2012 Shutterstock; *bottom right:* hydrocephalic skull of
25-year-old man (courtesy Hunterian Museum at the Royal College of Surgeons).
Front cover design by David K. Landis (Shake It Loose Graphics)

Manufactured in the United States of America

*McFarland & Company, Inc., Publishers
Box 611, Jefferson, North Carolina 28640
www.mcfarlandpub.com*

Acknowledgments

I am especially indebted to the librarians who gave of their time and talent to help create this book. Ronald Sims, special collections librarian of the Galter Health Sciences Library of Northwestern University, could, at a moment's notice, find "lost" references. Mr. Sims also did his best to teach me how to navigate the Internet. Carol Jeuell, reference librarian for the Brenneman Library of the Children's Memorial Hospital, Chicago, was always able to track down obscure journal articles; she kindly provided me with a copy of *A Century of Surgery, 1880–1990* by Dr. Mark Ravitch. Candace Heise, reference librarian for the Sanibel Public Library, through intra-library loan opened to door to the world's great libraries and invariably found important reference books and journals.

Many colleagues in the United States and overseas reviewed manuscripts and made suggestions. Dr. Ann Felice Ramenofsky, professor emerita of anthropology at the University of New Mexico, gave sound advice on early cultures and Native Americans. Charles Bagwell lent his expertise on surgery during the Middle Ages, Beiman Otherson shared his references to Ephraim MacDowel and Charles Kinlock, two early American surgeons. Tom Holder, Keith Ashcraft and Harry Richter provided important material on esophageal atresia. Jay Wilson had suggestions on the current treatment of diaphragmatic hernia and Michael Gauderer translated and corrected the material on Bochdalek and Heidenhain in the diaphragmatic hernia chapter. Laurence Moss was helpful with the chapter on necrotizing enterocolitis and David Wesson commented on trauma. Alberto Peña provided material to bring the chapter on ano-rectal anomolies up to date. Dan Young of Glasgow, Scotland, sent the entire bibliography of James Nicoll, an amazing turn-of-the-twentieth-century Scottish surgeon. Mark Dickens at the School of Oriental and African Studies of Cambridge University explained how the Syriac Christians brought Greek medicine to Islam. Dr. Patricia Donahoe kindly provided the painting depicting the first operation performed under ether anesthesia at the Massachusetts General Hospital in Boston. Dr. Jud Randolph and Lewis Spitz read and commented on the twentieth-century chapter.

David Raffensperger translated articles from the German literature and Becky Raffensperger used her computer expertise to find long-lost journal articles. My wife, Susan Luck, also a pediatric surgeon, read and corrected manuscripts.

I am indebted to the late Dr. Mark Ravitch, a Hopkins-trained surgeon, veteran of World War II and an all-around gentleman of the old school, for his work on pediatric surgical history. His book, *A Century of Surgery, 1880–1980*, is a marvelous history of American Surgery during the late nineteenth and twentieth centuries.

I owe a special debt to Dr. Orvar Swenson, who at age 103 is still actively interested in pediatric surgery. Dr. Swenson worked with Dr. Ladd in Boston and is a founding member of the Surgical Section of the American Academy of Pediatrics. He is best known for his elegant work on Hirschsprung's disease, but he also had brilliant results with a wide variety of lesions such as tracheo-esophageal fistula, intestinal atresia, Wilm's tumor and genitorurinary problems. Dr. Swenson was an inspiration during my early years in pediatric surgery. It was a privilege to observe his masterly surgical technique after I came to the Children's Memorial Hospital.

Each of us is all the sums he has not counted: subtract us into nakedness
And night again, and you shall see what started on Crete four thousand
   years ago
The love that ended yesterday in Texas.

— Thomas Wolfe

Table of Contents

PART II: SPECIFIC CONDITIONS AND TREATMENTS

Introduction

Children's surgery was the stepchild of adult medicine and surgery until the second half of the twentieth century; however, from the beginning of recorded medical history, some physicians and surgeons paid particular attention to birth defects and childhood injuries.

Surgical texts in ancient Egyptian scrolls were prescriptions for the treatment of injuries. Egyptian stone carvings depict circumcision, the first "elective" operation. The removal of stones by an incision into the bladder was perhaps the first major operation performed in children. Later surgeons treated clubfeet, anomalies of the anus and genitorurinary tract, cleft lip and hernia. It wasn't possible to treat birth defects of internal organs until after the nineteenth-century miracles of anesthesia and antisepsis, but medical historians consider the ancient practice of leaving deformed infants to die as "savage." Was abandonment a form of gentle euthanasia or murder? We still haven't answered the question of what is best for severely deformed infants.

Medical knowledge traveled from centers in India and Greece through Constantinople to Persia and Islam and finally back to Italy during the Middle Ages. The ancient Chinese, Indians and Greeks understood the need for cleanliness in wound care, but this knowledge was lost during the Middle Ages. Surgical technique and instruments changed little over the centuries. Most operations were performed with a knife, scissors, hemostats, needle, thread and the surgeon's fingers. During my internship in 1953, we bored holes in the head with a handheld drill and cut across bone with saws that were little different from those used by the ancient Greek or Islamic surgeons. It wasn't until the latter part of the twentieth century that surgeons could peer into the body cavities and operate with miniature instruments guided by images on a video screen. At this time, surgeons, remote from the patient, can repair organs or remove tumors while manipulating a computer-controlled robot.

Interest in children's surgery grew in Europe during the late nineteenth century, but the great twentieth-century development of pediatric surgery took place mainly at the Children's Hospital in Boston. In the aftermath of the Second World War surgeons flocked to Boston to learn new techniques and then returned home with their newfound skills. Today, children's surgery flourishes all over the world.

As an indication of how recently these advances have come about, the first patient to survive ligation of a patent ductus arteriosus in 1938 is still alive. Likewise, the first infant to survive primary repair of an esophageal atresia and tracheo-esophageal fistula, operated upon in 1941, is alive today. The longevity of these two patients also demonstrates the scope of children's surgery — a lifetime cure.

I first became involved with pediatric surgery during the 1950s. I later became the

1

chief of surgery at the Children's Memorial Hospital in Chicago and a professor of surgery at the Northwestern Medical School. Eleven of the contributing authors are either retired or actively practicing pediatric surgeons on medical school faculties. Two of the contributing authors are consulting academic pediatricians with an interest in the history of medicine. One of our contributing authors is a nurse, who has been involved with pediatric surgery as well as the editing of surgical manuscripts for 30 years. Most of the contributors of this book are from North America, but there are some from the United Kingdom, India and China. All of us are committed to the care of children and recognize the importance of bringing this extraordinary history of the surgical treatment of children not only to the medical profession but also to historians and others interested in child care.

PART I

In the Beginning

CHAPTER 1

Aboriginal Surgery

The healing arts most likely grew out of an instinctive impulse to nurture a sick, helpless infant. Our early ancestors may have learned to care for wounds and the healing properties of plants by observing animals, especially our closest relatives, the great apes. Gorilla infants remain in close contact with their mothers for nursing and grooming during the first three years of life.[1] If the mother dies or is separated from her infant, other females care for the orphan. Mother orangutans express grief and will continue to groom a dead infant.[2] Dian Fossey has observed a young female gorilla consoling and licking the wound of an injured older male.[3]

Trauma was likely the first surgical "disease" to afflict our ancestors. Imbedded foreign bodies, thorns, cactus spines, a splinter of wood or the spine of a fish that penetrated skin caused pain and swelling and discharged pus until it was removed. The first pediatric patient may well have been a child who stepped on a thorn. He cried, his foot became swollen and pus drained from the wound. His mother washed his foot and with her lips sucked out the pus and the thorn. The swelling and pain disappeared.

Our human ancestors, migrating from Africa to the most distant parts of the earth, gathered plants for food and found herbs that relieved pain and soothed wounds. When the English arrived in New Zealand, the Maoris had a vast knowledge of medicinal plants to treat illness and injury.[4] There is also evidence, in parts of the world as far-flung as New Zealand and California, that ancient healers used flaked stone tools for surgery.[5] The first operation, a deliberate incision into human flesh, was probably made to remove a deeply imbedded foreign body.

The intrusion of a foreign object was thought to be the cause of disease by many cultures, especially among Native North Americans.[6] In ancient China the inscription for an epidemic disease shows a man in bed with the arrow of disease shooting into him, and in the Talmud the illness and death of Titus was attributed to an insect that crawled through his nose into his head.[7] The concept of object intrusion as a cause of disease was reinforced when men began hurling missiles at one another and arrows became imbedded in the body. The appearance of an *Ascaris lumbricoides* in the stool of a sick child or a two-foot-long guinea worm, *Dracunculus medinensis*, emerging from a blister on the leg would confirm the idea that foreign objects were the cause of human illness. Object intrusion was a better theory of disease than bad air or God's punishment in Western medical tradition. It is a concept we must remember when a toothpick perforates the intestine or a leaking hearing aid battery erodes through a child's esophagus.

Our human ancestors learned to remove imbedded foreign bodies by sucking with the mouth. This technique became an almost universal method of treating illness. Shamans sucked on hollow tubes, such as reeds, horns or bird bones, to remove disease.[8] The application of hot cups to the skin to produce suction is another method. When combined with scarification or an incision, cupping was an effective way to drain an abscess. The induction of vomiting and purgation are other universal methods to rid the body of a foreign agent causing disease.

Though the medical and surgical practices of ancient cultures demonstrate many similarities, there are regional differences. Observations by early European explorers were biased and often inaccurate but do provide some information about medical practices in cultures that had no written record.

Explorers, missionaries and anthropologists observed and recorded the medical practices of North American natives for nearly five hundred years. At the time of conquest, Indians used more than four hundred medicinal plants, including a cure for scurvy, coca leaves to relieve pain and chinchona bark for malaria.[9] Balsam of Peru, turpentine and other agents used in wounds prevented infections. *Lithospermum ruderale* (Puccoon), used for birth control, contains natural estrogens that interfere with ovulation.[10] Many Indian remedies found their way into the white man's folk medicine and even our pharmacopeia. Podophylin, a native remedy, is still used for venereal warts. The Cherokee Indians used the pulverized root of *Spigelia marilandica*, known as pinkroot, to effectively treat intestinal worms.[11] Down from the common cattail was used to dress burns and as padding for infants' cradleboards. Pads of cattail and mosses were also used as diapers.[12] Many herbs were used for several different complaints at all ages, but specific roots were used on the gums of babies during teething and herbal teas were used to treat infantile diarrhea.

The first Europeans to reach the New World remarked on the excellent health of the natives and the seeming absence of birth defects and deformities. They also noted the skill with which the Indians treated wounds and their ability to survive injuries, even gunshots in viscera that would have killed a white man. As a result of frequent bathing and the use of a sweat lodge, the Indians were clean. With no knowledge of asepsis, they kept wounds scrupulously clean and used washes, powders and poultices made of boiled herbs. Several tribes sutured wounds with sinews and needles made of fish bone, with wicks of cloth or bark for drainage. Others grafted detached scalps and repaired torn ears with sutures of human hair or deer tendons. They controlled hemorrhage with spiderwebs or the down from birds to form a coagulum. In addition to wound care, Indians drained abscesses and even empyema. Two examples of surgery witnessed by a European attest to the skill of Indian surgeons. Naiuchi, a Zuni medicine man, first gave a woman with a breast abscess a decoction of datura (jimsonweed) that put her to sleep. He then incised the abscess with a sharp bit of flint and broke up the loculations with his finger. The lady slept through the procedure. The other case was a nine-year-old girl with a curvature of the spine and a cold abscess that pointed in the left groin. The incision extended from the posterior crest of the ileum downward almost to the inguinal ring. The wound was cleaned with water and packed with piñon gum, squash seeds and mutton fat. She died, apparently of tuberculosis, several months later.[13]

Other natives combined herbs with alum to control hemorrhage, and tribes from Peru to Canada treated wounds with egg whites, herbs, honey, Balsam of Peru and other resins derived from tree sap.[14] The Northern Cheyenne in Montana still use the spores of a brown puffball, *Bovista plumbea* (Lycoperdaceae), for bleeding and others applied the spores to umbilical cords of newborn infants to prevent infection.[15] Modern scientists have discovered that extracts from Lycoperdaceae produce significant antibiotic activity against a variety of bacteria.[16]

Indian "specialists" were also adept at setting fractures and reducing dislocations. Ojibwa medicine men treated broken bones by first washing the limb with warm water and rubbing the skin with grease and a poultice of wild ginger. Perhaps the heat and massage relaxed the muscles, so the fracture could be reduced with a "quick jerk." The limb was then immobilized with wooden splints or wet rawhide, which formed a tough, hard cast when dried. Others applied wet clay that hardened to a form-fitting cast.[17] Havasupai fracture doctors also used a mixture of hot ashes and wet sand to relax the muscles before reducing the fracture.[18]

Though Indian healers successfully treated many colonists, the Europeans, especially the missionaries, dismissed the natives' healing skills because the shamans who healed with herbs and surgery were considered pagans, even satanic. The healing practices of the shamans were founded on ancient traditions that were totally unlike Christianity. Individualistic Native American beliefs were based on dreams, the spirits of animals, departed ancestors and the forces of nature.[19] The shamans' healing often involved chanting, drumming and feats of magic to battle evil forces. A seventeenth-century Jesuit missionary referred to a shaman as a "juggler."[20]

Shamans underwent prolonged training and separation from the tribe in order to obtain healing power. The route to becoming a shaman often started with a dream or a severe illness that involved hallucinations or a near-death experience. They retreated to special places for solitude, fasting and sleep deprivation to induce an altered mental state. Initiates in some tribes used drugs such as datura that produce first nausea and vomiting, then ecstatic dreams in color that leave a sensation of rebirth. An older shaman interpreted the dreams of the initiate to determine the source of his power.[21] For example, tribes in the western Great Plains believed that visions of the bear gave the power to cure serious wounds.[22] The initiate then spent an apprenticeship with an older shaman to learn the rituals for healing and the traditions and taboos that protected the tribe. Europeans dismissed the drumming, chanting, prayer and dancing as pure witchcraft, but rhythmic sensory stimulation induces a powerful psychological impact and even an altered state of consciousness resembling anesthesia.[23] Religious sects continue to use music and other repetitive activity to induce hypnotic states that appear to activate the body's healing systems.[24]

When there was no obvious cause for disease, such as a wound, snakebite or fracture, shamans claimed that a particular sickness was caused by an object "shot" magically into the victim's body by an enemy or some spiritual being.[25] The object might be a pebble, a snake, a worm or even a bit of leather that could be removed with incantations and by sucking the affected part. The shaman would produce an object, and if the patient got well, could claim a cure. This process of blaming object intrusion and treatment with suction may go back to the real thorns and spines that afflicted ancient man. Sucking was probably the earliest treatment for real foreign bodies and is a universal treatment for snakebite. If, as some say, "magic is the father of medicine," then surgery may well be the mother of magic.

During the early part of the twentieth century, George Hunt, a well-educated Native American, became an assistant to Franz Boas, a pioneer anthropologist. In order to expose the "fraudulent practices" of shamans, Hunt went through the initiation ceremonies and learned the shaman's methods. As a part of his initiation, Hunt learned how to suck a bloody ball of eagle down from a patient and claim that he had removed the cause of disease. To his amazement, the patient recovered. Hunt become a skilled healer and cured many patients.[26] We should not be surprised, since patients often spontaneously recover and every doctor understands the power of a placebo.

Some shamans were best at treating mental illness. When a shaman was called to treat a young woman who could neither move nor speak, he first worked his chants, drumming and incantations. Then, with the aid of two assistants, he dunked her underwater in a nearby stream. She soon struggled and walked away — cured. This case reminded me of an intern colleague at the Cook County Hospital who had a patient, "paralyzed" from the waist down. He listened to her story and examined her while she was still on a wheeled cart. When he found that her sensation was normal, he lifted up one end of the cart so the patient slid down and landed on her feet. She cussed out the intern and walked out of the hospital.

Some shamans were generalists, while others had specific power to cure certain diseases. The prospective patient or his family would give gifts to the shaman before the healing ritual. A Montana Gros Ventre shaman, Little Man, had received his curing powers from a bear, an old man and a coyote. When a boy named Jimmy became ill with pain in his right side, the family called the shaman, according to the following account:

> Little Man painted his body the way the bear had told him, sang his healing song four times and passed a bear claw through a smudge fire. He said, "Tell me wherever it hurts and I will work on it." Jimmy said, "Here on my right side." The old man said, "That's a bad place. I don't like to suck there because it might hurt your guts. But I will use this bear claw." So he asked the boy, showing him the bear claw, "Do you think you can stand this?" Jimmy said he could and Little Man said, "Well, make sure you can stand it." He told the old lady to hold Jimmy's hands down and me to hold his feet down. The boy wriggled and made faces when the claw went in at the side. When Little Man jerked it out, a cherry seed and some "rotten gut" came with it. Right after that he was well.[27]

A bear claw is an unusual surgical instrument but would be sharp enough to make an incision through the abdominal wall. Was this magic, or did Little Man drain an appendiceal abscess? Older children with undiagnosed appendicitis often develop localized abscesses in the right lower part of their abdomen. In some cases the abscess spontaneously resolves, and others are cured by simple drainage of the pus. Foreign bodies such as cherry pits or a calcified fecalith, which resembles a cherry pit, often cause appendicitis. This case may be an example of pure hokum, but it is just as likely that Little Man hypnotized the boy with his bear song and drained an abdominal abscess.

American Indians learned to fashion instruments from available materials. A hollow reed attached to an animal bladder was used to irrigate wounds, or to give enemas, and bird beaks were used as forceps to extract foreign bodies. The following is an example of how a medicine man combined magic with surgery to remove an imbedded arrowhead:

> Rattles Stones Like a Bell, a Mandan Plains shaman during the mid-eighteenth century, received his doctoring powers from the crane. Another shaman, Cherry Necklace, had tried to remove an arrowhead stuck in the bone of a wounded warrior, but the man was in so much pain that he wouldn't go to sleep. The first shaman then consulted Rattles Like a Bell, who had two dried crane heads with the lower jaws attached and a stuffed crane. The shaman tied one of the dry heads around the patient's neck and painted his face red. He sang his medicine song, which put the wounded man to sleep. While he was singing, the crane came alive and walked around the wounded man. As the man was going to sleep, he heard the crane calling "Konix" and the medicine man answering "Konix" from the other side of the room. When he was asleep, the crane walked up to him and stuck his bill in the wound, using his bill as pinchers. After pulling several times, he succeeded in extracting the arrowhead. Matter and blood came out of the wound. The "doctor" then led his patient to the river to bathe, while the people in the village watched.[28]

This story also rings true. The hypnotic singing put the willing patient in a trance, allowing removal of the arrow point. Both the sandhill and the whooping cranes are magnificent birds that were once common throughout the West. Their long, strong bills could certainly be used as forceps. Bathing the man in the river was a good way to irrigate the wound.

We know nothing about the incidence of birth defects in Native Americans or how deformed infants were treated. Some observers claimed that the Indians abandoned deformed infants, but there is considerable evidence that Indian families were very careful of their children. In some tribes, due to their nomadic lifestyle, sick or aged relatives were left to die. A deformed child who could not keep up might also have been left behind.[29] The Sioux, by contrast, felt that a child was a great gift to be cherished.[30] The Cheyenne Elders, only two or three generations from the Indian massacres of the 1800s, remember that children were loved and protected. Mothers covered their infants with their own bodies to shield them from the soldiers' guns, and the rare child with a cleft lip or clubfoot grew to adulthood. There is also a Navaho tale of the Stricken Twins, one blind and the other lame, to illustrate the need for compassion. The blind twin carried his lame brother, who acted as his brother's eyes.[31]

Other ancient societies in different parts of the world expressed their fascination with birth defects by depicting deformities in amulets and statues.[32] One of the great stone statues on Easter Island had two heads, and in the Musée de Tahiti there is a carving of conjoined twins and a rock drawing of a woman delivering conjoined twins.[33] Other statues illustrate umbilical hernia, cleft lip and hyperthyroidism.[34]

North American Indians did not perform major amputations or trephinations, but skulls with holes indicating deliberate surgical trephination have been found in other parts of the world. Most of these operations were done in the Andes during the era of the Inca Empire. The Incas used a slingshot that threw an inch-and-a-half diameter stone, and a club with a bronze head, to bash the skulls of neighboring tribes. A collection of Inca skulls at the San Diego Museum demonstrated a variety of depressed skull fractures possibly due to hurled stones or war clubs. There were also skulls with small, round holes, suggesting an arrow wound or trephination with a drill. The absence of osteomyelitis in the skulls of survivors suggests the Indians used some form of antisepsis to prevent infection.[35] All evidence points to trephination as being a deliberate attempt to relieve the effects of trauma rather than to "let out evil spirits" as some have suggested.

An experienced Inca surgeon would have known that a depressed skull fracture causes coma with weakness or paralysis on the opposite side of the body. The next step would be an attempt to elevate the fracture with a lever. When this didn't work, the surgeon made a hole in the skull next to the fracture so he could introduce an instrument beneath the broken, depressed bone. This is exactly the procedure done today. It would not take a great step of imagination to believe that our ancient surgeon then opened the skull to release a blood clot. The finding of trephined children's skulls suggests that the operation was used to treat convulsions. In any event, the Inca surgeon appeared to treat his patients rationally. The oldest specimens of trephinated skulls date from as long ago as 3000 B.C.E., a time when the stone-headed ax was a favored weapon. Further evidence that trephination was used to treat real disease is suggested by Romanian shepherds who opened the skulls of sheep suffering from the staggers to remove the larva of Multiceps multiceps, a parasite.[36]

The Inca surgeon had to cut through the scalp with a sharp stone knife, possibly using extracts of coca leaves as a topical anesthetic. He could have controlled bleeding with pressure or with plants containing tannic acid. The surgeon chiseled away the outer and inner tables of the skull while avoiding injury to the dura mater. An alternative technique was to drill holes with a stone drill, twirled between the hands, and then connect the holes by chiseling the bone. Any modern surgeon who has drilled holes in the skull with a handheld drill and burr and then connected the holes with a Gigli saw knows that this is not an operation to be undertaken lightly. Among the Incas, the survival rate after trephination was approximately 75 percent, since 55 percent of trephinated skulls show complete and 16% demonstrate incomplete healing.[37] There are also skulls with multiple healed openings, indicating operations at different times with survival.

This cursory review of the literature reveals little about children's surgery in ancient times. It does suggest, however, that children were treated with love and respect and that a child with a wound or a fracture would be well cared for. Our ancient forebears had by trial and error discovered ways to prevent infection and relieve pain, and there were "specialists" who cured disease with their hands. At the time of conquest, the medicine and surgery of Native Americans was in many ways superior to that of Europeans. Unfortunately, the ridicule of the conquerors and missionaries together with devastating new diseases such as smallpox undermined the natives' faith in their traditional healing practices.

CHAPTER 2

Egyptian Papyri and Ritual Surgery

The first written records and stone inscriptions depicting surgery were found in Egypt. The Edwin Smith papyrus describes wound care as early as 3000–2500 B.C.E. The manuscript, made of papyrus, a reed that grows along the Nile River, was printed in pictorial signs or hieroglyphs. Other early Egyptian medical papyri indicate that the early doctor-priests used incantations, prayers and amulets to cure disease.[1] There were also conventional practitioners who used a wide range of drugs prepared from plants, animals and metal compounds. Thus, it is likely that Egyptian practice grew from the same combination of the supernatural and empiric medicine found in other ancient cultures.

This surgical treatise makes no mention of children but does provide our first recorded description of wound care. The papyrus was transcribed a thousand years after it was first written and appears to be incomplete. An American, Mr. Edwin Smith, found the papyrus at Luxor, Egypt, in 1862; James Henry Breasted of the Oriental Institute at the University of Chicago translated the hieroglyphs. Volume 2 of the translation consists of facsimiles of the original document on one page with a "clean" version on the facing page. Volume 1 contains the English translation with voluminous commentaries and interpretations. The general introduction provides the best references.[2]

The author of the papyrus systematically recorded a rational approach to 48 individual cases, suggesting that he was a surgeon. He described, for the first time, the meninges and the convolutions of the brain, the articulation of the mandible, the ribs, vertebrae, and recognized blood vessels. He knew that the brain controlled the motions of the body and recognized the importance of the pulse and the role of the heart in blood circulation.

The section on head wounds starts with a simple skin laceration penetrating to the skull and ends with a compound, comminuted skull fracture that exposed the brain. The treatments of fractures of the nose, maxilla, and zygoma and a dislocation of the mandible are rational and exhibit a good knowledge of anatomy. The author described wounds of the lip, chin and throat, crushed cervical vertebrae, clavicular fractures, injuries to the shoulder and humerus, fractured ribs, and last, a sprain of the spinal vertebra. The discussion of each case starts with the diagnosis and proceeds logically through examination and treatment.

In some cases, such as the open fracture of the skull, the surgeon predicted a fatal outcome and said "an ailment not to be treated." He did recommend keeping the patient upright to avoid pressure on the brain. In other cases that were possibly curable, he said "an ailment with which I will contend." All of the cases except for a tumor and an abscess of the breast appeared to be injuries due to falls or battle. The wounds were classified as soft tissue only, penetration to bone, perforation through bone, compound fracture and a "smash" that caused a compound comminuted fracture, including penetration to the brain.

The author used a form of adhesive tape to approximate simple flesh wounds, and in the case of a gaping wound of the eyebrow he said, "Thou shouldst draw together for him his gash with stitching." On the first day, the author applied fresh meat, perhaps to control hemorrhage; on the following days, a mixture of honey and grease was applied with lint.

Honey is mildly bacterostatic, and the author also used a decoction of willow leaves containing salicin that may have had a mildly antiseptic effect. For infected wounds, he used a solution containing salts of copper and sodium, similar to the normal saline soaks used today. The author immobilized fractures with medicated compresses, linen bandages and padded wooden splints.

In Case Twelve, we can see his perfectly rational approach to a patient with a broken nose, as well as the stilted language of the translation:

> If thou examined a man having a break in the chamber of his nose, and thou findest his nose bent, while his face is disfigured and the swelling which is over it is protruding, thou shouldst say concerning him; One having a break in the chamber of his nose. An ailment which I will treat. Thou shouldst force it to fall in, so that it is lying in its place, and clean out for him, the interior of both his nostrils with two swabs of linen until every worm of blood which coagulates in the inside of his two nostrils comes forth. Now afterward thou shouldst place two plugs of linen saturated with grease and put into his two nostrils. Thou shouldst place for him two stiff rolls of linen, bound on. Thou shouldst treat him afterwards with grease, honey and lint every day until he recovers.

The author was acquainted with children, because he likened the sensation of the brain in a patient with a comminuted fracture of the skull to the throbbing and fluttering of the weak place in the infant's crown before closure of the fontanel.

The Papyrus Ebers, dating from about the same time as the Edwin Smith papyrus, is a collection of remedies for internal ailments, diseases of the eye and skin problems. The sections concerning women and children include incantations, amulets to prevent disease and prescriptions for drugs.[3] The treatment for rectal prolapse included myrrh, frankincense, coriander, oil, and salt all boiled together and then applied to the "hinder part." Mostly, however, the magician-doctors relied on charms such as appeals to Horus to heal sick children. On the other hand, for a burned child the appeal to Horus is combined with a salve made of gum and ram's hair.[4]

The early Egyptian surgeons used bronze instruments, a great leap forward over stone tools. The temple at Kom Ombo, an ancient settlement on the east bank of the Nile twenty miles north of Aswan, is dedicated to Horus, a healing god. On one wall of the temple, there are carvings illustrating forceps, scalpels, hooks, saws and a speculum.

There are also illustrations of birth defects such as umbilical and inguinal hernia, clubfeet and dwarfs in statues and tomb reliefs. Though there was a royal proctologist (known as the herdsman of the anus), imperforate anus — an obvious anomaly — wasn't mentioned. There is little suggestion that the ancient Egyptians performed elective surgery, but they had knowledge of wound care and used an early form of antisepsis to prevent infection. They were also the first to use stitches to close wounds.[5]

Circumcision and Ritual Surgery

A carving from the tomb of Ankn-ma-hor at Saqquara in Egypt, dated approximately 2400 B.C., illustrates circumcision on teenage boys, the world's oldest depiction of a surgical operation.[6] Was this a religious rite of passage or was the operation performed for medical reasons? One medical indication for circumcision is an infected, swollen, painful foreskin that can't be retracted. Urination may be difficult. When warm soaks to the penis don't work, a small slit in the dorsum of the foreskin allows it to be retracted. It would only be a minor step to excise a part of the foreskin to prevent future problems.

Another explanation for circumcision follows from the mutilation of captured warriors in ancient Egypt.[7] At first an extremity was amputated, but if the prisoner survived, he was unfit for labor. The alternative, total castration by removal of the penis and testicles, carried too high a mortality rate. As a result, orchiectomy and later only circumcision marked these slaves. Eventually all descendants of slaves, including the Jews, were circumcised. By the time of the Jewish exodus from Egypt, circumcision had been adopted as a Jewish ritual. At some point in time, the operation was done in eight-day-old infants instead of older boys.[8] Moses Maimonides, the great twelfth-century Jewish physician, scholar and theologian, discussed circumcision in his commentary on the Mishneh Torah, saying: "The foreskin is regarded as an abomination, for which the gentiles are condemned in Scripture, as it is said, 'For all the nations are uncircumcised' [Jer. 9:25]. The patriarch Abraham was not called perfect until he had circumcised himself, as it is said, 'Walk before Me; and be perfect. And I will make My covenant between Me and you' [Gen. 17:1–2]. Whoever neglects the covenant of our ancestor Abraham, and retains the foreskin or artificially obliterates the marks of circumcision, even if he has acquired much knowledge of the Torah and practices good deeds, will have no portion in the world to come."[9] In his *Guide for the Perplexed*, Maimonides says circumcision is necessary to decrease sexual lust.[10]

Christians and Muslims adopted circumcision, and both male circumcision as well as excision of the clitoris in girls came to be practiced throughout much of the world, even in aboriginal Australia.[11] In Ottoman Turkey, circumcision of the Sultan's sons was an occasion for great festivities lasting 15 days.[12] There are detailed descriptions as well as lovely painted miniatures depicting the circumcisions of the sons of Mehmet in 1582 and the four sons of Ahmed III in 1720. The royal surgeons circumcised thousands of boys from poor families before operating on the Princes. The ceremonies took place in a special courtyard of the great Topkapi Palace in Istanbul overlooking the Bosporus. Fountains with running water at the windows of the courtyard provided a sense of tranquility and dulled the boys' cries. Led by the royal eunuch, two men marched each boy to the courtyard. The foreskin was cut with curved scissors between ligatures, and the wound was dressed with ashes or egg yolks boiled in rosewater. The Sultan demonstrated his power by providing days of sport, music and fireworks and gave gifts to the poor boys. Even today, in Istanbul one can see young boys, dressed in robes and crowns, going with their families to the circumcision ceremony.

Through the years, "congenital phimosis" and the "adherent prepuce" became diseases requiring surgical treatment. By the nineteenth century the operation was performed to treat bedwetting, masturbation, urinary infection, neurosis and even epilepsy. Today, circumcision remains the most common pediatric operation, demanded by parents and performed for the prevention of cancer and AIDS. Circumcision stands as an enduring symbol of the historic relationship between religion and medicine. It was probably the first "elective" operation, and from its beginnings only specialists — whether priests, blacksmiths or surgeons — performed the operation.

Another ancient form of ritual surgery, self-mutilation by amputation of a finger, is depicted in rock art.[13] The practice, which may have originated as a form of punishment or a way to protect children from evil, appears to have been most common in Australia and North America. When a Crow Indian died his near relatives sacrificed a finger, and when the tribe experienced high mortality from sickness or war men hacked off all but their thumbs and enough fingers to shoot a bow or gun. The amputations were performed through the first or second joint, by either running a sharp knife around the joint or striking with a tomahawk.[14]

The most extreme form of genital mutilation, castration, was used as punishment and a way to mark enemy captives. The lack of a beard and presence of a feminine voice made it easy to recognize slaves. Castration evolved into a way for rulers to have docile watchmen for the king's women. Since castration drove out sexual desire, princes and nobles used eunuchs to guard the harem. The word eunuch means "guard" or "bed keeper" in Greek. The avoidance of sexual sin and temptation also led to self-castration; St. Origen and St. Francis were self-imposed eunuchs.

The Sultans and Caliphs considered that removal of both the penis and testicles produced the safest eunuchs to watch over their harems. Since this operation carried a higher mortality rate, those whose testes and penis were removed were more valuable. The great eunuch factories of North Africa, often operated by Coptic monks, gathered thousands of boys every year and sold the survivors in markets all over Asia Minor. The helpless boy was tied down on a board and restrained with a collar around his neck. The operator then seized the penis and testicles and with one swoop of a razor-sharp knife slashed away the boy's manhood. A tube was placed in the urethra and the wound was packed to control hemorrhage.[15] Eunuchs often held prominent positions in courts, and in China young boys underwent the operation voluntarily.[16] Castration was also used to preserve a boy's singing voice. When Rome became a music center with the establishment of opera, eunuchs were in great demand and well-intentioned parents even allowed their children to be castrated to sing in church services.

The Edwin Smith papyrus provides a glimpse of how surgery progressed from the most ancient times. Surgeons had learned some anatomy, control of bleeding, suturing and wound care that may have inhibited infection. It is difficult for us to believe, but in all likelihood ritualistic surgery contributed to the surgeon's knowledge. At this stage in history, however, there has been no mention of surgery in children or the correction of birth defects.

CHAPTER 3

Biblical and Talmudic Accounts of Pediatric Conditions, Malformations and Diseases

JUDA JONA, M.D.

Ancient Hebrew texts, the Torah (the Five Books of Moses), the Mishnah, the Talmud, and other early sources, mention various deformities and conditions that classify a person as a "deviation" from the norm. Such a distinction places that person, if he is a member of the priestly tribe (Kohan), in a category that makes him unfit for service in the Holy Temple. These blemishes and malformations are mostly those visible to the public, and from their enumerations we may glean some insight into the extent to which the Hebrew sages recognized and classified them. In Leviticus 21:7, it is clearly stated that a priest who carries a deformity (*moom*) may not serve in the Holy Temple regardless of whether the deformity was from birth and permanent or transient or was acquired at some later point. Certain deformities may also preclude the priest from entering the Temple grounds altogether, and/or partaking from the usual portions of the sacrificial animal (the Korban) that belong to the priests. The donated portion of harvested products that the public is required to share with the priests (Troomot) is also forbidden for that blemished priest.

The second reason the Hebrew texts (Deuteronomy 25: 5–10) give for recognizing deformities and injuries pertains to the reproductive deficiencies of an individual, both male and female. Such recognition was used to nullify or prevent a marriage or in fulfilling the obligation of a Levirate marriage (*yiboom*). A Levirate marriage is the obligation of a brother of a man who dies without having children to take in marriage his widowed sister-in-law without an "official" wedding ceremony. Ordinarily, all other persons are strictly prohibited from taking a sister-in-law in marriage. The purpose of a Levirate marriage is to maintain the name of the deceased brother through closely related offspring. When either of the parties is sterile and cannot reproduce, however, there is no obligation for a yiboom. In the same vein, a person with a deformity that puts into question his or her true gender and that makes him or her sterile is prohibited from marriage within the Jewish community.

The third reason to recognize a deformity, especially in newborns, revolves around the issue of survivability. Any woman who gives birth to a living baby is considered impure (*niddah*) for a prescribed period of time. This bars her from conjugal relations and from

15

participating in any ceremonies in the Temple. The Hebrew sages recognized various deformities in babies that they proclaimed to be non-viable, and so the mother would remain pure after such a birth.

General Body Appearance

The general appearance of the priest, if unusual in proportions, size, and so on, will preclude him from Temple service but not from partaking in offerings.

A priest with unusually small stature, such as a dwarf or a midget (*na'nas*), is clearly mentioned in the Talmud (Bechorot 45/6), and also in the commentary on Leviticus 21:16–24 (Emor Sifra 3/95c).[1] Such an afflicted priest cannot serve in the Temple but may eat from the offerings.

A similar situation occurs when a priest is unusually large or tall. This condition was particularly prevalent among the ancient inhabitants of Canaan, as noted in Deuteronomy 3:11. The term "Kipe'ach" applies to these "giants" (Mishnah Bechorot 7:6 and Talmud Bechorot 58/b). In addition, among the general public marriage between two extra-short or extra-tall persons is clearly discouraged. If such a marriage occurred, divorce was encouraged by the rabbis.

Another condition recognized by the sages that affected general appearance was gynecomastia, the development of large mammary glands in men.[2] If it occurred in a priest, this condition made him unfit for service in the Temple.

Head and Face Deformities

Specific head abnormalities that preclude a priest from Temple service are generally those that are visible to the eye and involve the cranium. Those mentioned in the Talmud (Bechorot 43/b) are *kilon*, a pointed top of the head that is shaped like a keg cover; *liftan*, where the head is wide on the top and narrow lower down; *makban*, a hammer-like head shape with frontal prominence; and *segalgal*, a deformity presenting as a perfectly rounded head. This condition was thought to occur only in Babylon, since the Talmudic sage Hillel stated that there were unskilled midwives in Babylon who did not know how to shape the newborn head (Talmud Shabbat 31/a).

Various eye and eyebrow deformities, at times pathological or just profoundly unsightly, also excluded a priest from service in the Temple. Leviticus 21:18 says that he whose nasal bone is depressed or missing and whose eyes almost touch each other is to be excluded from Temple service and from partaking in the offerings. The meanings of many of the other deformities mentioned in Leviticus are obscured today, but the principle of negative impact on the priest's appearance prevails. Talmud Niddah 23/b clearly describes a Cyclops (a baby with only one eye in the middle of the face). This indicated a non-viable condition and the mother remained pure after giving birth. The rabbis went on to mention, however, that if a newborn has only one eye positioned on one side, the baby is regarded as viable and the mother as impure.

Hand, Foot and Limb Deformities

Congenital hand malformations and those incurred as a result of injuries or poor healing are also among the categories that barred a priest from service. Specifically mentioned is a poorly healed fracture (Talmud Bechorot 45/a). On the same page, the occurrence of extra digits in one or all limbs is discussed. Even in those days, this was recognized as a common anomaly. However, the significance of supernumerary digits caused much debate among the sages. According to Rabbi Yehuda (Talmud Bechorot 45/a), a person with extra digits is "fit" (*kasher*) to serve in the Temple, but the sages overruled him and called such a person unfit.

Non-symmetrical limbs are another type of defect mentioned. This condition, hemi-hypertrophy, could be congenital, as elaborated by Rashi in Leviticus 21:18, or could exist as a consequence of overuse of a limb, with excessive muscular growth.[3] This deformity affected a person's general appearance and prevented a priest from serving.

A newborn missing a single limb (foot or hand) is considered viable and the mother is impure for the prescribed duration following such a birth (Talmud Niddah 23/b). Deformities of the lower extremities, and especially abnormal feet, were particularly emphasized in exempting a priest from Temple service, keeping in mind that the priests perform the Holy Service barefoot. Most notorious among these deformities was clubfoot. Leviticus 21:18 describes a limping person who may be exhibiting a hollowed mid-foot along with crooked toes. The Rambam (Maimonides) explains this as one who walks on his heel and toes, with the forefoot arched upward and the toes turned inward, which is a typical clubfoot appearance. In addition, pigeon toes and an acquired bunion are described in Hilcot Bet Hamikdash 8:13.

Deformities of Internal Organs

The ancient Hebrew texts mention several deformities of internal organs as well. Esophageal atresia is clearly mentioned in Talmud Niddah 23/b, stating that if the esophagus in a baby is obliterated (*atoom*), the child cannot survive. Interestingly, this prognosis remained dire until well into the twentieth century. On the other hand, a perforated or open (*nakoov*) esophagus may present a chance for survival of the baby, though no remedy is offered. This distinction was primarily important for observing the purity status of the mother.

Asplenia, either acquired or due to congenital absence, was not considered a threat to life (Mishnah Chulin 3:2).[4] In Talmud Sanhedrin 21/b, Rabbi Yehuda said in the name of Rav that Adoniya, the son of King David, procured 50 runners to run before his chariot. Rabbi Yehuda believed Adoniya had their spleens eliminated (shrunk) using medications, so that they could run faster.

Imperforate anus was likewise known to the Talmudic sages. The recommendation given in Talmud Shabbat 134/a was to rub the perineum with oil and cut at the most transparent site with the pointed end of a barley grain. This could be done for a covered anus and/or a very low anal atresia. Use of metal, especially iron, instruments was prohibited in this situation, because of the inflammation it might provoke (Talmud Chulin 77/a).

The lodging of foreign bodies in the esophagus or pharynx, a common occurrence in children, was recognized as a most dangerous event. For a pharyngeal object, it was permitted to desecrate the Sabbath in order to remove the object because of the threat to the individual. For deeply lodged esophageal foreign bodies, only magical incantations could be offered.[5]

Genital Issues

Hypo/epispadium, undescended testicles (UDT), and intersex anomalies have a strong impact on the reproductive capabilities of males and females. Much is written in the Torah, Mishnah and Talmud concerning the appearance of these problems and the prohibitions that follow them, especially the way they affect priestly service in the Temple. In addition, these anomalies can lead to nullification or even prohibition of a marriage within the Jewish community. Finally, they can affect Levirate marriage for both the man and the woman.

Hypo- and epispadius is a malformation of the external genitalia that is most commonly recognized in males but can be present with less functional aberration in females. In Talmud Yevamot 76/a, by decree of Rava the son of Rav Huna, it was written that a priest who urinates from two locations is unfit for service in the Temple. Rosner (p. 219) assumed that such an anomaly could be described as either a urethral fistula or hypospadius. The decree could also be applied to a Levirate marriage. Since the rabbis assumed that he who ejaculates anywhere but from the glans would not be fertile (that is, "cannot shoot his sperm like an arrow"), such a male was not to marry or give a yiboom. Elaborating further on the same anomaly, Talmud Bechorot 44/b mentions that a male may have two channels, one for urine and the other for semen. If there is a connection between them, the man may be sterile and all restrictions therefore apply.

Undescended testicles (UDT) are mentioned in Talmud Bechorot 44/b, which states that the term *mero'ach ashach* (which also appears in Lev. 21:20) refers to someone who is missing one or both of his testicles. Rabbi Akiva, however, interprets the term to mean "he who has a space between his testicles," or a bifid scrotum. This condition primarily affects priests who cannot serve in the Temple or visit the place but may eat from the Temple offerings. The term *meshuban* (Mishnah and Talmud Bechorot 44/b) refers most likely to a person who has extremely large testicle(s). This can easily be assumed to mean the presence of a hydrocele or a hernia. This condition also prohibited a priest from service or visits in the Temple. If a man's penis was unusually large, he fell into the same category as one with enlarged testicles. Deuteronomy 23:2 describes one whose glans is missing and who is therefore prohibited from marrying an Israelite woman because he is assumed to be sterile. Talmud Yevamot 8/b emphasizes that if even a sliver of his corona remains, he may marry. The Rambam (Maimonides) permits all to marry if the glans is absent due to an illness or is congenitally absent. Rabbi Shmuel agrees that if the cause is congenital, then in all instances the man may marry (Talmud Yevamot 75/b). However, if the absence of the glans is due to injury or is self-inflicted, the man cannot marry.

Androgyny and hermaphrodism are clearly mentioned in Mishnah/Talmud Niddah 28/a. The text states that if a mother delivers a baby whose sex is unclear, a question is raised as to the amount of time the mother must observe "unclean" days in the postpartum period. This period differs with male and female newborns. The text further states that if as an adult an androgyne brings forth a white emission (probably sperm) or a red emission (probably menstrual blood) or both, he/she may not enter the Holy Temple, as would a regular man or woman. In Talmud Chagiga 4/a, androgynes are excluded from the obligation of going to Jerusalem (Aliyah L'Regal) and visiting the Temple, as is required by all males three times a year (Exod. 34:23).

The male genital abnormality known as *toomtoom* describes a baby whose sex is unclear at birth. However, if he/she is operated on and found to be a boy and later noted to be sterile, he cannot give yiboom (Talmud Yevamot 83/b). It is unclear if the toomtoom is also excluded from the obligation of visiting the Temple three times a year, because if he is "opened" (operated on) he may be found to have bilateral cryptorchidism and therefore be regarded as a male. In general, he would have all male religious obligations, but if he is a firstborn he is not entitled to a double portion in his father's inheritance.

Regarding female genital anomalies, there is mention in Talmud Bechorot 45/a of a prostitute in whom a double vagina ("two doors") was found. More significant is the case of the Eyelonit, a female phenotype with primary amenorrhea (most likely Turner's Syndrome). Deuteronomy 25:6 mentions the fact that since the primary purpose of Levirate marriage is to produce an heir for the deceased husband, if the widow is an Eyelonit and cannot bear children there is no need for yiboom. This is based on the explicit statement in the Torah regarding the yiboom "...she should bear–give birth." In addition, because of her sterility, her deceased husband could have dismissed her from their marriage without an official divorce decree (get), meaning that the initial marriage was never sanctified (Talmud Yevamot 2/b).

Monstrosities or Teratology

In order to consider the product of the womb a human being, it must have a human face, even if the rest is not recognizable as human. For a humanoid face, the rabbis in Talmud Niddah 23/b required a forehead, eyebrows, eyes, cheeks and chin. Ears, nose and mouth are not among the requirements. The one with no forehead, who is thought to represent anencephaly, is also mentioned with the preceding deformities. Newborns and children with spinal abnormalities were recognized in the Torah (Lev. 21:20). In Talmud Niddah 24/a, a crooked or split spinal column is described. This same Talmudic discourse mentions a newborn whose lower body and legs may be missing or underdeveloped (a deformity known nowadays as caudal regression) and who may fall under the category of non-viable offspring in order to exclude the mother from having to observe the obligatory impure period after birth. When a priest has a hunched back or a similar deformity, he is not allowed to serve.

Parasitic and Conjoined Twins

An unusual case of a parasitic twin is described in Talmud Niddah 25/b. The parasite is called sandal, a name given to a flatfish, such as sole. The text states that the parasitic twin was always seen with an otherwise well-formed and viable twin. However, Yerushalmi Talmud (Niddah 3:50/d) states that the well-formed twin baby was considered non-viable for the purpose of the mother's purity.

Talmud Menachot 37/a deals with conjoined twins where both appear viable at birth. At the time of the Mishnah, Rabbi Yehuda HaNasi issued an edict that the father of firstborn conjoined sons must pay twice the required five shekelim (five for each boy) in order to redeem them from the priest (Num. 18:16). Later rabbinical writings (Ralbag in 1547, Shuvat Ya'akov in 1739, Chesed Shlomo in 1773 and others all the way into the modern era) dealt mostly with the ethical issues of such twins.

CHAPTER 4

Pediatric Surgery in Ancient India

V. RAVEENTHIRAN, M.D.

India, a cradle of ancient civilization, has virtually forgotten her ancient history of medicine.[1] Archeological excavations at Mohenjo-Daro and Harappa reveal details of the Indus valley civilization that flourished during India's Bronze Age (circa 2500–1700 B.C.E.).[2] Nothing is known about the health-care system prevalent in this civilization. Arguably, access to plenty of nutritious food, an unpolluted environment and a general state of peace could have contributed to infrequent disease. However, it is also plausible that Aryans, who invaded the Indus valley between 2000 and 1500 B.C.E., might have destroyed the native medical system to prove their supremacy. Aryans, a tribe of Indo-European ancestors, developed their own code of life known as the Vedas.[3] Among the four Vedas, Atharvana contains sections pertinent to health care. This section is called Ayurveda (from Ayush, which in Sanskrit means "longevity," and Veda, which means "code").

Ancient Hindus considered it a sin to write Vedas in any media.[4] Generation after generation, the Vedas were transmitted secretly by word-of-mouth among selected clans of Aryans. Transmission through each generation unwittingly introduced additions, omissions and redactions to the original text that could not be traced in the absence of a written master copy. An unremitting succession of foreign invasions (including the Greeks, Mongols, Arabs, Moghals, British, French and Portuguese) and the resultant sociopolitical calamity that prevailed over several millennia meant that Aryans could not keep up the chain of continuity of knowledge. Consequently, most books of the Vedic period (circa 2000–1200 B.C.E.), including Ayurvedic texts, are lost or are only available in a distorted form.[5]

With the rise of Buddhism in the post–Vedic period (circa 600–200 B.C.E.), the cultural focus shifted from theology, superstition and secrecy to the wider well-being of humanity.[6] Buddhist monks who did not care for the sentiments and superstitions of Hindu Brahmins began to write useful texts in the form of palm-leaf manuscripts and stone engravings. One such monk, Nagarjuna (circa 150–250 C.E.), compiled the scattered verses of Ayurvedic texts available to him.[7] The three major compendia of Ayurveda that we find today — *Sushruta Samhita*, *Charak Samhita* and *Vagbhata Samhita*— are thus redactions of redactions collected by Nagarjuna.

While the *Charak Samhita* and *Vagbhata Samhita* are concerned with medical illnesses, the *Sushruta Samhita* records ancient India's surgical heritage.[8] *Samhita* in Sanskrit means "compendium," and the three texts are named after their respective authors. Most Western historians place the author *Sushruta* between 1200 and 600 B.C.E.[9] He learned the art of surgery at Kasi from the Holy Lord Dhanvantri.[10] Dhanvantri is regarded as a demigod of medicine in Hindu mythology, as is Asclepius for Greeks and Imhotep for Egyptians. Kasi, located on the banks of the River Ganges, had a reputable university that dated back to the establishment of the world-famous Nalanda University of the Buddhist era.

Sushruta was obviously not the first surgeon of ancient India.[11] He frequently cited passages from the books of Prajapati, Ashvins, Indra and Devodasa, which are now lost. Thus, the collective wisdom found in the *Sushruta Samhita* goes back to incalculable antiquity.

The Sushruta Samhita and Pediatric Surgery

Sushruta divided his portion of the Ayurveda into eight subspecialties: Salya Tantra (surgery including traumatology), Shalakya Tantra (otorhinolaryngology and oral surgery), Kaya Chikisa (internal medicine), Bhuta Vidya (the science of children, though often mistranslated as "exorcism"), Kaumara Bhritya (pediatric care), Agada Tantram (toxicology), Rasayana Tantra (the science of rejuvenation) and Vajeekarana Tantram (sexology).[12] In Western countries, pediatrics did not become a separate specialty until the late nineteenth century, but Sushruta identified pediatrics as distinct from adult medicine and considered anyone below 16 years of age as a child. Those less familiar with Sanskrit tend to translate *Bhuta* as "demon," but the word also means "child."[13] Vidya, which means "science," makes no sense when used in combination with the word "demon." Therefore, *Bhuta Vidya* must mean "Pediatric Medical Science." Similarly, *Kaumara Bhritya* likely means "Pediatric Nursing" (*Kaumara* means "childhood;" *Bhritya* means "care" or "nursing"). Unfortunately, books on Bhuta Vidya have long been lost.

Sushruta also defined the viability of a fetus long before modern experts set 28 weeks as the time when lung maturity enables the fetus to breathe on its own: "For four months after the date of fecundation, the faetus remains in a liquid state, and hence its destruction or coming out of the womb goes by the name of abortion. In the course of the fifth and sixth months the limbs of the foetus gain in firmness and density, and hence, its coming out at such a time is called miscarriage (sic)."[14]

Sushruta meticulously described human anatomy under the section "Sarirasthanam" of his samhita.[15] He gained his anatomical knowledge through the dissection of pediatric corpses. Hindu holy scriptures dictate that any dead human being must be burned rather than buried, but infants younger than two years and firstborn male children were exceptions to this rule.[16] Adult corpses in ancient India being unavailable, anatomical dissections could only be done on the buried corpses of children. This probably explains why Sushruta counted more bones than his Greek counterparts; he may have counted the unossified parts of a child's bones separately, leading to an excess of 60 bones.[17]

Sushruta was aware of the circulatory system centuries ahead of William Harvey.[18] He called arteries *dhamani* and veins *sira*. He pointed out that in placental circulation fetal and maternal blood never mix; nutrients cross the placental membrane by transudation.

Sushruta outlined the theory of crossing over of paternal and maternal genes and maintained that a child is formed by half *pitrika* (paternal factors) and half *matrika* (maternal factors).[19] An embryo's sex was said to be determined by the domination of pitrika or matrika. When both were equally dominant, the result was believed to be a hermaphrodite.

Sushruta's discussion of organogenesis in an embryo is an intellectual treat:

Saunaka says that probably the head of the foetus is first developed since the head is the only organ that makes the functions of all other organs possible. Kritaviryya says it is the heart that is first developed since the heart is the seat of Manah and Buddhi [mind and intellect]. The son of Parasara says that the development of the umbilical region of the foetus must necessarily precede [that of any other part of its body], inasmuch as it is through the umbilical cord that an embryo draws its substance from its mother's body. Markandeya says that the hands and feet of a foetus are first to be developed since they are the only means of movements in the womb. Sabhuti Gautama says that the development of the trunk is the earliest in point of time, since all other limbs and organs lie soldered to and imbedded in that part of the body. But all these are not really the fact. Dhanvantari holds that the development of all the parts of the body of an embryo goes on simultaneously; and they cannot be perceived or detected in their earlier stages of development in the womb owing to their extremely attenuated size.[20]

Sushruta clearly distinguished between three different types of congenital disorders.[21] *Adivala pravritta* (genetic or familial disorders) stemmed from defective semen or ovum; *janmavala pravritta* (congenitally acquired disorders) resulted from improper conduct by the mother during her pregnancy; and *sahaja* (sporadic malformations) occur through unexplained causes. Sushruta has recorded several congenital malformations, including cleft palate, cleft lip, hemangiomas, congenital deafness, achondroplasia, congenital cretinism, intersex disorders such as congenital adrenal hyperplasia, upper limb malformations such as meromelia, undescended testis, congenital stricture urethra and kyphoscoliosis.

He describes surgical correction for some of them, such as the suture of split lips using bolsters. However, he attributes the majority of these malformations to the mother's improper conduct; excessive talkativeness, for example, caused cleft palate, and extramarital coitus caused virilization of the newborn. Children with gross malformations were considered a source of shame and abandoned in the wilderness, and so Sushruta does not describe the surgical correction of malformations. Abandonment of anomalous children was common among ancient people; according to Greek mythology, beautiful Aphrodite was ashamed of her son Priapus, who was born with a hunchback, disproportionately large penis, dark complexion and large tongue. She abandoned Priapus in the wilderness to be raised by shepherds.[22]

Sushruta did describe several afflictions of childhood such as inguinal hernia, hydrocele, phimosis, paraphimosis, rectal prolapse, soft tissue abscesses, splenomegaly, ascites, greenstick fractures, congenital syphilis, congenital leprosy, tubercular lymphadenopathy of the neck, facial palsy in newborns (probably due to obstetric trauma) and sacrococcygeal teratoma.[23] Sushruta believed that prolonged withholding of urine caused scrotal hydrocele, but he seemed to grasp the concept of urine reflux from the bladder to the ureters:

> The urinary ducts (ureters) pass close by the large intestines (pakvasaya) and constantly replenish the bladder and keep it moist with that waste product of the system in the same manner as rivers carry their contributions of water into the ocean. These passages or ducts (which are two) are found to take their origin from hundreds of branches [or mouths, tubuli uriniferi], which are not visible to the naked eyes, on account of their extremely attenuated structures.... The vayu in the bladder, coursing in its natural downward direction, helps the full and complete emission of urine; while coursing in a contrary direction, it gives rise to various forms of maladies such as prameha [urinary tract infection] or strangury.[24]

There cannot be a more accurate description of vesicoureteric reflux than this. Similarly, Sushruta described a condition called *vadha gudodaram*, which is remarkably similar to the modern description of Hirschsprung's disease.[25] Sushruta considered some of these disorders incurable, but he described palliative operations such as a sigmoid colostomy to relieve Hirschsprung's disease.

Sushruta also described caesarian section, vesicolithotomy, urethral strictures and rhinoplasty, but his most important contribution to our history of pediatric surgery was his description of extracting bladder stones through a perineal incision. This may have been the first elective pediatric operation:

> A person of strong physique and un-agitated mind should be first made to sit on a level board or table as high as the knee-joint. The patient should then be made to lie on his back on the table placing the upper part of his body in the attendant's lap, with his waist resting on an elevated cloth cushion. Then the elbows and knee-joints [of the patient] should be contracted and bound up with fastenings (sataka) or with linen. After that the umbilical region [abdomen] of the patient should be well rubbed with oil or with clarified butter and the left side of the umbilical region should be pressed down with a closed fist so that the stone comes within the reach of the operator. The surgeon should then introduce into the rectum, the second and third fingers of his left hand, duly anointed and with the nails well pared. Then the fingers should be carried upward towards the rope of the perineum i.e. in the middle line so as to bring the stone between the rectum and the penis, when it should be so firmly and strongly pressed as to look like an elevated granthi [tumor], taking care that the bladder remains contracted but at the same time even.
>
> An operation should not be proceeded with nor an attempt made to extract the stone in a case where, the stone on being handled, the patient would be found to drop down motionless with his head bent down and his eyes fixed in a vacant stare like that of a dead man, as an extraction in such a case is sure to be followed by death. The operation should only be continued in the absence of such an occurrence.
>
> An incision should then be made on the left side of the raphe of the perineum at the distance of a barleycorn and of a sufficient width to allow the free egress of the stone. Several authorities recommend the opening to be on the right side of the raphe of the perineum for the convenience of extracting the stone from its cavity so that it may not break into pieces nor leave any broken particles behind, however small, as they would in such a case be sure to grow larger again. Hence the entire stone should be extracted with the help of a forceps, the points of which are not too sharp.
>
> After the extraction of the stone, the patient should be made to sit in a cauldron full of warm water and fomented, thereby. In doing so the possibility of an accumulation of blood in the bladder will be prevented; however, if blood be accumulated therein, a decoction of the Kshiira-trees should be injected into the bladder with a urethral syringe.[26]

At the end of this description he added: "children are more frequently afflicted by bladder stones, as they take less water and as they indulge in daytime sleep; but it is easier to do the operation in children as the bladder is superficial and thin in them." The success of this operation probably prompted Abillsaibial (800 C.E.) to translate *Sushruta Samhita* as *Kitab-i-Susrud* in Arabic.[27]

Throughout his Samhita, Sushruta emphasized the differences between adult and pediatric surgery and warned that metal instruments should not be used in a struggling child, as they may penetrate deeper than the intended level. Instead he advocated sharp-pointed instruments of soft materials, such as bamboo strips, blades of *khusa* grass, crystals and broken glass, to make incisions (*bhedanam*) in children.[28] When children were frightened by the knife or other instruments, he advised the surgeon to use sharp fingernails to make quick incisions of abscesses and to use nails as forceps for extraction of foreign bodies. Alkali and cauterization had been recommended in adults for hemostasis, but he prohibited their use in children. Bloodletting by venesection was commonly used in adults, but the application of a leech was used in children. Anal fistulae of adults were cauterized using alkali, but pediatric anal fistulae were treated by a gentler medicated seton.

Wine and strong decoctions of Indian hemp or datura were used to anesthetize adult patients, but for children he advised toys and distraction rather than drugs. Sushruta gave meticulous instruction to calculate drug dosage in infants and children when necessary; the dose of a drug should be increased by one *rati* per month until one year of age and thereafter by one *masha* per year of age. Exact modern equivalents of measurements such as rati and masha are not known. In breast-fed newborn infants, Sushruta recommended that drugs intended for a child should be administered to the mother and excreted in her milk. For older infants, he advised that the mother's breast be plastered with a paste of the drugs so that the infant could unknowingly consume them while breast-feeding.

Several sections of the *Sushruta Samhita* contain incomplete descriptions of disease, perhaps because of lost text. Sushruta mentioned frothing of saliva as a disorder peculiar to infants, possibly a sign of esophageal atresia. Also, his description of blood-mixed mucoid stools and an intermittent cry in infants may have been referring to an intussusception. Sushruta may also have been referring to an appendiceal abscess when he said that a tundi (umbilical abscess) was incurable.[29]

There is considerable evidence to suggest that ancient Hindu surgeons operated on infants and children to drain abscesses and remove bladder stones, as well as performing rhinoplasty and possibly even a colostomy for Hirschsprung's disease. The *Sushruta Samhita* shows considerable sophistication of medical knowledge for its day, stretching back into Indian antiquity.

CHAPTER 5

Traditional Chinese Medicine

JIN-ZHE ZHANG, M.D.

Traditional Chinese medicine's five-thousand-year history is an important part of China's ancient civilization. Legends such as Fu Xi inventing nine types of needles and Sheng Nong tasting hundreds of herbs show that Chinese medicine can be traced to remote antiquity, when there were no written records. Surgeons were illiterate but passed on their craft to students by practice and oral teaching. There is, however, archeological and X-ray evidence suggesting that ancient surgeons deliberately opened the skulls of human beings during the New Stone Age with stone or bronze instruments. It appears that surgery developed in China in the era of hunting and gathering, long before Confucian doctors or written language.

The "Tian Guan," a chapter in the classic book the *Zhou Li*, written in 600 B.C.E., recorded that chief doctors were government officials in charge of health administration and the collection of herbs to cure disease. There were specialists in diet therapy, surgery, internal medicine and veterinary medicine. During the Han Dynasty (600–300 B.C.E.), the first Chinese history book, the *Zuo Zhuan,* or *Chronicle of Zuo*, recorded the "Pathogenesis of Six Climatic Factors" (6 Qui), or the yin, negative; yang; positive; wind; rain; darkness; and brightness. The *Shi Ji*, records of the grand historian, chronicled achievements of the legendary doctor Bian-que, who first made diagnoses by feeling the pulse. Bian-que's real name was Qin Yue-ren, and according to the dates of his birth and death, it may be that his name was fabricated to represent all the famous doctors of that time. Many of the official records of medicine during the Spring and Autumn of the Warring States Period (600–300 B.C.E.), written by Ban Gu in the official record, the Han Shu, have been lost. Fortunately, the book *Prescriptions for Fifty-two Diseases*, written on bamboo slips, was unearthed at the Mawangdui tomb near Changsha City in 1972. This text describes surgical techniques for problems such as knife wounds, neonatal tetanus and the treatment of anal fistula.

Three famous doctors are recorded in the *History of the Eastern Han Dynasty* and the *History of Three Kingdoms*, before the third century C.E. The first, Zhang Zhong-jing, the Sage of Medicine, wrote *Treatise on Cold Damage and Miscellaneous Disease*. This volume was lost, but Zhang's student Wang Shu-he recompiled the material during the Jin Dynasty (260 C.E.) into *Synopsis of Prescriptions of the Golden Chamber and Treatise on Cold Remedies*. Zhang Zhong-jing may have been the first to develop the idea of targeted treatment in his work *Pattern Identification and the Classical Formula*.[1] At about the same time, another of his students, Du Du, wrote *Infant Fontanel Prescriptions*, the first book on pediatrics in China. Its primary focus was on fevers and infectious diseases.

The second of the famous doctors, Hua Tuo, addressed as the Originator of Surgery, may well be the first surgeon in history to recommend elective laparotomy to cure disease.[2] In "Fang Shu Lie Zhuan" from the *History of the Later Han Dynasty*, he wrote: "For those patients with diseases in the interior, and the drug or acupuncture is unable to reach, the body should be cut open to remove the disease accumulations. If the disease is in the intestine, the latter should be also cut to remove the bad contents. The wound should be sutured and an herb paste applied. The wound would heal in four to five days and the patient will recover in a month."

Hua Tuo used an herb, Mafo powder, in wine as an anesthetic. He also developed the "Five Animal Exercises," a system of physical exercise still popular in China. During the early years of the Three Kingdoms Period, he was a military surgeon, but because of his pride he left the army, was arrested and was killed in jail. His *Book in a Blue Bag* was burned, but his student Wu Fu wrote *Hua Tuo's Prescriptions*.[3]

Dong Feng (220 C.E.), China's foremost medical ethicist, never accepted a fee but asked for apricot seeds as payment for curing a disease. In time, a prosperous apricot orchard surrounded his house. The phrase "the spring of apricot forest" is still used to praise a skilled, ethical physician.

During the Tang Dynasty in the seventh century, when scientific medicine developed, the most prominent doctor was Si Miao, considered the god of herbal medicine. His encyclopedia of medicine, *Essential Prescriptions Worth a Thousand Gold*, included chapters on internal medicine, surgery, gynecology, pediatrics, ophthalmology, otorhinolaryngology, medical ethics, pharmacology, eubiotics, diet therapy, detoxification, first aid, acupuncture and massage.[4] He listed fifty-three hundred prescriptions and diagrammed all aspects of the human body with illustrations of meridians and acupoints. His chapter on medical ethics was the Hippocratic oath for Chinese physicians.

In 1000 C.E., Lin Yi and others compiled the four classics of traditional Chinese medicine during the Northern Song Dynasty; these are *Synopsis of Prescriptions of the Golden Chamber, Treatise on Cold Damage Diseases, Huangdi's Internal Classic* and *Shennong's Materia Medica*. Later, in 1578, Li Shi Zhen wrote *Compendium of Materia Medica*, and Wu Qian and others compiled the *Golden Mirror of Medicine* in 1742. These are still classics in traditional Chinese medicine.

These thousands of years of Chinese medical literature contain only scattered, short notes relating to surgery in children. Eunuchs during the Han Dynasty described castration, *qi sui jing shen*, of boys at seven years of age. Most eunuchs survived, attesting to the skill and technique of the surgeons. The symptoms and treatment of inguinal hernia, described as *chang ji*, or intestinal impaction, were described in the bamboo slip book *Prescriptions for Fifty-two Diseases*. Wei Yong-Zhi, whose biography was recorded in *History of the Jin Dynasty* during the third century, had a cleft lip. The doctor who repaired the lip advised that Wei neither talk nor smile and take only a liquid diet for a hundred days. He was cured. Chao Yuan Fang mentioned neonatal omphalitis and tetanus in *Treatise on the Pathogenesis and Manifestations of Disease* (610 C.E.). He also described the symptoms of bladder stones in children: "Pain took place in the urethra and urine dripped out. Patients suffered intolerable urgency and cried for death."

There are descriptions of erysipelas, pernicious vomiting and neonatal tetanus in *Key to Therapeutics of Children's Diseases*, written by Quian Yi during the Song Dynasty (1000 C.E.). Descriptions of syndactyly, cleft lip, dwarfism and disabled limbs were also found in *Comprehensive Comments on Child Health*. According to this book, the harelip could be repaired, but the scar could not be removed. In the fifteenth century, Zeng Shi Rong, a pediatrician in the Yuan Dynasty, wrote in his book *Hao You Xin Shu* (A book of children): "...subcutaneous nodules appear behind the ear and side of neck. At first, they may be single, but soon increase up to ten or more around the neck like a chain of beads of different size. Subsequently, some become swollen and rupture with purulent drainage. Mild ones heal spontaneously, but others, called sinuses, continue to discharge throughout the child's life."

Xu Yi, a physician who practiced during the Ming Dynasty in the sixteenth century, appears to have understood the cause and prevention of omphalitis and neonatal tetanus. Xu Yi also said that at birth, before being divided, the umbilical cord should be charred with a *moxa* roll soaked with sesame oil. After it was divided, the cord was wrapped in soft silk and thick cotton and was prevented from being wetted with urine.

Wang Ken-tung, another Ming Dynasty physician, in his book *Wai Ke Zhung Shen* (Book of surgery and external diseases) described intussusception in a five-month-old baby with a mass the size of a plum or an egg in his abdomen. If on the left side, it was called *xuan qi*; on the right, *pi qi*. These infants had dark faces and staring eyes and passed dark, bloody stools, and their lips, nose, hands and feet were cold. They were unable to eat and died. During the same era, Sun Zhi-Hung said that a baby born with no anus was unable to pass stool and would die in ten days. He recommended cutting open the anus with a lancet to reach the bowel and then inserting a finger-like silk roll soaked in sesame oil. The wound was treated with herbs until it healed.

Confucian scholars played an important role in developing Chinese medicine. According to the ancient philosophy in *Yi King, the Book of Changes*, everything in the universe was divided into yin and yang, positive and negative. All substances were divided into five elements symbolizing the changing balances of forces in the Ba-Gua, or eight diagrams. The traditional Chinese doctor applied the terms *yin-yung* and *wu-sing* to all anatomical and physiological terms. The Confucian scholars were atheists who believed that life came from nature and the body born of parents was unchangeable. It was not permitted to "damage" the body, and therefore the study of anatomy, surgery and the repair of congenital anomalies was forbidden. Confucians claimed that the best doctors were those who prevented disease. Common doctors treated disease mostly with personalized homeopathy, and they derided poor doctors who treated the worst or out-of-control disease with ordinary medicine.

Acupuncture, a peculiar and poorly understood form of therapy, was described in detail in Huangdi's *Internal Classic* and called the Miraculous Pivot. In ancient times, doctors had no understanding of the circulatory or nervous systems but believed that there should be routes that connected all parts of the body. By their experience and observation, they found 12 main channels plus 2 more, called *ren mai* and *du mai*, and many transverse connecting channels, named *luo*. There are 350 special points, termed *shu-xue* or *xue*, where needling of the skin would cure disease. This process is called acupuncture. Another method of treating disease at special points is called moxibustion, which is the burning of moxa, an herb roll, to warm the skin. These two methods have been used in China for more than two thousand years, up to the present day. Although there is no scientific proof that they work, acupuncture and moxibustion have become popular methods of treatment all over the world.

During the 1970s, acupuncture was used in China as anesthesia for surgery and medical experts sought a scientific explanation for its effectiveness. The author of this chapter was diagnosed with cancer of the stomach and had a Billroth II gastrectomy performed under acupuncture anesthesia. Needles were inserted into special points on the ear and on both sides of the abdominal incision. A rhythmic electrical stimulation was done instead of turning the needles by hand. During the four-hour operation, I felt no cutting pain, only as if a heavy mass were being pressed on my abdomen. My greatest discomfort came from lying on a hard, narrow board for the six hours it took for preparation and the operation. As a result of this experience, when I returned to the practice of pediatric surgery I used acupuncture anesthesia in 1,474 operations in children.[5] Initially, the child was put to sleep with intramuscular sodium pentothal, but in place of local infiltration with Novocain or an epidural block we used acupuncture. Although all the operations were successful and the analgesic effects of acupuncture were as good as an epidural block or local infiltration, later on we used conventional anesthetic techniques. In the future, doctors should not neglect acupuncture (*jing-luo*).

Chairman Mao Tse-tung, the great founder of the New China, said: "Traditional Chinese medicine is a great treasure house that should be explored scientifically." Ten universities of traditional medicine and hundreds of modern research institutes are studying these practices, which have a history of thousands of years. In China there are herbal drugstores even in small villages, and Chinese medicine has attracted interest in many developed countries.

In modern pediatric surgery, both doctors and parents are impressed with the idea of reinforcing the healthy qi and eliminating pathology with homeopathy. With this practice, the ill child will enjoy adequate rest and nutrition. Herbs are also used successfully to treat some common postoperative complications such as stomatitis, unknown fevers, idiopathic distention, constipation, diarrhea or dyspepsia. When no organic pathology is found, the use of simple herbs often provides dramatic relief of symptoms.

As a specific example, the conventional treatment of an anal fistula involves cutting open the tract. Postoperative bleeding and pain often causes parental anxiety. The traditional Chinese method was to open the tract gradually with a paper wick containing corrosive drugs and soothing herbs. We now insert a rubber band instead of the paper wick, just like a seton for a deep abscess. The band cuts through the tract in three to five days with no pain or bleeding.[6] Another idea from traditional medicine is the use of short, padded wooden splints instead of plaster casts to immobilize limb fractures. The splints allow a combination of immobilization with early movement to promote rapid healing while avoiding muscular atrophy.[7]

Chinese pediatric surgeons can make more contributions to the world of modern medicine from the vast field of Chinese traditional medicine.[8]

CHAPTER 6

The Ancient Greeks
and Hippocrates

Homer's *Iliad,* a tale of men at war when gods walked the earth, whether a myth or based on actual events, connects the history of medicine and surgery from religion and magic to Hippocrates.[1] The *Iliad* opens with a "burning wind of plague" brought by the angry gods who shot arrows from the sky to cause the soldiers to feel "transfixing pain." The armies of Agamemnon sickened and died. Here is the ancient concept of object intrusion as a cause for disease. We see the concept of "sucking" to treat wounds when Makhaon, a surgeon and son of Asklepios, the god of healing, draws an arrow from the wounded Menelaos and sucks the wound clean of blood. Menelaos recovered to fight another day.[2] Homer also described rational wound treatment when a common soldier excised an arrow from the thigh, washed away the blood and applied a powder of the "bitter yarrow root" that dulled the pain and clotted the blood.[3]

In the centuries between the *Iliad* and Hippocrates, Greek philosopher-scholars studied natural sciences to lay the foundation for modern medicine. By the fifth to fourth centuries B.C.E. there were medical schools and temples of healing located near clean water and pure air and away from plague-ridden cities. The patients rested, wore clean clothing and were purified with bathing. The emphasis on cleanliness suggests that the ancient Greeks understood the role played by dirty water and air in causing disease. Patients were "cured" and Greek physicians accumulated a wealth of practical knowledge based on observation. They learned some anatomy from the study of wounds and came to believe in natural rather than supernatural causes for disease. For example, epilepsy, known as the "sacred disease," was thought to have a divine cause, but Hippocrates claimed it was no more sacred than any other disease and had a natural cause.[4]

The *Corpus Hippocraticum* has perhaps the best clinical descriptions of disease until the publication of *The Principles and Practice of Medicine* by Sir William Osler in 1892. The various books in the *Corpus* appear to have been written over a period of at least a hundred years by several authors in a collection of papers and case histories from the medical library at Cos.[5] However, there is a suggestion that Hippocrates was a real physician, because Plato refers to a teacher of medicine at Cos named Hippocrates while speaking with a student, Protagoras.[6]

The Hippocratic theory of disease is that the body is composed of blood, phlegm, yellow bile and black bile. Pain or disease happens when these elements are out of balance. For example, if the vessels of the head overfill, the patient has a headache radiating to the neck; when he gets up, he is dizzy. The treatment was to shave the patient's head, make an incision in the forehead and sprinkle the wound with salt. If the brain suffered from bile, the treatment was cold compresses and instillation of celery juice into the nostrils, with a diet of thin gruel, honey, cabbage and laxative foods. If there was a thick, purulent nasal discharge, the patient was to have a vapor bath of vinegar, water and marjoram, good treatment for a sinus infection.

Aphorisms, or the sort of hints that clinicians pass on to students during hospital rounds, are scattered throughout the work. Hippocrates correlated various children's diseases with age when he said that babies suffered aphthae, vomiting, coughs, terrors and inflammations of the navel. While cutting teeth, they have irritation of the gums, fevers, convulsions and diarrhea. Older children have infections of the tonsils, curvature of the spine, stones, worms, scrofula, warts and swellings of the ears. Those approaching puberty suffer from the preceding maladies, protracted fevers and nosebleeds.[7]

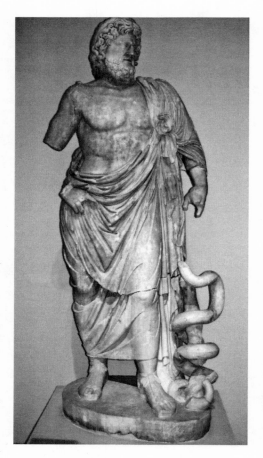

The Greek god of medicine in ancient Greek religion, Asklepios was the son of Apollos and the Trikkaion Princess Coronis. The serpent twined around the staff brought healing herbs to the physician. Asklepios become so skilled as a healer that Zeus killed him with a thunderbolt for fear that he could prevent death. Greek temples of healing were named *Asclepium*. This statue was originally in the temple of Asklepios at Epidaurus and is now in the National Archeologic Museum in Athens, Greece.

In chapters on geography, climate and diet, Hippocrates says that in cities facing cold winds children suffer from dropsies in the testicles (hydrocele) while they are little, which disappear as they grow older. In summer there are epidemics of dysentery and quartan fever, and children are highly subject to hernias. He says that drinking mineral-laden water causes bladder stones in children and recommends diluted wine. Boys with bladder stones had violent pain on urinated and pulled at their "privy parts." These symptoms are similar to those described in the *Sushruta Samhita*.

Hippocrates listed symptoms, not diagnoses, but it must have been mumps that caused boys and young men to have soft swellings by both ears and painful inflammations in the testicles that subsided spontaneously.[8] Here are the clear day-by-day observations of a teenage girl with acute fever, dysentery and dehydration:

A maiden was seized with an acute fever of the ardent type. Sleeplessness; thirst; tongue sooty and parched; urine of good color, but thin.

Second day. In pain, no sleep.

Third day. Copious stools, watery and of a yellowish green; similar stools on the following days, passed without distress.

Fourth day. Scanty, thin urine, with a substance suspended in it which did not settle; delirium at night.

Sixth day. Violent and abundant epistaxis; after a shivering fit followed a hot, copious sweating all over; no fever; a crisis. In the fever and after the crisis, menstruation for the first time, for she was a young maiden. Throughout she suffered nausea and shivering; redness of the face; pain in the eyes; heaviness in the head. In this case there was no relapse but a definite crisis.[9]

He also describes the course of septicemia leading to septic joints: "In infants, a cough with stomach upset and continuous fever in the second month indicates generally that there will also be swellings in the joints twenty days after the crisis. If the material from above settles below the navel in the lower joints, it is good. But if in the upper ones, it does not similarly resolve the disease unless there be festering. Festering in the shoulder for infants of that age makes them "weasel-armed."[10] Another case describes a four-month-old infant with pain and swelling around his navel, fever and vomiting who wasted away from what could have been an infected urachal or an omphalo-mesenteric cyst. This case history clearly noted the infant's depressed skull fontanelle, a clear indication of severe dehydration.[11]

Hippocrates may have differentiated cancer from benign cysts when he said that abdominal swellings that were big, hard and painful indicated a danger of death in the near future but that soft, painless swellings were more chronic. He knew that collections of pus in the lower abdomen, possibly appendiceal abscesses, that came to a point were more favorable than those that turned inward. He said favorable pus was white and smooth, uniform and least evil smelling. Pus of the opposite character was the worst.[12] Hippocrates knew that a little blood mixed with yellow sputum at the beginning of pneumonia was a very favorable sign of recovery, but if a patient brought up black bile with sputum he was likely to die.[13] The black bile could have originated from a liver abscess that had ruptured into the pleural cavity.

Hippocrates accurately described intestinal obstruction in patients who passed neither air nor food and who vomited, first phlegm, then bile, then feces, and had pain, abdominal distention and later fever. Treatment consisted of moist fomentations, sitting the patient in a tub of hot water with a suppository of honey and bull's gall, followed by an enema. Then came what might be the first suggestion of reducing an intussusception by blowing air into the rectum with a smith's bellows. If the treatment succeeded, the patient was to be given honey and new wine. If not, fever came on and the patient died. In another passage, Hippocrates describes a boy who had been sick with fever and vomiting black bile for 11 days, who passed feces after an enema. Hippocrates doesn't say if the boy survived.[14]

The descriptions and treatments for pneumonia, lung abscess and empyema are some of the best clinical descriptions ever made:

In pneumonia the following happens: there is violent fever, and the patient's breathing is rapid and hot; he is distraught, weak and restless, and beneath his shoulder-blade he suffers pain that radiates toward his collar-bone and nipple; he has a heaviness in his chest, and is deranged. In some patients, there is no pain until they begin to cough. The patient first expectorates white frothy sputum and his tongue is yellow; as time passes, the tongue becomes dark. The patient suffers these things for at least fourteen days, at the most twenty-one; he coughs, first copious frothy sputum, and then on the seventh or eighth day a thicker sputum. On the twelfth to the fourteenth days, it is copious and purulent. If the patient stops coughing purulent sputum by the sixteenth day, he recovers, but if the sputum becomes "sweetish" his lung is suppurating and the disease will last for a year. If the sputum has a foul taste, the disease is mortal.[15]

The foul sputum probably was an indication of a putrid lung abscess, indeed a mortal disease, especially in men who vomited and aspirated during an alcoholic stupor. Hippocrates treated pneumonia with the root bark of the caper plant, pinches of mustard, silphium juice, warm baths and sweet wine. Until the advent of antibiotics, these measures were as good as any.

Until the Empyema Commission of the First World War made its recommendations, patients died with a pneumothorax when doctors opened the chest too soon. Hippocrates waited until the pus was thick and the mediastinum was fixed. He determined which side the pus was on by shaking the patient while applying his ear to the chest. If the pus was too thick to make a splashing sound, he wrapped the chest with wet cloth and operated on the side that dried first, an indication of local heat.[16] This sounds crude and possibly inaccurate, but I know of a surgeon who didn't examine the chest and operated on the wrong side because the X-ray was reversed. To drain an empyema, Hippocrates cut the skin between the ribs with a bellied scalpel, the blade wrapped with a piece of cloth to avoid penetrating too far into the thorax. He drew off the pus once a day until the tenth day, when he filled the pleural cavity with warm wine and oil and inserted a hollow tin drainage tube, which was removed a bit at a time until the incision closed.[17] If the pus was white, the patient would recover, but if it was muddy and evil smelling, the patient would die.[18] The evil-smelling pus may have been a mixture of aerobic and anaerobic organisms.

In a chapter on wounds of the head, Hippocrates discusses the anatomy of the skull and various types of injuries. He gives special attention to children, saying that the skull bones of young children are thinner and softer and when they are wounded, the skull suppurates more readily than in older people. For comparable wounds, younger children die sooner.[19]

He differentiates sharp incised wounds of the scalp from contusions with skull fracture that are more likely to suppurate and take a long time for the crushed tissue to separate. If he couldn't determine the presence of a fracture line by visual inspection, he advised probing the wound to distinguish normal sutures from fractures. He would also extend incisions to better examine the skull and warned against trephining near suture lines. He didn't operate on depressed fractures, especially multiple fractures radiating from a depression. Perhaps he thought the brain was already decompressed.

The trephining instrument was a sharp-toothed, circular bronze saw twirled with a cord, which was plunged into cold water to avoid overheating and drying the bone. At times, he saws only through the outer table and at other times through to the "membrane," or dura mater. In this case, he frequently examines the cut to avoid injury to the dura mater and tries by to-and-fro movements of the saw to lift up the bone. He never mentions cutting through the dura mater but once referred to "drawing" blood with the trephine, and in another passage he advised trephining to let out serum.[20] It seems as if he was trephining to remove infected, sequestrated bone, rather than evacuating a hematoma.

Here are three case histories of children in whom the operation was intended to drain pus either from the subdural space or from the skull:

> The boy, wounded in the head with a potsherd by another child, became feverish after twelve days. The explanation: the woman who washed the wound rubbed the area around it and it took a chill. The lips of the wound puckered and the skin all around it grew thin. He was trephined without delay, but no pus ran off. It was expected that he would fester beside the ear, at the jaw, on the left side [that was the side of the wound]. As it happened, that failed to fester, and the right shoulder quickly developed an abscess. He died around the twenty-fourth-day.[21]
>
> An eleven-year-old boy was struck on the forehead above the right eye by a horse. The bone did not seem sound and a little blood squirted out of it. He was trephined extensively down to the diploe. And he was cured, despite this condition of the bone, which was festering. On the twentieth day a swelling began by the ear and fever and shivering. And in the daytime, the

swelling and pain were greater. He became fevered, beginning with shivering. His eyes and face swelled. He was affected more on the right than the left side of the head, but the swelling spread also to the left. Finally the fever was less continuous. He survived after being cauterized, purging it with medicine for drinking and treated with plasters on the swelling.[22]

The child, whose skull was laid bare on his forehead, had fever on the ninth day. The bone became livid. The child died. Also the children of Phanias and Euergus; when their bones became livid and they became feverish, the skin stood away from the bone and pus gathered below. When they were trephined a thin serum came out of the bone itself, like fig juice, slightly yellow, foul-smelling, deathly. And it occurs in such cases that there are vomiting and convulsions at the end, and some cry shrilly; some are paralyzed; if the wound is on the right side, paralysis on the left, if on the left, the right.[23]

In the chapters on surgery, fractures and joints, we are eyeball-to-eyeball with a master clinician and a brilliant orthopedic surgeon who is speaking from a detailed knowledge of anatomy and wide experience. The author, presumably Hippocrates, emphasizes gentleness and cleanliness and splints injured extremities in their natural, functional position. The many references to the gymnasium and wrestling suggest that most fractures and dislocations were sports injuries.[24]

For the initial treatment of closed fractures, Hippocrates recommends soft wrapping with linen bandages, applying firm pressure to the site of injury, with less pressure above and below. The second layer of bandage was moistened with cerate, a mixture of wax liquefied in oil of roses. The idea was to drive edema away from the fracture so that by the seventh day after the injury the swelling was reduced and the bones were mobile and ready for "adjustment." The fracture is then reduced with a combination of traction, manipulation and splinting.

For fractures of the humerus, Hippocrates placed a rod under the armpit. Then a strong man pulled down on the elbow, bent at a right angle, while the surgeon adjusted the bone with the palms of his hands. The arm was then splinted and secured to the chest with a broad band. To prevent inward deviation, a thick compress was placed between the humerus and the ribs. For both bone fractures of the forearm, Hippocrates makes a point of splinting the elbow in flexion with the arm pronated. For fractures of the femur, he anticipated the modern orthopedic table by constructing an oak plank with supports for the body and a post between the legs at the crotch. Broad ox-hide straps were attached to soft wrappings around the foot and connected to a windlass, which applied traction. When the leg was fully extended, the surgeon manipulated the bones with his hands and the dressing was applied while the leg was still in traction. The ingenious Hippocratic version of the Thomas splint consisted of soft leather circlets at the crotch and ankle with loops into which were placed bent wooden rods that maintained traction and allowed inspection of the wound. It was, in fact, a primitive Ilizarov apparatus that maintained continuous traction and immobilization.

If the bone in a compound fracture could be replaced, the only change in treatment was to apply cerate with pitch to the wound. Pitch, made from coal tar or a resin from conifer trees like balsam of Peru, has bacteriostatic properties. The dressings were moistened with an astringent wine. One passage says that these wounds heal just like ordinary fractures, and another says that "purification"— or the discharge of pus — will take place and the wound will "cicatrise" more rapidly than usual. Hippocrates describes reducing complicated compound fractures by inserting iron rods into the wound; one levered up the distal bone and another applied pressure to the proximal fragment. He warned that this procedure should only be done on the first or second day to avoid more inflammation and spasm. In severe compound fractures with splintering or when the bone was denuded and the soft tissues became necrotic, the bone would "come away" with suppuration within 40 to 60 days. He considered resection of denuded bone but then said the bone would spontaneously extrude without surgery, though the limb would be shortened.[25]

Dislocation of the shoulder must have been a common sports injury, because Hippocrates describes the signs and symptoms in great detail and gives several methods of reduction with traction on the arm and lateral pressure on the head of the humerus. One was the familiar "dirty sock" method, in which the patient lies on the floor and the surgeon sits with his foot in the patient's armpit to apply counterpressure while pulling on the arm. The arm is then bandaged to the side of the chest with a compress in the axilla to keep the head of the humerus in its socket.

Men with recurrent dislocated shoulders were barred from sports and were considered useless in warfare, but the treatment of recurrences with white-hot cautery irons inserted through the skin to scar and tighten tissues around the joint seems drastic.[26] Hippocrates warned against inserting the irons into the axilla because fire is "hostile" to nerves and because there is a large blood vessel in the neighborhood. He said that an unreduced dislocation in an adolescent or one that occurred in the womb causes the arm to shorten, a conditioned termed "weasel-armed." Children who have "deep suppuration" of the shoulder joint also become "weasel-armed."

"Hump-back" is his term for kypho-scoliosis in children, a condition that results in poor development of the chest cavity and shortness of breath when the defect is above the diaphragm. When the deformity is mild, these patients remain in good health until old age, but most are short-lived.[27]

Hippocrates said the leg in children with congenital dislocations of the hip joint becomes flaccid and atrophic and they crawl about miserably on the sound leg, supporting themselves with the hand on the sound side.[28] In a later passage, he says that the displaced head of the thighbone is sustained by "soft and yielding flesh," or a "friction cavity." The joint eventually becomes painless; these patients can walk without a crutch and bear weight on the injured leg. When the thighbone has been displaced since birth, however, or was forcibly put out during adolescence, it undergoes necrosis and sometimes chronic abscesses. This may refer to the aseptic necrosis of the head of the femur seen in adolescents. Yet another passage refers to bilateral outward displacement of hips at birth or from disease that causes defective growth of the entire body, except the head. Hippocrates relates this and deformities to "irregular movements and contractures of the uterus." This obscure suggestion by Hippocrates was confirmed centuries later, when F. Douglas Stephens correlated a number of birth defects, such as torticollis, dislocated hip, clubfoot and ano-rectal anomalies, with intrauterine pressure.[29]

Hippocrates' classic description of clubfoot is worth reading in the original:

> There are certain congenital displacements which, when they are slight, can be reduced to their natural position, especially those at the foot-joints. Cases of congenital club-foot are, for the most part, curable, if the deviation is not very great or the children advanced in growth. It is therefore best to treat such cases as soon as possible, before there is any very great deficiency in the bones of the foot, and before the like occurs in the tissues of the leg. Now the mode of club-foot is not one, but manifold; and most cases are not the result of complete dislocation, but are deformities due to the constant retention of the foot in a contracted position. The things to bear in mind in treatment are the following: push back and adjust the bone of the leg at the ankle from without inwards, making counter-pressure outwards on the bone of the heel where it comes in lie with the leg, so as to bring together

the bones which project at the middle and the side of the foot; at the same time, bend inwards and rotate the toes all together, including the big toe. Dress with cerate well stiffened with resin, pads and soft bandages, sufficiently numerous, but without too much compression. Bring round the turns of the bandaging in a way corresponding with the manual adjustment of the foot, so that the latter has an inclination somewhat towards splay-footedness. A sole should be made of not too stiff leather or of lead, and should be bound on as well, not immediately on to the skin, but just when you are going to apply the last dressings. When the dressing is completed, the end of one of the bandages used should be sewn onto the underside of the foot-dressings, in line with the little toe; then, making such tension upwards as may seem suitable, pass it round the calf-muscle at the top, so as to keep it firm and on the stretch. In a word, as in wax modeling, one should bring the parts into their true neutral position, both those that are twisted and those that are abnormally contracted, adjusting them in this way both with the hands and by bandaging in like manner; but draw them into position by gentle means, and not violently. Sew on the bandages so as to give the appropriate support; for different forms of lameness require different kinds of support. A leaden shoe shaped as the Chian boots used to be might be made, and fastened on the outside of the dressing; but this is quite unnecessary if the manual adjustment, the dressing with bandages and the contrivance for drawing up are properly done. This then is the treatment, and there is no need for incision, cautery or complicated methods: for such cases yield to treatment more rapidly than one would think. Still, time is required for complete success, till the part has acquired growth in its proper position. When the time has come for footwear, the most suitable are the so-called "mud-shoes," for this kind of boot yields least to the foot; indeed, the foot rather yields to it.[30]

This passage more than any other in the entire *Corpus*, or perhaps in any medical literature up until the nineteenth century, indicates the author's regard for children, together with an appreciation of the child's growth and development.

Hippocrates recommended making no attempt to reduce compound dislocations of joints for fear of gangrene but dressing the wound with warm cerate and compresses steeped in wine. The patient would be deformed and lame, but would survive.[31] This advice sounds strange until we remember that tremendous force is required to cause a compound dislocation and that a forcible reduction without benefit of anesthesia would cause more soft tissue and vascular damage. It wasn't until the Korean War in the 1950s that surgeons learned to repair damaged blood vessels and salvage limbs that would otherwise become gangrenous. We may further ask why Hippocrates did not perform an immediate amputation in such cases but waited for demarcation of gangrene. Then he amputated through a joint and left remaining dead tissue to slough spontaneously. This may have reflected a desire to avoid further pain and to preserve as much limb length as possible.

In the section on surgery, there is one cryptic reference to abdominal trauma, in a child who died on the fourth day after being kicked in the belly and liver by a mule. In another case, Hippocrates described opisthotonos and spastic fixed jaws in a patient who developed tetanus after injuring his thumb. The patient died on the third day.

Volume 8 is devoted almost entirely to elective operations, philosophy and instructions to students on arrangements for good light, cleanliness and potable water in the operating room.[32] Hippocrates advised prospective surgeons to serve in the army.[33] Hippocrates ligated bleeding vessels and treated edema in children with dropsy by making multiple small incisions with a scalpel.[34] He also describes what might be a sure-fire way to treat prolapse of the rectum:

If the rectum prolapses, support it with a soft sponge, anointed with medications, and suspend the patient upside down for a short time and it will go in. If it prolapses further, encircle the body with a band and run a strip down around the back. Then press the rectum in with a soft sponge in warm water in which you have boiled saw-dust of lotus and apply. Squeeze out the sponge and then run the strap down between the legs and tie it up at the navel. When the person wishes to go to stool, let him sit on as narrow a night-stool as possible; if it is a child, he should sit on a woman's feet leaning against her knees. During defecation let him extend his legs, since in this position, the rectum is least likely to prolapse.[35]

Finally, there is the Oath, that short statement of morals and ethics recited at least once by every physician. Very little is known about the oath's origins, except that it appears to be genuinely Hippocratic, though possibly altered by centuries of translation and interpretation.[36] Was it required of members of a guild or upon graduation, or was it administered to new students? In those days, there was no real graduation as we know it and little evidence for a guild of physicians, other than their associations with various schools. Some of the wording, such as the vow to treat children of a teachers healer's as his own brothers, to share his livelihood with a healer's teachers and to teach his teachers' children, suggests that it was an oath taken by students indentured to a teacher or school.

This might explain those enigmatic injunctions against cutting for stone and abortion. Abortion was common in Greek society as a means of population control and is even mentioned in the *Corpus*. We know that the Greeks were expert surgeons and certainly understood the terrible pain endured by those who suffered with bladder stones. There was no obvious reason why they should not have performed the operation. The best explanation is that students were to leave these procedures to the experts. Another explanation might be that the oath was altered in translation during later years, when the Catholic Church was opposed to abortion and surgery.

There are reports that the Greeks, especially Spartans, put puny or ill-formed infants to death in a chasm under Mount Taygetus.[37] How do we reconcile this practice that was designed to produce vigorous, strong children for the public good with Hippocrates' concern for infants and children with orthopedic deformities? Could it have been a different time, or did the patients of Hippocrates come from a different social stratum? There is no way of knowing, but once again we must remember that many "puny and ill-formed" infants suffered from birth defects for which there was no treatment until modern times.

How can we evaluate Greek classical medicine of the fifth century B.C.E.? Hippocrates replaced chanting shamans and the supernatural with a theory of medicine based on a reasonable, though faulty, physiology. He did this through careful clinical consideration of the patient's history and visible, palpable and audible physical signs. In surgery, with emphasis on cleanliness and the use of wine and other bacteriostatic medications, his wound care was superior to any other until the age of Lister. We may say that a child with an injury, pneumonia or a deformed extremity would have fared better under the care of Greek doctors on the island of Cos than at any other time until the twentieth century.

For many centuries the original works of the Greeks came down, sometimes erroneously, through the filter of Galen. Those twin evils religion and politics prevented the skill and knowledge of Hippocrates from being passed to succeeding generations of physicians until the Renaissance.

CHAPTER 7

The Alexandrians and Galen

Alexandria, a city named for Alexander the Great, became a famed center of learning with a large collection of books and manuscripts. Herodotus and Erasistratus, Greek physicians at Alexandria, by dissecting human bodies and doing vivisections on live criminals discovered and named many anatomical structures such as the ventricles of the brain and the mitral valves. With the rise of the Roman Empire, many Alexandrian-trained Greeks went to Rome.[1]

A Roman scholar, Aulus Cornelius Celsus, recorded most of what we know about medical knowledge from Hippocrates to the beginning of the Christian era in *De Medicina*, written in elegant Latin. Celsus lived during the reign of Emperor Tiberius (14–37 C.E.).[2] Unfortunately, Celsus had little influence on medicine until he was rediscovered during the Renaissance.

Celsus described operations unknown to Hippocrates and listed many new medications for wound treatment such as the salts of copper or iron, alum, pine resin, turpentine and herbs boiled in wine or vinegar. Honey was often added when a soothing medication was required. One prescription to "eat away fungus flesh" contained copper scales, frankincense, soot and verdigris; when combined with honey, this prescription "cleaned ulcers."[3]

Celsus advised practitioners that it is impossible to save a patient with wounds of the base of the brain, the heart and other internal organs. His accurate description of the fading pulse, pallid and cold skin, sweating and death after a heart injury suggests he had firsthand knowledge of surgery.[4] He was also familiar with the radiation of pain to the clavicle in splenic injuries and knew that kidney pain spreads to the groin and testicles. These observations were still important in the days when we diagnosed a ruptured spleen or kidney on clinical grounds.

Celsus controlled bleeding with dry lint covered with a sponge soaked in cold water or by pouring vinegar into the wound. When that didn't work, he recommended seizing the blood vessel, tying around the wounded spot and cutting across the vessel. Some creative young surgeon invented the ligature when he seized a gushing artery with his fingers and had an assistant tie a string around the vessel. The next step was to use pincers or forceps to grasp the vessel before applying the ligature. Celsus cleaned wounds with bacteriostatic medications and then took the radical step of closing the wounds with a fibula. This was a thorn or a pin inserted through the skin from one side of the wound to the other. A thread wound around the ends of the fibula as a figure eight brought the edges of the skin together. Celsus cautioned that the more stitches, the greater the inflammation and advised leaving part of the wound open as an outlet to drain "humours."

The treatment of infected wounds, gangrene and foreign bodies with topical medications, drainage and excision of necrotic tissue was as good as anything up until the antiseptic era. Celsus' treatment of human and animal bites with incision, suction, the application of salt solutions and caustics was unchanged until the era of antibiotics. Celsus recognized the futility of treating hydrophobia due to the bite of a mad dog but suggested throwing the patient into a tank of water and forcing him to drink.[5] He recommended constriction above a serpent's bite, incision and suction with a cup. If a cup wasn't available, it was safe for a man to suck the wound, because the poison was harmless if swallowed. Celsus' recommendation to apply half of a freshly killed chicken to the bite made little sense, but one cannot argue with his advice to have the patient sip strong wine with pepper.[6]

Any physician practicing in a cold climate where newsboys go without mittens or overshoes will recognize this description of frostbite:

> Ulcers are also produced in winter by the cold, mostly in children, and particularly on their feet and toes, sometimes also on the hands. There is redness with moderate inflammation; sometimes pustules arise followed by ulceration; the pain is moderate. The itching is greater; at times humour exudes, but not much. In the first place, the ulcers are to be fomented freely with a hot decoction of turnips, or if these are not to be had, some kind of repressant vervaine. If there is not yet an open ulcer, copper scales as hot as can be borne are to be applied. If there is already an ulceration, then apply equal parts of alum and frankincense pounded together with the addition of wine or pomegranate-rind boiled in water. If the skin has become detached, in that case also soothing medicaments do good.[7]

Celsus also recognized the synergistic infectious gangrene, "cancrum oris" or "noma" seen in the mouths of infants and children even today in Africa. A tomb inscription by the Roman writer Martial (40–104 C.E.) describes this terrible disease and the sadness of the child's parents:

> Candace, the daughter of Aeolis, lies buried in this tomb; Little Candace, Whose seventh winter was her last. Alas for the guilt and the crime of it! Thou, passer-by, who art quick to weep may lament here, not the shortness of life, but something sadder than death, the way death comes. A dreadful canker wasted her face and settled on her tender mouth and consumed her very lips. Before they were surrendered to the smoky pyre. It had to come with so ill-timed a flight, fate should have come by another path, but death hastened to close the channel of her charming speech, lest her tongue might have power to bind the stern goddesses.[8]

The treatment included washing the nurse's breasts and rinsing the child's mouth with honey, saffron, myrrh, alum and wine, or concentrated mulberry juice. If that didn't work, they used a caustic such as copper ore.

Celsus gives away his identity as a gentleman-scholar when he modestly describes afflictions of the "privy parts." He suggested applications of hot water or olive leaves boiled in wine when the penis swelled with inflammation and the foreskin couldn't be drawn back. If these measures didn't work, he recommended notching the foreskin with a scalpel to release the edema fluid.[9] This recommendation could have been for a poor little boy with an infected paraphimosis or for one who caught his foreskin in a zipper and couldn't pee.

Celsus implied that any physician may treat a preexisting wound, but only surgeons should cure by making an incision, such as for drainage of an abscess or to remove dead bone from infected wounds. When there was spontaneous drainage of pus from between two ribs, he advised resecting a segment of rib above and below the fistula. There is a suggestion of a subphrenic or liver abscess that had ruptured into the pleural cavity when he described a fistula that passed through the transverse septum separating the intestines from the lungs.[10]

He performed tonsillectomy by "scratching around with a finger" or excision with a scalpel, followed by a vinegar rinse to stop bleeding.[11] He may be responsible for the still-prevalent belief that "tongue tie" causes speech problems. He grasped the tongue with a forceps and incised the membrane beneath the tongue, using great care to avoid the blood vessels. He was skeptical of the operation because some patients who could easily protrude their tongues still couldn't speak.

Celsus referred to two lesions in the neck, between the trachea and the skin: One was filled with a fluid like honey; another contained hair and bits of bone: Both were contained in a capsule. It was thought that these were goiters, but they sound more like thyroglossal duct and dermoid cysts. They were treated with caustics to eat away the skin together with the capsule for drainage of liquid matter; solid material was "turned out with the finger." Then he said: "But treatment with the knife is shorter. A linear incision is made over the middle of the tumour down to the tunic; then the morbid pouch is separated from the sound tissue, and the whole removed along with its covering. Next the wound is washed out with vinegar to which salt or soda has been added, and the margins brought together with one suture." There was no better treatment for these cysts until surgeons learned to remove a portion of the hyoid bone in the twentieth century.

Umbilical hernias were treated by forcing the intestine inside, then ligating the base of the sac with a flaxen thread. The excess skin was burned away with caustics or the cautery. He warns that infants and old men shouldn't be operated on, but that children between 7 and 14 years are most suitable for treatment.[12] Celsus describes the anatomy and surgical treatment of inguinal hernia, but in young children he advised bandaging before considering the knife.

The description for the removal of bladder stones by perineal lithotomy is practically the same as that in the *Sushruta Samhita*. It was done during the spring in boys between the ages of 9 and 14 years. The surgeon, after carefully paring his fingernails, pressed the stone down to the perineum with a finger in the rectum and a hand on the hypogastrium. He cut down through the neck of the bladder and removed the stone with a scoop; afterward, the boy was placed in a bath of strong vinegar and salt. When the bleeding stopped, he was placed in a tub of warm water. After Hippocrates warned against cutting for stone, why did Greek surgeons do the operation? Did physicians traveling with Alexander the Great's army learn the operation from Indian surgeons? An Indian raja gave Alexander a girl, a philosopher, a magic cup and a physician.[13] Alexander's physicians could not save him, and he died on his way home from India in 323 B.C.E.

Celsus treated obstructions of the vagina that occurred "even in the mother's womb" by excision of the membrane, avoiding the urethra and inserting a roll of wool dipped in vinegar into the vagina. Later, a lead tube was used to keep the vagina open. Although this could have been a simple imperforate hymen, the extensive treatment sounds more like it was a type of vaginal atresia.[14]

Syndactyly was said to occur either before birth or later, after the fingers adhered to one another following an ulceration of the adjacent surfaces (probably from a burn). The adherent fingers were divided with a knife and separately enclosed in a plaster until healed. Celsus makes no mention of obvious birth defects such as imperforate anus or cleft lip. Was there a stigma attached to these defects and the parents didn't bring children affected by them to the surgeon, or were they considered too lethal to treat?

The question of what happened to deformed infants is found in the works of another distinguished physician, Soranus. Born in Ephesus in Asia Minor sometime during the first century C.E., Soranus was trained in Alexandria and practiced medicine in Rome during the rule of Trajan (98–117 C.E.) and Hadrian (117–138 C.E.). Soranus was a generalist, but his best-known work, on the diseases of women and children, influenced child care for the next fifteen hundred years. T. N. K. Raju, a neonatologist, considered Soranus, who eloquently wrote about childbirth and care of the infant, to be the world's first perinatologist.[15]

The first decision after the birth of a baby was whether the infant was worth keeping: "Now the midwife, having received the newborn, should first put it upon the earth, having examined before-hand whether the infant is male or female, and should make an announcement by signs as is the custom of women. She should consider whether it is worth rearing or not."[16]

The decision to keep the baby depended on the child's being born at the due time and to a healthy mother. The baby had to have a vigorous cry, because those with a delayed cry were weak. The baby also had to be perfect, with his ears, nose, pharynx, urethra and anus free from obstruction. His joints had to bend and stretch and he had to respond to painful pressure and pricks. If the baby wasn't perfect in every way, he wasn't worth keeping. This reflected the decree of Romulus, the founder of Rome, that all male infants who were not monsters or otherwise malformed were to be reared.[17]

Soranus explains how to ligate and divide the umbilical cord to prevent hemorrhage and warns against bathing the newborn in cold water or wine. Sprinkling with salt was acceptable, but he preferred to clean the baby with honey and olive oil or the juice of barley and then wash him with warm water. The nurse also cleaned mucus out of the nose and ears and washed the eyes with olive oil. Soranus then advised dilating the anus with the little finger to aid in expelling meconium. This is still good advice! What better way to diagnose intestinal obstruction in the newborn?

After the bath, the midwife put the baby down "gently on her lap" and swaddled him with cloth to keep him warm. After the newborn was swaddled and put to bed on a soft straw mattress, Soranus advised withholding food for two days and then offering a feeding of barley water or honey boiled in water. Since maternal milk, for the first 20 days, was too thick and unwholesome, he preferred a wet nurse, or goat's milk with honey. The wet nurse had to be between 20 and 40 years of age, in good health, with medium-sized soft breasts. She should be self-controlled and sympathetic and speak Greek, so the baby would hear the correct language. There was a great deal of advice on how to maintain the health of the wet nurse, how to test the milk and what to do if the milk stopped flowing, and how to care for the child up until the time of weaning, walking and teething. Soranus treated gum inflammation associated with teething by giving the child soft fat to chew or through the application of honey and linseed poultices to the gums. He said lancing the gums with the knife was harmful.

After this long discourse on the care of normal infants, Soranus recommend poultices to the throat for tonsillitis and treating thrush with honey or an assortment of fruit juices and herbs mixed with honey. There were also remedies for itching, coughing, and fevers. For diarrhea, he recommended giving juice of the plantain as an enema to the infant and a constipating diet to the wet nurse. As usual with all ancient medical writers, Soranus said nothing about the results of treatment. He ends his book on child care by leaving to the realm of philosophy the age at which a child is "handed over to a pedagogue" for his education.

In his discussion of pregnancy, Soranus said the state of the soul of the woman produces changes in the fetus. He discussed the conduct of childbirth and recommended embryotomy or morcelation to deliver the baby and save the mother if the infant's head was too large or if there was hydrocephaly.[18]

The writings of Celsus and Soranus represent the high point of surgery from the beginning of man's earliest wound care until the nineteenth century. During the first century C.E., a surgeon trained in the Alexandrian school could treat wounds, broken bones and dislocations with considerable skill. He could drain an empyema or an abdominal abscess and remove superficial tumors. He might also operate upon a child with an incarcerated hernia or a painful bladder stone with some degree of success. He could correct a clubfoot with bandaging about as well as a modern orthopedic surgeon.

Dr. Guido Majno, a pathologist, has shown the effectiveness of many ancient wound medications against bacteria.[19] Copper salts, known to the Greeks as copper rust, inhibited bacterial growth. Honey is bacteriostatic and, boiled together with copper oxide, was especially effective. A mixture of animal grease or oil with honey also prevents bandages from sticking to wounds and does not inhibit wound healing. Vinegar, another universal remedy, contains acetic acid, which inhibits fungi as well as bacteria. The antiseptic power of wine depends not on alcohol but on polyphenols, complex versions of phenol. When boiled with other ingredients, polyphenols become more concentrated. Even animal dung, when heated and dried, contains ammoniacal compounds inhibitory to bacteria. Some natural plant remedies, especially the sap of trees such as balsam of Peru, are soothing as well as antiseptic. The Greeks also came close to solving the problem of pain during surgery with opium, mixed with alcohol.

Galen

Galen, the most famous physician of the Greco–Roman period, was born in 129 C.E. in Pergamon, a city on the coast of the Aegean Sea in what is now Turkey. Pergamon had an excellent school and a library second only to that of Alexandria. The pillars of Pergamon's ancient library are still standing, on a hilltop with a magnificent view of the surrounding countryside.

Galen studied philosophy, mathematics and literature until he was 17 years of age, when his father had vivid dreams about his son studying medicine. The boy first studied, in Pergamon, at the temple of the healing god Asklepios, famous for medical teaching. Remnants of this temple still stand next to a freshwater spring that was so essential to Greek healing and surgery. At age 19, Galen traveled and continued to study until he arrived in Alexandria. There he was exposed to the great scientific tradition of the earlier Greek anatomists and teachers. At age 28, he returned to Pergamon to be surgeon to the gladiators. He claims to have gotten the job because he eviscerated an ape and challenged the other surgeons to repair the damage. When the surgeons refused, Galen did the job. There is no mention of how he returned the guts to the abdomen, but perhaps by then the poor ape was in shock.[20]

Galen was the "team physician" to gladiators when athletes fought lions and tigers and went at each other with bare knuckles, swords and spears. They suffered animal bites, gashes, fractures, dislocations and major head injuries. Galen used Hippocrates' methods for reducing fractures and dislocations but was more advanced in his method of suturing muscles and tendons. He avoided inflammation by the liberal application of "astringent wine."[21] We

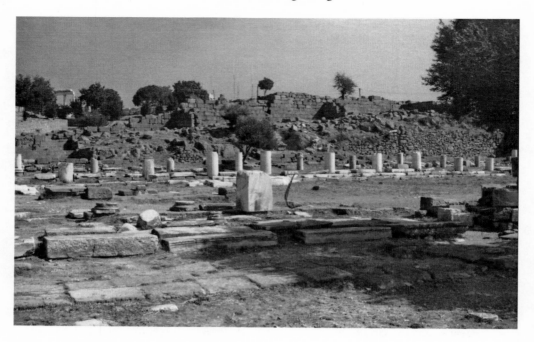

The remains of the Library of Pergamon, where Galen first studied medicine, are high on a hill, overlooking the surrounding countryside.

can assume that this wine wasn't the mild drink favored today but something nearer to the strong, resin-flavored Greek wine retsina.

Galen would have had little opportunity to treat children, except for young athletes. One of his most famous cases was a boy who was struck on the sternum and developed an abscess that had to be opened twice. Here is the case history: "As, however, the spacelus [necrosis] of the sternum was believed by everyone to exist, and as the movements of the heart were visible on the left side, no one dared to move the diseased bone. Because they thought opening of the thorax would be necessary. But I promised to take away the bone without opening of the thorax; I exposed the place, and removed the diseased bone especially from that spot where the upper end of the pericardium and the heart seemed exposed, because the pericardium was necrotic."[22]

This was a heroic piece of surgery. Galen had to know enough anatomy to stay within the anterior mediastinum, avoiding the pleural cavities; he also understood the necessity of removing diseased bone. Modern cardiac surgeons face the same problem when a sternotomy incision becomes infected.

After four years in Pergamon, Galen went to Rome, where he became physician to the Emperor; after success with his distinguished patient, his fortune was made and he treated many others of high social rank. He also dissected apes and dogs for the instruction of medical students and to amuse the aristocracy. In one of his public dissections, Galen demonstrated the relationship between respiration and vocal sounds by ligating the intercostal muscles until the pig stopped squealing. Then, when Galen removed the ligatures and breathing recommenced, the pig again took up its loud squealing. [23] Galen returned to Pergamon for three years during an epidemic of plague in Rome and avoided going to war against the German barbarians with the Emperor. Most of his time was spent lecturing,

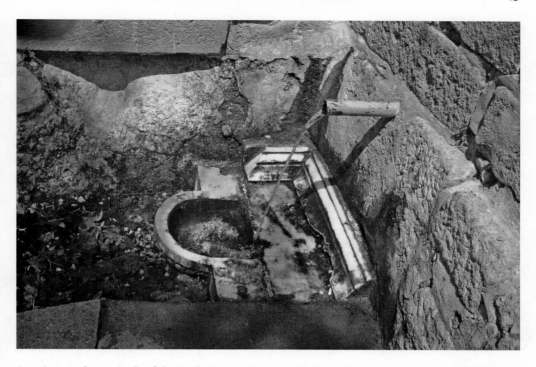

A spring on the grounds of the Asclepium at Pergamon, where Galen may have treated gladiators after he returned from his medical studies at Alexandria. Fresh, clean water was essential to Greek medical treatment and for wound care. Cleanliness and the use of natural antiseptics was common practice by the earliest surgeons.

writing and arguing theories of medicine with other physicians. His writing, partly auto-biographical, has long discourses on the education of a physician and arguments pro and con on the various theories of medicine.[24]

Galen is often criticized for basing his anatomy on animal rather than human dissections, but he explicitly stated that he was using animals that most resembled humans. The Barbary ape was his favorite animal. We should forgive him, because the Romans forbade human dissection. Furthermore, we still test new drugs in animals, even though mice and rats don't respond exactly like humans. In addition, the essentials of anatomy are similar between many animals and humans. Most of us learned laparoscopic surgery by practicing on pigs. We can also forgive him for another major error. It would take some fifteen hundred years before William Harvey corrected Galen's mistaken belief that venous blood originated in the liver, arterial blood carried air and blood crossed the interventricular septum of the heart.

Galen did not have the tools of modern science but did his best to explain disease. Inflammatory reactions are warm, so it is easy to understand his idea that an abscess "boils" its way through the skin or that leprosy is caused by black bile. Galen was a talented observer and we still use his words to describe some lesions. For instance, he correctly used the term "ecchymoses" to describe a black-and-blue mark on the forearm. He knew it was an inconsequential hemorrhage through blood vessels in old, fragile skin. Perhaps it was his observation of closed wounds that led to his idea of "laudable pus." Some of the wounds he had closed with sutures undoubtedly became red, painful and swollen. At the same time, the patient became restless and feverish and often died. If pus drained after Galen opened the wound, the patient might survive. Patients whose contaminated wounds were left open to freely drain were less likely to develop sepsis. We no longer speak of "laudable pus," but we talk about "good" drainage and are often happy to find and drain a pocket of pus in a sick patient.

Galen's greatest legacy was to record the teachings of Hippocrates and the other famous Greek physicians. He wrote widely on surgical topics, most importantly on his attempts to understand inflammation and tumors; in treatment, he followed Hippocrates. Galen wrote little specifically on child care and then mostly repeated Soranus. According to some translations, Galen described atresia of the urethra, hydrocele, paraphimosis, hermaphroditism, umbilical anomalies, and various infectious disorders of childhood.[25] During the latter part of his life, he traveled in search of "healing earths" and may have visited the island of Milos in the Aegean Sea, where there are deposits of kaolin, bentonite and sulfur that are still used in medications.

In one of his works, *On the Usefullness of the Parts of the Body*, Galen's philosophy was almost religious when he explained that only a thoughtful creator could have designed each part of the human body for its intended function.[26] Although he was not a Christian, this may partly explain why his works were accepted so uncritically during those many centuries of domination by the Catholic Church. Through the ages, Galen's writings were translated into Arabic, back to Greek, then into Latin and every European language.

Galen died in Pergamon at age 70 at the end of the second century C.E. He remained unmarried and left no successor or heir.

CHAPTER 8

From Galen to the Crusades

Within three centuries after Galen's death, the Roman Empire was reduced to a fraction of its former power by a combination of decadence, internal strife and war on the frontiers. The Huns, Goths and Franks to the north carved out kingdoms, which would become the countries of Europe. To the east, the Sassanid Persians challenged the Roman army. One Emperor after another was assassinated, leaving the central government in disarray.[1] During those centuries of Roman decline, Christianity was in the ascendancy. In 313 C.E. Emperor Constantine converted to Christianity, and by the early fifth century Christianity became the official state religion. In 330 C.E., Constantine split the empire when he made Constantinople the capital. During the ensuing centuries, there would be one dominant church, one language, one social system, and no salvation for humanity outside the church. Monastic schools replaced secular education; these in turn became cathedral schools and eventually the great universities of Europe.

Traditionally, Romans thought of disease as a sign of divine displeasure, to be treated by prayer, magic and home remedies administered by slaves or the father of the family.[2] Despite enthusiasm for Greek culture, the Romans never really accepted Greek medicine and downplayed medical education. The practice of surgery may have fared better; a trove of fine bronze surgical instruments was excavated at Pompeii, a city destroyed by volcanic ash during the first century C.E.[3] On the other hand, Roman hygiene and sanitation in the form of baths and sewage disposal was unequaled until modern times. They also understood the need to place their cities away from unhealthy marshes.[4]

Rome also enacted the first laws for the protection of children. During the reigns of the Emperors Nerva, Trajan, Hadrian and the two Antoines, infanticide was discouraged and homes were established to care for abandoned children. Constantine ordered magistrates to allow poor families to sell their newborn infants in order to save them from death by exposure.[5]

Since the beginning of mankind, medicine and especially surgery had been groping away from the supernatural toward a rational explanation for disease. The rise of Christianity swept away this search for the truth and pushed medicine into the darkest of dark ages. The Gospels viewed disease as God's punishment, devil possession or magic. St. Luke, possibly a Greek-trained physician, who accurately described disease should have known better than to say: "There met Him a certain man, who had a devil now a very long time" (Luke 8:27). St. Paul dismissed the wisdom of the Greeks as "foolishness" and claimed that all knowledge except that which resulted in the salvation of man was useless.[6] Even the principle of cleanliness and bathing, a cornerstone of Greek and Roman medicine and essential to surgery, were dismissed when Jerome said that he who is washed in the blood of Christ need not wash again. Paula, a nun and companion of Jerome, told her nuns that a clean body and clean clothing betoken an unclean mind.[7] More and more, the treatment of disease came to depend on miracles, the exorcism of devils, martyrs' bones and fragments of the Cross.

A sick man was said to be more urgently in need of a priest ministering to his soul than a physician attending to his physical needs. When he visited a monk or a shrine and was cured, it was considered a miracle and the "patient" converted to Christianity. The saints became associated with specific diseases, often related to their own life experiences. Diseases of childbirth as well as those of children became known as St. Margaret's disease. Damian and Cosmos, two martyrs from Asia Minor, eventually became the patron saints of surgery. The names of at least 130 saints were associated with various diseases.[8]

Perhaps out of the natural impulse to help the sick and injured, or from the Christian admonition to aid the sick and poor, monks and nuns took over the care of bodily as well as spiritual ills. During the fourth century, St. Basil organized a hospital for the sick, with separate buildings for lepers. Early Christian communities appointed a widow to care for the sick.[9]

The Roman Church took up the healing of the sick in earnest when St. Benedict founded a monastery on Monte Casino in southern Italy in 529 C.E. The Benedictines cultivated scientific medicine by establishing schools, libraries and herb gardens, and most important, they collected ancient medical manuscripts. Eventually, monasteries developed into specialized medical centers and schools. Monastic medicine reached its height during the tenth century, but the Council of Rheims in 1219 forbade monks from practicing medicine outside the monastery.[10]

The church also prevented the clergy from practicing surgery because contact with blood was contaminating. Some monks defied the pope and developed considerable surgical expertise, but in 1215, at the Fourth Lateran Council, Pope Innocent III expressly forbade the clergy from performing any surgical procedure. The council also stated that before a physician could look after the bodily needs of a patient a priest must attend to his soul.[11]

During the early Middle Ages, a remnant of Greek culture and medicine remained in southern Italy and secular schools that taught philosophy, literature and medicine did not entirely disappear. Jewish physicians at times were called upon to treat kings and popes. Itinerant, often poorly trained surgeons treated infections and minor wounds; others specialized in treating broken bones, hernias and bladder stones. During the reign of the Frankish King Theodoric in 590 C.E., one lay surgeon named Reovalis was called to see a small boy whose case was "hopeless." Reovalis incised the boy's testicles and restored him to health.[12] This procedure could have been the drainage of a hydrocele.

The fall of the Roman Empire brought the consolidation of tribes and nomads into towns and then cities and nations. Crowding and lack of sanitation in cities increased the incidence of contagious disease and brought on the epidemics of bubonic plague, or the Black Death, that decimated Europe during the Middle Ages. Christian prayer, relics, amulets and charms were useless against the plague, which was considered God's punishment for the sins of humanity. The plague tried men's faith and the church sought scapegoats to explain the pestilence. The Jews in particular were persecuted.[13]

The incessant civil wars and conflicts between cities and states prompted a continued need for surgeons. Violence and a disregard for life assumed greater heights with the Roman Church's obsession to subjugate the Eastern Church and win back the Holy Land from Islam. Kings, Princes, lords, knights and their retinues, with hordes of camp followers, marched off to gain riches, glory and salvation in the Crusades. On their way to the Holy

Land, they killed thousands of Jews and heretics and fought among themselves. From 1096 to 1270, the Crusades ravaged entire countries; during the sack of Jerusalem, the Christian Crusaders butchered seventy thousand civilians. In 1212, thirty thousand children, none older than 15, led by a shepherd boy, set off with the Pope's blessing on a crusade to free the Holy Land. It ended with the boys being sold into slavery and the girls sent to brothels. This episode is surely the blackest stain on humanity and the low point in society's concern for children.[14] Perhaps the Children's Crusade was one of those aberrations that strike adolescents from time to time, but during the Dark Ages thousands of unwanted children in Gaul, Germany and Britain were exposed, left to die or sold into slavery. Despite the teachings of the church, poor children who were old enough to work were regarded as little more than chattel until well into the nineteenth century.

The teachings of Christ about children, the importance of the Madonna and the Christ child, and the belief that even the unborn child has a soul fostered a new attitude toward children, though it did not always work out in practice. The fathers of the church denounced infanticide, abortion and the practice of abandoning babies. Clement of Alexandria said that man is more cruel to his children than to animals; Barnabas, a contemporary with the Apostles, said, "Thou shalt not slay the child by abortion nor destroy it after birth." Mothers were allowed to leave unwanted children in the churches. In 787, the Archbishop of Milan created the first hospital for foundlings, who were trained for a trade and released at eight years of age. During the ensuing years, more foundling homes were built in association with churches.[15] Little or nothing was written about the medical care of infants and children during the Middle Ages; when ill, they were looked after by midwives and wet nurses.

The improved weaponry of medieval warfare brought another dimension to surgery. Gunpowder, the Chinese combination of saltpeter, charcoal and sulfur for fireworks, was first used by the English against the French at the battle of Crècy in 1346.[16] Cannons, first used as siege weapons to knock down castle walls, were soon firing shells, firebombs and canisters against ranks of soldiers on the battlefield. By the sixteenth century, well-disciplined units used handheld muskets and pistols to mow down opposing armies. Surgeons once faced with slashes, fractured skulls, broken bones and arrow wounds now had to deal with cannonballs and bullets that could tear a man in half or smash his bones and leave necrotic, infected tissue. Even if they had access to the works of Galen, there was nothing in ancient medical literature to guide them in treating bodies smashed with cannonballs. Fortunately for suffering humankind, the teachings of the Greek physicians were saved and translated and finally seeped back into Europe from those most unlikely sources, the Eastern Mediterranean and Islam.

CHAPTER 9

Byzantium to Baghdad

Greek philosophy and medicine continued in the eastern portion of the Roman Empire because Greek was the language of Christianity. Syriac Christians translated Greek scientific literature into their language as early as the fourth century.[1] Greek physicians continued to practice in Constantinople, where there was a repository of ancient documents. Christian and Jewish physicians in Pergamon and Alexandria taught medicine and preserved the works of Galen and Hippocrates.

Oribasius (325–403), who studied at Alexandria and later became a court physician to Emperor Julianus at Constantinople, had sound advice on the care of children. He said that frightening a child would lead to convulsions and epilepsy and that children under the age of 14 were not to be bled. He described three varieties of what he called hydrocephalus: one with fluid between the scalp and the pericranium (which may have been a hematoma), one with fluid between the pericranium and cranium, and one with fluid between the cranium and the cerebral membranes. We can wonder how he would have known about intracranial fluid collections, except by autopsy or trephination. None of these conditions are what we now term "hydrocephalus," illustrating how difficult it is to interpret the ancient physicians. Oribasius also described hypo- and epispadius of the penis, together with a surgical treatment. His suggestion that boys and girls should have genial, humane tutors whose praise and encouragement will inspire them to excel was remarkably modern.

Aetius of Amida (527–565), a lord high chamberlain at the Byzantine court, described the restriction of speech by a tight frenulum, as well as umbilical hernia, tonsillitis and otitis.[2] The sixth-century physician Caelius Aurelaianus accurately described the incessant coughing and hemoptysis of tuberculosis and recommended diet, fresh air, steam inhalations and a sea voyage for treatment. He also described auscultation of breath sounds and percussion of the abdomen to distinguish intestinal distention with air from fluid.[3]

The seventh-century physician Paul of Aegina, named for his birthplace on the island of Aegina, was the last of the great Byzantine physicians who recorded and preserved what was known of medicine and surgery at that time. His *Epitome*, seven well-organized books that summarized the work of Oribasius, Galen and the Alexandrians, was translated into Arabic and later into Latin. Paul, who studied and taught at Alexandria just prior to its destruction by a Muslim army, was an important link between the Greeks and Europe. He is known for describing the delirium, vomiting of bile, abdominal distention, pain, diarrhea, trickling of blood from the nose, thirst, restlessness and convulsions that are symptoms of the plague. One can foresee the plague, he said, when animals perish, suggesting that he understood the role of rats as carriers of disease. For treatment, he recommended aloes, ammoniac perfume and myrrh in fragrant wine.[4]

Paul's writings on pediatrics follow Soranus and Oribasius, but he had more to say on several surgical conditions. He opened the occluding membrane of imperforate anus with a scalpel, then irrigated the wound with wine. Vaginal atresia is clearly differentiated from an imperforate hymen, and after exploration with a probe he excised the membrane with a scalpel and packed the vagina. He noted three types of hermaphrodism in males and one in females and recognized strabismus as a spastic condition of the eye muscles, which he treated with a visor-mask.[5]

Paul quoted another surgeon, Antyllus, in recommending tracheotomy for inflammations of the throat and palate. The patient's head was bent back and an incision was made at the third or fourth tracheal ring, just as we do today. The surgeon knew when he had entered the trachea by the whizzing noise and loss of the patient's voice. Paul also described the sensation of palpating an arterial aneurism as a sort of "sound" that disappeared on pressure. He ligated the artery above and below the aneurism with a double thread, closed the wound with ligatures and applied a compress soaked with wine and oil. He also used the ligature to tie off vessels during the removal of scrofulous glands in the neck and during thyroidectomy. Healing by first intention and use of the ligature were signal achievements, but he also made free use of cautery, bleeding and cupping. He abandoned thoracotomy for empyema in favor of cauterizing the chest wall. He removed the testicle when operating for a hernia.[6]

A large portion of Paul of Aegina's writings was translated and incorporated into the textbooks of Arabian authors. The material, often repeated verbatim, was later translated into Latin and eventually reached Europe.

The story of how Greek culture and the ancient medical manuscripts became woven together with alchemy and astrology to become Arabian medicine and were reborn in Christian Europe a thousand years later is worthy of *A Thousand and One Arabian Nights*. Skilled physicians with knowledge of Greek medicine were in demand at court, where sultans paid for cures with bags of gold or beheaded the physician when he failed. There was also intrigue, beautiful slave girls and miraculous cures of the Sultan's favorite wives. This history is clouded by the difficulty of translating anatomical and pathological terms and the fact that names of places changed at the whim of rulers. To make things more confusing, some historians used the original names of people and places, others the Latinized forms.

Fortunately, historians and theologians have studied this period in depth. Allen O. Whipple, a famous American surgeon who served as Surgeon in Chief of Columbia-Presbyterian Hospital in New York during the 1950s, wrote a monograph on the role of the Nestorian Christians in the history of medicine. Dr. Whipple, best known for his operation for cancer of the pancreas, was born in Iran of missionary parents and in 1959 studied ancient medical schools and hospitals in the Middle East. His work sheds light on this interesting but poorly understood era in medical history.[7]

Greek scientific thought had spread abroad in many different directions as Greek armies captured and then abandoned foreign lands. Greek became the language of science and government from Persia to Egypt. After the first century C.E., Christianity spread through Mesopotamia and Syria. Common people continued to speak their own languages and translated the Bible into their own vernacular. In the earliest period of Christianity, the Syrian Church translated both the Old and New Testaments into Syriac, an Aramaean dialect. This ability to read and translate Greek was important in the preservation and transfer of medical documents.

The process of biblical translation also resulted in a controversy over the nature of Christ.[8] The Syrian Church established schools for the teaching of theology and medicine in Nisibis, a frontier town between Roman territory and Damascus, and later at Edessa. An Aramaean monk named Nestorius taught that Mary was not the mother of God and that the spirit entered Jesus after birth.[9]

Nestorius was Patriarch of Constantinople from 428 to 431 but was condemned as a heretic and expelled from Edessa. The King of Persia welcomed the Nestorians to the city of Jundi-Shapur in western Persia. Medical teachers and physicians brought along their translations of Hippocratic and Galenic medical texts. The Nestorian Christian Church, with Syriac as its language, established itself in Persia. The school at Jundi-Shapur became a magnet for Christian, Jewish and Greek physicians, who mingled with Indian and Persian doctors. The school and hospital at Jundi-Shapur, based on Greek tradition, became a world-class medical center.

In the seventh century, the Prophet Mohammed (570–632) brought forth a new monotheistic religion that rapidly replaced paganism in the Middle East. Islam's conquest of Persia brought the followers of Mohammed to the university at Jundi-Shapur and into contact with the Nestorian and Jewish physicians who had preserved the Greek traditions. One of the Prophet's physicians who studied in Persia and settled in Mecca divorced his wife, who later remarried and had a son born with an imperforate anus. The boy survived an operation and later grew up to be extremely cruel and bloodthirsty, perhaps because he had suffered through childhood with fecal incontinence. Later, he developed a carcinoma of the stomach. His Christian physician confirmed the diagnosis by tying a bit of meat to a string and passing it down his throat. On the physician's withdrawing the string, the diagnosis was confirmed because a swarm of worms adhered to the meat.[10]

After an intermediate period of warfare and expansion, Islam under the Abbasid Caliphs settled in Baghdad, not far from Jundi-Shapur. The Abbasids developed a thirst for knowledge and established hospitals and universities. By the middle of the eighth century, the Caliphs invited Christian and Jewish physicians to teach and to translate the old medical books from Greek and Syrian into Arabic.[11] As the influence of Islam spread, medical and teaching centers arose in Damascus, Cairo, Córdoba and Toledo.

The classic period of Arabian medicine began with Abu Bekr Muhammed ibn Zakariya al Razi, known in the West as Rhazes. Born in 865 C.E., Rhazes spent the first years of his life writing poetry and studying music. On his first trip to Baghdad, he visited the Muqtadiri hospital, where a physician showed him a fetus with two heads. Rhazes returned the next day and, moved by the misery of the hospital patients, began to study medicine. After five years he continued his studies in Persia, and in 918 he returned to be the Chief Physician and teacher at the hospital in Baghdad.[12] His extensive writings included a monograph on the diseases of children, with descriptions of hydrocephalus, spina bifida, urinary calculi and umbilical hernia, essentially the same conditions described by earlier authors.[13] His best work was on measles and smallpox; he also introduced animal gut as a ligature and described the reaction of the eye to light. He was considered the Arabian Hippocrates because of his careful clinical observations, attention to diet and hygiene and use of simple drugs. Rhazes was also a chemist, or rather an alchemist, because he attempted to transform base metals into gold. In the process, he also discovered medical uses for several mineral salts.

Avicenna, an Arabian physician born a hundred years after Rhazes, memorized the Koran and studied rhetoric and astronomy. At the age of 16 in the year 1000 C.E., he commenced the study of medicine in Baghdad. Avicenna was as much a philosopher and politician as a doctor and as a result fell in and out of favor with the court and several times had to flee for his life. He wrote on astrology, mathematics and music as well as medicine, but there was nothing new in his treatise on children and infant hygiene. He mainly followed the Greek authors and Rhazes.[14]

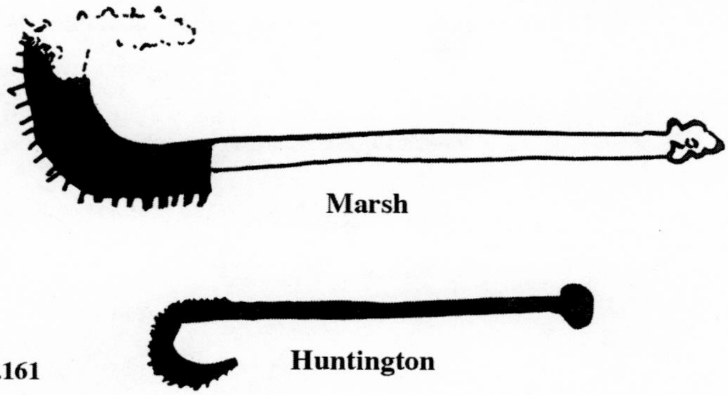

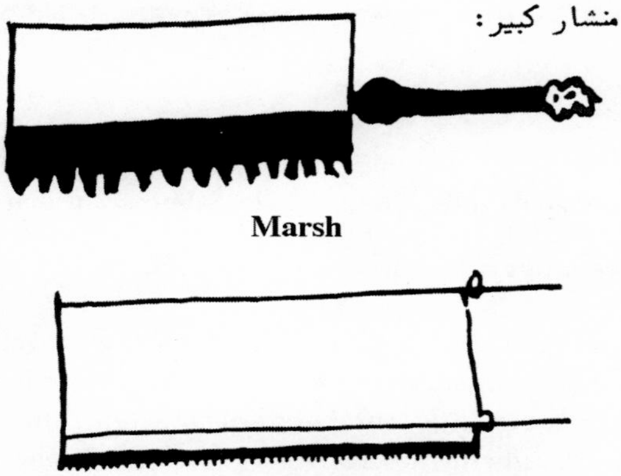

In the year 709, Arab forces crossed the Strait of Gibraltar and spread throughout the Iberian Peninsula. The Spanish Arabs created an atmosphere of religious tolerance and learning, where Christian, Jewish and Arab physicians worked together in harmony. The arts and sciences flourished in the Spanish cities of Córdoba, Granada, Seville and Toledo. Religious tolerance and academic freedom lasted until Their Catholic Majesties Queen Isabella and King Ferdinand defeated the last of the Arab rulers in 1492 at Granada.

Abd al Rahman, who became the Caliph of Cordoba in 929, estab-

صورة منشار صغير:

Marsh

Fig.161   **Huntington**

صورة منشار كبير:

Marsh

Fig. 162   **Huntington**

Saws for cutting bone used by Albucasis made of bronze or iron. Amputations were performed for severe injury and for senile gangrene. Bone saws have changed very little over the centuries.

lished a university that was for centuries the center of learning in Europe.[15] During this golden age of Spanish-Arabian harmony, a surgeon named Albucasis wrote one of the most remarkable and oft-quoted surgical textbooks of all time. Known in Arabic as Abu al-Qasim Khalaf ibn Abbas al-Zahrawi, he was born near Córdoba, Spain, in 1013 and died in 1106. His book *On Surgery and Instruments*, comprising approximately one-fifth of his entire medical work, is available in a handsome English translation.[16] The author's purpose was to revive the art of surgery as taught by authors from Hippocrates to Paul of Aegina. In addition to reviewing the ancient works, Albucasis drew on his own experience as a practical surgeon to describe specific operations and instruments in great detail. He utilized a tonsil guillotine, the concealed knife for opening abscesses in nervous patients, scissors, syringes, a lithotrite and a table for reducing fractures. He used animal gut as a suture and devised a paste consisting of flour and egg white that hardened to form a cast for fractures. During the second half of the twelfth century the book was translated into Latin, and for the next five hundred years it influenced European surgery.[17]

The book opens with a lucid discussion of the advantages of the cautery and special instruments to cauterize specific lesions. We regard the "red hot iron" as a barbaric instru-

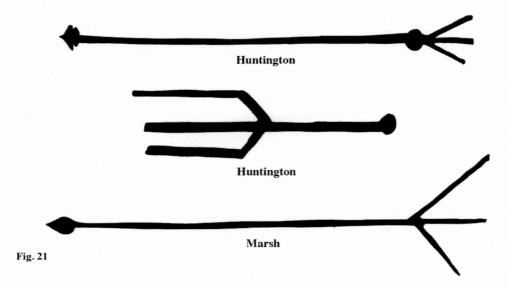

Huntington

Huntington

Marsh

Fig. 21

Three-pronged cautery irons used by Albucasis, which would have been thrust, white-hot, into the shoulder joint to scarify and tighten the tissues to prevent recurrent dislocation. This technique was originally described by Hippocrates.

ment, but Albucasis used it with great delicacy, much as we would use a needle-pointed electrosurgical instrument or the laser. At first glance, his use of the cautery for headache or sciatica makes little sense, until we remember that in certain pain syndromes the injection of a local anesthetic into a "trigger point" often relieves the pain. Albucasis either cauterized or ligated the temporal artery for "throbbing" headaches. At one time, when I had problems with my hospital administration, I developed severe headaches, relieved by finger pressure or an ice cube on the temporal artery. Ligation of the artery completely stopped the headaches, proving the effectiveness of this ancient method.

For epilepsy in a boy, Albucasis used a fine-pointed cautery, applied to the occiput and each frontal prominence. Unfortunately, he does not give us any long-term results of this treatment. His treatment of ingrown eyelashes required steady hands and great care: "Put the patient's head on your lap and mark upon the eyelid the shape of a myrtle leaf, beginning near the lashes. Then apply cotton wool soaked in egg white. Then heat a cautery of this form and burn over the shape marked out, slowly with many small strokes till the whole surface of the skin marked out to the shape of the myrtle leaf be cauterized. The eyelid will contract, drawing the lashes away from the eye."[18]

Albucasis used the cautery for everything from harelip to toothache and sciatica. When he was cauterizing "scrofulous" tumors, the surrounding tissues were protected from the heat by inserting the hot iron through a hollow cannula. To drain a liver abscess, he used a remarkable hollow, sharp-pointed trocar that would cut, cauterize and allow drainage of the pus. In later years, surgeons seared the entire wound or amputation stump to control bleeding, but Albucasis first stopped the bleeding with finger pressure on the artery and then put several olivary-shaped cauteries in the fire until they were very hot. He promptly removed his finger and applied the cautery until the artery was sealed. If the cautery didn't work, he tied a ligature around the artery or applied a tight bandage.

Albucasis describes several specific indications for cautery in children. He treated "humpback," possibly tuberculosis of the spine, by cauterizing the most prominent vertebra with a circular iron; he warned against the cautery if the condition was due to a nervous spasm. The idea behind cauterization for hernia was to produce extensive scar tissue to obliterate the hernia sac and the canal. The boy being operated on lay upon his back while the surgeon reduced the intestine and omentum back into the abdomen. Then, with assistants, sitting on the patient's legs and chest, the surgeon marked a semicircle pointing upward at the lower end of the hernia. A slender, white-hot cautery emitting "sizzling sparks" was inserted to the pubic bone. The wound was then dressed with butter and the boy kept in bed for 40 days. One can only guess at the intense initial pain, but as in a third-degree burn, the nerve endings would have been immediately deadened. We can hope that the boy was given a good dose of opium and wine prior to the operation.

Albucasis also described a lengthy, difficult operation for hernia, in which he dissected the layers around the hernia sac and then incorporated the sac and all its layers, including the testicular vessels, with four sutures. He then removed the testicle. This operation would have been longer and possibly more painful than the cautery. Instead of simple drainage of hydroceles, he dissected and removed the sac with a knife or cautery. He treated varicoceles by ligation of the testicular veins.

Albucasis observed that hydrocephalus occurred in small infants and that the head would grow so large the child could not sit upright. The disease was fatal. He preferred not to treat these infants when the fluid was beneath the bone and the sutures were separated, but he describes incising the skin with a T-shaped cautery and draining the fluid. The wound was then dressed with bandages soaked in oil and wine.

When an infant was born with an imperforate auditory meatus, Albucasis cut away the membrane with a slender knife and kept the passage open with a medicated plug. He also opened an obstructed urinary meatus in a boy, at the time of birth, with a sharp scalpel and kept the opening patent with a lead sound. He also describes tonsillectomy, excision of "scrofulous" neck nodes and suture ligature of umbilical hernia in children. Albucasis had a good understanding of male psychology when he referred to boys who at puberty developed an "abhorrent" female-like breast. The treatment was to make a semicircular incision on the breast and dissect away the excess tissue, pack the wound with a cicatrizing compound and sew the wound edges. Except for the scar-forming compound, this is essentially the same operation performed for gynecomastia today.

It is with circumcision that we learn of his sensitivity to the pain and apprehension of his patients. Albucasis said that since circumcision is the result of our deliberate action, we should plan the very best operation and the easiest way that leads to safety. He also pointed out that the "Ancients" (being Greek) made no mention of circumcision and that the operation done by barbers and common practitioners with a razor was unsatisfactory and sometimes amputated the tip of the penis. He used a bit of psychology before the operation:

> ...make the boy imagine that all we are going to do is tie a ligature at the tip of his penis and leave it for another day. Then amuse him and cheer him as much as you can, according to his intelligence; then stand him upright before you and hide the scissors in your sleeve or under your foot and do not let the boy's eye chance upon that or any other instrument. Then with your hand take hold of the tip of the penis, blow into the foreskin and draw it back until the glans penis is exposed and cleanse from it all the unclean matter that has collected. Then ligate the indicated place with a double ligature and a second right around beneath; then take hold at the site of the lower ligature with thumb and forefinger, very firmly, and cut between the ligatures [with a scissors]; then quickly push back the skin and draw out the glans penis; let a little blood flow, then wipe it with a piece

of soft cloth, then sprinkle the ashes of dried gourds or else fine white flour. Apply on top of the powder a piece of linen with egg-yolk cooked in rosewater, beaten up with oil of roses.[19]

The instrument used in this case was a modern-type hinged scissors, suggesting that Arabian surgeons were the first to use this instrument rather than shears. Note that Albucasis didn't use the cautery for circumcision. You can almost hear him tell his students not to use the cautery for fear of burning the penis. Almost a thousand years later, there was a case report of a boy who lost his entire penis after a circumcision performed with an electrocautery unit.

The symptoms of bladder stones, the optimum age for operation and the technique of perineal lithotomy are so similar to previous descriptions that we are again led to believe there was a connection to Indian surgeons. Albucasis adds a few new tricks. First, he notes the association of rectal prolapse due to the boy's straining to urinate against a blocked urethra and he has the boy jump from a height in order to lodge the stone at the outlet of the bladder immediately prior to surgery. If the stone was too large to remove through the perineal incision, Albucasis crushed it with a special rough-jawed forceps. He also had a new instrument to remove stones impacted in the urethra. This was "a drill of the finest steel with a triangular point" and a wooden handle. The drill was gently pushed through the urethra until it touched the stone. By twirling the drill, the stone was penetrated and broken up, and then it was washed out with urine. The forceps and drill anticipate lithotripsy.

Albucasis recognized three types of inter-sex abnormalities. One case, in a female, must have been a true hermaphrodite, because the clitoris was enlarged to the size of a male penis and there were testicle-like structures. His treatment was complete amputation of the clitoris. He is less clear in his description of intersex abnormalities in males. One form may been a severe form of hypospadius, but he still recommended amputation of the penis.

His discussion of imperforate anus is similar to that of Paul of Aegina when he says that the midwife should perforate the membrane with her fingernail or a sharp knife, taking care to avoid the sphincter muscles. The wound is kept open with wool dipped in oil and wine or a lead tube.

Albucasis was much bolder in advising limb amputation for gangrene and even after the bites of venomous serpents. He cut through normal tissue above the gangrene with a broad knife and protected healthy tissue with linen while he sawed through the bone. He cauterized specific vessels and used styptics to control bleeding. His treatment of open wounds with wine and resins, trephination for head injuries and methods for reducing fractures and dislocations follow his predecessors.

It is worthwhile looking at his treatment of compound fractures, especially because in later years a compound fracture was an indication for amputation. When bones protruded through the skin, Albucasis reduced the fragments to their proper position, using a metal lever as described by Hippocrates when necessary. He chiseled or sawed away sharp splinters of bone and when the bones were replaced in their proper position, he dressed the wound with "sharp wine." After applying splints, he left the bandages loose to allow drainage. He wisely observed that a wound that remained unhealed after many days and continued to drain contained loose bone fragments that had to be removed.

One of his cases demonstrates a patient's fortitude and the persistence of an obviously great surgeon. The patient was a 30-year-old man who had multiple chronic draining sinuses in his leg for two years. The draining pus was evil smelling and the man was wasted, jaundiced and near death. With a probe, Albucasis determined that the sinus tracts communicated with one another and led to bone. He cut down and removed what appeared to be all the diseased, dead bone. When the wound refused to heal, he repeated the operation twice more until he had chiseled and sawed away all the diseased bone. New bone grew, the wound healed and the man was cured.[20]

Albucasis is far and away the most well-rounded surgeon we have yet seen. It is easy to criticize his extensive use of the cautery and for employing those ancient remedies bloodletting and cupping. He was, after all, handicapped by a lack of knowledge of anatomy, since the Muslims, like the Christians, forbade human dissection.

We can also see he had a concern for children and cared for a variety of birth defects. One of the first acts of the Prophet Mohammed was to prevent pagans from burying female newborn infants alive and from sacrificing children to the gods. Whether Albucasis' concern for infants with birth defects was an extension of a basic Muslim philosophy or a result of the tolerance and liberalism of the Spanish Muslims, he helped improve the lot of children.

Serafeddin Sabuncuoğlu, a surgeon practicing in central Anatolia (now Turkey), wrote a textbook of surgery, *Cerrahiye-i Ilhaniye*, in 1465. This textbook was in part a faithful translation of *On Surgery and Instruments* by Albucasis. We can say that in a sense, Arabian surgery found its way back to Byzantium. Serafeddin Sabuncuoğlu went beyond Albucasis, however, since his book describes new techniques for the drainage of hydrocephalus and he used a hollow canula instead of a solid plug to stent the urethral meatus. He also observed the frequency of bilateral hernias in children and made more detailed descriptions of intersex anomalies. Most important, he stressed the need for a "master surgeon" to operate on infants with imperforate anus in order to avoid damage to the sphincter muscles. This suggests that he was operating on more complex lesions instead of a simple membrane.

According to S.N. Cenk Buyukunal and N. Sari, who reviewed the original handwritten copies, this textbook with its beautiful illustrations may very well be the first atlas of pediatric surgery.[21]

CHAPTER 10

Salerno and the Universities

The European reawakening to Greek and Arabian medicine came through Salerno, a small city on the southwest coast of Italy, not far from Monte Cassino. The south of Italy had never been completely abandoned by Greek-speaking people, and Salerno had been a Roman health resort for hundreds of years. The medical school at Salerno was probably founded by monks from Monte Cassino, but Jewish and Muslim physicians were involved with the school from its beginning. The teaching staff included at least one woman, Trotula, who was mainly interested in gynecology and obstetrics.[1]

Constantinus Africanus (1020–1087) was the key figure in bringing medical knowledge from the Muslims to Salerno. A native of Tunisia, Constantine the African first came to Salerno as a merchant. He fell ill and after consulting an Italian doctor, probably a monk, decided that Italian medicine was inadequate. Constantinus returned to Carthage, where he studied medicine and collected medical manuscripts. According to legend, he journeyed to Persia and India to learn medicine before returning to Salerno, where he converted to Christianity and translated the works of the great Muslim physicians as well as Hippocrates and Galen into Latin.[2] These translations became the basis for medical learning and teaching at the medical school in Salerno.

Another avenue for the transfer of medical knowledge to European physicians opened when Alfonso VI of Castile conquered Toledo, an important center of Muslim learning. There, in libraries filled with manuscripts, Gerard of Cremona (1114–1187), a Lombard who had learned Arabic, translated many scientific documents, including the works of Albucasis.[3] The Crusaders returning home from their adventures in the Holy Land brought an appreciation for the civilization they had tried to defeat and also contributed to medical knowledge.

The combination of these events led to a revival of medicine and surgery and a new interest in medical writing. The first book to come out of Salerno is known as the *Bamberg Surgery* because it was found in Bamberg, a town in Germany. The book was little more than a collection of notes and excerpts from earlier books about the treatment of wounds and common surgical conditions. The *Bamberg Surgery* does, however, describe a soporific sponge soaked in hyoscyamus and poppy for surgical anesthesia.

A more organized book of surgery appeared in 1170, written by Master Roger Frugardi, a student and later a teacher at Salerno. This offered mostly a simplified version of Greek and Arabian surgery, with one important addition on intestinal wounds. A thin, hollow tube made of elder wood was placed inside the wounded intestine, presumably as a stent, so the sutures would not obstruct the lumen. The intestinal wound was then sutured with silk thread and a sharp needle, the intestine was cleaned of dirt and the bowel returned to the abdomen. The patient was placed on a plank and "shaken" so the intestine would slide into its normal position.

The surgeons in Salerno treated goiter with dried seaweed (for the iodine) and then, "with the aid of a hot iron, passed setons through the thyroid gland."[4] During the next one hundred years, Roger's students added to his work and created the *Surgery of the Four Masters*, which became the authoritative textbook of Europe. Unfortunately, this book promulgated the idea that wounds should be treated with ointments and poultices to encourage the formation of pus and, in comparison with the Arabian surgeons, had little to say about children.

Other scholars as well as physicians benefited from contacts with Arab and Jewish thinkers in Spain. The exchange of ideas between Christians, Muslims and Jews in intellectual centers such as Toledo led to the idea that learning was universal, without respect to religion or race. Latin-speaking intellectuals then came together in cities all over Europe to establish universities. Initially, there was a certain amount of intellectual freedom, but the universities soon became the bulwark of the church and the instruments of Kings. Both Pope and ruler needed men trained in law and theology to become canon lawyers and bureaucrats, the first civil servants of the church and state. There was no place for real study of the natural sciences or for disputation, since according to the church, "we are called by God not to acquire wisdom or dazzle mankind, but to save our souls."[5] The teachers were for the most part clerics and the curriculum consisted of the liberal arts, philosophy and theology.

Medicine in the universities was closely allied with philosophy and students spent more time discussing astrology, fine points of philosophy and alchemy than seeing patients. A diagnosis was more likely to be made by casting a horoscope than by examining a sick patient. The bedside medicine of Hippocrates and Galen gave way to idle speculation. Treatment consisted of elaborate, useless prescriptions including such nonsense as oil of a scorpion. The administration of drugs was influenced by the planets and stars. Medical men paid little attention to children; perhaps it is fortunate that their care was left to wet nurses and midwives.

Not only did the church forbid clerics from performing surgery, but also the care of wounds and the draining of boils were deemed beneath university-trained physicians. These mundane chores were left to semi-trained laymen or monks who had left the church. Barbers "let blood" for a variety of ailments, pulled teeth and treated burns, and a few set fractured bones. Another class of surgeons specialized in bladder stones, hernia, needling cataracts and the repair of amputated noses. Some of these surgeons were in families who handed their skills down from father to son; others went from village to village, just ahead of the angry relatives of deceased patients. The barber surgeons gained respect on the battlefield, however, during the unending wars of Europe. When Henry V invaded France in 1415, the Surgeon in Chief of the army, William Morstede, had a second-in-command and 12 assistant surgeons to care for an army of thirty thousand men. He had his own bodyguards, a chariot and two wagons and could impress as many assistants as required. The king paid his chief surgeon 250 pounds per year for his services, a tidy sum.[6]

The barber surgeons gradually sought recognition and over time became more influential. A Barbers' Company was organized in London in 1308 and was established by ordnance in 1376. As a result of royal patronage, the company was given a charter in 1462. In 1540, King Henry VIII signed a charter establishing the Guild of Barbers and Surgeons. This organization later became the Royal College of Surgeons.[7]

A few university-educated clerical physicians sought training in surgery in spite of the church. These surgeons, who had access to Latin translations of the Greeks and Arabians, wrote textbooks that guided European surgery for several centuries. The first truly wide-ranging university in Europe was established in Bologna, which began mainly as a school of canon law that attracted students from all over Europe. So well known did this university become that in 1220 Pope Honorius III said the rulers of the Christian people came from Bologna.[8] The school of medicine was founded by students and faculty who came north from Salerno.

Hugo of Lucca (1160–1257), first a student and then a teacher at the university, was appointed city physician in 1214 and in 1218 went on Crusade with the Bolognese contingent.[9] Perhaps as a result of his experience in battle, Hugo became especially skilled in the treatment of arrow wounds and skull injuries. In one case, he successfully treated a man who had the side of his skull and part of his brain slashed away with a sword. In another, Hugo debrided a necrotic, foul-smelling lung in a patient who had been wounded in the chest. Hugo left no written text, but his son and disciple, Theodoric, wrote one of the most important surgical textbooks of the Middle Ages.

Theodoric was a Dominican friar who studied at Bologna and learned surgery from his father. He became the Lord Bishop of Cervia, minister to the church of Botanto and confessor to Pope Innocent IV. Theodoric wrote his textbook toward the end of his life, in 1267.[10] He often referred to Galen, Hippocrates and Rhazes but contradicted these authors by citing his own experience. His most remarkable advice, repeated throughout the book, was to be gentle, debride wounds of all dirt and foreign material and wash wounds with strong, boiled wine. He preferred to close wounds with bandages and didn't disturb the dressings for three to five days, unless there was pain. In this way, he achieved primary healing. He closed facial and eyelid wounds with sutures, perhaps recognizing that the excellent blood supply to the face allowed for good healing. He controlled hemorrhage with pressure, bandages and, when needed, the ligature; he treated open fractures with dressings soaked in wine. It is hard for us to believe ancient surgeons could suture intestinal wounds and close the abdomen, but like many others before him, Theodoric washed the intestine with "hot dark wine" and closed intestinal wounds with the narrowest needles and delicate thread made from fine silk or the intestines of animals. To close the abdominal wall, he relaxed the muscles by hunching the back to make the belly concave.

Theodoric recognized that even poorly reduced fractures in children undergo molding and with growth become normal when he said that fractured bones in children readily "return to their normal state" because their bones are softer. Like Albucasis, Theodoric operated on "fatness of breasts in males" because it was contrary to nature for males to have breasts like women. He operated on umbilical and inguinal hernias but also treated small inguinal hernias with a compress of strong astringents, bound up tightly with a bandage. The patient was then kept on his back and on a liquid diet for 40 days. The bandage was kept in place for another 40 days. If this didn't heal the hernia, an operation was indicated.

Theodoric was one of the first to specifically mention hernias in children: "Very often, wise women cure their children without medications, since they recognize the onset of the disease and apply a truss and keep the child from groaning, yelling and excessive movement."

Theodoric's insistence on cleanliness is seen when he put patients to be operated on for bladder stones on a liquid diet and enemas for two days prior to the operation. He also bathed his patients up to the umbilicus before the operation and irrigated the wound with hot vinegar and water or hot wine afterward. He was the first to mention suturing the wound above the narrow bladder neck.

He mentions the "soporific sponge," a sponge with a mixture of opium and the juices of a half-dozen other plants boiled up together and dried on it, which was soaked in water and inhaled by the patient until he fell asleep. Theodoric's surgery reflects his high status in the church, since he advises specific prayers and exorcisms to be said along with the treatment of wounds. His use of drugs is confusing, and although he differs on some points, he mainly follows the "authority" of Galen. Theodoric clearly had experience with children and mentions for the first time trusses for children's hernias, the treatment of choice until the twentieth century. There is no indication that he treated other birth defects. His main contribution was his insistence on cleanliness, boiled wine to irrigate wounds and healing by first intention, without pus.

Despite Theodoric, most surgeons in Europe believed that if a wound didn't suppurate, the poison was absorbed internally. If the wound didn't produce pus spontaneously, they probed, poked and applied compresses soaked in various medications until the wound became infected and drained pus. A French surgeon, Henri de Mondeville, was the most ardent advocate of wound healing without suppuration during the Middle Ages, but his work was ignored.

France took over the leading role in medicine and surgery at the end of the thirteenth century when civil war in Italy led to the decline of the Italians. Lanfranc, a cleric and university trained, studied in Bologna before fleeing to France and becoming a professor of surgery in Paris. He must have been a "rebel priest," since he fathered several children and disobeyed the popes by doing surgery. Lanfranc treated hernias with trusses and operated for bladder stones only as a last resort. He is most important for bringing the science of surgery to Paris.[11]

The most important French surgeon at the end of the thirteenth century was Henri de Mondeville (1260–1320), a cleric who studied at the universities of Montpellier and Paris and then learned surgery from Theodoric in Bologna. De Mondeville returned to Paris to teach anatomy and surgery. He had extensive surgical experience in the military campaigns of France as well as a large practice. He was a royal body surgeon to King Philip the Fair and later his successor, King Louis X.[12] De Mondeville's position at court may have kept him from trouble with the church, since he bitterly condemned the separation of medicine from surgery. He soundly ridiculed the doctors of medicine who preferred to speculate and engage in abstract reasoning instead of doing practical work. He was also critical of the illiterate, rustic, stupid surgeons who learned operations from their ancestors but who didn't understand the principles of medicine.[13]

Between 1306 and 1320, de Mondeville worked on a textbook of surgery that stressed anatomy, but since he never dissected a human body, he taught with highly inaccurate pictures. He wrote on wounds but never finished his work because, he said, "to the shame of his Royal Majesty," he had "lost a lot of time at court and following the armies in the wars with England." The most important part of his book, and at the time the most controversial, was his insistence on using Theodoric's treatment of wounds to avoid suppuration. This entailed the immediate removal of foreign bodies and dirt, the control of hemorrhage, by ligature if necessary, cleansing with wine and closing the wound with compresses soaked in hot wine, held in place with bandages. De Mondeville used sutures when necessary and supported the patient with rest, nourishing food and wine. His colleagues violently opposed his methods with disdain, shameful words and even threats.[14]

In a swipe at doctors and in recognition of pediatric surgery, de Mondeville said: "The surgeon has a hand in human life long before the doctor does, when he rectifies nature by coming to the aid of some at the moment of birth who came into the world without an anus, without vulva, without any egress of urine."[15] He also quotes a woman who cured her two-year-old child's hernia by keeping him in bed for a month and giving him small doses of wine. Unusual for his time, de Mondeville blamed nature rather than God. He was also critical of those who thought God, rather than the surgeon, was responsible for the cure.

Henri de Mondeville advised surgeons to study hard, take care of the poor for charity, and be honest and open-minded. He tried without success to reconcile theory and practice and to unite medicine and surgery. It is unfortunate that his colleagues ignored and ridiculed this eminent, well-educated man. His book remained in manuscript form and was not printed until the nineteenth century.

Jehan Yperman (1260–1330) is in the topmost rank of all surgeons up to the time of Lister. Yperman was from Ypres, a Flemish city in Belgium, which was a center for textile manufacture. The city was the scene of many battles, in his time as well as in the world wars of the twentieth century. Yperman may have gained his interest in medicine from his mother, who was a nurse. He studied medicine and surgery in Paris and was a cleric, but he never took holy orders. Thus, he was one of those rare individuals who had university training but whose performance of surgery was not restricted by the church. He knew French and Latin but wrote his textbook of surgery in Flemish.

Yperman practiced in his native city for 30 years. In 1304, the city agreed to pay him four pounds a year for his services to the poor in l'Hôpital del Belle. He was required to live near the hospital to be on hand for emergencies. Unlike other prominent surgeons of his day, Yperman did not serve at the court of a King or the Pope but was a surgeon to the people. Perhaps this is why he had so much experience with children. He also led the surgical corps when the city went to war.[16]

Yperman's textbook *La Chirurgie* is dedicated to God the Father, Son and Holy Ghost, and to the Virgin Mary, "by the saints Cosmos and Damien, glorified martyrs for the Lord, and by St. Luke, glorified attendant of our Lady Mary." He frequently quotes earlier works of surgery, but mostly he followed the teachings of Lanfranc and Theodoric on wound care. Yperman's book commences with practical anatomy and injuries of the head. There is a mixture of science and superstition when he says that a bloody discharge and pus from the nose indicates torn meninges and death happens at the appearance of the next new moon. He also says head wounds heal faster in children because they are endowed with vitality conferred by the Lord. When the brain was exposed by an injury, Yperman shaved the head, removed all bone spicules and then dressed the wound with oil, tar, wax and gum resins, all boiled together. This ointment promoted granulation tissue and scarring that drew the wound together. He trephined the skull by placing the patient's head between his knees and scraping away bone to expose the dura mater to release pus or blood. The wound was then dressed with warm wine.

It still seems unbelievable that surgeons in the Middle Ages, without anesthesia, relaxation or intravenous fluids, were able to treat wounds of the intestine. Yperman honestly says that wounds of the jejunum and rectum are fatal but that perforations of the duodenum or ileum can be cured by resecting and then suturing the edges of the perforated intestine over a smooth tube of elder bark. One would think that there must be some error in translation, because the duodenum lies deep within the abdomen and even today a duodenal repair is liable to leak. Yperman replaces the intestine but leaves the abdominal wound open until the intestine heals. He says: "If the abdominal wound closes before the other and the intestinal wound suppurates, the suture line will come apart and both the intestines and the abdomen will distend with toxic matter and gas. This is a treacherous situation and you must recognize it at once and re-open or the patient will die. The bark tube will be passed per rectum."[17] His advice to leave the abdomen open and his advice to reoperate could have come from a current surgical journal.

Yperman closed wounds of the face, ears and hands with small, sharp, triangular needles threaded with fine waxed silk or linen thread, indicating his interest in obtaining fine scars. He must have been among the first surgeons to close cleft lips in children. First, he cut the edges of the cleft, to raise a flap of skin and leave a raw edge. Next, he placed sutures inside and outside. He then passed a needle from one side of the defect to the other a "good distance" away from the sutures. Threads were wrapped around the ends of the needle to take tension off the suture line. The wound was then dressed with a plaster of egg white and oil of roses. He also repaired clefts in the nostrils.

Yperman was correct when he said children frequently inherit their parents' defects. We can forgive him for thinking that other defects were the result of the mothers' fantasies during the "procreative act." Harelip is in that category, but some claimed it was due to something the mother ate during her pregnancy, such as a rabbit. Even today, grandparents especially may blame the mother for an infant's birth defects.

Yperman understood the natural course of umbilical hernias in children because he knew some would close spontaneously. He hurried the process by reducing the intestine and bandaging a pad of lint soaked in vinegar over the hernia. Up until a few years ago, when parents demanded that something be done for their child's umbilical hernia residents would use a similar tactic and strap a coin over the umbilicus. When all else failed, Yperman grasped the hernia with a forceps, pushed the intestine back into the abdomen and applied a clamp across the base. He then tied two strong threads around the sac above the clamp. When the infarcted tissue fell off, he dressed the wound with an ointment. He treated inguinal hernias in children with a truss and said: "If the patient is a baby, with a recent hernia use a pad and the bandage and this medication. Take a fistful of royal fern, sedum and comfrey, fennel and prunella. Soak the pile in wine, then give the patient a spoonful twice a day. Keep the truss snugly in place until the herniated viscera stay in the abdomen. The opening will close in about eight weeks. If this fails, you have to operate." Yperman also used doses of "minced herb Robert in wine," perhaps to sedate the child so he wouldn't push out the hernia.

Yperman never used the cautery for hernias but dissected away the spermatic vessels and sutured the hernia sac, leaving the testicle in place. The sutures were left long outside the wound and eventually came away. The patient had to stay in bed for 40 days and had to refrain from straining and sexual activity and avoid fattening, gas-forming foods.

It is unfortunate that Yperman's work was lost for several centuries. He was an unknown away from the universities, who wrote in his native language instead of Latin. He was one of the few medieval surgeons to irrigate wounds with wine, use the ligature and achieve primary wound closure without suppuration. His work on infantile hernia and cleft lip suggests that he had an interest in and experience with pediatric surgery.

Unlike Jehan Yperman, Guy de Chauliac practiced surgery at the center of Christian power and wrote in fluent Latin. Perhaps for these reasons, rather than his surgical skills, he has been considered the most influential surgeon of his time and of succeeding generations.

Guy de Chauliac was born to a peasant family in a tiny village at the end of the thirteenth century. A wealthy family recognized his talents, and with their help he studied at Toulouse and later at the University of Montpelier. He took holy orders and qualified as a master of medicine in 1325, when he was about 25 years old. The faculty did not teach surgery; he may have apprenticed to a "free" surgeon or to his anatomy teacher in Bologna.

De Chauliac was in Paris sometime after the death of de Mondeville and settled in Lyon in about 1330, where he was connected with a religious chapter.[18] In 1342, when Clement VI became pope, de Chauliac was called to Avignon, where he had access to Latin translations of Galen and works by earlier medieval surgeons.

During the plague epidemic of 1348, de Chauliac served as the Pope's personal physician. Unlike many physicians who fled the city, de Chauliac remained and treated the victims. During the second great epidemic of 1360, he contracted the disease and developed an abscess in his groin, which was drained and cauterized. He survived after a six-week illness. De Chauliac recognized the contagiousness of the plague and advised the Pope to keep a fire burning and to accept no visitors.[19]

After Clement, de Chauliac was physician to Popes Innocent VI and Urban. He also held ecclesiastical positions at Rheims and the cathedral at Lyon until his death in 1370.

How did de Chauliac practice surgery against church edicts under the noses of the popes? He also observed dissections of the human body in Bologna at a time when the study of anatomy was forbidden. The answer may lie with the rise of the state and the weakness of the Avignon Papacy. In 1230, Frederic II, Holy Roman Emperor and King of Sicily and Jerusalem, issued an edict requiring physicians to study human anatomy.[20] Philip the Fair of France, who moved the papacy to Avignon, was an adversary of the Popes, who at the time were more concerned about raising money and fighting heresy than whether or not a priest was doing surgery. Perhaps the Popes and Bishops preferred a well-trained physician-priest-surgeon to an illiterate barber surgeon when they needed an operation.

Guy de Chauliac's book, *La Grande Chirurgie*, published in 1363, near the end of his career, would become the unchallenged authority on surgery for two hundred years. In the preface, he thanked the Lord for giving him a long life and the knowledge and art of medicine. He said one should strive for a cure except when the disease was incurable, like leprosy, or if the patient couldn't stand the treatment, such as an amputation. He also advised against over treatment and used the example of bleeding hemorrhoids, which he said were a kind of phlebotomy to drain off the humors that caused ascites. His reasoning was wrong, but he was aware of the relationship of ascites with hemorrhoids even if he didn't understand portal hypertension.[21]

De Chauliac described how the professors at Bologna dissected criminals who had been decapitated or hanged by first opening the abdomen and removing the viscera. On succeeding days, the thoracic organs, the head and finally the muscles and nerves were studied. He also said one can study muscles and nerves in bodies dried by the sun. This study of anatomy was imperfect, followed Galen and probably did little to advance the practice of surgery.

The book extensively quotes previous authors from Hippocrates to Albucasis and de Mondeville and adds a few new ideas. De Chauliac's detailed directions for the care of head wounds include the removal of bone spicules from the brain, the drainage of subdural blood and pus and the use of instruments in elevating depressed skull fractures. He quotes Albucasis' description of depressed skull fractures in children as resembling a dented copper pot.

De Chauliac used wine, vinegar or warm oil to cleanse wounds and controlled hemorrhage with pressure, hemostatic stitches and catching a vessel with a hook and then applying a ligature. He closed facial wounds with sutures and with needles applied through the wound with encircling threads. Once again, we see the use of a monofilament, non-irritating method of closure to obtain a fine scar. Any modern surgeon who reads de Chauliac's treatment of abdominal wounds, suturing the stomach and intestine, restoring the bowel to the abdomen and suturing all layers of the abdomen while an assistant holds in the bowel with both hands cannot fail to be impressed.

De Chauliac's review of the cautery is as extensive as that of Albucasis and leads one to believe it was not as barbaric as we once thought. For amputating a dead limb, de Chauliac either cut through a joint or sawed bone, then applied the "red hot" cautery or boiling oil to staunch the bleeding. He improved on the treatment of fractures with a system of ropes and pulleys to provide traction. His treatment of hernias included manual reduction, trusses and surgery to block the canal with sutures and removal of the testicle. He suggested an innovation in the treatment of hernia by mentioning the "passage of a gold wire that pleats the canal." The monofilament, metallic wire would be less likely to extrude than silk or linen.

De Chauliac mentions tongue tie, tonsillectomy, hydrocephalus and strabismus in childhood, which he said was treatable with eye exercises by having the baby follow a candle or bright objects. He may have been referring to mastoiditis when he described draining fistulas from diseased bone behind the ears. The treatment was to chisel away bone down to the meninges and apply detergents or ointments of rose oil and honey.

His operation for a cataract sheds light on the fortitude of the patient, the outdoor operating room, astrology and the role of religion:

> For mature cataracts — a young willing patient, he is healthy and not over anxious. The weather is clear, the hour is 9 am, the moon is increasing and not in Aries. The opposite eye is covered with a bandage and he is seated on a narrow bench, his legs straddling it as if he was in a saddle. An assistant sits behind him and holds tight his head. The surgeon has prepared himself by chewing seeds of fennel, garlic or aromatic herbs. He sits astride the same bench, slightly higher. The patient thrusts his hands under his own thighs and the surgeon's knees snugly embrace those of the patient. He will use his left hand to needle the right eye and his right hand for the left eye. He holds open the lids on the operated side and gently exhales three or four times into the open eye to warm the cataract and to loosen it. He asks the patient to turn his eye inward and to stare at his own nose and to hold it so. Then with a prayer to God the surgeon introduces the needle far enough under the conjunctiva so he can see it clearly. With care to avoid veins, he directs the point of the needle through the cornea so he can see the tip, which he pushes to the center of the pupil or just above the center. He catches the cataract and pushes it down and holds it there long enough to recite the Pater Noster or the Miserere three times. If after release the cataract rises, he repeats the maneuver. When it remains below and there is no need to re-couch it, he withdraws the needle.

De Chauliac's *La Grande Chirurgie* summarized a thousand years of surgery since Galen. Progress was slow and incremental, but a sick or deformed child had a fair chance of being treated rather than being abandoned to die. A skilled surgeon could operate on a low imperforate anus, hernia, cleft lip, urethral obstruction, some intersex abnormalities, strabismus, clubfoot, and perhaps some cysts of the neck. A child with broken bones, dislocated joints and wounds might fare as well at the hands of a surgeon during the Middle Ages as now. The operations for tongue tie, fistula in ano, gynecomastia and tonsillectomy have changed very little since the thirteenth century. The masterpiece of surgery up until this time was the perineal lithotomy for the removal of bladder stones. All surgeons, from the time of the ancient Indians, indicated that the operation was successful in children.

La Grande Chirurgie circulated in manuscript for a hundred years and was printed in 1478, only 24 years after the invention of the printing press. It was translated from Latin into other languages and remained the surgical authority for two centuries until it was overshadowed by the works of Ambroise Paré.[22]

CHAPTER 11

The Anatomists

During the next two hundred years, except for the study of anatomy, there were few, if any, advances. The treatment of wounds actually deteriorated, possibly because many surgeons encouraged the formation of "laudable" pus in wounds.

Most historians claim that prohibitions against dissection of the human body by all the world's religions retarded the progress of surgery. In reality, a study of the anatomy of animals combined with observation of patients provided surgeons with enough basic anatomy to operate on surface lesions and wounds. They knew the difference between arteries and veins and the locations of the great vessels that were likely to be wounded or involved in tumors. All the surgeons who wrote textbooks knew about the diaphragm that divided the chest from the abdomen, the location of the spleen and liver, the membranes surrounding the brain and the layers of the inguinal canal. They knew enough osteology to set fractures and reduce dislocations without the benefit of X-rays. Surgeons gained this knowledge by long experience. There was, however, no organized teaching of anatomy to medical students. Without a working knowledge of the human body, physicians were happy with astrology, magic and prayer to cure disease.

Some doubt exists that the Papacy actually forbade human dissection for the study of anatomy. It could have been a misinterpretation of Boniface VIII's bull in 1300 against cutting up and cooking bodies to make it easier to send the bones home from the Crusades for burial.[1] During the fourteenth and fifteenth centuries, as the stranglehold of the church on society loosened, there was a growing thirst for knowledge. The voyages of Columbus and Magellan proved that the world was round. Copernicus showed that our world was not the center of the universe. The schools in Venice, Salerno and Bologna were allowed to dissect the corpse of one executed criminal a year. A professor read from the podium while a barber or surgeon dissected the body, but because of rapid putrefaction there was little time for real study. There were no new discoveries because whatever was found was made to conform to the teachings of Galen.[2]

It was a professor of anatomy and surgery at the University of Bologna, a man known as Mundinus or Mondino (1275–1326), who revived systematic human dissection. Mundinus graduated from the University of Bologna in 1290 and practiced medicine and surgery there until his death. He performed actual dissections and apparently had more than the allotted one body a year. Some of his students were even accused of body snatching. One of his assistants, a woman, became adept at injecting arteries and preparing anatomical demonstrations. Mundinus' dissection manual, *Anathomia*, which included clinical surgery, was used by students until the time of Vesalius. Unfortunately, the book adhered to Galen's teachings and added little new information to either anatomy or surgery.[3] It would be another 250 years before Andreas Vesalius challenged Galen and initiated the modern study of anatomy.

Vesalius (1514–1564) was born in Brussels, then a part of the Hapsburg Empire. He was a fourth-generation physician. His grandfather was the Royal Physician to Emperor Maxmilian, while his father was an apothecary to Maxmilian and later a valet to his successor, Charles V. Vesalius first studied the arts at Louvain and then attended lectures on Galen's theories at the University of Paris. He was not happy with this instruction and along with fellow students exhumed bones from the Cemetery of the Innocents for study.[4]

When war broke out between France and the Holy Roman Empire, Vesalius returned to the University of Louvain, where he first assembled a complete human skeleton. He went with a friend to a place where those who had suffered the death penalty were displayed in public: "I came upon a skeleton like that of the brigand which Galen records having seen. The birds had stripped the flesh from Galen's one, and I think they had picked this one clean as well, for a year ago his body had been merely charred as if it were roasted over a straw fire, and tied to his stake provided the birds with such a tasty meal that the bones were completely bare and bound together solely by ligaments." Vesalius untied the skeleton from its post and secretly carried it to his home.[5]

His graduation thesis was on the works of Rhazes the Arabian physician. Vesalius then went to Padua to continue his medical work and graduated in medicine with "highest distinction." He was appointed professor of surgery and anatomy in 1537, the day after his graduation at the age of 25. Unlike his predecessors, Vesalius did his own dissections, with students crowding around the table. He believed that the only way to teach was by hands-on, direct observation. Vesalius may have made some of the early drawings of his dissections himself, but most of the illustrations for his books were made by Jan de Calcar, thought to be a student of Titian. It was during Vesalius' intense period of anatomical studies in Padua that he realized Galen had based his anatomy on animals and not humans.

Vesalius' book, *De Humani Corporis Fabrica* (On the fabric of the human body), published

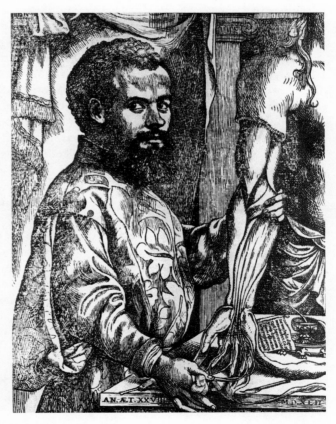

Andreas Vesalius was the first professor to perform his own dissections, rather than merely lecturing while a barber surgeon dissected. This portrait first appeared in the Fabrian of 1543.

in 1543, is one of the most important and lucid books in medical history. Originally there were seven books in Latin, covering every aspect of human anatomy down to terminal vessels and nerves. Vesalius was keenly critical of his forebears, especially Galen, when he found discrepancies between his own human dissections and their descriptions. He had the book published in Basel, where Protestants and liberal Catholics lived together in relative peace, thereby hoping to avoid theological controversy. Even so, because he claimed that Galen was wrong the book aroused a storm of protest. One professor, in a letter to Charles V, wrote: "I implore his Majesty the Emperor to punish, severely as he deserves, this monster born and reared in his own home, this most pernicious exemplar of ignorance, ingratitude, arrogance and impiety, to suppress him completely, lest he poison the rest of Europe with his pestilential breath."[6]

Fortunately, Vesalius was a man of independent means and had powerful friends at court, and the church was involved with insubordinate Protestants and the advances of the Turks on Vienna. Soon after publication of *De Humani Corporis Fabrica*, Vesalius became royal physician to Emperor Charles V, and for the next 11 years Vesalius traveled with the court. During this time, he treated the Emperor for gout and asthma, and performed surgery. In 1544, while with the Imperial army, he took care of a gunshot wound to the shoulder of the Prince of Orange, who died.[7] Vesalius had better luck with empyema; three of four patients whom he drained via an incision over the tenth rib survived.

Because of his work on anatomy, especially of the azygos vein, Vesalius was drawn into an academic controversy about where to perform venesection for the treatment of pleurisy. Hippocrates had claimed that stagnant blood should be taken from the same side as the disease, while the Arabs drew blood from the opposite side. When a Paris faculty member sided with Hippocrates, he was declared a heretic and banished. The argument went as far as the Pope and the Emperor. Vesalius wrote a long letter discussing the relationship of the azygos vein to the pleura and essentially agreed with both sides.

At that same time, new plants, including herbs, thought to have medicinal value came to Europe from the Americas. Vesalius wrote an essay on an herb known as china root but which might have been nothing more than sasparilla, a flavoring for soft drinks. It did not cure syphilis and didn't help the Emperor's gout or asthma. At one point, Vesalius was so depressed by vitriolic attacks on his work that he burned all his manuscripts.

When Charles V abdicated, Vesalius continued in the court of his son, Philip II. Vesalius' career ended with his death in a shipwreck at the age of 50, during a pilgrimage to the Holy Land. The exact circumstances surrounding this voyage are subject to debate. Some claim he performed an autopsy on an aristocrat, whose heart was still beating, and the Inquisition then sentenced him to death, but Philip II commuted the sentence to a pilgrimage.

In publishing *De Humani Corporis Fabrica*, Vesalius made full use of the new printing press and the reproduction of illustrations. The book was copied, pirated and widely used. Vesalius opened the way for his students and followers to new discoveries and to the discipline of pathological anatomy. He had little to say about children, but in his discussion of the styloid process he mentioned tying a peg or a stick to the side of the wrist to prevent children from becoming left-handed.[8]

In the 1543 edition, Vesalius described a small boy with a head twice the normal size. The child had been carried from door to door by a beggar woman and put on display by actors.[9] In the 1555 edition, Vesalius said he thought this boy was similar to a two-year-old girl, whose head had grown in seven months to the size of a man's head. In this child, water had accumulated within the ventricles of the brain (a case of true hydrocephalus) and not between the dura and the brain, as described by the ancients.[10]

This same edition includes a rather humorous explanation for the passage of ingested foreign objects through the gastrointestinal tract, a common problem in pediatric surgery. In his discussion of the size of the lower end of the stomach, he tells of a Spaniard who, while making love to a lady, noticed her pearl necklace. He gave her the "sexiest of all possible workouts" so she would sleep soundly. He then undid the necklace and swallowed the pearls, the jeweled cross and even the string. The jewels passed through his gastrointestinal tract and he recovered the necklace.[11] In another bit of anatomizing, Vesalius explained the "brilliant design of the channels that convey urine to the bladder." He correctly observed that it was the oblique entrance of the ureters through the wall of the bladder that prevented reflux, even when the bladder was tightly distended.[12] This principle of oblique insertion is the basis of reimplantation of the ureters to prevent urinary reflux, an important operation in children.

Andreas Vesalius influenced the history of surgery in one more important way. When Henry II was mortally wounded during a joust with the Count of Montgomery, Vesalius met Ambroise Paré, a lowly barber surgeon in consultation at the bedside of the dying King. This episode led the leaders of the surgical College of St. Côme to admit Paré to membership despite the fact that he did not write a thesis in Latin and he was a Protestant. The college could not deny membership to man who had been surgeon to a King.[13] Paré became one of the most celebrated surgeons of his day, particularly famed for his treatment of wounded soldiers. Had he not met the eminent and well-connected Vesalius when he did, the history of surgery might have unfolded very differently.

CHAPTER 12

Ambroise Paré

PRAVEEN GOYAL, M.D., *AND* ANDREW WILLIAMS, M.D.

> In 1536 when Francis the French king sent a puissant army beyond the Alpes, many were wounded on both sides with all sorts of weapons but chiefly with bullets. When he ran out of the scalding Oyle which was being used by others for treating gunshot wounds, Paré applied a digestive made of the yolke of an egge, Oyle of Roses, and Turpentine. To his surprise he found the results with his new remedy beyond expectation.
>
> — *The Workes of Ambrose Paréy*[1]

Ambroise Paré (1510–1590), famous for his treatment of wounded soldiers, is one of the most written about and best-known surgeons of all time.[2] This leading surgeon of the Renaissance also treated children and wrote about their diseases. His fame is due to his treatment of wounded soldiers, but little is known about his treatment of children.[3]

Paré's fascinating life story shows talent overcoming adversity. Born in the French town of Laval, Paré did not receive formal teaching and had little knowledge of Latin and Greek. However, his limited education could not stop his quest for learning. He learned his art from firsthand experience, initially with an apprenticeship to a barber surgeon. One of Paré's tasks was to hold the kicking legs of a patient undergoing a perineal lithotomy for bladder stones.

Paré was so impressed with the surgeon's dexterity that he went to Paris in 1533 to perfect his own surgical skills. He was a house surgeon at the famous Paris hospital Hôtel-Dieu. Some historians suggest that his inability to afford the examination fees for admission to the barber surgeons led him in 1536 to take the position of surgeon to the Mareschal de Montejan in the French army.[4] Paré had no salary but was paid whatever his patients thought he was worth. His

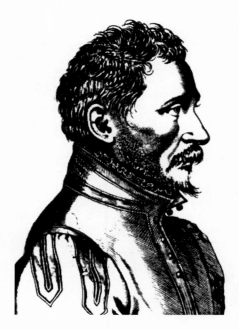

Ambroise Paré in middle age. The motto "Labor Improbus Omnia Vincit" translates to "Ceaseless Labor Overcomes All Things."

first campaign was to Turin, where the French army was forced to retreat. In all, Paré served as an army surgeon in 17 military campaigns. He passed the examination in 1541 and subsequently was appointed as head of the French College of Surgeons in 1567.

Paré's contributions to the field of surgery remain well acknowledged centuries later. In the twentieth century, G. Keynes described Paré as being "the emancipator of surgery from the dead hand of dogma."[5] Paré's ability to incorporate understanding of anatomy into the art of surgery makes him stand apart from empiric surgeons.[6] He is best known for his revolutionary treatment of gunshot wounds.[7] At the time, gunshot wounds were thought to be poisoned or "envenomed"; standard treatment was to pour boiling oil into the wound, while bleeding was controlled with the red-hot iron. Surgeons kept huge cauldrons of boiling oil over wood fires during battle. There were so many casualties during the retreat from Turin, however, that Paré ran out of oil. In desperation, he applied a mixture of egg yolk, oil of roses and turpentine to shattered arms and legs and broken heads. The next day, his patients treated with boiling oil were feverish and in great pain, but those treated with the new mixture had slept well and were free from pain and inflammation. Paré also reintroduced the ligature to control bleeding, a vast improvement over hot iron.[8]

As a result of his success with war wounds, Paré became famous, and four successive French Kings appointed him Surgeon in Chief to the royal household. Paré could not write in Latin, but he learned enough to translate *De Humani Corporis Fabrica* into French. Paré had consulted with Vesalius at the deathbed of King Henry II, and as a result, the surgical College of St. Côme could no longer deny him membership because he could not write a thesis in Latin. Paré went on to become one of the leaders in the College.

Paré's influence on pediatric surgery and child health care remains largely unrecognized. Still's *History of Pediatrics* cites Paré's interest in the care and feeding of infants: "One is apt to think of Ambroise Paré in connection with battlefields and wounds rather than sucking infants."[9] Still, however, omitted Paré's treatise on the management of congenital and acquired disability in his seventeenth book, *Traitant des Moyens et Artifices d'Adiouster Ce Qui Defaut Naturellement au par Accident*.[10] Paré treated children with a range of deformities, including hydrocephalus, congenital dislocation of the hip, squint, anal atresia, trauma, and urinary bladder stones.[11] Where unsure, he would seek a second opinion

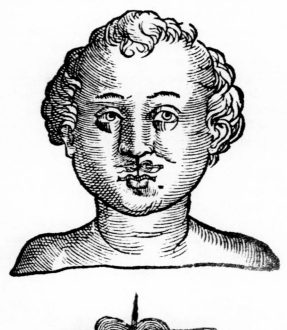

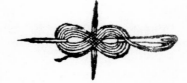

A needle passed across the wound left after freshening the edges of a cleft lip would have caused less tissue reaction than sutures. A figure-of-eight thread around the needle closed the wound. This technique was used by Paré and Jehan Yperman.

irrespective of the social status of the patient.[12] His treatments were mainly conservative. As an example, he would wait to see if a child would pass a bladder stone, but when surgery was required Paré performed perineal lithotomy with the usual method.

In 1552, Paré proposed pincers for removal of superfluous digits in the young but cautioned: "...each hand hath five fingers onely: whatsoever more or lesse is against nature, if there will be fewer, it is a fault not to be helped by art but there will be more that is for the most part helped by the art."[13]

Paré was the first to suggest the conservative management of clubfoot using the orthopedic boot rather than surgery. This less invasive treatment is in line with modern opinion.[14] He speculated, however, that the condition was caused prenatally by the mother sitting with her legs crossed or postnatally by the mother holding the child with its feet pressed inward, a view not held in modern practice.[15]

Paré wrote with sympathy and compassion about disability. He invented various appliances, such as a padded metal jacket for scoliosis whose design was used for centuries afterward.[16]

Paré also made good use of others' discoveries, irrespective of their source, where they clearly benefited the patient. One such example is a speaking aid.[17] With regard to intersex abnormalities, Paré described the clinical features of hermaphrodism. He also attempted to classify these abnormalities to determine gender and whether or not the patient was impotent.[18] Paré advocated the use of trusses for hernia treatment, and was against surgery except for incarcerated or strangulated hernias. He attributed hernias in children to their continual crying and coughing and kept the child seated in his cradle for 30 or 40 days in addition to wearing the truss.[19] Guy de Chauliac and contemporary surgeons removed the testicle during hernia surgery, and this may have been why Paré was opposed to surgery for hernias.[20] He also mentioned a case where the intestine had run out of the wound during an operation for umbilical hernia and the child died.

Paré was refreshingly fierce in condemning quackery, despite being limited by the medical and scientific understanding of his age. He did not hesitate to expose fraudulent medical practice such as using unicorn horn as a therapy for childhood eczema.[21] He was equally dubious of other nostrums such as mummy and bezoar but was almost as credulous as his peers concerning the efficacy of theriac (a complicated distilled and fermented drug used as a preventive as well as a curative medication against "venoms"). He listed at least three formulas for its preparation.[22] On the other hand, he recognized the possibility of a child's exposure to maternal medication through breast milk.[23] Paré attempted to attribute an unexplained infant death to teething, although this may be one of the earliest descriptions of SUDI (Sudden Unexpected Death in Infancy).[24]

Ambroise Paré is usually remembered for his remarkable contributions to military surgery. However, he also clearly saw children in his practice and advanced the art of surgery in children. Paré's observations and use of logical thinking set him apart from the ordinary barber-surgeon, as well as his more empiric colleagues. Believing that "experience without reason is like a blind man without a guide," he incorporated the concepts of sixteenth-century medicine into his practice.[25] He educated the surgeon to practice within the context of known medical understanding. This aim of creating the "learned surgeon" improved not only surgical care but also the reputation of surgery itself: "With which the Chirurgion being provided and instructed shall not onely know by what means to find out a remedye, but also, lest he may seeme to mocke any with vaine promises, he shall discerne what diseases are uncurable, and therefore not to be medled with."[26]

Paré's writings are an outstanding example of a desirable model of personal and professional surgical practice, based in this case on his superb technical skill, integrity, wide experience and quest to integrate surgery. [27] Paré's humility in recognizing his own limitations and those of surgery, and in seeking a second opinion when clearly in his patient's interests, is exemplary. Paré's remark "Je le pansay: Dieu le Guarit" emphasized his core belief that cures were not his but God's, who was working through Paré by employing his surgical art. Thus, Paré should be seen as more than an exceptional surgeon. His words and practice remain both challenging and inspiring.

CHAPTER 13

Some New Birth Defects

During the sixteenth and seventeenth centuries, four men in Switzerland elevated the art of surgery and contributed to the surgical care of children. The first was Felix Wurtz of Zurich, who was born in 1512 and died in approximately 1575. He apprenticed to a barber surgeon at the age of 14, then studied in other centers, including Padua, perhaps when Vesalius was teaching anatomy.[1] He did most of his work in Basel, where he was the head of an "honest burgher family" and a member of the Shearers' Guild. Perhaps his interest in children's surgery arose from his own son, who was crippled and too disabled to work. In 1563, he published *Practica der Wardartzney* in German. An English edition, *An Experimental Treatise of Surgerie in Four Parts*, was published in 1632. This book, which dealt with wounds, gunshots and fractures, condemned probing and other meddlesome interventions that inhibited natural healing. Wurtz anticipated asepsis when he warned surgeons not to breathe into wounds and to keep the wounds clean. He recommended pure cloth dressings with wine or water and salt and used sutures only to replace flaps. Unlike his contemporary Ambroise Paré, he didn't ligate blood vessels but used a plaster with turpentine, rosin, mastic and amber. It seems that Wurtz, for all his practical experience, was not familiar with — or perhaps didn't believe in — ligatures.

One incident in his life indicates his standing with his fellow surgeons and his failure to use the ligature. Wurtz suffered with such severe headaches, exacerbated by bright light, that he begged his colleagues to cut his left temporal "pulse vein" (the temporal artery). He said: "...but I continued still with my lamentations, hoping that one or other would take pity on me." When a fellow surgeon agreed, the operation was done, with all the Master Surgeons gathered around Wurtz's bed. When the artery was divided, the wound bled "vehemently" but stopped spontaneously. Wurtz praised the Lord for delivering him from his pain.

Wurtz appears to have been a pediatrician as well as a surgeon. His fame in pediatric surgery derives from his *Children's Book*, published after his death in 1612 by his brother Rudolph.[2] This addendum to Felix's surgical work deals with the nutritional management of young children, skin and eye diseases, "cramps," orthopedic injuries and deformities. He wrote that congenitally deformed feet were caused by frights, strange sights or carelessness of the mother. He used bandages and splints for treatment but never mentioned actual surgery.

Pierre Franco, a provincial surgeon of lowly origin and a contemporary of Paré, was one of the great surgeons of the Renaissance. He was born around 1500 and his only education was an apprenticeship to a herniotomist. Franco began as a "cutter," with even lower status than a barber surgeon. He certainly had no medical education or even instruction in surgical theory, sharing a non-academic origin with Paré. Judging from Franco's work, he must have performed anatomical dissections and by the time he wrote his second book of surgery he had learned Latin and some Greek. Franco was born in Provence, but because of persecutions against Protestants he fled to Berne and later Lausanne in Switzerland, where Calvinism flourished. By 1556, when he published his first book, he had performed hernia operations for ten years in the pay of "very powerful lordships of Bern." Apparently, he was a city physician. In his first book, he called himself a hernia surgeon, but he was also a skilled lithotomist and cataract surgeon and he improved the operation for cleft lip. The English translation of *The Surgery of Pierre Franco* by Dr. Leonard D. Rosenman includes Franco's biography, an excellent history of surgery during the Renaissance, as well as Franco's books.[3]

Franco's work on hernia surgery opens with a detailed discussion of the anatomy of the peritoneal cavity, the intestines, the cremasteric muscle, the dartos and the course of the testicular vessels and vas deferens. His usual operation started with strapping the patient to a board or a cot in the head-down, feet-up position that facilitates reduction of intestine into the abdominal cavity. Franco then pinched the skin between his fingers to reduce incisional pain. Instead of opening the groin, he made a high scrotal incision to reduce bleeding. While an assistant held up the testicle, Franco dissected the sac and all layers including the testicular vessels and vas deferens up to the groin. There he applied a right-angle clamp and doubly transfixed and ligated all structures with a silk thread. He mentions that the pressure of the clamp anesthetized the distal structures, so that the application of a cautery only "warms the patient comfortably." This operation removed the testicle but, despite its crudeness, would have cured an indirect hernia, which is most common in young people. He then made an incision lower in the scrotum for drainage and left the ends of the sutures dangling outside the wound until they spontaneously came away. If the omentum was adherent in the hernia sac, he ligated, divided and cauterized the omentum before returning it to the abdomen.

Franco's most important contribution to hernia surgery was saving the testicle in patients who had only one. He freed enough of the cord structures to apply his clamp "only moderately tightly," then passed a gold wire with one sharpened end, about the length of a finger and the diameter of a "fat pin," through the cord structures, avoiding the spermatic vessels and the vas deferens. The ends of the wire were then brought together like a ring to occlude the sac along with its covering layers. He then loosened the clamp, folded the wire and pinched down the ends. It was really a gold staple that closed the hernia sac and all its layers, except the spermatic vessels and the vas deferens. Franco said gold thread was as pliable as lead and the retained metal caused no discomfort. This truly amazing operation was anatomically correct; unlike a multifilament silk or linen suture, which harbored bacteria-causing infections, metal sutures remain in the tissues without becoming infected. In later years, sutures made of silver, stainless steel and monofilament plastics almost completely replaced fibers such as silk and cotton.

Franco also described the techniques and complications of hernia operations used by Guy de Chauliac and others. He had abandoned groin incisions because of increased bleeding and infections as a result of poor drainage. He also described a young man who had undergone two previous operations but had a recurrent fist-sized hernia. Franco cured the hernia with his operation.

Franco's method for dealing with incarcerated hernias, when the bowel was adherent to the sac, required remarkable surgical skill. He recommended early surgical treatment because, he said, when the scrotum turns blue or grey and the patient has a distended abdomen it is too late for an operation. His method was to open the scrotum and cord structures and insert a flat wooden dissecting rod between the intestine and the sac; he lifted the layers away from the intestine with hooks and cut up to the ring. He passed his finger around the bowel, separating it from the sac, and reduced the intestine into the peritoneal cavity, starting with the bowel closest to the ring. This is a difficult operation under the best of conditions. The steep head-down position must have been the key to reducing the bowel.

Franco also described a spherical mass that appears in the groin but doesn't descend into the scrotum and is softer. He claims to have treated many of these hernias in men, women and children of all ages. It is difficult to know whether he is describing small indirect hernias or the direct variety. In these cases, he made a groin incision in the direction of the "skin wrinkles" after pinching the skin long enough for it to become numb. He cut through the tissues until he saw the hernia sac and followed it to the ring, where he applied a stitch tie to the neck. He then sutured the tissues to close the wound.

After surgery, Franco advised tight bindings, bed rest and comforting medications; he also used a hollow sound to treat postoperative urinary retention and said that postoperative infections were "not infrequent." From his references to male infants and children of all ages it is apparent that he treated children as well as adults.

He distinguished hydroceles from hernias by grasping the upper scrotum and squeezing the mass downward rather than up toward the abdomen. He also said: "If you hold a flaming candle on one side of the tensed scrotum, you will clearly see through the watery mass; that is a sure sign that there is no irreducible intestine or omentum in it. You must be certain of that, because an error can lead to a fatal outcome."[4] We still use transillumination to distinguish hydroceles from hernias and testicular tumors, but with a flashlight rather than a candle.

Franco knew that many bladder stones form in the kidneys and may be trapped while descending through the ureters, but he also said that in children stones often form in the bladder. Franco introduced the "master's twist," the maneuver of pointing a curved metal catheter toward the groin on approaching the bladder neck to push an obstructing stone back into the bladder. He was also the first to discuss the difficulty of capturing the stone with his fingers in the rectum. At times, he said his fingers became so exhausted that he had to stop the operation and return a few days later to complete it. In the meantime, he irrigated the bladder with a syringe to "subdue the discomforts and mild inflammation." He also placed a silver grooved director in the urethra to find the stone and used scoops or forceps to remove it. For patients too old or debilitated to withstand stone removal at one sitting, he stopped the operation and left the wound open, covered with bandages. The stone often passed spontaneously through the incision in the bladder neck and appeared in the dressings. Franco invented several instruments to facilitate stone removal, including a retractor introduced into the rectum for pulling stones down to the bladder neck.

One of his most remarkable patients was a two-year-old child in whom Franco could not push a stone, the size of a hen's egg, to the bladder neck through the perineal incision. He said: "The patient had been tormented by his symptoms and his parents said that they preferred his death to a lifetime of suffering. Added to that was my own foolish embarrassment at my failure to remove the stone. I faced his stubborn parents with the idea of a supra-pubic approach, because the stone could not be brought down for a perineal route for removal." Franco then pushed the stone up from below, made an incision just off the midline above the pubis and removed the stone.[5] The very sick child recovered. This has to be one of the most amazing cases in the history of pediatric surgery. Any surgeon who has had to "break scrub" and talk to frightened parents during the course of a difficult operation can understand the scene. Later surgeons who attempted to remove bladder stones through a supra-pubic incision encountered difficulty when they opened the peritoneum and the intestines eviscerated.

Pierre Franco did more than two hundred operations for cataracts and claimed to have cured nine out of ten of his patients.[6] His technique was essentially the same as that used by Guy de Chauliac, but Franco provided more details about the operation and its complications. He stressed the importance of knowing when the cataract was "ripe" for couching and said he caused his patients little suffering.

Franco also published a description of bilateral cleft lip, or "hare's teeth," in 1556.[7] When the gap was too wide to close easily, he made incisions inside the mouth, through the muscles, but left the skin intact to reduce tension. He usually sutured the wound directly but also described passing needles through the tissues and holding the wound with wrappings of thread around the needles, similar to the technique of Jehan Yperman. Franco also described a "sutureless" innovation that involved gluing patches of cloth on each side of the wound and then suturing the cloth. In either case, he reinforced the wound closure with pads and bandages to relieve skin tension. Franco was highly critical of those who, for religious reasons, ascribed birth defects such as cleft lip to "God's reward" and left the child untreated. He then mentioned the removal of extra digits and other defects that left the patient with a long and useful life.

Pierre Franco was also an obstetrician who performed postmortem caesarian sections and used a variety of instruments to dilate the cervix for difficult deliveries. For his time, he was a most accomplished surgeon despite his humble beginnings.

Guilhelmus Hildanus Fabricius, also called Fabricius Hildanus or Fabry, was a German Swiss who lived from 1560 until 1634. He had to give up his academic education when his father died, but Guilhelmus apprenticed to a surgeon and then practiced in Geneva with Jean Griffon, who performed nose replacements.[8] After that, Fabry traveled, presumably to practice, in Lausanne, Cologne and Holland. In 1613 he was in Lausanne, where two thousand people, including two of his daughters, died of the plague. At the age of 55, in 1615, he settled in Berne, where he did most of his surgery and publishing. He wrote on hernias and bladder stones and published 600 case histories, of which 150 were observations on diseases of children. His special concern for the suffering of children may have arisen from the deaths of four of his own. Unlike Franco, Fabry hardly ever operated on hernias in children but used trusses and bandages and strengthening the body with "internal cleansing."

He was one of the first to mention the major defect of the abdominal wall, what is now termed "omphalocele." On July 18, 1609, a baby was born whose "liver, intestine, stomach and spleen were hanging out on the abdominal wall." The child lived only a few hours and there must have been an autopsy, because Fabry's report indicated that the hepatic vein was split and that the other organs were normal. There was no mention of a membrane covering the organs, but because the liver was outside the abdominal cavity, this must have been an omphalocele instead of a gastroschisis.

In 1593, Fabry incised a closed anus in a six-day-old boy and maintained the opening with ointments and a lead rectal dilator. The boy recovered and was known to have lived in good health for at least 19 years. In another report, Fabry described a male infant with a closed anus who passed feces with urine from his urethra. After consultations, the doctor decided not to operate and the infant died with a distended abdomen and a fever on his seventeenth day. At autopsy, they discovered the rectum was connected to the bladder. Fabry also described a child with an encephalocele; several cases of hydrocephalus, which he thought were incurable; and a newborn infant with a lump on his sacrum the size of a goose egg and covered with thin skin that drained water. The infant died at four days of age, clearly from a draining meningomyelocele. Fabry's case records also included girls with vaginal atresia and a child with an absent vagina, who was incontinent because her urine drained directly through what must have been a uro-genital sinus.

Fabry operated on several children with hemangiomas, including one the size of a peach on a boy's nose and another the size of a plum. He commented that he had to work fast to remove the entire tumor and used caustics to control bleeding. Another of his firsts was a woman who had suffered from a huge tumor with blisters that enveloped her arm and drained a clear yellow fluid. This must have been a lymphangioma, a condition not previously described.

Peter P. Rickham, who founded the world's first neonatal surgical unit at the Alder Hey Hospital in Liverpool during the 1950s and later was Chief of Surgery at the children's hospital in Zurich, claimed that Johannes Fatio should have the honor of being considered the world's first pediatric surgeon.[9] Fatio, who lived from 1649 until 1691, was descended from Italian Protestants who sought refuge in Basel, Switzerland. He apparently wanted university training, but at the time academic physicians still did not do surgery. He apprenticed to a barber surgeon and at the age of 23 became a member of the barber surgeons' guild. He later took a doctor's degree at the Protestant University of Valence in the Dauphine and returned to Basel in 1678. He was not recognized as a qualified physician because the medical hierarchy refused to recognize a foreign degree. Despite this setback, during the following 13 years he had a successful surgical and obstetric practice in Basel and the professors consulted with him on surgical cases.

His remarkable book, *The Helvetian Reasonable Midwife*, had a chapter on diseases of neonates and infants. In the first paragraph, he advised midwives to take a few drops of wine and blow into the mouths of newborn infants who did not breathe, while pinching their nostrils. This was an example of mouth-to-mouth resuscitation. He successfully operated on boys with peno-scrotal hypospadias by passing a trocar from the glans penis along the shaft of the penis to the opening. He then passed a lead tube through the new channel into the bladder, where it was left for 16 days. He strapped the opening closed with bandages. He also operated on hydrometrocolpos, nevi and hemangiomas. He described

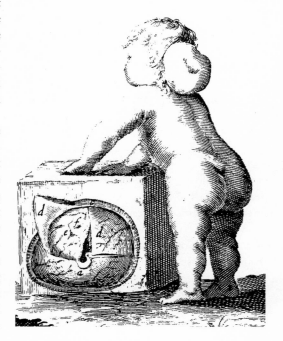

A baby with an encephalocele, a hernia of the meninges from a defect in the skull, drawn by Job van Meekeren, a fifteenth century barber surgeon who lived in Amsterdam.

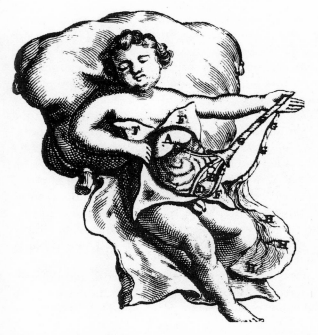

A drawing of an infant with an omphalocele, from the casebook of Job van Meekeren. Note the presence of the umbilical cord at the top of the sac containing intestine.

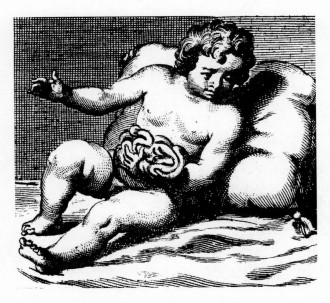

An infant with a gastroschisis, also drawn by Job van Meekeren. The exposed intestine without a sac differentiates this gastroschisis from an omphalocele. It is interesting that the baby is holding his intestine in his hands — just as one would do who had suffered a traumatic evisceration.

many pediatric conditions, including the "setting sun" appearance of the eyes in babies with hydrocephalus. He distinguished between the common umbilical hernia, which he said rarely required treatment, and omphalocele, or prolapse of the abdominal organs outside the body at the time of birth. According to Rickham, "In those days many children with exomphalos were born with rupture of the membranes and prolapse of coils of the intestine. Fatio returned the gut carefully into the abdomen and closed the defect by continuous strapping." This is truly an amazing statement. Though nothing is said about the survival of these infants, the method of treatment was entirely correct.

In 1689, Fatio made what may be the first separation of conjoined twin sisters.[10] The twins were born to a 42-year-old mother and were joined at the umbilicus by a narrow tube of skin. After consultations with local surgeons and professors, Fatio separated the twins in the presence of "distinguished members of the city of Basel."

The twins were joined from the xiphoid process to a single umbilicus. Fatio tied umbilical vessels to the navel and then transfixed and tied the bridge between the two infants with a silken cord and divided between the two ties. The ligature fell off on the ninth day and both infants recovered. Not until the twentieth century would another set of conjoined twins be separated.

While Fatio was active in Basel, the city council, dominated by old families, rich merchants and factory owners, became intolerably corrupt. Bribery was common. In 1690, Fatio became a leader in a citizens' committee that opposed the city council. After an armed confrontation, Fatio worked out a liberal constitution that gave voting privileges to all citizens. The deposed Lord Mayors reacted, again seizing power, and at sword point imprisoned Fatio in a city tower. Despite his popularity with the people and his surgical skills, the council tortured Fatio and then had him beheaded in the public square. The ousted members of Parliament placed his head on a spike and stuck it on the roof of the Rhine Gate, perhaps as a warning that surgeons shouldn't meddle in politics.

For the first time in our history we find descriptions of gastroschisis, omphalocele and spina bifida in the same city, during the same century, by the two surgeons Fabry and Fatio. This was not an isolated phenomenon; in Amsterdam, another center of medical learning, Job Janszoon van Meekeren (1611–1666) left behind a casebook with detailed drawings of infants with gastroschisis, omphalocele and encephalocele. Van Meekeren's teacher, anatomist and physician Nicolaes Tulp (1593–1674), was the first to name spina bifida.[11] Von Meekeren was also the first to describe the elastic skin of what we know as Ehlers Danlos Syndrome in a 23-year-old man.[12]

We have noted the apparent absence of deformities in primitive societies, and although writers from the time of Hippocrates observed other external birth defects, they made no mention of infants born with their abdominal organs outside their bodies. It is hardly likely that all infants with these obvious, dramatic abdominal wall defects were put to death without the knowledge of a physician. It is even more unlikely that careful observers from Galen to de Chauliac would not have commented on such obvious human defects. Almost all of these authors noted enlarged heads, which may have been due to hydrocephalus but were just as likely to have been collections of fluid or blood due to birth trauma. The encephalocele, a large collection of fluid on the back of the skull, is another new phenomenon, as is spina bifida. Here we have the appearance of what seem to be entirely new birth defects appearing in Europe during the seventeenth century.

We must remember that during this period and for a century or more previously Europe was the scene of almost continuous warfare involving the increased use of cannons, guns and tools, all of which required a tremendous increase in the mining, smelting and refining of metal. The by-products of this industrial activity could have contained teratogens that triggered these new birth defects. The introduction of tobacco from the New World could have been another factor.

Gastroschisis, the evisceration of the intestine onto the abdominal wall with no amniotic covering, is particularly interesting from an environmental standpoint. Most pediatric centers didn't see more than one of these patients a year until the 1970s, when the reported incidence of gastroschisis increased in all almost all parts of the industrial world. It is not unusual nowadays for pediatric surgical centers to report on series of a hundred or more cases. Could this increased incidence stem from the almost universal use of toxic chemicals such as pesticides and herbicides? Given that question, the apparent appearance of new birth defects in the war-torn seventeenth century is a bit of history that deserves more attention.

CHAPTER 14

Return to Padua

Three famous medical men have strong connections to Padua: Hieronymous Fabricius ab Aquapendente, William Harvey and Giovanni Battista Morgagni. Fabricius and Harvey were teacher and student at the University of Padua for a portion of their lives; Morgagni taught at the same university nearly a century later. All three were responsible for major innovations in our understanding of medical science.

Fabricius (1537–1619) made contributions to human anatomy and embryology as well as medicine and surgery. He was born in Aquapendente, a small Italian village, and at the age of 17 commenced his study of medicine at the University of Padua, where his professor Gabriele Fallopio had succeeded Vesalius. Fabricius graduated with a doctorate in medicine and philosophy in 1559 and commenced to practice medicine and surgery. In 1565 he was appointed to the chair of anatomy and surgery; he was primarily interested in anatomical research. In 1594, the Senate of the Republic of Venice erected a large amphitheater for the demonstration of anatomy and named it for Fabricius.[1]

Fabricius Aquapendente lived to the ripe old age of 82, much loved by his students and patients. His most important surgical contribution was to revive tracheotomy, an operation that had been performed by the Greeks and Arabians but was abandoned during the Middle Ages for fear of injuring the carotids or the jugular veins. According to Fabricius, of all the operations performed on man for cure, tracheotomy was the one that gave prompt relief to those at the point of death. He said the operation was not indicated if the trachea was filled with pus, as in pneumonia, but was only done for obstructions above the pharynx, in the mouth, throat or tonsils. When the patient's suffocation could not be relieved by other means, his head was bent backward and the surgeon drew a straight line in ink from the larynx to the sternal notch in the middle of the anterior neck. He then made a transverse incision between two tracheal rings, three or four rings below the larynx in order to be far away from the seat of disease. Fabricius separated the muscles that lie on the trachea with hooks and, with the trachea exposed, cut deeply enough to enter the cavity. He then inserted a short, straight cannula with two wings. After three or four days, the cannula was removed and the wound sutured. The operation is performed today in almost exactly the same manner.

Fabricius' most important contribution to the study of anatomy was his paper "De Venarum Ostiolis," published in 1603, in which he described the valves of the veins. He thought the valves prevented blood from pooling in the extremities and aided the ebb and flow of blood from the heart. He also believed his discovery lent support to Galen's theory about the circulation of the blood. When we consider that dissections were performed on fresh and sometimes semi-putrid cadavers in a deep amphitheater by candlelight, it is amazing that the professor or his students could find valves in veins. It is doubtful that many of today's medical students dissecting in brightly lit laboratories have observed venous valves.

William Harvey was born at Folkestone, England, on April 1, 1578, during the reign of Elizabeth I, while Sir Francis Drake was on his voyage around the world. Harvey studied at Kings' School in Canterbury, then Caius College in Cambridge, where he graduated with a B.A. degree in 1597. He then entered the University of Padua, where he studied anatomy under Fabricius Aquapendente and graduated with a doctorate in medicine at the age of 24 in 1602. William Harvey became warm friends with Fabricius and it is likely that Harvey's studies in Padua led to his work on blood circulation. Upon his return from Padua, he entered the College of Physicians of Cambridge and graduated in 1604. He became a Fellow of the College in 1607 and was appointed to St. Bartholomew's Hospital in London. He soon became the physician in charge at St. Bartholomew's and was responsible for ministering to the poor without pay.[2]

At the age of 37, Harvey commenced giving the Lumleian lectures on anatomy, during which he explained his ideas on the circulation of the blood. Harvey was appointed as Physician Extraordinary to King James I in 1618; at the King's order, Harvey accompanied the Duke of Lennox on a three-year tour of France and Spain during a time of war and plague. Harvey wrote that he had never seen such misery, desolation, poverty and famine and that it was time to leave off fighting and war. In 1632, he became physician to Charles I, and during the English civil war Harvey attended the wounded and settled in Oxford, the headquarters of the King.

William Harvey's book, *De Motu Cordis* (The circulation of the blood), was published in 1628 and dedicated to Charles, King of Great Britain, France and Ireland.[3] This 72-page book gave a clear account of the action of the heart and the movement of blood around the body in a circle. Harvey completely and finally disproved Galen's theory that blood originated in the liver and that the heart produced heat, the lungs cooled the blood and the arteries contained air.

In explaining why arteries could not carry air, Harvey used the examples of fetuses, dolphins and whales, who had no access to air. He understood fetal circulation, including the role of the foramen ovale in shunting blood from right to left, but knew that the foramen was closed in adults. By observing the formation of the heart in the chick embryo he was able to describe how the ductus arteriosus "dries up" and ceases to exist in the adult, just like the umbilical vein.[4] These early embryological observations would lead centuries later to our understanding of fetal circulation, so important in treatment of diseases of the newborn infant. He also observed how in the fetus, blood returning from the placenta through the umbilical vein bypasses the intestines.

To obtain proof of how the blood circulates, Harvey dissected living animals, fish, frogs and serpents, to observe how blood flowed in the arteries in diastole and systole, as well as the synchrony of the contraction of the auricles and then the ventricles. He demonstrated how a partially occluding ligature caused a limb to become swollen with blood and that after the immersion of the limb in cold water release of the ligature allowed cold blood returning to the heart to change the pulse rate. He also opened the chests of animals to ligate the vena cava near the heart and then demonstrated that an artery in the neck was empty, but the veins were full. In another demonstration, in the presence of King Charles and many notables, Harvey divided the exposed internal jugular vein of a doe to demonstrate a gush of blood from the head side but only a few drops of blood from the lower portion, rising up from the chest.[5] As final proof of his dissecting skill, he described the lacteals in the mesentery, the cysterna chyle and their connection to the subclavian vein, saying, "Milky fluid is chyle, being carried away from the intestines to all parts of the body for their nourishment." The professors who still taught Galen's theories of anatomy were critical of Harvey, and his practice suffered.

William Harvey established the relationships between physicians and surgeons when he ruled that a surgeon may not trephine the head, pierce the body or dismember or do any major operation on the body without the direction of a doctor. He clearly felt that surgeons were subservient to physicians. After the civil war, William Harvey retired to London, where he died in 1657.

Our knowledge of disease took another great leap forward with the publication of *On the Seats and Causes of Disease* in 1761. The author, Giovanni Battista Morgagni, was a 79-year-old professor of anatomy at Padua. Born in 1682, Morgagni attended the University of Bologna medical school and graduated in 1701. He immediately began to practice medicine and write on anatomical subjects. In 1715, the Senate of Venice appointed him professor of anatomy at Padua, the same position once occupied by Vesalius and Fabricius Aquapendente.

Morgagni lectured and demonstrated anatomy in the old amphitheater with its steep balconies where his predecessors had taught anatomy for more than 150 years. He did more than study anatomy; he kept careful clinical histories and correlated the patients' symptoms with abnormal findings at autopsy. After nearly 50 years of teaching, Morgagni organized his notes on over seven hundred autopsies into five books, starting with the head, then the thorax, the abdomen, surgical and traumatic disorders, and finally a supplement on miscellaneous diseases.[6]

In book 1 on diseases of the head, Morgagni, like his predecessors, defined several types of water in the head as hydrocephalus, but he differentiated fluid between the skull and skin from fluid within the cranial cavity. He had cured "hydrocephalus," fluid beneath the skin, without the surgeon's knife in an infant and described children with subdural fluid after trauma. He had also dissected fetuses in whom he found intracranial fluid but no brain, or anencephaly. Another infant, who died immediately after birth, had only a small portion of cerebellum; the rest had been "destroyed by water." Morgagni described many similar cases of "monstrous hydrocephalus" that he had personally observed, as well those seen by other authors. He understood the relationship between hydrocephalous and spinal meningocele, saying that sometimes, as the "watery tumor" on the spine increased in size, the size of the head diminished. He had never seen a case of true intracerebral hydrocephalus cured.

Morgagni ended his discussion with a case history of a large, strong, well-nourished ten-month-old boy with a tumor over his sacrum that had grown since birth to "fist sized." The tumor was soft and contained water that "shone through the parietes" in several places. The boy's legs were weak and his feet distorted, typical for children with low meningomyeloceles. Morgagni advised the family to do nothing, but being "ignorant country people," they took the child to a surgeon who incised and drained the fluid. "From the time the child was cut upon, he never ceased to cry and weep, though he had been cheerful before. He trembled in his whole body and his face, which before was smooth and well colored, began to wrinkle and pale." The child died on the third day after the operation.[7]

Morgagni gave a classic description of otitis media and mastoiditis that progressed to meningitis in a 12-year-old boy.[8] After a bout of smallpox, the boy suffered pain in his right ear, deafness and purulent discharge. When a swelling appeared behind his ear, a surgeon incised the skin and a large quantity of pus, identical to that which drained from the ear, "issued forth." The boy then suffered convulsions, delirium and pain in his head. At the autopsy, Morgagni found green pus that communicated from the meatus auditorium through the temporal bone to beneath the cerebrum and down the spinal canal. Until the introduction of antibiotics in the middle of the twentieth century, otitis media, mastoiditis and meningitis were major killers of children. Family doctors regularly lanced eardrums to drain pus during home visits.

In book 3, *Diseases of the Belly*, we find a number of conditions related to children. Intussusception, especially in association with intestinal worms, appeared common.[9] Morgagni had this to say: "For when one part of the intestine enters within the part next to it, the portion of the mesentery, that is annex'd thereto, must enter in at the same time. Wherefore, if it stay there for any considerable time and a constriction comes on, the motion of the blood, through its vessels, being retarded, it will swell to such a degree, as to hinder the intestine that has entered in, from receding and likewise prevent the passage of matter, and the circulation of the blood is entirely precluded." These patients "vomited excrement" and their intestines at autopsy were distended with flatus. He also described intestinal volvulus and "morbid appendages" or diverticulae in the ileum. This could have been a reference to Meckel's diverticulum.

Morgagni cited several references in the literature to infants with imperforate anus and added his description of infants in whom surgeons had attempted operations on high lesions. He claims that an infant in whom the rectum was encountered the distance of "two joints of the little finger of a moderately sized man" survived but later died of a different disease. There were also histories of women who passed feces via their vagina or bladder. Morgagni wrote: "But if there is no exit at all, to the abdominal faeces, a doubtful method of cure ought to be preferred to the certain death of the infant."[10] Imperforate anus remains a difficult lesion to treat and even with all our modern technology a cure is still doubtful.

It is difficult to sort out references to children and birth defects in the old literature because they are not separated from adult diseases. Morgagni's book 4 tells of a 25-year-old man who died 13 hours after suffering two sword thrusts to his upper abdomen. At the autopsy, there were wounds of the lung and stomach and a "broad" wound of the diaphragm. The stomach had passed up into the chest through this traumatic diaphragmatic hernia. Next, Morgagni describes cases of diaphragmatic hernia with portions of the stomach or intestines drawn into the chest in patients who had not suffered trauma. One was an old man who at autopsy had a defect in the mid-anterior part of the diaphragm just below his xiphoid cartilage, with a part of the colon in the chest. This we now call a hernia through the foramen of Morgagni. There was also the case of a young man who had no respiratory difficulty but died with intractable vomiting. His stomach was "turned up almost to the clavicles," occupying the entire right chest. The right lung was absent. Morgagni also refers to an infant of two months who was sick from birth and at autopsy had almost all his intestines herniated through a foramen just to the left of the esophageal hiatus. He describes dissections of fetuses in which the stomach, spleen, a part of the liver and the intestine were in the left chest. He also noted that the left lung had only one "lobule." These are excellent descriptions of infants who had foramen of Bochdalek diaphragmatic hernias, including the all-important hypoplastic lungs commonly found in these infants.[11]

Like his predecessors back to Hippocrates, Morgagni was fascinated by congenital genitourinary defects. He considered the difficulties that adults with chordee and hypospadius have with intercourse but unlike previous authors offered no surgical treatment. He performed autopsies on women with vaginal obstructions at various levels, as well as on a girl whose urethra had been dilated by a surgeon on the assumption that it was the vaginal opening. Most puzzling were Morgagni's cases of "double bladder" in girls. In one case he wondered how watery fluid could accumulate in the totally separate doubled bladder without a ureteral orifice. He described it as proceeding from the "matrix" and having two layers. The girl also had menstrual irregularities, so one has to wonder if this wasn't an example of a fluid-filled septate vagina rather than a double bladder.[12]

Three hundred years before neonatology evolved as a specialty, Morgagni took a great interest in the diseases of newborn infants: "You see, how very wide, and, at the same time, an almost unbeaten track, lies open to investigate the diseases of new-born infants, I mean by an attentive and accurate observation in dissection after death, as well as while they are living, if the foolish love of parents did not withstand." He went on to say that the bodies of infants have many peculiarities and that it was important to compare the symptoms of children while living with the findings at autopsy.[13] Although he didn't realize the cause, he observed the sunken fontanels of infants who were about to die due to collapse of the brain in severe dehydration.

Paré and others had described "monsters" who looked like frogs or toads because the mother had handled a frog while pregnant. At first glance, this would appear to be another fancy common to the Middle Ages, but Morgagni's description proved that the "toad" was really an anencephalic fetus. The cranium was small and "not the least trace" of a brain was found; there was only fluid. The head was situated on the shoulders, the ears were low set, the mouth was gaping and the lower part of the body was also distorted. He reviewed other, similar cases and asked if these "monsters" were not due to some horrible spectacle seen by the mother but then said he did not understand why these things happened. In his section on monsters, Morgagni described infants with omphalocele, conjoined twins and cardiac anomolies. He said these disorders destroy a great part of the human race and that because physicians could not take histories from children they could not provide remedies. He did make some astute clinical observations, such as advising the use of a long teat of a goat that would extend beyond the cleft to feed infants with cleft palates. Remarkably, he knew that the usual jaundice of the newborn was self-limiting unless the intestinal feces were white, indicating that bile didn't flow into the duodenum. Here was the differential diagnosis between biliary atresia and non-obstructive jaundice.

Morgagni anticipated the surgical morbidity-mortality conference where the autopsy is used to demonstrate surgical mistakes. The case was a nine-year-old boy who had been troubled with a bladder stone for six years. The surgeon who operated on the boy had a great deal of difficulty, "tortured the boy to a violent degree" and was able to extract only a portion of the stone. The boy died and at autopsy Morgagni found that the bladder was lacerated and a part of the stone remained. He was highly critical of the surgeon, mainly because he had operated without palpating the calculus.

Morgagni's discussion of bladder stones included a teenage girl who had inserted a hair-bodkin into her urethra and bladder. A stone formed around the object and the girl suffered intense pain along with pus discharged from a sinus tract. After lingering in misery, she died. At autopsy, the stone encasing the needle filled the bladder and the kidneys and ureters were filled with pus. This was a common occurrence, since Morgagni knew of other cases in which surgeons had been able to extract the needle with a curved hook introduced into the urethra. He assumed it was due to a "salacious humor" that the girls introduced objects into their urethras.[14]

Morgagni described many internal diseases and put medicine on sound scientific principles, but the practice of surgery — hampered by the lack of anesthesia and still plagued with infections — changed little. Fortunately, during the eighteenth-century, in which Morgagni lived, English surgeons attained great skill, a concern for children and respectability.

CHAPTER 15

The Eighteenth Century

On November 9, 1737, Queen Caroline of England was seized with severe abdominal pain and vomiting. She vomited the brandy, snakeroot and Daffy's elixir administered by the court physicians. Next, they removed 12 ounces of blood and gave her an enema. The queen suffered through another bleeding, more enemas and blistering; when these remedies failed, two more physicians bled her a third time. Finally, John Ranby, house surgeon to the King, was allowed to palpate the royal abdomen and found a strangulated umbilical hernia. That evening, the surgeons lanced the umbilicus and let out a small amount of "matter," but not enough to relieve her obstruction. After several days of intense suffering, the strangulated hernia burst and excrement poured out on the bed and floor. The Queen died on November 20. John Ranby, the surgeon who operated on her, served the royal family for many years and was the first master of the company of surgeons that later became the Royal College of Surgeons of England.[1]

Umbilical hernia, a common birth defect, resolves spontaneously or can be corrected with a simple operation. Queen Caroline's hernia probably reopened after one of her many pregnancies. This sad history illustrates the status of surgery during the early eighteenth century, but three English surgeons — William Cheseldon, Percival Pott and John Hunter — rank high among contributors to surgery in children.

Sir Zachary Cope, famous for his book on the acute abdomen, delivered a lecture on William Cheseldon to the Royal College of Surgeons in 1952. Cope wrote a short biography of Cheseldon to draw attention to the surgeon who played a decisive role in separating surgeons from barbers.[2] In addition to his other achievements, Cheseldon (1688–1752) was compassionate and did his best to alleviate the pain of surgery for the many children he operated upon.

His experience with a broken arm during childhood may have directed Cheseldon toward a career in surgery. In 1703, at the age of 15, he was apprenticed to a surgeon on the staff of St. Thomas Hospital in London. Apprentices were paid as much as three hundred pounds a year to assist with the dressing of wounds and at operations in the hospital and the surgeon's private practice. Cheseldon studied anatomy with William Cowper, a well-known anatomist. After serving a seven-year apprenticeship, Cheseldon passed the examination to become a barber surgeon but did not have a hospital appointment.

When Cowper died, Cheseldon taught anatomy, and in 1713, at the age of 25, he published *Anatomy of the Humane Body*. This text, illustrated with Cheseldon's own drawings, remained in print for a hundred years. It included descriptions of operations and some physiology, so it really was a text of surgical anatomy.[3] His lectures and textbook were so popular that he took students and surgeons away from the public lectures and dissections given at the Barber Surgeons Hall. At one point, the barber surgeons prevented Cheseldon from obtaining the bodies of executed criminals for his dissections, an incident that likely led him to press for a bill passed by the House of Commons to separate the surgeons from the barbers and to form a new Corporation of Surgeons in 1745.[4]

Cheseldon also published *Osteographia, or Anatomy of the Bones,* with 56 plates. He used the skeleton of a 20-month-old child to illustrate the differences between children and adults. He noted that in infants the skull is larger in proportion to the rest of the body and described the presence of cartilage at the extremities of limb bones. He also described the soft spongy bone with thickened periosteum in children who died with rickets.

In 1718, when he was almost 30 years old, Cheseldon was appointed to St. Thomas Hospital, where he took care of injuries, removed nasal polyps, operated for

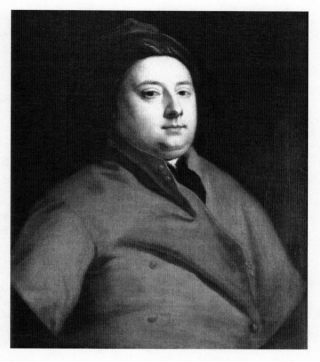

William Cheseldon brought perineal lithotomy for the removal of bladder stones to the peak of perfection during the eighteenth century. He operated with great speed to reduce pain in his young patients. This portrait by Jonathan Richardson, 1720s or 1730s. Courtesy and © Hunterian Museum at the Royal College of Surgeons).

breast cancer and in one case tapped a woman's belly to remove several gallons of blackish, viscid water. The character of the fluid makes it sound more like he tapped into an ovarian cyst rather than ascites. He made frequent amputations for "carious" bone, probably tuberculosis.

One of his more amazing cases was that of a 73-year-old woman with a "rupture of her navel" that burst in a fit of vomiting. She had 26 inches of "mortified" gut hanging out. Cheseldon removed the gut, which had adhered to the edges of the hernia. She then "voided her excrements" through the bowel and lived for many years. Another remarkable case was a rupture of the intestine into the scrotum in a man who had overstrained himself at work. Cheseldon made a "large wound" at the bottom of the abdomen, easily reduced the intestine, drained a quart of water from the scrotum and resected a piece of omentum that was adherent to the hernia sac, avoiding the spermatic vessels. The man developed erysipelas but recovered and was cured.[5]

William Cheseldon brought the operation for bladder stones to a peak of perfection while showing a measure of compassion for the intense pain and suffering endured by his patients. Early in his career, he attempted the supra-pubic approach to the bladder because he was concerned about injuring the rectum in very young children. His first patient, a seven-year-old boy, developed an abscess three weeks after the operation because the incision was too small. It was necessary to open the skin with a "gentian tent" to allow the urine and pus between the bladder and skin to escape. The boy survived, and a week later Chesel-don operated on three more boys: "Richard Smith of London, aged 11, Joseph Reynolds, 12, William White, 9, both living in Southwark, were cut May 22nd, 1722. Joseph Reynolds never complained during the operation and they were all easy soon after. In these three there was nothing remarkable during the whole cure; the urine in Reynolds and White came all the right way in about three weeks; but in Smith [who was of a weak constitution] in a month and it was two months before he was perfectly cured; but the other two much sooner."[6]

Cheseldon abandoned the supra-pubic approach because injury to the peritoneum allowed the intestines to eviscerate and urine drained poorly. He then approached the bladder through a lateral perineal incision, using a staff or guide in the urethra:

> I first make the incision as long as I can, beginning near the place where the old operation ends, and cutting down between the musculus accelerator urinae and erector penis and by the side of the intestinum rectum: I then feel for the staff, holding down the gut all the while with one or two fingers of my left hand, and cut upon it in that part of the urethra which lies beyond the corpora cavernosa urethreae, and in the prostate gland, cutting from below upwards, to avoid wounding the gut; and then passing the gorget very carefully in the groove of the staff into the bladder, bear the point of the gorget hard against the staff, observing all the while that they do not separate, and let the gorget slip to the outside of the bladder; then I pass the forceps into the right side of the bladder, the wound being on the left side of the perineum; and as they pass, carefully attend to their entering the blad-der, which is known by their overcoming a straitness which there will be in the place of the wound; then taking care to push them no further, that the bladder may not be hurt, I first feel for the stone with the end of them, which having felt, I open the forceps and slide one blade underneath it, and the other at top; and if I apprehend that the stone is not in the right place of the forceps, I shift it before I offer to extract, and then extract it very deliberately.

He then suture-ligated bleeding vessels with a "crooked needle" and applied very loose dressings that allowed free drainage of urine. An apprentice once timed the operation at one minute and 15 seconds and noted that Cheseldon used only five instruments. It often appeared to observers that he was distressed by the pain he was forced to inflict on his patients. One time, he offered a sweetmeat to a child if he would hold perfectly still and not cry out during the operation. The boy didn't utter a peep and insisted on his reward when the operation was finished.

Cheseldon's mortality among his patients with bladder stones varied by age; there were three deaths in 105 under ten years of age and four deaths in 64 patients between 10 and 20 years of age. Twelve died of the 41 patients between the ages of 20 and 80. Cheseldon's method remained essentially unchanged for a century. The mortality rate of 4 percent in patients under 20 years of age, without anesthesia or antisepsis, is astounding. The free drainage of urine from the wound apparently discouraged infection and the speed with which Cheseldon operated would have minimized bacterial invasion of the tissues.

Cheseldon was as well known for eye surgery as he was for stone removal. One of his patients was a 13-year-old boy who had been blind since birth with congenital cataracts. After operations on each eye, the boy was astounded by bright colors and was delighted by his restored sight. Cheseldon said: "I have couched several others who were born blind, whose observations were of the same kind; but they being younger, none of them gave so full account as this gentleman."[7]

Cheseldon's inquiring mind and interest in children led him to try a splint used by bone-setters in the treatment of fractures. He had first learned to correct the position of a congenital clubfoot with adhesive plaster but became dissatisfied because the foot swelled and the leg atrophied. He then remembered how his own fractured arm had been immobilized with bandages dipped in the whites of eggs and wheat flour. This bandage, replaced every two weeks, held club feet in position without undue constriction.[8]

His compassion and kindness was remembered in verse. One of his portrait painters wrote this: "With anxious skill supplied the best relief / And healed with balm and sweet discourse his grief." Another, written by a former child patient, contained these lines: "But by such ceaseless racks before, / And such intestine tortures bore; / That e'en a child I wished to die. / The work was in a moment done, / If possible without a groan; / So swift thy hand, I could not feel / The progress of the cutting steel." The poet ended with these lines: "As I from youth to age have past; / In this memorial first shall stand/His mercy by thy saving hand; / And above all the race of men, / I bless my God for Cheseldon."

Every medical student knows or should know the name of Percival Pott. Pott's puffy tumor is the scalp edema that overlies osteomyelitis of the skull and is a sign of an underlying abscess; Pott's disease is tuberculosis of the spine; and the Pott's fracture is a fracture through the distal fibula with lateral dislocation of the astragalus on the tibia.

A student and contemporary of Cheseldon, Pott apprenticed in 1729 at age 15 to Edward Nourse, an assistant surgeon at St. Bartholomew's Hospital. After passing the examination, Pott was admitted to the Company of Barber-Surgeons and practiced surgery in London. He later became surgeon to St. Bartholomew's and gave classes in anatomy and surgery. While recovering from a fractured leg incurred when he fell from a horse, Pott embarked on the career in medical writing that led him to be so well remembered.[9]

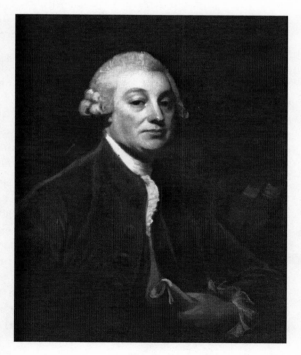

In one of his works, he described congenital inguinal hernia in newborn infants. Later, William Hunter would claim that he had first observed the hernia in newborns and that Pott plagiarized his material. The controversy didn't affect Pott's career, because Pott had enormous clinical experience and developed the most fashionable surgical practice in London. In one of his most significant works, *A Treatise on Head Injuries*, Pott recognized the lucid interval that precedes coma in extradural hematomas. He used the trephine to explore for intracranial hematomas much as neurosurgeons used exploratory burr holes in the days prior to CT scans.[10] Though he had no way of knowing the etiology of tuberculosis, he described the

Percival Pott, who first described scrotal cancer in chimney sweeps. His work led to the first child labor laws in England. The portrait is by George Romney, 1788 (courtesy and © Hunterian Museum at the Royal College of Surgeons).

cough, enlarged cervical lymph nodes, joint swellings and spinal deformities of what he termed "scrophula." He perfectly illustrated the carious destruction of vertebral bodies causing spinal curvature, lumbar abscess and paralysis of the lower extremities that occurred so often in young children. He also understood that attempts to straighten the spine with splints or braces were of no use but that prolonged rest might result in a cure. His classic description of tuberculosis of the spine would have been enough to ensure a place for him in surgical history.

Percival Pott's article on cancer of the scrotum in chimney sweeps, published in 1775, is one of the first descriptions of an occupational cancer.[11] It also appears to be the first detailed clinical description of a cancer in children. The cancer first appeared as a painful, ragged, ill-looking sore with hard rising edges on the inferior part of the scrotum. It was known as a "soot wart." The lesion invaded the dartos and the testicle and spread through the spermatic cord to the inguinal glands, from which it then invaded the abdomen and became "painfully destructive." Pott observed that removal of most of the scrotum before the cancer invaded the testicle was the only chance for a cure. He had seen healing after removal of the testicle and scrotum with patients leaving the hospital seemingly well, but then they returned with the same disease in the other testicle and in the inguinal glands. Here we have a classic description of local invasion and lymph node metastasis of a cancer.

Pott thought the disease stemmed from soot in the rugae of the scrotum as a result of the child's occupation. He wrote: "The fate of these people seems singularly hard; in their early infancy, they are frequently treated with great brutality, and almost starved with cold; they are thrust up narrow, and sometimes hot chimnies, where they are bruised, burned and almost suffocated; and when they get to puberty, become peculiarly liable to a most noisome, painful and fatal disease."

It was not until 1840 that Parliament passed an act forbidding boys under the age of 21 to climb chimneys. The law was not enforced until 1875, and as late as 1892 there was no decline in the numbers of cancer cases. The disease seemed to be peculiar to England, perhaps because of the type of coal burned and the lack of protective clothing. The chimney sweeps' disease provides insight into the attitudes of society toward poor children, who in those days were worked in mines and factories until they died.

On the Continent, especially in Paris, medical students could dissect cadavers rather than listen to a lecture while the professor dissected. In England, the shortage of cadavers did not allow students to do their own dissection. The brothers William and John Hunter, by refining "grave robbery" to obtain bodies, changed the way anatomy was taught in London.

The Hunter brothers were born to a poor family and raised on a farm in Scotland. William studied divinity at Glasgow but changed to medicine in 1737. He went to London to be a resident student under William Smellie, an obstetrician, and studied anatomy at St. George's Hospital. A courtly gentleman, William Hunter became a wealthy, fashionable obstetrician in London and founded a school where he taught anatomy to the most successful surgeons of the day. His most important work was the illustrated *Anatomy of the Gravid Uterus*.

John Hunter (1728–1793) was ten years younger than William. Unlike his brother, John had no formal education and was unable to read or write until he was a teenager. Instead, he spent his time roaming the woods, studying nature. He worked for a while as a carpenter and at the age of 21 went to London to assist his brother in the anatomy school.[12]

John was an immediate success at dissecting and demonstrating anatomy, but his main job was to procure enough bodies — men, women, fetuses or newborn babies — so that each student had his own cadaver. John liked to drink, was at home in the pubs and was on good terms with low-life thieves who snatched bodies from graves for a living. The body snatchers fought pitched battles with friends and relatives over the bodies of executed criminals, but the usual way to obtain a body was to dig into a fresh grave, break open the head of the coffin and slide the body out. Throughout his career, even after he became a successful surgeon, John Hunter was involved in grave robbing.

In addition to his study of human anatomy, John Hunter dissected and compared the anatomy of animals from fish to an elephant. He may have been more interested in natural science and experimental work than in surgery. His only formal surgical training was a summer spent at a hospital for retired soldiers as a surgical pupil to William Cheseldon, who was semiretired. Hunter spent another summer with Percival Pott at St. George's Hospital. During the winter, Hunter returned to the anatomical laboratory to continue his studies and teaching. He dissected the cranial nerves, made serial studies of chick embryos, studied the internal structure of the testicle and, most important for pediatric surgery, proved that the testicle normally completed its descent into the scrotum by the eighth month of intrauterine life. This work, which included a description of congenital hernias, led to a conflict with Percival Pott.[13]

By 1760, John Hunter had dissected over a thousand corpses but had little surgical experience. William arranged for him to join the army as a surgeon. During the Seven Years' War with France, John served on Belle Isle and in Portugal. At the time, army surgeons opened wounds to extract musket balls and performed amputations on manure-soaked fields of battle. After he observed several soldiers whose wounds had healed with little inflammation and without surgery, John Hunter left most wounds alone for nature to heal. He also brought the wounded back from the battlefield to where conditions were better.

While in Portugal, John Hunter continued his work on natural science with studies of the regeneration of lizards' tails. In 1763, at the end of the war, he returned to civilian life and took up dentistry to earn money. At the time, the gentry had rotten teeth as a result of using excess sugar in their tea. Hunter became interested in transplantation; after he implanted a human tooth into a cock's comb and a testis into the same rooster's belly and found regeneration of blood vessels, he transplanted teeth from corpses into his patients. When his patients didn't like the idea of having a tooth from a cadaver, he advertised for living donors. Poor children lined up to have their teeth extracted and implanted into the mouths of the gentry, a craze typical of the eighteenth century that exploited the poor.[14]

In 1776, John Hunter was elected to the Royal Society for his work in natural history and anatomy, an indication of his major interests. It was not until the next year that he passed the examinations for the Surgeons Hall. With his brother's help, John was appointed to the surgical staff of St. George's Hospital and commenced seeing patients on a regular basis.

After the death of Percival Pott, John Hunter became the most sought-after surgeon in London. He is best known for curing popliteal aneurism by proximal ligation of the femoral artery. Hunter demonstrated collateral circulation by ligating the carotid artery of a stag and observing how the antler became cold and stopped growing. A week later, when the antler became warm, Hunter killed the stag, injected the arteries, and demonstrated the collaterals.[15] Hunter's first patient, operated on in 1785, was a coachman with a huge popliteal artery aneurism, with swelling of his leg and foot. Hunter made an incision on the anterior, inner part of the thigh, across the inner edge of the sartorius muscle, and applied four ligatures to the femoral artery. The ends of the ligatures were left hanging out of the wound, which was closed with adhesive tape and linen bandages. The patient left the hospital and returned to driving coaches with no complaints about his leg, which appeared to be normal. He died 15 months later, perhaps of pneumonia. Hunter obtained and dissected the leg, which demonstrated no signs of gangrene.

Hunter was also known for his work on venereal diseases after he inoculated himself with gonorrheal pus from a patient who also had syphilis. He observed the course of the disease in himself and treated the symptoms with mercurial ointments.

John Hunter had many interests, including the Irish Giant, attempted resuscitation of hanged men, and birth defects such as hermaphrodites. His casebooks with histories of three young patients provide insight into his pediatric practice. On March 21, 1787, he saw Sandie Boswell, son of James Boswell, Samuel Johnson's biographer. The boy had an inguinal hernia with an undescended testicle that prevented the application of a truss. Sandie couldn't attend the academy for fear of being hurt, so Hunter made him read and examined him until the family could find a tutor. Hunter was somewhat of a generalist, since he also cared for Mrs. Boswell during her attacks of hemoptysis due to tuberculosis and treated Mr. Boswell for his attacks of gonorrhea.[16]

Hunter's most famous patient was Lord Byron, the poet, who was born with a deformed foot. The father had abandoned Byron's mother, who was in a "pitiable state, penniless and without friends, nursing a deformed infant." Hunter's diagnosis was contraction of the Achilles tendon, which drew up and twisted the right foot. He prescribed an orthopedic boot and inoculated the infant against smallpox.[17] Ever since Byron's death, there has been speculation over the exact nature of his lameness. Some thought he suffered with a clubfoot, while others claim he had mild spastic monoplegia from a birth injury. The appliance Hunter used to treat him was made to fit inside a shoe or boot and extended to just below the knee.[18] If the deformity was an ordinary clubfoot, John Hunter likely would have applied a bandage of the type used by Cheseldon, rather than prescribing an orthopedic boot.

Another pediatric case suggests Hunter was a bit of a psychologist and understood the ways of children. The patient was a 12-year-old boy who, after being cured of rheumatic fever with tepid sea baths, feigned a limp and pain in his knee. Hunter advised putting the boy to bed, with a bowl of grapes across the room. The family watched from a keyhole as the boy got out of bed and walked across the room to the grapes without a limp.

John Hunter had an irascible tem-

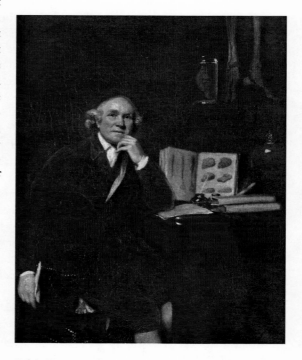

John Hunter, the great anatomist surgeon, posed with an open anatomy book. The portrait was painted by Joshua Reynolds, 1786 (courtesy and © Hunterian Museum at the Royal College of Surgeons).

per and toward the end of his life suffered angina pectoris. He collapsed and died after losing his temper during a surgical meeting at St. George's Hospital. The autopsy demonstrated lesions in his aorta compatible with his self-induced syphilis.

Hunter taught a number of outstanding physicians and surgeons, including Edward Jenner, who in 1796 inoculated an eight-year-old boy against smallpox using material from the blisters of cowpox. This was the most important medical discovery of the eighteenth century. Hunter's most enduring legacy is the Hunterian Museum at the Royal College of Surgeons in London, which still exhibits specimens preserved in jars and deformed skeletons from his collection.

The eighteenth century saw little progress in the general care of infants and children. The lot of poor children was especially grim. Mortality rates in foundling homes in Dublin, London and Paris varied from 80 to 99 percent but fell to 60 percent in babies who were breast-fed. Infant formulas included broth, bread, tea, wine, sugar and small beer. Young women sometimes abandoned their own illegitimate children to become wet nurses for pay.

In 1767 London physician George Armstrong published *An Essay on Diseases Most Fatal to Infancy*, and in 1769 he established the first pediatric hospital in England. It was the only institution that accepted the children of poor parents. Thirty-five thousand children were admitted and treated during the 12 years that Armstrong's Dispensary for the Poor Infant existed. It eventually closed for lack of financial support.

Armstrong's essay said that the best doctor for a sick child was an old woman. He described the common diseases of childhood and also described an infant who died at three weeks of age with "watery gripes"; at autopsy, the infant's stomach was filled with curdled milk, the pylorus was firm and the intestines were empty. Dr. Armstrong said: "...it looked as if the disease had been chiefly owing to a spasm of the pylorus." Undoubtedly, this was a case of congential pyloric stenosis. Dr. Armstrong also stressed the importance of keeping infants warm to preserve them from catching cold. This is especially necessary advice today, when we operate on babies in air-conditioned operating rooms.[19]

Nicolas Andry's book *Orthopedia, or the Art of Preventing and Correcting Deformities in Childhood* was first published in French and in 1743 translated into English. Andry (1658–1742) coined the word "orthopedia," meaning "straight child"; the frontispiece of his book, illustrating a crooked tree tied to a stake, continues to be the international symbol of orthopedics.[20]

Born in Lyons, Andry studied for the priesthood and then medicine at Rheims and Paris. In 1701, he was appointed to the faculty of the College of France in Paris, where he became dean of medicine in 1724. His first medical work, *An Account of the Breeding of Worms in Human Bodies*, describes microscopic studies of human parasites. His microscopic work led him to think that diseases such as smallpox were caused by microorganisms, but he also concluded that spermatazoa were a unique parasite.

In *Orthopedia*, Andry recommended exercise and correct posture to prevent and correct orthopedic deformities. He used a neck brace to keep the head straight and manipulation to treat deformed feet in the young, but used splints and massage for older children.[21] High-heeled shoes made the bodies of children crooked, and he said children had to sit upright with their backs straight to prevent a protuberant belly. He was absolutely correct in his treatment of congenital torticollis of the neck by massage with warm wine and oil, together with gentle movements of the head, measures that prevent the need for surgery when applied during early infancy. The book addressed other problems as well, such as teething, rectal prolapse, smallpox and measles.

Andry treated umbilical infections with spikenard and turpentine or a mixture of strong red wine with the ashes of burned cloth. Here he was one of the few in the eighteenth century to use medications with antiseptic properties. This suggests he was familiar with earlier writers such as de Mondeville. A reference to "bronchocele" in Andry's works evidently meant tuberculous lymph nodes, or the "King's Evil." He mentioned finding enlarged glands in the mesentery at postmortem examination, which he also attributed to tuberculosis. His treatment was mineral water with Epsom salts.

He used progressively tightened ligatures to remove supernumerary digits but advised that when bone was present the patient should not be subjected to surgery, "because cutting it could kill the child." He also warned against cutting and stitching harelips in infancy because the operation could cause death when performed too soon after birth. Instead, he suggested waiting until the child was five or six years old. He also warned against an operation for cleft lip if the parts could not be easily joined and said that one should only treat birth-marks on the face if they could be easily ligated.[22] These admonitions suggest that Andry was sufficiently realistic to realize the dangers of surgery or that, being a physician, he held the view that surgery and the shedding of blood was still an inferior branch of medicine.

Like many others of his time, Andry believed the imagination of the mother influenced the development of birth defects and that the shape of a child's head and face depended on the parents' upbringing. He gives sound advice in *Orthopedia,* which seems directed more to parents than to physicians.

The eighteenth century ended with war and rebellions, good for surgeons but not con-ducive to good health in children.

CHAPTER 16

The Nineteenth Century

The beginning of the nineteenth century, with the senseless slaughter of the Napoleonic wars, was not auspicious for surgery or children. A steel knife had long since replaced a flake of obsidian, but the craft of surgery was still cruel and primitive. Fortunately, the nineteenth century would see dramatic changes in all aspects of medicine and surgery. The art of diagnosis had previously depended on sight and touch, but the new skills of percussion and auscultation allowed clinicians for the first time to diagnose internal disease with considerable accuracy. By the end of the 1800s, the magical roentgen ray brought the interior of the body into plain view. For centuries, children who went "under the knife" suffered great agony and must have thought their pain was God's punishment for some terrible misdeed. The discovery of ether, widely known as "an American dodge," brought blessed relief, and by the century's end antisepsis — the great discovery by Joseph Lister — ushered in the modern era of surgery.

The nineteenth century also saw new hospitals built exclusively for children. The numbers of books and articles written about pediatric surgery indicated a growing interest in the correction of birth defects. Most important, stories about poor and abused children by Charles Dickens and Victor Hugo brought about laws to curb the worst abuses of child exploitation. Out of the Crimean War came saintly Florence Nightingale and modern nursing care, without which pediatric surgery would be impossible. George Frederic Still, a professor of pediatrics at Kings' College and physician to the Great Ormond Street Hospital in London, admirably summarized the many wonderful advances in child care during the nineteenth century.[1]

Hospitals for Children

Midwives and nurses cared for sick children at home, and foundling homes often associated with monasteries or a cathedral looked after abandoned, unwanted children. The death rate in these institutions was high, possibly because more attention was paid to salvation of souls than to a child's physical well-being. Children could be admitted to adult hospitals, but most physicians felt frustrated because there was little they could do for sick infants. The movement for separate children's hospitals began in 1769 with George Armstrong's Dispensary for the Infant Poor in London. Unfortunately, Dr. Armstrong was unable to win support for his efforts and the dispensary closed.[2]

France led the way in the care of children, commencing with the Foundling Hospital of Paris, known as "La Couche," which opened in 1636. It was taken over by St. Vincent

De Paul in 1640, and in 1670 the French government took control of the home, which became the center of an extensive system of infant welfare in France. In 1785, an investigation ordered by King Louis XVI found that in the Hôtel-Dieu, the prime hospital of Paris, eight or nine children with contagious diseases were stacked in a single bed. The investigators ordered that children should have their own beds and be separated from adults.[3]

The Hôpital des Enfants-Malades was founded in 1802, during the tenth year of the French Republic, while Napoléon Bonaparte was the prime consul.[4] The Conseil General Des Hôpitaux decreed that a former orphan's home was to be used exclusively for the care of children under 15 years of age. There were three hundred beds, with 59 staff members, including two physicians and a surgeon. Initially, the contagious disease wards were separated from the rest of the hospital by gardens and courtyards. The hospital soon became a teaching center for physicians, including Bernard Marfan, Paul Broca and Armand Trousseau, who performed the first tracheotomy in Paris in 1831.[5]

The next children's hospitals were opened in St. Petersburg, Russia; in Vienna, Austria; and then in almost every medical center in Europe. In 1852, Charles West founded the Hospital for Sick Children, Great Ormond Street, in London. This institution had an autopsy room for the study of disease, and from its inception some of the most gifted pediatricians in medical history worked at this hospital. Today, it is one of the world's best centers for pediatric surgery. The Children's Hospital of Philadelphia, the first in the United States, opened in 1855, and in 1869 the Boston Children's Hospital was established with 20 beds.[6] Children's hospitals became centers not only for the care of children but also for teaching and research in association with medical schools.

Advances in Diagnosis

Leopold Auenbrugger, a Viennese physician, opened the way to improved diagnosis with percussion of the chest to demonstrate differences in sound over areas of fluid or lung consolidation.[7] His observations were based on his correlation of findings in the living patient with the autopsy. The duller the sound and the more extensive the area of dullness, the more severe the disease. He said the total absence of sound over an entire pleural cavity was generally a fatal sign. Many of Auenbrugger's colleagues ridiculed his observations, but gradually the entire medical profession realized the value of chest percussion. At one time, medical students spent many hours perfecting their percussion skills in an attempt to emulate the great clinicians who could demonstrate a patch of infiltrated lung or a small pleural effusion before the X-ray. Medical students once learned to detect small amounts of peritoneal fluid by the sign of "shifting dullness" in the abdomen.

R. T. H. Laennec, the most talented French clinician of the nineteenth century and Physician in Chief at the Necker Hospital in Paris, applied the flared end of a hollow wooden tube to the patient's chest and put the other end in his ear. With this simple but elegant stethoscope, he identified heart sounds and learned to distinguish the sound of air passing through a diseased lung from normal air: "The cylinder applied to the chest of a healthy person who sings or speaks produces a sort of vibration which is more distinct in some places than others. The signs afforded by mediate auscultation in the diseases of the lungs and pleura are derived from the changes presented by the sound of respiration, by that of the voice and coughing within the chest and also by the rhonchus as well as certain other sounds which occasionally are heard in the same situation."[8]

Like Auenbrugger, Laennec correlated his findings in living patients with the autopsy. Chest auscultation developed into a fine science and remained an important diagnostic tool until well into the last half of the twentieth century. Every contact with a patient included a careful examination of the heart and lungs — on bare skin, not through the patient's clothing. By making a game of auscultation in small, frightened children surgeons could demonstrate that they were not ogres, and occasionally one would find a heart murmur or an asthmatic wheeze in a child with a hernia. Surgeons also loved to demonstrate the changes in intestinal sounds in children with appendicitis or intestinal obstruction to interns and medical students. This practice also continued well into the twentieth century, until the advent of CT technology. Now, nurses and technicians carry stethoscopes draped around their necks as a sort of badge and physicians rely on imaging studies.

On November 8, 1895, William Conrad Roentgen, a physicist at the University of Würzburg, noted bright fluorescence from crystals of barium platinocyanide on a screen that had been exposed to a mysterious ray. Roentgen used his own hand to demonstrate how bones and flesh produced an image. On December 28, 1895, he presented his discovery to the Medical Society in Würzburg; the paper was translated and appeared all over the world.[9] The equipment used to produce X-rays was in every physics laboratory, and soon doctors everywhere used the new technology to examine patients. Within a year, E. P. Davis in Philadelphia used the new "ray" in a three-day-old infant and demonstrated a fetus in utero in a pregnant woman.[10]

X-rays were especially useful in showing fractured bones and foreign bodies. One of the first reports indicating its clinical value was the case of a boy who had choked and apparently swallowed a nail. When the nail couldn't be extracted from his esophagus, an X-ray showed the nail in a bronchus.[11] Roentgen received the Nobel Prize in physics in 1901 but refused to give a lecture and never published. He lived until 1923, long enough to see the results of his wondrous accidental finding.

Anesthesia

Long ago, one of our ancestors became tipsy and "felt no pain" after drinking fermented fruit juice. This fortuitous discovery led to the use of alcohol for the relief of pain. It was especially effective when mixed with opium and other herbs, but the dose required to dispel the pain of surgery was nearly lethal. Mandragora, an extract from the mandrake plant, is a narcotic and when mixed with wine and opium produces insensibility. This mixture was used until the Middle Ages and must have been partially effective but unreliable. It would have been especially dangerous in children. Without an effective remedy for pain, surgeons operated with great speed. However, even Cheseldon, who could remove a bladder stone in less than two minutes, relied on strong men to hold the patient still. We can scarcely imagine the agony suffered by children during those few minutes when the knife cut into their flesh.

The discovery of nitrous oxide, an anesthetic gas still in use, was as fortuitous as the discovery of alcohol. Humphrey Davy, who later became Sir Humphrey for his chemical discoveries, was a precocious boy with a taste for science. At 17 years of age, he apprenticed to a surgeon in Penzance, England, and became interested in chemistry. This interest led him to Bristol and an institution established for the purpose of investigating the medical powers of various gases. There he and his associate engineer James Watt experimented with nitrous oxide, originally as a cure for hangover. Davy noted that nitrous oxide, also known as laughing gas, relieved pain, but the gas was used for parties rather than as an anesthetic.[12] A Massachusetts dentist named William Morton and his partner, Horace Wells, used Davy's laughing gas to relieve dental pain. When one of Wells' patients died from the gas, Wells committed suicide.

Morton attended Harvard Medical School, where students inhaled the fumes of sulphuric ether to become intoxicated. While under the influence of ether, the students felt no pain. Morton tried ether first on a dog, then on himself, then on a patient. When he, the dog and the patient all recovered without any ill effects, Morton — while still a medical student — requested an opportunity to demonstrate ether during an operation at the Massachusetts General Hospital. John Collins Warren, the senior surgeon, agreed but almost went ahead with the removal of a tumor without the anesthetic because Morton was late. When he finally arrived, Morton gave ether to the patient, who slept through the operation. The spectators were amazed and Dr. Warren said, "Gentlemen, this is no humbug." The date was October 16, 1846.

There is controversy over who first used ether as an anesthetic, but if it had not been for John Collins Warren (1778–1856), the profession would not have accepted ether so rapidly. Dr. Warren was the eldest son of John Warren, a surgeon in the Revolutionary War

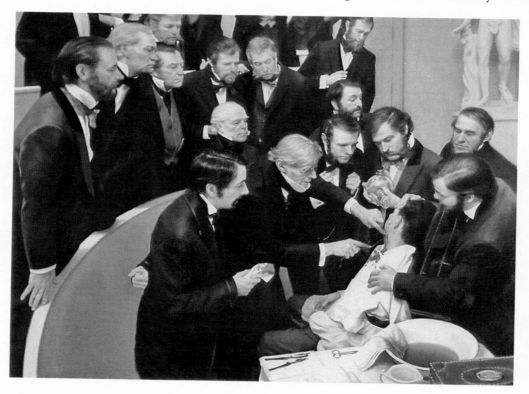

John Collins Warren performing the first operation under ether at the Massachusetts General Hospital. After removing a tumor from the patient's jaw, without pain, Dr. Warren said, "Gentlemen, this is no humbug." This painting by Warren Prosperi, posed by current hospital staff members, hangs in the Ether Dome of the Massachusetts General Hospital (courtesy Patricia Donahoe, M.D. and Massachusetts General Hospital).

and a founder of Harvard Medical School. In 1799, John Collins went to England to be a pupil of William Cowper and Astley Cooper. Collins was a dissector at Guy's Hospital for a year, then spent a year in Edinburgh, where he took his M.D. After that he studied medicine and chemistry in Paris, and so he was well known on both sides of the Atlantic. In 1802, he returned to Boston to take over his father's practice. In 1815, he became a professor at Harvard and was a founder of the Massachusetts General Hospital. In 1811, he helped found the *New England Journal of Medicine.* He was 70 years old at the time of his first operation under ether. It is fortunate for all of us that he accepted a new, untested technology.[13] The Ether Dome in the Bullfinch Building of the Massachusetts General Hospital has since been preserved as a national landmark.

None other than Oliver Wendell Holmes, professor of anatomy and poet, suggested the name "anesthetic" for the new miracle gas. This was, however, not the first time ether had been used as an anesthetic. Crawford Long, a doctor in Athens, Georgia, had used ether to remove a tumor from a boy named James Venable in 1842. Dr. Long's achievement was not widely known, but when the distinguished surgeon John Collins Warren published his experience with ether in the *Boston Medical and Surgical Journal* the news quickly spread around the world.[14]

A mixture of sulfuric acid with alcohol, ether could be manufactured in any chemistry laboratory. It was simple to administer and so safe that any physician could quickly learn the technique. The job of giving the anesthetic was often relegated to medical students and interns. This remained common practice well into the twentieth century. (When we interns in the class of 1954 gave too little ether, the patient moved and the surgeon yelled. If we gave too much, respiration slowed and became shallow long before the heart stopped. Except for the smell and postoperative vomiting, ether was an almost perfect anesthetic.)

The great neurosurgeon Harvey Cushing, while a second-year Harvard medical student at the Massachusetts General Hospital, gave ether to a patient with a strangulated hernia. The woman died on the operating table in front of the class, and Cushing blamed himself despite the presence of gangrenous intestine.[15] When he was a fourth-year student in 1895, he and fellow student Amory Codman devised the ether chart, a record of the patient's temperature, pulse and respirations during surgery. At the time, there was no way to determine blood pressure, but several years later, when Cushing saw the Riva-Rocci pneumatic instrument for recording blood pressure at Pavia in Italy, he brought the device to the United States.[16] Cushing's recordings of the pulse, respiration and blood pressure would be the only intra-operative monitoring used for the next 50 years.

James Young Simpson, a surgeon and professor of midwifery at Edinburgh University, had tried hypnosis to relieve pain during surgery and childbirth. It worked for a few operations but was useless for childbirth. After a London surgeon named Liston used ether for surgery, Simpson tried it for delivering babies. Unfortunately, ether smells bad and irritates the lungs, so Simpson and his assistants sniffed a variety of drugs to find a better anesthetic. They became giddy and then unconscious when they inhaled the fumes of chloroform, a compound discovered by chemists in France and Germany in 1831. Simpson used chloroform on a doctor's wife, who was so thrilled with the painless delivery that she named her baby Anaesthesia. On November 15, 1847, Simpson gave chloroform to a four-year-old boy who underwent excision of a bone in his forearm. The operation was a complete success.

Chloroform was less expensive than ether, more agreeable to patients, and required only a pocket handkerchief to administer. Some objections to the use of chloroform arose, however, when doctors claimed the drug would cause lung complications and death. The main objection to it came from the church, based on the biblical injunction to bring forth children in sorrow. Simpson answered the dead hand of religion with his own Bible verses. The objections came to an end when Her Majesty Queen Victoria gave birth to a son while under the influence of chloroform.[17]

These early anesthetics began as recreational drugs used to satisfy man's eternal quest to escape from the trials of daily living. Nowadays, if a group of students had "ether frolics" the police would soon be on hand for a drug bust.

Pediatric Surgical Literature

The rise of children's hospitals that concentrated care and the discovery of anesthesia stimulated interest in the surgical problems of children. For the first time, books and articles appeared that were devoted exclusively to pediatric surgery. Again, France led the way.

In 1844, Paul Guersant (1800–1869) instigated the first pediatric surgical unit at the Hôpital des Enfants-Malades, and in the same year he published the first textbook of pediatric surgery. The book, *Notices sur la Chirurgie des Enfants*, translated into English in 1873 as *Surgical Diseases of Infants and Children*, reviewed the surgical cases at the Hôpital des Enfants-Malades.[18] This remarkable book covers the full range of pediatric surgery from children "mutilated by the wheels of machinery or crushed on the streets" to all the external birth defects and tumors. Guersant noted the ability of fractured bones to heal and mold, as well as the delayed healing in children with rickets or tuberculosis. He performed over a thousand tonsillectomies with the knife, scissors or tonsiltome and stopped bleeding with a white-hot iron or perchlorate of iron. Only three children lost blood. Children with rectal polyps were given enemas; when they pushed out the fluid with the polyp, the polyp was grasped and ligated. He treated 140 patients under 20 years of age with bladder stones, of whom 21 died. He drained hydroceles with the tip of a lancet and injected alcohol at 36 degrees centigrade. The alcohol was removed after three to four minutes and the scrotum was bandaged.

Professor Guersant treated burns with cold water and then cerate of glycerine dressings. If the burn was infected, he used chlorinated soda covered with cornstarch to produce crusts. Chlorinated soda, a strong antiseptic similar to Carrel-Dakin solution, suggests that Guersant anticipated antisepsis.

He operated on infants with cleft lip at birth by paring the edges and closing the wound with an ingenious needle that had a turn screw attached to threads on the ends. Turning the nuts on the needle brought the flaps together. He treated hernias in the early months of life with a truss but also described the case of an 11-year-old girl who had a prolapsed ovary in the hernia. He admitted mistaking the ovary for a cyst, which he ligated and removed. The child died two days later with peritonitis. Guersant punctured low anal imperforations with a trochar and kept the wound open with a gum elastic tube, or he pulled the rectum down to the skin with a blunt hook and sutured the bowel to the skin. When the rectum could not be found, he performed either a Littré type of colostomy, six to eight inches above the inguinal ligament, or an Amussat left lumbar, extra-peritoneal colostomy. He performed 60 tenotomies for strabismus and also mentioned clubfeet, tracheotomy for foreign bodies in the airway, cancer of the testicle and encephalocele.

Guersant was truly a surgeon for the whole child. His book, based on his own extensive experience, is sensible and practical. His decision to close cleft lips at birth anticipates the current practice of correcting as many birth defects as possible at the time of birth, and his use of an antiseptic chlorinated soda water on infected burns was far advanced for his day.

Athol A. Johnson, surgeon to the Great Ormond Street Hospital in London, presented a series of three lectures on surgery in childhood that was published in the *British Medical Journal* in January of 1860.[19] In his introduction, Mr. Johnson said there were no books on the subject and that the surgical afflictions of childhood had been largely ignored by physicians. He first addressed congenital malformations and noted the change from killing malformed babies to what he called "heroic treatment." He illustrated this change by telling of two women who in 1812 were tried in court for drowning an infant with a malformed cranium.

He said that some malformations, such as atresia oris, or fusion of the lips in a newborn, and imperforate anus, required immediate lifesaving surgery at birth. One such case was a 23-day-old girl with an imperforate anus, who passed tiny amounts of stool through a fistula in the back wall of the vagina. The infant was sick and "pining away," straining constantly and evidently suffering much from the difficulty in passing feces. Mr. Johnson passed a probe into the bowel through the fistula and then made an incision a little in front of the coccyx until he reached and opened the bowel. He then secured a large gum elastic catheter into the bowel. "There was no great amount of hemorrhage; faeces came away freely; no bad consequences followed and the child throve very well." He followed the child for some months, and when she last was seen Mr. Johnson could pass a "pretty large instrument" into the rectum without difficulty.

He then went on in his lecture to review the recent literature, noting that when stool issues from the penis and the rectum ends higher in the perineum a colostomy is indicated. He recounted the histories of patients who had lived for many years with a colostomy, including a woman who had married and borne four children. The Littré operation, which placed the artificial anus in the groin near the iliac crest, was preferable to a prolonged search for the bowel in the perineum. The case histories recounted in these lectures are among the first in our history that tell of long-term results of treatment.

Mr. Johnson went on to discuss vaginal atresia, cleft lip and congenital joint dislocations, referring to his own experience and the recent literature. He particularly warned about operating on tumors or cysts of the skull that could be encephaloceles containing brain. He then illustrated the pathology of spina bifida and meningomyelocele, using a specimen from an infant who had died at five months of age to illustrate the fixation of spinal nerves to the sac. He mentioned two cases, treated by Sir Astley Cooper, who had lived for 28 and 29 years in good health. One case was treated with compression and the other by needle puncture, aspiration and compression. Suture, excision and ligature of meningomyeloceles had all been followed by death, but there were patients who lived many years with no treatment or with simple compression. Johnson also referred to other surgeons, including Daniel Brainard of Chicago, who had injected iodine into the sac, which then shrank with the application of colloidion.

The lectures included references to the incidence of hernia in children, perhaps the first use of statistics in pediatric surgery. Johnson quoted Malgaigne, stating that 1 in 20 males under 1 year of age were ruptured, but that by age 13, only 1 in 77 had a hernia. Mr. Johnson's personal experience included 54 males and ten female children with inguinal hernias. He also quoted the Truss Society as saying that over the course of 28 years they had gathered 2,775 cases of umbilical hernias in girls but only 664 in males. There had been only one case of a child with a femoral hernia at the Great Ormond Street Hospital.

Despite the enthusiasm for surgery by earlier authors, English surgeons during the nineteenth century used trusses to treat hernias. Mr. Johnson said: "...it is in early life especially that a radical cure of hernia may be hoped for and confidently expected, if methodical pressure is maintained for a certain period. In umbilical and inguinal hernia, there is a strong natural tendency of the openings to contract — and the abnormal channel will become blocked up." The special truss for infants encircled the pelvis with a softly padded metal spring that applied pressure against the entire hernia canal with a lower portion passed under the perineum. The truss could be modified to avoid pressure on an undescended testicle. He also pointed out that incarceration and strangulation could take place at any age and noted infants varying in age from 17 days to 14 months who required surgery for strangulation.

Mr. Johnson acknowledged that over the years he had had become more conservative in surgery for chronic conditions of the bones and joints. He must have been referring to tuberculosis, since he said that nursing care, fresh air and a nourishing diet did as much good as surgery. He concluded his lecture series by saying that those who worked at the Great Ormond Street Hospital had a trust to contribute to the general knowledge of the diseases of children. Mr. Johnson's content and method of presentation were impressive by any standards. Who today could delve into all aspects of children's surgery, from eye to anus and everything in between?

John Cooper Forster at 37 years of age published *The Surgical Diseases of Children*, the first textbook of pediatric surgery in the English language, in 1860.[20] Mr. Forster, whose father and grandfather were general practitioners, entered Guy's Hospital at age 18 and in 1847 took the London M.B. He obtained the gold medal in surgery, and in 1849 he became F.R.C.S. by examination. Forster was a colleague of such medical notables as Sir James Paget and Jonathan Hutchinson.[21]

One of the first surgeons to dis-

The first gastrostomy for a lye stricture in a child, performed by John Cooper Forster. Gastrostomy and colostomy were the only abdominal operations described in his textbook, *The Surgical Diseases of Children*. The stomach is sutured to the abdominal wall. It is likely that gastric juices would have leaked to the outside, had the child survived.

cuss anesthesia in children, Forster said that chloroform was so safe, there was no justification for inflicting pain on children. He advised that it be given on an empty stomach to prevent vomiting and emphasized the importance of good nursing in postanesthesia care.

Mr. Forster described trauma and surface lesions but dismissed the alimentary tract as the province of physicians. In his book there is an illustration of cancrum oris, a frightful disease that caused necrosis of rthe face, first encountered in Roman times. There were one or two of these cases a year at Guy's Hospital, and all were fatal.

Like Guersant, Mr. Forster operated on cleft lips in newborn babies for the mother's peace of mind and to improve the child's nutrition: "I should have no hesitation in

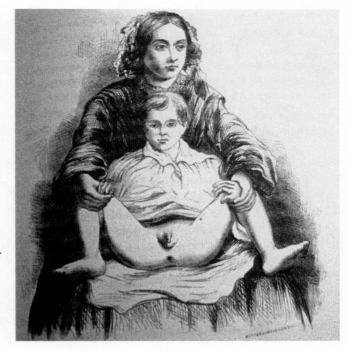

A nurse holds a child for a perineal lithotomy to remove bladder stones. The incision would be between the anus and the scrotum. This is the same operation described in the *Sushruta Samhita* and used by Cheseldon and others through the nineteenth century.

operating immediately after birth, so as to avoid the shock to the mother occasioned by the sight of her child. The operation has been performed successfully within 7 hours after birth."

Mr. Forster performed tracheotomies for diphtheria and for the removal of foreign bodies from the airway. He did the first gastrostomy in a four-year-old child with a lye stricture of the esophagus, who had been unable to swallow liquids and was nearly unconscious at the time of surgery. The patient died when the stomach separated from the abdominal wall and feeding spilled into the peritoneal cavity.

Mr. Forster continued to publish on pediatric topics in *Guy's Hospital Reports*. Between 1857 and 1866, he reported on his results with the Cheseldon operation for bladder stones in 162 children up to 15 years of age, with only four deaths. In 1872, he reported the remarkable case of a 13-year-old boy with extensive burns, whom Forster treated by grafting more than one hundred pieces of skin. He felt that wounds of any size should be skin grafted.[22]

Like his contemporaries, he used trusses for inguinal hernias and recommended splinting, rest, fresh air and cod-liver oil for joint infections. Infantile syphilis was considered a surgical disease, which he treated by rubbing mercurial ointment on the abdominal wall. He, too, recommended the Littré colostomy for high imperforate anus.

Forster's book demonstrates how few changes there were in children's surgery, even after the introduction of anesthesia. Gastrostomy and skin grafting for burns were the only new operations. He was, however, one of the first surgeons to emphasize the importance of nursing care in the postanesthetic period and after tracheotomy.

Mr. V. A. J. Swain, honorary consulting surgeon to the Queen Elizabeth Hospital for Children in London, provided an account of pediatric surgical patients treated by Robert W. Parker, who was a surgeon to the East London Hospital, Shadwell, from 1876 until 1902. Before that, Parker had been a resident medical officer at the Great Ormond Street Hospital.[23] Parker described his patients in a series of notebooks illustrated with sketches that add a close, personal view of pediatric surgery during the latter part of the nineteenth century. There are cases of clubfoot, genu recurvatum, spina bifida with hydrocephalus, talipes equines, amniotic bands, and infantile paralysis, two cases of sarcoma of the low limb and two cases of "cancrum oris." One figure illustrates severe bilateral talipes equinos varus with this notation: "Fred Bardell, 5 months. Admitted 1889, on January 18th, under chloroform Mr. Parker separated Achilles and Tibialis Anticus tendons. Feet put in plaster of Paris. January 26th, feet to be worked in water and rubbed every morning. Flexible splints applied. February 10th. Great improvement, feet in very good position. Sent home in plaster to be removed in a fortnight. August. Feet much improved and a pair of boots ordered."

An illustration of cancrum oris shows a child who, after measles, developed a black spot with swelling on his lower lip. The gangrene spread despite the application of acid nitric of mercury and carbolic acid until the entire side of the face and the eye were lost to gangrene. The child died after six days. There is also a drawing of an infant with bilateral cleft lip and palate, brought to the hospital at two days of age because he wouldn't take food. He was fed with a syringe and tube but lived only 14 days.

One of the drawings in Mr. Swain's paper shows a hospital ward in the Shadwell hospital in 1878 with a high ceiling, tall windows, a row of crib beds and nurses carrying small infants. High on a wall at one end of the ward is the inscription "My Lord knows that children are tender." Nurses in those days required courage and great tenderness to look after some of their patients who had terrible, hopeless diseases.

CHAPTER 17

Pediatric Surgery
in the Age of Lister

Joseph Barron Lister, born in 1827 to a Quaker family in Upton, England, decided at an early age to become a surgeon. He attended University College in London at the age of seventeen, took a B.A. degree and then qualified in medicine at University College Hospital.[1]

On December 21, 1846, while a freshman student, Lister observed Robert Liston performing a thigh amputation with the patient under ether. This was the first operation under ether in England.[2]

As a house surgeon in London, Lister was profoundly disturbed by the terrible suffering of septic patients; he was responsible for treating cases of hospital gangrene by scraping away the slough and applying a caustic chemical. He described the progress of the disease in a case that defied this treatment and demonstrates his early interest in the chemical treatment of wounds:

> The only exception to this rule was a very stout woman, in whom the disease attacked an enormous wound of the forearm caused by an accident that raised a very large flap of skin. In that case the caustic application removed indeed the pain and the extensive inflammatory blush; but when the slough separated, a small brown spot was seen at one place among the otherwise healthy granulations, and this spread with astonishing rapidity over the entire sore. The treatment was tried again and again with the same result, till the deep structures of the limb having become seriously involved, Mr. Erichsen resolved to amputate. On the evening before the day of the operation, I again put the patient under chloroform, and after scraping the sore very thoroughly, allowed the liquid caustic to lie in pools upon it for a quarter of an hour to destroy as effectually as possible all material in the sore that might otherwise infect the amputation wound. With a similar object, I washed the skin of the limb with soap and water including the shoulder, where it had been decided to perform the amputation. The stump healed perfectly kindly.[3]

In September 1853, Lister went to Edinburgh to observe James Syme, the Surgeon in Chief at the Royal Infirmary. Syme, the world's most outstanding surgeon, attracted students from all over the world because of his operative and teaching skills.[4] Lister soon became Syme's devoted friend, and in 1856 he married Dr. Symes' daughter Agnes. Four years later Lister was called to Glasgow as surgeon to the Royal Infirmary. There he continued research that led to his most famous discovery, antisepsis. His writings from early on in Glasgow demonstrate his interest in children:

> I had a very satisfactory case the other day, giving me the first opportunity of using to advantage on the living body an instrument which I made some time ago for extracting

foreign bodies from the ear. Children often put in objects of a rounded shape, such as small stones, beads, etc., and when they are nearly as large as the meatus auditorious, it is extremely difficult to get them out. Attempts with forceps only push them further in and thus, the irritation is increased, and inflammation, it may be fatal inflammation, is induced. The instrument I have contrived is a hook with the lower end curved that can be passed between the wall of the canal and the foreign body, then turned and withdrawn with the object. The patient was a little girl who had put in a large iron bead two days before. She could not sleep the night before I extracted it, but next night, she slept well.[5]

While an assistant surgeon to the Royal Infirmary, Lister published his first clinical paper. The patient was a six-year-old girl whose legs became deathly pale following scarlet fever. One leg turned gangrenous; Lister performed an above-the-knee amputation and dissected the amputated leg. He found an organized clot in an inflamed popliteal artery that extended into the anterior tibial artery. In typical fashion, he used this case to discuss blood coagulation.[6]

Most of Lister's practice in Glasgow was orthopedic trauma or complications of tuberculosis, such as joint infections and psoas abscesses. Prior to the introduction of antisepsis, compound fractures, osteomyelitis and joint infections required amputation. A few surgeons had success in salvaging limbs after excision of joints, but excision of the wrist joint was unsuccessful until 1865, when Lister reported on 15 patients in whom he had excised the wrist joint for tuberculosis or trauma. Eight of these patients were children or teenagers.[7]

The idea for successful wrist joint excision came to him when a 17-year-old boy who had fallen down a mine shaft presented with a compound dislocation of the wrist: "The articular ends of the radius and ulna protruded interiorly for about an inch and a half through an irregular wound. I sawed off the exposed portions of the bone and placed the limb in a splint. At the end of five months, his hand was nearly as supple and strong as the other."

Lister then studied the anatomy of the wrist joint, in order to preserve the nerves and tendons to the fingers while removing the carpal bones and all involved cartilage in patients with tuberculosis of the joint. He said this about preserving function: "...to save a hand from amputation, and restore its use-fullness is an object worthy of any labor involved in it."

Until 1865, all hospitals were unsanitary and had few facilities, such as running water. Lister's ward in the Glasgow infirmary often had to be closed because of postoperative pyemia and hospital gangrene. Attempts to improve cleanliness with soap and water and open windows did little to prevent infection. Most surgeons accepted the idea that these diseases were due to overcrowding, dirt and pollution of the air, but some, accustomed to "a good old surgical stink," hardly noticed the sickly odor that pervaded the wards.[8]

A few surgeons, such as Ignaz Phillip Semmelweis in Vienna, realized that simple hand washing could reduce the incidence of puerperal fever. Sadly, Semmelweis was not only ignored but also ridiculed. There were scattered attempts to prevent wound infections by the application of substances such as alcohol, tincture of benzoic and coal tar products. In 1865, Lister learned from the work of Louis Pasteur that putrefaction or wound suppuration was a form of fermentation caused by microscopic "beings" carried by the air. After careful study, Lister decided to exclude air and microorganisms from the wound with carbolic acid. His article "A New Method of Treating Compound Fractures, Abscesses, Etc." appeared in the journal *Lancet* in 1867.[9]

The first patient on whom Lister used the carbolic-acid method, an 11-year-old boy named James G., was admitted to the Glasgow Royal Infirmary on August 12, 1865, with a compound fracture of the left leg caused by the wheel of an empty cart passing over the limb a little below the middle. A probe passed into the wound went some inches beyond the site of the fracture. Lister's house surgeon applied lint dipped in carbolic acid over the wound. When carbolic acid irritated the skin, he applied a dressing soaked in a solution of 1 part carbolic acid in 20 parts of olive oil. After six weeks the bones were firmly united, and two days later the "sore" was entirely healed. Four of Lister's original 11 patients with compound fractures treated with carbolic acid were children, usually with terrible injuries. The right leg of a "fine intelligent" boy seven years of age was run over by both wheels of a crowded omnibus. The boy was in shock from blood loss, his tibia was broken, the skin wound extended from the knee to ankle and muscles were contused. With the boy under chloroform, the entire wound was irrigated with carbolic acid, the skin flaps replaced but not sutured, and the bone positioned with the leg extended. Despite extensive sloughing of the wound and exposed bone, Lister persevered in saving the limb with applications of carbolic and nitric acid. After many months, and many debridements, the wound healed.

He also applied his antiseptic technique to the treatment of abscesses and infected joints. Two of the patients he treated in 1867 were children. One was a five-year-old boy with a psoas abscess reaching from the umbilicus to mid-thigh. After draining a "pound of pus," Lister wiped out the interior of the wound with a rag dipped in carbolic acid and applied a carbolic dressing. He also used carbolic acid to treat an infected ankle joint in a boy after draining pus and later reported that the ankle was free from pain and drained only a small amount of clear liquid.[10] In August of 1867, Lister presented a penetrating wound of the thorax, a gunshot wound and the case of a boy whose arm had become entangled in machinery to the British Medical Association:

There was a wound six inches long and three inches broad, and the skin was very extensively undermined beyond its limits, while the soft parts were generally so much lacerated that a pair of dressing forceps introduced at the wound and pushed directly inwards appeared beneath the skin at the opposite aspect of the limb. From this wound several tags of muscle were hanging, and among them was one consisting of the tri-

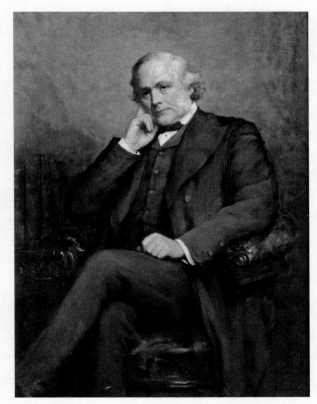

Joseph Lister, who revolutionized surgery with his discovery of antisepsis, was also known for his gentleness, especially with children. Once while Lister was making rounds, an urchin on the ward said, "It's us wee yins he likes best and next it's the auld women." This painting is unsigned (courtesy and © Hunterian Museum at the Royal College of Surgeons).

ceps in almost its entire thickness; while the lower fragment of bone, which was broken high up, was protruding four inches and a half, stripped of muscle, the skin being tucked in under it. Without the assistance of the antiseptic treatment, I should certainly have thought of nothing else but amputation at the shoulder joint; but, as the radial pulse could be felt and the fingers had sensation, I did not hesitate to try to save the limb and adopted the plan of treatment described above, wrapping the arm from the shoulder to below the elbow in the antiseptic application, the whole interior of the wound, together with the protruding bone, having previously been freely treated with strong carbolic acid.[11]

This wound, which would tax today's surgeons, healed. In those days, the healing of a wound this severe without infection was miraculous.

In 1869, Lister replaced James Syme as professor of surgery at the University of Edinburgh and became Chief Surgeon to the Royal Infirmary. He continued to teach, lecture, do research and carry on a busy practice while propagating the antiseptic method. His students, house officers and visitors who came to see his technique became enthusiastic followers, but the profession at large ignored Lister and ridiculed his germ theory. In 1877, he accepted the call to become professor of surgery at Kings' College in London so he could convince more surgeons to follow his antiseptic technique.

After many frustrating years the profession recognized his great work and Lister was showered with honors. Throughout his life, he continued to do research in bacteriology, chemical antiseptics, anesthesia, and especially absorbable, sterile catgut ligatures. He introduced heat sterilization and was the first to demonstrate that ligatures could be cut short and left in the wound. In adults he operated on cancers of the breast, tongue and penis and diseases of the bones and joints, placed skin grafts on open wounds and treated incarcerated hernias. His practice in Edinburgh must have included large numbers of children, because he said there were often two or three children in a bed.[12]

Throughout his writings, he fondly referred to his pediatric patients: "I opened in a little, sickly, dwindled child a conjoint psoas and lumbar abscess, associated with spinal disease. I emptied the extensive cavity by free incision in the lumbar part, and dressed with gauze. Within a week of opening the abscess, the discharge was only a few minims of serum per idem and the boy had already picked up wonderfully in general health."[13] After Lister removed a rib and drained 30 ounces of pus from an empyema in a six-year-old boy, treated with antiseptic dressings, he said, "I was delighted to see, on coming back after a fortnight's absence, how plump the emaciated little fellow had become."

Joseph Bell, best known for being Sir Arthur Conan Doyle's model for Sherlock Holmes, was a colleague of Lister at the Royal Infirmary in Edinburgh and was one of the first surgeons to adopt the antiseptic technique. Dr. Bell was especially interested in surgery on children, had a gentle touch, and in 1887 was appointed surgeon to the first surgical ward in the Royal Edinburgh Hospital for Sick Children.[14]

While he was Syme's house surgeon, Bell invented a pipette to suck thick secretions from tracheotomy tubes in children with diphtheria. Bell himself developed the disease while using his pipette.[15]

His textbook *A Manual of the Operations of Surgery for the Use of Senior Students, House Surgeons and Junior Practitioners* describes a number of operations for children.[16] Tuberculosis of the joints was the most common surgical problem. Of this subject, Bell said: "In our cold climate, so cursed by scrofula and especially among the children of the laboring poor, such joint diseases are very prevalent. Treatment of these joint diseases with bed rest, a good diet and cod liver oil might result in a cure, but the joint will become ankylosed." Amputation of the limb was quick and easy but left the child with an artificial leg. Bell's operation for tuberculosis of joints was removal of the articular cartilage and all diseased tissue back to healthy bone. This was a long, tedious operation that often left a shortened but still useful limb. Bell preferred excision, except for the hip joint, where excision carried a 40 percent mortality rate.

For cleft lip, he excised the mucosa and sutured the cut edges with metallic sutures. He also did tonsillectomies, recommended circumcision for intractable bed-wetting, and advised the use of a truss for inguinal hernias. He manually reduced incarcerated hernias by the use of warm baths, the inverted position and, when necessary, chloroform anesthesia. If the hernia couldn't be reduced, Bell advised an early operation, which consisted of cutting through all the layers to the sac. If the intestine was pink and glistening, he returned the bowel to the abdominal cavity and closed the internal ring with catgut sutures. Gangrenous bowel was left outside in the hopes that an intestinal fistula would form. He observed that most hernias recurred after an operation. He also treated children with hydroceles, clubfeet, tuberculosis of the lymph nodes and large numbers of burns.

Dr. Bell claimed no case had died on his wards from an operation or within three months of one and that all deaths had been cases of hopeless burns. These results are skewed somewhat because cases of intussusception, rectal atresia and peritonitis were considered terminal and weren't operated on.[17] Of his young patients, he said: "Had I four times the number of beds at my disposal, I could fill them all in a week with cases of spinal and hip joint disease. Only the very worst can be admitted, where psoas abscesses have to be opened or hip abscesses drained or joints to be excised. Scraping and excision of the swollen and suppurating glands of scrofulous children are daily duties. A depressing lot of cases, some will say; but for the child's marvelous good nature and infinite fun once they recognize you mean friendship, their exuberant vitality renders it almost impossible for a child to die if only you can avoid shock and hemorrhage."

In 1895, Dr. Bell's house surgeon reported on the most recent 93 ward admissions. One child with severe burns died of pneumonia and gastrointestinal bleeding. The duodenal ulcer found at autopsy that may have been one of the first stress ulcers identified in a child. A common operation was the drainage of pus in children with otitis media or mastoiditis. There were still many operations for complications of tuberculosis and even syphilitic gummas. Except for operations to correct curvature of the tibia due to rickets and tenotomy for clubfoot, there were few "elective" operations. Hernias were still treated with trusses. The eight deaths were due to infections such as meningitis, tubercular peritonitis or pneumonia.[18]

Joseph Bell was far ahead of his peers with his keen insight into the psychology of children, as demonstrated in his *Notes on Surgery for Nurses*:

> Never deceive a child, tell it honestly that the dressing or movement you are going to make will hurt ... but also that you will hurt it as little as possible, and it will help you loyally. Don't make favorites; children are much sharper than you think, and a quiet child may soon get a sore heart if you take less notice of it than of the more cheerful one in the next bed. You must always have the one great rule to guide you about sick children — that they don't cry or moan for fun, but because they are ill and in pain, or from a nameless weariness if not in actual pain. Healthy children may yell and scream as an evidence and result of an original iniquity, but sick children don't ... if once you get a child's confidence and love it, it is marvelously loyal and utterly trustfull.... Adults can read and amuse themselves, but a child's convalescence will often be much hastened by toys, cheering words, and fun of the mildest type. The stages in sick children are more rapid. Death is imminent before you are aware; yet if staved off, recovery is like a miracle. They stand loss of blood very badly, and yet they remake blood very quickly.[19]

During his presidential address to the British Association for the Advancement of Science in 1896, Lister told how the introduction of anesthesia 50 years earlier had revolutionized the practice of surgery. Lister discussed the recent discovery of roentgen rays, but most of his lecture was on Pasteur's work in bacteriology and his treatment for rabies. Lister discussed the identification of the staphylococcus and streptococcus bacteria that caused erysipelas, the tubercle bacillus and the discovery of an antitoxin for diphtheria. He himself made many original observations in the field of bacteriology and had almost single-handedly demonstrated how germs caused infections in surgical wounds.

During the later part of the nineteenth century, acceptance of the germ theory and Lister's antiseptic technique led to more advances in the fight against infection. Steam sterilization was used for instruments and linens; gowns replaced bloodstained frock coats, and surgeons vigorously scrubbed their hands and the patient's skin with chemical antiseptics. Surgeons had also learned to cover their faces and hair with caps and masks. These advancements led to new operations in children when surgeons addressed the problems of hypertrophic pyloric stenosis, intussusception, appendicitis, hydrocephalus and spina bifida.

Lister's most valued trait was his invariable gentleness and sympathy. Once a small urchin in the wards, following Lister with his eyes, confided in a bystander, "It's us wee yins he likes best and next it's the auld women."

After being summoned to treat Queen Victoria for an axillary abscess, Lister was made a Baronet in 1883 and a lord in 1897. In London, a monument in his honor bears a single word: "LISTER." Although asepsis has almost supplanted Lister's work, we still swabbed the stump of the appendix with carbolic acid and alcohol during the 1960s and an over-the-counter preparation containing phenol is still one of the best remedies for itching insect bites. A few of us continued to irrigate traumatic wounds with antiseptics at least until the early twenty-first century.

Lister never opened an abdomen, but abdominal surgery — which became one of the great triumphs of the twentieth century — originated with a suggestion by Edinburgh surgeon John Bell. Bell suggested it might be feasible to remove an ovarian cyst by opening the abdomen. One of his students — Ephraim McDowell of Danville, Kentucky, deep in the American wilderness — had been with John Bell in Edinburgh from 1793 to 1794. McDowell never took a medical degree but became a skilled physician. In 1809, he was called away over the mountains to see a farmer's wife who was thought to have a long overdue pregnancy. McDowell diagnosed an ovarian cyst and said the only hope was an operation to remove the cyst. The patient, Jane Crawford, agreed and rode horseback 20 miles to Danville. McDowell described the operation as follows: "I opened her side and extracted one of the ovaria which from its diseased and enlarged state weighed upwards of twenty pounds; the intestines as soon as an opening was made run out upon the table and remained out about thirty minutes and, being Christmas Day, they became so cold that I thought proper to bathe them in tepid water previous to my replacing them; I then returned them, stitched up the wound and she was perfectly well in twenty-five days."

During the operation, the patient sang psalms. According to McDowell's nephew, a medical student who assisted, the surgeon opened and drained the ovary and ligated the pedicle prior to its removal.[20] The country's most prominent doctors denounced McDowell's operation, but he is remembered as one of the great surgeons of America. H. Bieman Otherson, a pediatric surgeon from Charleston, South Carolina, has written that McDowell had all the compassion, personal cleanliness and courage of a great surgeon. The logo of the Southern Surgical Association includes a bust of McDowell.[21]

McDowell and others performed a few more ovarian resections, but it remained for another Edinburgh-trained surgeon, Lawson Tait (1845–1899), to literally "open up" the belly. Like most of Britain's surgeons at the end of the nineteenth century, Tait didn't believe in the germ theory and never used the antiseptic technique. He did, however, boil his instruments and sponges, use only freshly laundered linen and keep scrupulously clean. Influenced by James Simpson, the Edinburgh surgeon who discovered the anesthetic effects of chloroform, Tait took an interest in the diseases of women. Shortly after leaving Edinburgh, he had removed ovarian cysts from five women, four of whom survived. In 1881, at the International Medicine Congress in London when he was 37 years old, Tait described many operations for the removal of ovaries, gallstones, ruptured ectopic pregnancies and uterine myoma.[22]

The impressive array of physicians and surgeons in attendance and the program presented by the British Medical Association's Section of Diseases of Children in 1898 illustrate the growing importance of surgery in children. Joseph Bell, surgeon to the Royal Edinburgh Hospital for Sick Children and President of the section, presided over the meeting. There were physicians from Berlin and Paris as well as William Osler, then Chief of Medicine at Johns Hopkins. Pioneer neurosurgeon Sir Victor Horsley and orthopedic surgeon Robert Jones discussed surgical treatment of tuberculosis of the spine. Horsley recommended removing diseased bone and irrigating with antiseptics, while Jones favored splinting with immobilization. There were papers on the surgical treatment of clubfoot, dislocation of the hip during acute fevers, tendon grafting in children with infantile paralysis and harelip. Harold Stiles, another Edinburgh surgeon, discussed mastoid and middle ear infections. Perhaps the most remarkable papers were those by James Nicoll of Glasgow on surgery for spina bifida and one by Sutherland and Chene on the drainage of spinal fluid from the ventricles of the brain to the subdural space in children with hydrocephalus. This remarkable group of papers illustrated the rapid advance in children's surgery after Lister's discovery of antisepsis. In contrast to the optimism and progress in these surgical diseases, the papers on rheumatic fever, congenital syphilis and pneumonia were mainly concerned with diagnosis. Little was said about the treatment of these diseases that within a halfcentury would be eliminated by antibiotics.

CHAPTER 18

Prelude to the Twentieth Century

During the latter part of the nineteenth century, French and German scientists established the scientific basis for modern medicine and surgery. I can only skim over a few of those who worked on pathology, bacteriology and physiology who are most pertinent to my story. Claude Bernard at the Sorbonne developed a scientific theory and his work on pancreatic and liver metabolism led to the term "mileu interior," or internal homeostatis.[1] Berlin pathologist Rudolph Ludwig Karl Virchow worked on the cellular basis of cancer and described pulmonary embolism and metastases to the supraclavicular lymph node that is still known as "Virchow's node."[2] Carl von Rokitansky of Vienna developed the autopsy into the ultimate diagnostic tool and described many new syndromes.[3] In Berlin, Robert Koch discovered the tubercle bacillus and stated the postulates necessary to prove that a specific bacterium is the cause of a disease. His postulates are no longer entirely true but were important to the development of microbiology.[4]

Koch's students included Emil von Behring, who discovered the diphtheria antitoxin in 1901; August Wasserman, who devised the serological test for syphilis; and Paul Ehrlich, who discovered Salvarsan, the first effective therapy for syphilis. By identifying the three major blood groups and later the Rh factor, Karl Landsteiner made blood transfusion safe and practical.[5] In France, while working at the Pasteur Institute in 1897, Edmond Nocard demonstrated that an antitoxin produced by animals induced passive immunity against tetanus in humans.[6] One of the most famed human and scientific stories of the twentieth century was of the isolation of radium by Marie and Pierre Curie that led to use of radiation for treatment of cancer.[7]

German surgeons, led by Theodore Billroth, pioneered surgery of the gastrointestinal tract by successful removal of portions of cancerous stomach and intestine. They also bypassed pyloric obstruction and treated duodenal ulcers by anastomosis of the stomach to the small intestine. In Bern, Switzerland, Theodore Kocher (1841–1917), who led the way in thyroid surgery, recognized the effects of hypothyroidism following complete removal of the gland. These phenomenal advances in surgery of the gastrointestinal tract and the thyroid gland resulted in German domination of surgery during the early part of the twentieth century.

The names of nineteenth-century German surgeons are still in everyday use. We speak of the Billroth I and II type of gastric resection, the Heineke-Mikulicz pyloroplasty, the Kocher hemostat and the Payr clamp for transecting the stomach. The Kuttner dissecter, a bit of balled-up cotton held in a hemostat, is still a useful surgical tool. A patient tipped head down is in the Trendelenburg position, and the Trendelenburg sign indicates a congenital dislocation of the hip. Frederich Trendelenburg, professor of surgery at Leipzig, is also remembered for his interest in removing pulmonary emboli.

Richard von Volkmann went beyond Lister's antiseptic methods when he introduced preoperative shaving and scrubbing of the surgical site. "Volkmann's ischemic contracture" is the term still applied to the necrosis of forearm muscles and fibrosis of nerves following a supra-condylar fracture of the humerus with vascular damage. The operation for hypertrophic pyloric stenosis is named for Conrad Ramstedt, the common kidney tumor of childhood is named after Max Wilms and the Meckel's diverticulum is named for Johan Freidrich Meckel, a German anatomist.

Students of surgery flocked to the German centers from the late 1800s until the beginning of the First World War. German became the universal language of science and medicine, and German surgical journals disseminated the new surgery to the world. In a letter to Harvey Cushing written in 1895, William Stewart Halsted advised: "It is very necessary nowadays for a medical man to have a thorough knowledge of German so that he can read medical German quite as well as English. You probably know that there is little if any scientific work done in this country in medicine and that most of it is done in Germany."[8]

The transfer of surgical knowledge from Germany to the United States started with a few well-trained surgeons who left Germany for the New World. Two of the most prominent were Christian Fenger and Willy Meyer. Fenger, born in Denmark, studied with Billroth and Rokitansky before coming to the United States in 1877. He became a pathologist and then a surgeon at Cook County Hospital in Chicago, where he established a "school" of surgery.[9] The Mayo brothers and others from the Midwest visited his clinics and learned European techniques. He encouraged students like John B. Murphy, one of the founders of the American College of Surgeons, to study in Europe. Another Chicago surgeon, Nicholas Senn, was born in Switzerland and moved to the United States but returned to Munich for medical study. Senn became Chief of Surgery at the Rush Medical School and was the author of major surgical textbooks. Willy Meyer studied with Trendelenburg and in 1884 moved to New York. Dr. Meyer did the first gastroenterostomy for pyloric stenosis and introduced many new techniques to the United States. His main interest was in thoracic surgery; he was President of the American Association for Thoracic Surgery from 1918 to 1920.[10]

Abraham Jacobi, a pediatrician, was as interested in surgical as medical problems. Dr. Jacobi obtained his M.D. from the University of Bonn in 1851 and after being imprisoned for his political views left Germany for New York. He became a professor of childhood diseases and established the first department of pediatrics in a general hospital at Mount Sinai. He wrote extensively on childhood diseases, including *Sarcoma of the Kidney in the Foetus and Infant.* As a tribute to Dr. Jacobi, the American Medical Association and the American Academy of Pediatrics in 1963 established the Jacobi award for excellence in pediatrics.[11]

At a time when few opportunities existed for postgraduate medical education in the United States, many doctors went to Germany to further their education. In 1889, when Dr. Charles Mayo visited the Continent, German surgeons were scrubbing their hands and cleaning their nails before surgery. Some even wore boiled white cotton gloves. Here was the beginning of asepsis, rather than antisepsis.[12] During the following years, one or another of the Mayo brothers visited their German counterparts annually. After graduating from Yale and Harvard and interning at Bellevue Hospital in New York, William Stewart Halsted spent from 1878 to 1880 studying and attending clinics in Germany and Switzerland.[13] He knew Woelfer, who had performed the first gastroenterostomy, and Mickulicz of pyloroplasty fame and was friends with Volkman. In later years, Halsted visited Germany at least once a year and became an honorary member of the German Surgical Society.[14] He especially admired and appreciated Theodore Kocher's work on goiter. Halsted probably learned his meticulous attention to hemostasis and the use of fine silk ligatures from Kocher. He also arranged for his own residents to work in German clinics and for young German surgeons to work in his laboratory at Johns Hopkins.

The most enduring result of Halsted's visits to Germany was his residency system of training surgeons that combined clinical work with laboratory experience. After four years as Halsted's resident at Johns Hopkins, Harvey Cushing visited surgeons in England and attended clinics in Germany and Switzerland during 1900 and 1901. While working in Kocher's laboratories, he established the relationship between intracranial pressure, the pulse and systemic blood pressure.[15]

On almost every page of the minutes of the early years of the American Surgical Association, there are references to German surgeons.[16] During the meeting in 1900, in a discussion of perforating duodenal ulcers and gastric surgery, there were references to Mikulicz, Kocher, Pagenstecher and others. In 1903, Mikulicz was a guest and discussed surgery of the small intestine and cancers of the colon. In 1906 Trendelenburg described his method for closing extrophy of the bladder, and in 1907 the honored guest was Professor Kuster from Marburg, Germany, who discussed spinal anesthesia. These exchanges of information came to an abrupt halt with the onset of World War I in 1914.

Harvey Cushing left us with one of the best descriptions of surgery during the First World War because he not only served with our army later in the war but in 1915 also was a volunteer with the British army during the second battle at Ypres, when there were thousands of casualties. He operated on many men with head wounds and in one case extracted a fragment of metal from deep in the brain with an electromagnet. Cushing recorded these experiences, as well as his second tour of duty from May of 1917 until the end of the war, in *From a Surgeon's Journal*, 1915–1918.[17] Cushing eloquently described the pathos of war, his many hours at the operating table (often only a mile or two away from the fighting), the mud, rain and cold, as well as the humor of hospital work in France. He was involved in almost every major battle of the war, either as a front-line surgeon or as a consultant. His cryptic surgical notes always included something personal about his patients. During the Passchendaele battles, one day started with: "Winter, E. 860584, 7th Borderers, 17th Div. Penetrating cerebellar, sitting down, helmet on. Blown into the air. Unconscious for a time, does not know how long. Later crept back to a trench — legs wobbly — dizzy — etc."

Cushing, a member of a research committee in France, mentioned Alexis Carrel's studies of antiseptics in war wounds, as well as his work in determining the most effective dosages of tetanus antitoxin and developing a serum to prevent gas gangrene. There were also studies on the use of intravenous saline for resuscitation of the badly wounded. Early in the war, surgeons in the Canadian army treated soldiers in hemorrhagic shock with whole-blood transfusions, and American surgeons learned to store refrigerated, citrated whole blood for as long as 48 hours.[18]

The limitations of surgery at the time are illustrated by one of the saddest episodes in the history of medicine. Revere Osler, the only child of Sir William Osler, Regius Professor of Medicine at Oxford and the former Chief of Medicine at Johns Hopkins, suffered shrapnel wounds to his abdomen, chest and leg. Some of the best American surgeons, including Harvey Cushing and George Crile, arrived at the aid station in a driving rain. The surgeons gave Revere Osler a transfusion and opened his abdomen to find holes in his colon and mesenteric vessels. He died shortly after the operation.[19]

CHAPTER 19

Children's Surgery
Comes of Age

The British, French and Germans had well-established hospital surgical training programs while in the United States anyone with a medical degree could learn surgery on the job. The situation improved when the American College of Surgeons, founded in 1913, set basic standards for the education of surgeons. The American Board of Surgery, established in 1936, further set criteria for residency programs. There were other specialty boards, but it was not uncommon for general surgeons in those days to operate on all areas of the body in patients of all ages. A surgeon might start the day with removal of a gallbladder, then repair a hernia in a child, do a pyloromyotomy and end by removing a tumor from the spinal cord. The idea of general surgery as an all-encompassing specialty retarded the development of pediatric surgery until well after World War II. In 1951, when I was a student at the Presbyterian Hospital in Chicago, I held retractors for a surgeon who started the day with a mitral commisurotomy, followed by a gastric resection, and a pediatric hernia, and ended with the application of a body cast for a fractured vertebra. He did the full gamut of pediatric and adult surgery.

The idea of specialization in pediatric surgery was not even considered in the United States, though a few surgeons were interested in and wrote about children's surgical problems. One of these authors, Edmund Owen, Senior Surgeon to the Great Ormond Street Hospital in London, did tracheotomies for infants with croup, drained empyemas by resecting a small segment of a rib and treated intussusception by "kneading" the abdomen under chloroform anesthesia along with the injection of air or water by rectum. An operation was a last resort. Owen operated on children with cleft lip and spina bifida, performed tonsillectomies and recommended trusses for hernias. He drained appendiceal abscesses but would only remove the appendix if it was easy.[1]

Perhaps the first textbook of pediatric surgery illustrated with radiographs was by Edouard F. Kermisson (1848–1927), a professor of pediatric surgery and orthopedics at l'Hôpital des Enfants-Malades in Paris. Professor Kermisson discussed the embryology and pathology of the omphalomesenteric duct and fistulas in the neck as well as orthopedic deformities and spina bifida. He treated Pott's disease of the spine with a full-body splint.[2]

In the United States, the first surgical textbook devoted to children was *The Surgery of Childhood*, published in 1910 by De Forrest T. Willard. It was mainly concerned with fractures and orthopedic deformities.[3] This book also had excellent illustrations of chest and bone X-rays. Willard recommended exercise and deep breathing for chest deformities, the Halsted or the Bassini operation for hernias and air reduction with a hand bellows for intussusception. If that failed, the child was operated on. Willard cited one operation for an omphalocele, but the infant died. Another text, *Surgical Diseases of Children,* in two volumes by S.W. Kelley and first published in 1909, recommended fresh air and cod-liver oil for tuberculosis and syrup of iron iodide for syphilis.[4] There was also a section on that ancient, terrible destruction of the face cancrum oris, as well as many pages devoted to cysts, superficial tumors, abscesses, empyema and fractures.

The memoirs of Harvey Cushing, during his time as a student extern at the Boston Children's Hospital in 1893, also provide a look at children's surgical work. Cushing did a "septic phymosis circumcision," applied casts, braces and splints, and learned the difference between valgus and varus deformities of the legs.[5]

Even in children's hospitals, the attending surgeons often treated adults to make a living. One exception was Dr. Vaclav Kafka, who became the Surgeon in Chief at the New Children's Hospital in Prague, Czechoslovakia.[6] Dr. Kafka treated six thousand cases of congenital dislocation of the hip and continued to practice until 1946; he may well be the first purely pediatric surgeon.

James Henderson Nicoll in Glasgow and Harold Stiles of Edinburgh became interested in children and did exceptionally clever work. Nicoll graduated from the University of Glasgow in 1886 and then took a four-year apprenticeship with Sir Frederick Treves, famous for draining King Edward VII's appendiceal abscess. On his return to Glasgow, Nicoll operated on children with cleft lip, hernia, tonsils and even spina bifida in the outpatient dispensary of the Children's Hospital. Nicoll did some of the early work on pyloric stenosis and has been called the Father of Day Surgery.[7]

Harold Stiles, surgeon to the Royal Edinburgh Hospital for Sick Children, made detailed studies of internal hydrocephalus and tried various operations for congenital pyloric stenosis. By 1908, he had performed 84 operations for pyloric stenosis, with a mortality of 53.6 percent. In 1910, he divided the muscle and closed serosa over the mucosa. The infant died, but it was essentially the same operation as performed by Ramstedt in 1911.[8] Stiles' method of performing a ureterosigmoidostomy by tunneling the ureter through the wall of the bowel was the standard method of urinary diversion for many years.[9]

While working as an honorary surgeon to the Royal Edinburgh Hospital for Sick Children, Stiles commenced the first modern treatment for infants with inguinal hernia in about 1910. The procedure was taken up by his followers, John Fraser and most enthusiastically Miss Gertrude Herzfeld, the first woman pediatric surgeon. Gertrude Herzfeld (1890–1981) graduated from the University of Edinburgh in 1914 and after several hospital appointments joined the staff of the Children's Hospital.[10] Because there was a shortage of hospital beds, children with hernias were operated on in the outpatient department. Since the babies weren't separated from their mothers, breast-feeding could continue and the patients gained rather than lost weight after surgery. The wound was covered with a bit of tape and wound infection was not a problem. The operation, a simple ligation of the hernia sac, could be done in a few minutes. It was said that Miss Herzfeld once performed six hernia operations in 54 minutes.[11] These Scottish surgeons were doing outpatient surgery 50 years before it became routine in the rest of the world.

In the aftermath of the First World War, Europe suffered terrible economic and political turmoil. There were few advances in surgery on the Continent, but two Americans, William E. Ladd of Boston and Herbert Coe of Seattle, along with Denis Browne of London, established pediatric surgery as a distinct specialty.

William E. Ladd (1880–1967) is recognized the world over for his enormous contributions to pediatric surgery and as the founder of the specialty in the United States. Ladd graduated from Harvard Medical School in 1906 and, after training in general surgery, held appointments at the Boston City Hospital and the Children's Hospital. Prior to the First World War, Ladd did general surgery and gynecology, but he was especially fond of the charity work he did at the Boston Children's Hospital.[12]

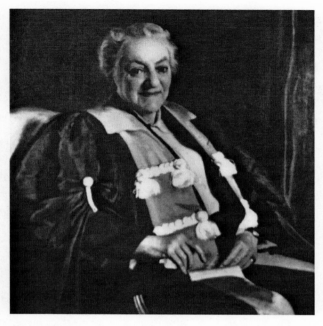

On December 6, 1917, the SS *Mont Blanc*, a French cargo ship loaded with explosives and bound for Europe, collided with a Norwegian ship in the harbor of Halifax, Nova Scotia. The explosion obliterated five hundred acres of the city and caused thousands of injuries. Children on their way to school were especially hard hit. Dr. Ladd led a volunteer group of Boston doctors and nurses who worked for more than a month in

Gertrude Herzfeld, a pioneer woman pediatric surgeon who practiced during the early twentith century in Edinburgh, Scotland. Dr. Herzfeldt advocated outpatient surgery long before the practice became popular in America (courtesy H. Beiman Otherson, Jr., M.D., of Charleston, South Carolina).

a makeshift hospital treating all types of wounds. When he returned to Boston, Dr. Ladd took on the entire spectrum of pediatric surgery, including cleft lip and palate.

It has been part of our medical folklore that Dr. Ladd's experience treating injured children in Halifax was a deciding event in his career. Recently, however, a handwritten letter from Dr. Ladd to Dr. Gerald Zwiren, a pediatric surgeon from Atlanta, Georgia, came to light that indicates Ladd's interest in children's surgery began long before the Halifax disaster. An extract from that letter, written on March 28, 1963, states: "From 1908 I had been on the visiting staff of the Children's Hospital, the Infants and the Boston City Hospital. All this work was entirely charity; I, like most other surgeons of the time, did most of our pay operating in numerous small hospitals widely scattered. A very unsatisfactory arrangement. The Children's was my very first and most permanent love. As soon as it became feasible after the First World War, I devoted myself exclusively to pediatric surgery and have never regretted it."[13]

Dr. Ladd is best known for his pioneering efforts in the treatment of esophageal atresia, congenital defects of the gastrointestinal tract and Wilms' tumors. One of his most important contributions was the recognition of the peritoneal bands causing duodenal obstruction in infants with anomalies of intestinal rotation. Prior to his work, surgeons would treat the volvulus but didn't recognize the duodenal obstruction.

Dr. Ladd served as Surgeon in Chief at the Boston Children's Hospital from 1927 until 1945. His textbook *Abdominal Surgery of Infancy and Childhood*, coauthored with Robert E. Gross and published in 1941, remains a classic in surgical literature.[14] Many of its chapters still apply today. The book represents the personal experience of the authors in the treatment of thousands of children, along with the pertinent literature. Many chapters, such as those on biliary atresia, omphalocele and congenital diaphragmatic hernias, accurately depict these diseases and their successful treatment for the first time. There are detailed instructions on pre- and postoperative care, along with the remark that the survival rate in surgical conditions improved when the surgical service took over the complete care of the infant or child. The book is well illustrated and the material is presented so that general physicians and surgeons could use it as a guide to the treatment of common conditions. In the preface, the authors state: "This does not imply that Pediatric Surgery should always be set apart as a separate specialty, but it does indicate that infants and children can obtain improved surgical care if an appropriate number of men in each community will take a particular interest in this field and give it the attention which it rightfully deserves."

Dr. Ladd trained many of the pediatric surgeons who led the specialty during the mid-twentieth century. In 1954, the Section on Surgery of the American Academy of Pediatrics honored Dr. Ladd by establishing the Ladd Medal to be given to outstanding pediatric surgeons. One of the more poignant episodes in the history of pediatric surgery occurred when Dr. Ladd suffered a fractured hip in 1967. Dr. Hardy H. Hendren, one of his distinguished successors at the Boston Children's Hospital, held Dr. Ladd's hand as he was anesthetized. Dr. Ladd died later that year at the age of 87.[15]

Dr. Herbert Coe, who graduated from the University of Michigan at the age of 17 in 1904, returned to Seattle and joined the staff of the Children's Orthopedic Hospital. In 1919, he went to Boston to observe surgical work at the Children's Hospital there. He then returned to Seattle, where he became the first surgeon in the United States to restrict his practice to children's surgery.

Dr. Coe saw the need to establish a meeting place for surgeons interested in children. He was a visionary, but surgical organizations scoffed at his ideas. The surgical hierarchy was afraid that any subspecialty would weaken general surgery. After many years of diligent correspondence and persuasion, Dr. Coe convinced the American Academy of Pediatrics to allow a small group of surgeons to organize the Section on Surgery. Dr. Coe was chairman of the section from 1948 until 1954.[16]

Sir Denis Browne (1892–1966) graduated from medical school in 1915, joined the Australian Armed Forces and immediately went to Gallipoli, where he contracted typhoid fever.[17] He served in France for the duration of the war and

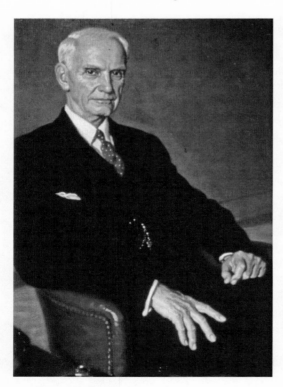

William E. Ladd, the surgeon in chief of Children's Hospital, Boston, from 1925 to 1945 (Children's Hospital Boston Archives, Boston, Massachusetts).

then took surgical training in England. Browne made history when he did up to 25 tonsillectomies a day while he was a casualty surgeon at the Great Ormond Street Hospital. When Browne became the resident medical superintendent of the hospital, he took on the full scope of pediatric surgery, from clubfeet to cleft lip and palate.[18] He studied the anatomy and physiology of almost every congenital defect and made innovative contributions to cleft palate repair and malformations of the anus and external genitalia. He performed primary anastomosis rather than enterostomy after the resection of necrotic intestine, and introduced new and better treatment for intestinal atresia. He was also a pioneer during the early days of pediatric cardiovascular surgery.[19]

Denis Browne was one of the founders and the first President of the British Association of Pediatric Surgeons, the premier pediatric surgical organization. After his death, his widow and the trustees of BAPS established the Denis Browne Gold Medal to be awarded to the most distinguished pediatric surgeons. Denis Browne and William Ladd established the meccas of pediatric surgery that became the training grounds for the surgeons who led pediatric surgery into the second half of the twentieth century.

Pediatric surgery could not have moved forward without advances in other areas. The intravenous needle and parenteral fluid therapy have become as important in the care of a sick or injured child as a scalpel. It is difficult to believe how early surgeons successfully treated babies with pyloric stenosis or intestinal obstruction with only rectal "clysis" and subcutaneous fluids. The clinical descriptions of these diseases emphasized the wizened appearance, sunken eyes and dry skin symptomatic of severe dehydration. The first attempts to correct dehydration consisted of the rectal administration of fluids such as milk, wine, beef broth and even whiskey. During the nineteenth century a few physicians treated cholera patients with intravenous saline solutions, but this therapy was not accepted for many years.[20]

The first attempt to give parenteral fluids was by subcutaneous injection, and as late as the 1950s we still inserted long needles into the subcutaneous tissues of the axilla or back. The subcutaneous saline created huge swellings, but the fluid was gradually absorbed into the circulation. At first intravenous fluids were given to adults twice a day through a cannula sutured into a vein, but in 1923 Rudolph Matas of New Orleans introduced the concept of a continuous saline drip in adult patients with prolonged vomiting due to abdominal sepsis or intestinal obstruction.[21]

James L. Gamble, working in the laboratories at the Johns Hopkins University in the 1920s, demonstrated that death in animals with experimental pyloric obstruction was due to the loss of water, sodium and chloride.[22] Clinical and experimental research by Gamble and others led to a realization of the importance of restoring fluid and electrolytes in sick infants and children. Surgeons now had to learn the difference between intra- and extracellular fluid, daily electrolyte requirements, and formulas for the replacement of lost fluids. The term "milliequivalent" became commonplace, and one of the most frequently asked questions on rounds was, "How are the 'lytes?"

There was an early appreciation of the need for plasma or whole blood in the treatment of burns and other major trauma. E. I. Evans and his associates included plasma with saline and maintenance fluids in the treatment of burns.[23] Surgeons also became aware of the "third space," or fluid sequestered in the peritoneal cavity or the intestinal lumen and lost to the circulation in children with intestinal obstruction or peritonitis. This was one of the main differences in children with surgical as opposed to medical problems, and one not well appreciated by pediatricians.

Severe mechanical problems existed in the delivery of intravenous fluids to small infants. Despite immobilization, needles would slip out of small veins and the fluid would infiltrate. It was necessary to "cut down" on veins and insert metal cannulas until someone had the idea of attaching a bit of plastic tubing to the metal cannula. Unfortunately, peripheral "cut-downs" were often performed at the patient's bedside with less than optimum sterile conditions. After a day or two, the vein became infected or clotted. Until the advent of micro methods for determining serum electrolytes, it was necessary to take at least five milliliters of blood for analysis, usually by sticking the femoral vein at the groin. A few pediatricians and surgeons became adept at inserting small needles into the scalp veins of infants, but the cutdown was necessary for practically every infant who required an operation until well into the 1960s. The development of methods for the percutaneous insertion of soft plastic catheters finally replaced the peripheral cut-down. The increasing ease of giving intravenous fluids, together with micromethods for determining electrolytes in sick infants, took all the mystery out of fluid therapy.

The spectrum of disease in children dramatically changed within a few years after the Second World War. By 1950, entire hospitals existed for children with tuberculosis and rheumatic fever. Medical students could easily find patients with congenital syphilis and gonorrheal ophthalmia in the pediatric wards of charity hospitals. By the end of the decade, penicillin had essentially eradicated rheumatic fever, syphilis and gonorrhea; it was difficult to find a child with tuberculosis or mastoiditis for teaching purposes.

Contagious disease hospitals had been filled with children devastated by poliomyelitis, but in the summer of 1956 we interns and residents of Cook County Hospital in Chicago, along with thousands of doctors all over the country, took part in the first mass program to protect children from polio with the inactivated poliovirus vaccine developed by Jonas Salk at the University of Pittsburgh. The elimination of these ancient diseases allowed physicians to turn their attention to birth defects and cancer. In the wake of the war and its aftermath, a question arose that is still debated: Did all the chemicals that seemed so beneficial to mankind and the radiation released by our quest for energy increase the incidence of childhood cancer and birth defects?

Some of the most exciting advances in pediatric surgery, the correction or palliation of congenital cardiac defects, took place in a ten-year period prior to and just after World War II. First came ligation of the patent ductus arteriosus by Robert Gross in 1938, then resection of coarctation of the aorta by Clarence Crafoord in Stockholm, then the Blalock-Taussig subclavian–pulmonary shunt and the Potts aorto-pulonary shunt for infants with tetralogy of Fallot, and finally Brock's pulmonary valvotomy for pulmonary stenosis.[24]

Phenomenal advances in open heart surgery, with the first closure of atrial septal defects under hypothermia and then the correction of ever more complicated intracardiac defects with the heart-lung machine, are beyond the scope of this book. For a while, cardiac surgery was part of the allure of pediatric surgery, but as time went on the surgery of congenital cardiac lesions became a specialty in itself.

At the end of the war in 1945, Boston was the epicenter of pediatric surgery. Robert E. Gross, appointed Surgeon in Chief in 1947, and Orvar Swenson, who had worked out the cause and treatment of Hirschprung's disease, attracted surgeons from all over the world. Those surgeons returned home to establish centers of excellence in the surgical treatment of children.

The classic textbook by Robert E. Gross, *The Surgery of Infancy and Childhood*, published in 1953, defined pediatric surgery.[25] Unlike previous texts, there were no chapters on tuberculosis, orthopedics, cleft lip or spina bifida and nothing on infectious diseases. Instead, there were exciting chapters on the surgery of premature infants, esophageal atresia, intestinal obstructions and rare anomalies such as duplications of the esophagus and gastrointestinal tract. The material on diseases of the heart and great vessels was brand-new and fascinating. The book covered the gastrointestinal tract from mouth to anus, cysts, sinuses and tumors of the neck, and anomalies of the genitourinary tract. The material on Wilms' tumors and neuroblastoma included the best results yet obtained for these childhood cancers. The material — with charts, diagrams, embryology, pathology, diagnosis, technique and the results of surgery — was clearly presented. It became the bible of pediatric surgery; residents carried the book into the operating room for immediate reference. The book made pediatric surgery seem so easy that every surgeon thought he could operate on babies.

In the very first chapter, Dr. Gross asked:

> What is children's surgery? It is a field that is impossible to define exactly; it is easier to tell what it is not. Children's surgery is not limited to an anatomical area of the body, such as the thorax or the abdomen. It is not the encompassment of diseases of a single system, such as urologic surgery. It has no standing as a circumscribed and well-defined field recognized by all physicians. It has no recognized programs of training, widely available in teaching centers throughout the country. There are no special boards which can certify those men who would like to practice this type of surgery. The field of pediatric surgery has little of the éclat which surrounds the well developed fields of special surgery which have sprung up in the last half century.[26]

In the years to follow, there would be more textbooks of pediatric surgery from around the world in every language. Among the first was one by Max Grob from Switzerland. His book included chapters on treating hydrocephalus with the Torkildson shunt, spina bifida, tonsillectomy, cleft lip and "lop ears" as well as diseases of the abdomen and thorax.[27] From Germany came the most extensive book on pediatric surgery ever published: the *Lehrbuch der Chirurgie und Orthopadie des Kindersalters*, in three volumes representing all the surgical specialties, was published in 1959.[28] These two books indicate the different direction taken by most European pediatric surgeons. In 1980, when the author visited Liverpool and Zurich, pediatric surgeons (unlike Americans) were caring for children with fractures, head trauma and hydrocephalus.

Willis J. Potts was inspired to become a full-time pediatric surgeon after reading the book by Ladd and Gross on abdominal surgery while he was on duty with the army in the South Pacific. He became the first pediatric surgeon in Chicago. Dr. Potts is known for designing atraumatic toothed forceps for vascular surgery and a dissecting scissors that is sharp on the outside for gently teasing apart delicate tissue. During a visit to the Boston Children's Hospital, he had an idea for anastomosis of the aorta directly to the pulmonary artery for treatment of cyanotic heart disease. Despite these achievements, his most enduring legacy is an almost poetic book, *The Surgeon and the Child*.[29] This is not a standard textbook of surgery but more of a guide for obstetricians and family doctors who were most likely to see a child with surgical problems. The tone of the book is set in the first chapter, "The Cry of a Child": "With no language but a cry, children are asking for better surgical treatment of their ills and are begging for more thoughtful attention to the congenital deformities it was their misfortune to be born with. The newborn infant has no words to demand his rights and is aided only by a couple of flustered parents, dismayed at the sudden misfortune of an unanticipated catastrophe. Many of the most severe ills, especially of infants, are emergencies which preclude thoughtful analysis by parents of the surgical care their children are about to receive."

Dr. Potts addressed in a thoughtful, empathetic manner the relationship between the surgeon and the child, and the impact of hospitalization on young patients. He said: "...the mystical heart of a child is a precious and beautiful thing. It is marred only by wounds of a thoughtless and not too intelligent world." At that time, and for the next 10 to 15 years, there were strict visiting hours when parents could visit their child, and children were kept in the hospital for at least five days for even minor operations. Dr. Potts described the pitiable child, standing in a hospital crib with a tearstained face crying, "I want my mommy." Potts was one of the first to insist on personalized care to soothe crying, sick children. His ideas eventually led to unrestricted parental hospital visits. Dr. Potts also addressed the still-unresolved issue of how to care for hopelessly deformed infants. He believed in providing the parents with an honest prognosis and letting the family decide what was best for their own child.

As the world recovered from the Second World War, Britain and many other European countries developed delivery systems that provided health care to all citizens, and in many areas complex pediatric problems were centralized in children's hospitals or university departments of pediatric surgery. This centralization enabled a few surgeons to gain immense expertise in the care of the most severe congenital anomalies and childhood cancers. Physicians in the United States, however, adamantly retained the fee-for-service method of payment and would not accept "socialized medicine." This system retarded the development of specialty centers to treat complex problems. General and specialty surgeons did not want to give up their children's practices to a new specialist, who claimed to take care of the entire child. Moreover, pediatricians were reluctant to give up pre- and postoperative care.

The chairs of university departments were convinced that their surgeons could take care of children. In fact, general surgeons together with the pediatricians provided adequate care for common surgical conditions, although general surgeons still used complicated adult-type inguinal hernia repairs. More than one child suffered testicular atrophy after a general surgeon "tightened up" his internal ring.

Most children were cared for in general hospitals where neonatal birth defects were very rare. A general surgeon might make a fine anastomosis in an infant with intestinal atresia but overlook a second, distal atresia or operate on a baby with pyloric stenosis and know nothing about fluid and electrolyte replacement. Postoperative complications and death were often attributed to bad luck rather than lack of skill. Pediatricians dominated children's hospitals and refused to admit that a specially trained surgeon had anything new or different to offer. They made the preoperative diagnosis, sometimes marked the incision site and took over complete care when the patient came off the operating table.

The surgeons and pediatricians at the Philadelphia Children's Hospital told C. Everett Koop that he was not wanted when he arrived in 1948 to become Surgeon in Chief.[30] The tide slowly turned, however, as babies born with tracheo-esophageal fistulas or intestinal obstructions survived under the care of pediatric surgeons. The pediatricians also noted how infants with inguinal hernias recovered more rapidly when a pediatric surgeon operated. Rather than treat babies with trusses until they were "old enough for an operation," regular pediatricians learned to trust pediatric surgeons with the operation.

New Technology

The care of newborn infants, especially premature or sick babies, changed very little until the middle of the twentieth century. As more babies were delivered in hospitals, the nurseries for newborns were geared primarily to care for healthy babies. At most, the infant who failed to breathe properly might be dipped in cold water, slapped on the bottom or given oxygen. By mid-century, some nurseries had specially heated incubators to maintain warmth for premature infants. Infants who required surgery were often kept on a pediatric ward with older children.

Surgeons, guided by the work of Ladd and Gross, gradually learned to cope with the fluid requirements of postoperative infants, and during the 1950s there was an increased understanding of the metabolic derangements caused by surgery. Peter Paul Rickham at the Liverpool Children's Hospital established a unit entirely dedicated to neonatal surgery. Rickham carried out analyses of water and electrolyte alterations and studied his patients' nutritional needs. He pointed out the dangers of overhydration and the necessity for special incubators to control atmospheric oxygen and humidity, as well as constant expert nursing care.[31]

The mortality rate for neonatal surgery decreased dramatically during the 1950s, but two vexing problems remained. Some infants died of respiratory failure and others simply withered away for lack of nutrition. These two problems were gradually overcome beginning in the 1960s.

As surgeons repaired more complex lesions in smaller babies, the combination of muscle-relaxing anesthetic agents, pain medication that depressed the respiratory system and painful incisions made it difficult for some infants to move air in and out of their lungs. Respiratory failure was an increasingly common cause for postoperative deaths. Endotracheal tubes used during anesthesia caused drying of tracheo-bronchial mucosa, edema and secretions that led to airway obstruction. Humidified air and oxygen helped, but increased oxygen tension damaged the retinas of premature infants.[32] Premature infants were also subject to spells of irregular respirations, and in some the lungs failed to expand. In 1963, the premature son of President John Kennedy died of respiratory distress syndrome because, even in the best of hands, there was no way to support his breathing.

There was a need for mechanical ventilatory support in postoperative patients. Anesthesiologists used hand-squeezed bags to deliver oxygen and anesthetic gases during operations, but short of staying at the bedside for hours or days, there was no way to provide long-term artificial ventilation to infants or postoperative patients. The Drinker respirator, better known as the iron lung, was introduced in 1928 for the treatment of respiratory muscle paralysis caused by poliomyelitis. The patient's body rested in this tank-like device with his head outside. Intermittent negative pressure inside the tank allowed the lungs to expand passively. This device was not suitable for postoperative patients or for small infants.

Ernst Trier Morch, a Danish anesthesiologist, fashioned a ventilator for anesthesia during the German occupation of Denmark during World War II. At the same time, this remarkable physician worked with the Danish resistance movement to help Jews escape from the Nazis. When Danish surgeons refused to allow Morch to organize a separate department of anesthesia, he immigrated to the United States and redesigned the positive pressure ventilator that he had invented in Denmark.[33] The Morch ventilator worked with a piston and a bellows to drive air and oxygen into the patient's lungs through an endotracheal tube or a special swivel adaptor connected to a tracheotomy tube.

Dr. Morch was Chief of Anesthesia at Cook County Hospital in Chicago while I was a surgical resident in 1958. His ventilator was lifesaving in patients with a crushed chest due to trauma and temporarily supported adults with breathing problems but was not satisfactory for infants. For a while, we used respirators designed for small laboratory animals to care

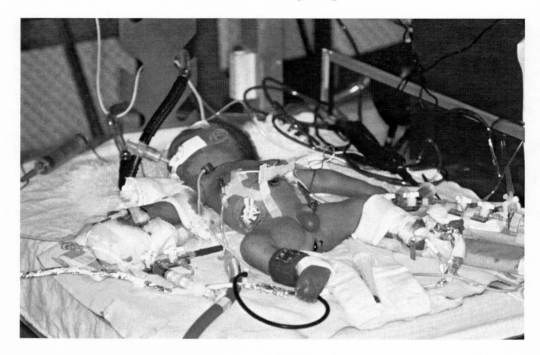

An example of modern technology in the neonatal intensive-care unit. This infant is lying in a heated open incubator and has an endotrachal tube in his mouth that is connected to a ventilator to breathe for him. The catheter in his chest wall leads to a large vein and is used for intravenous nutrition. There are leads taped to his skin to monitor his heartbeat, as well as numerous other tubes for intravenous medications. Note that he was circumcised at birth—the oldest elective pediatric operation.

for infants after cardiac surgery, until the Bird respirator introduced in 1955 became the first practical ventilator for children.[33] The long-term use of endotracheal tubes for ventilatory support in some cases traumatized the trachea, causing tracheal stenosis.[34] There were other complications as well, including oxygen toxicity, barotrauma, pneumothorax, and a new syndrome, broncho-pulmonary dysplasia. Some babies "fought" the ventilator and had to be sedated. This often led to difficulties in "weaning" the baby from the ventilator. Gradual improvements were made in the tubes and ventilators; surgeons spent increasing amounts of time at the bedsides of sick children adjusting valves, pressure and volume to optimize ventilation. It also became necessary to sample arterial blood to determine concentrations of oxygen and carbon dioxide. This led to the continuous monitoring of arterial blood and eventually to sophisticated devices that sensed oxygen concentration through the skin.

The increasing complexity of respirator care required intensive-care units, staffed with specially trained nurses and respiratory therapists, which were eventually separated into areas for newborn infants and older children. These intensive-care units were at first supervised by surgeons and anesthesiologists, but soon pediatricians took an interest in sick and premature infants. This led to the development of a new specialty, neonatology, in 1975. Surgeons who spent long hours in the operating room eventually had to share patient care, sometimes unwillingly, with this new breed of specialists.

Babies with severe intestinal abnormalities, especially those requiring the removal of long segments of bowel, would live for a few weeks when given routine intravenous fluids, but without oral nutrition they withered and died. We simply could not provide enough calories and protein for healing and growth. Older children with severe burns, inflammatory bowel disease and cancer also had severe nutritional problems. There were attempts to provide protein and calories to adult patients with intravenous amino acids, and in 1955 J. Garrot Allen, a surgeon at the University of Chicago, demonstrated equal growth in littermate puppies when fed either a normal diet by mouth or by intravenous glucose supplemented with plasma.[36] In 1968, surgeons at the Philadelphia Children's Hospital reported on a new method to provide enough calories and protein in the form of 20 percent glucose and amino acids through a catheter introduced through the external jugular vein into the superior vena cava.[37]

The ability to provide total intravenous nutrition, or hyperalimentation, revolutionized the care of critically ill infants and children. At first, the house staff mixed glucose and amino acid solutions on the wards. Stiff intravenous catheters sometimes perforated veins, or the catheter would find its way into the wrong vein or even the liver. Catheter infection, systemic sepsis, and venous thrombosis were major problems. These complications were overcome with the development of softer plastic catheters, meticulous sterile technique and localization of the catheter with X-ray control. Patients who required intravenous nutrition for long periods of time developed mysterious skin rashes, poorly healing wounds and vitamin deficiencies. These problems were traced to a lack of fatty acids, zinc and other trace elements and were overcome with intravenous lipids and packets of micronutrients and vitamins.

At first there were objections to long-term, indwelling catheters, but soon other physicians clamored to have central lines inserted in their patients for the administration of antibiotics, cancer chemotherapy and long-term steroid therapy. The catheters, inserted in the operating room under local or general anesthesia, obviated the daily pain and suffering of inserting intravenous needles into children. The call for an emergency insertion of a central line often came late in the afternoon. In the operating room, surgeons and anesthesiologists worked overtime to keep up with the demand. Soon there were nutritional specialists, central line "teams" to oversee catheter dressing changes and pharmacists who became expert at deciding on the right solution for individual patients. Surgeons became technicians who inserted the lines and ordered hyperalimentation in our own patients. A pharmacist or nutritionist would decide on the formulation. It was another technology introduced by surgeons but taken over within a few years by other specialists.

Ventilatory support and intravenous nutrition resulted in unforeseen ethical dilemmas. The introduction of these two miraculous technologies made it possible to artificially maintain life in babies who otherwise would have died of respiratory failure or malnutrition, and so the medical profession was forced to redefine death. Should the ventilator be turned off when an infant is hopelessly ill or brain damaged? Was it right not to provide intravenous nutrition to patients who would never be able to take oral nutrition? Was removal of an endotracheal tube death with dignity or euthanasia? Some physicians felt it was necessary to sustain life no matter what, and others thought parents should decide; but parents were often confused by physicians' conflicting advice.

When it first became possible to repair life-threatening birth defects, the decision to treat or not was between a physician and the parents. Often, in cases of multiple birth defects or mental retardation, the decision was not to treat. This decision-making process became more difficult as more physicians, nurses and the government became involved. As early as 1976, one author wrote that keeping hopelessly ill infants alive was medical deception and that the neonatal intensive-care unit was a medical milestone but a moral hazard.[38]

In 1982, an infant was born in Bloomington, Indiana, with Down's syndrome and a tracheo-esophageal fistula. The attending physician, together with the parents, decided that the most humane treatment was to let the infant die. State authorities used every legal means to force the family to have the patient treated, but the infant died anyway.

C. Everett Koop, a pioneering pediatric surgeon, was Surgeon General of the United States at the time; he disagreed with allowing the child to die. Soon afterward Congress added a "Baby Doe" amendment to child abuse legislation that essentially forced physicians and parents to treat deformed infants. As a consequence, federal agents descended on hospitals at the slightest suspicion of infant neglect. The American Academy of Pediatrics sued to have the law overturned, but the issue remains unresolved.[39]

An Independent Specialty

Widening interest in pediatric surgery led to the development of special organizations, starting with the Scottish Pediatric Surgery Club and the Section on Surgery of the American Academy of Pediatrics in 1948. The British Association of Pediatric Surgeons, established in 1953, became a gathering place for surgeons from all over the world to exchange ideas and to learn new techniques. As surgeons trained in Boston and London started departments in other centers, pediatric surgery gathered momentum. There was also an amazing exchange of young surgeons. Americans traveled to Liverpool and London for fellowships, while others visited and lectured all over the world. Surgeons from Europe and Asia visited pediatric surgical centers in the United States as observers, fellows or research assistants. They came to observe the work of Gross, Swenson, Koop, Potts and others, then returned to establish pediatric surgery in their home countries.

The visitors taught as much as they learned. Perhaps the best example of the "internationalizing" of pediatric surgery is the pioneering Japanese surgeon Morio Kasai (1922–2008). Dr. Kasai graduated from medical school in 1947 and by 1953 was an associate professor of surgery at Tohoku University. Biliary atresia, a type of obstruction of the bile ducts that affected infants, was considered inoperable by most surgeons. These babies suffered jaundice, terrible itching of their skin and enlarged livers, and most died before they were a year old. Most pediatric surgeons had given up treating these sad infants; there was such a sense of hopelessness that several surgeons condemned different operations as quackery. Dr. Kasai successfully treated these infants by carefully dissecting remnants of the bile ducts in the hilum of the liver, then suturing a loop of intestine to the liver. Dr. Kasai was a fellow in pediatric surgery with Dr. C. Everett Koop in 1959, but his operation was not recognized until 1968, when his startling work appeared in the *Journal of Pediatric Surgery*.[40] A few patients seemed to be cured after the Kasai operation; the symptoms were relieved in others and their lives were prolonged. Still other patients with biliary atresia eventually had liver transplants. The disease changed from being the darkest chapter in pediatric surgery to one with an optimistic outcome. Dr. Kasai received many well-deserved honors for his work, including the Ladd medal from the American Academy of Pediatrics and the Denis Browne Gold Medal from the British Association of Pediatric Surgeons.

These exchanges led to new pediatric surgical centers and pediatric surgical organizations in every country and region as well as international associations. These organizations, as well as new journals, were evidence that pediatric surgery had become an international independent discipline. In 1959, the *Revista Italiana di Chirurgia Pediatrica* was the first journal devoted to pediatric surgery. In the United States, pediatric surgeons had difficulty getting their work published in existing surgical journals. Stephen L. Gans, of Los Angeles conceived of a pediatric surgical journal, international in scope. First published in February 1966 with C. Everett Koop as editor, the new journal became an immediate success. By the end of the century, there would be more local, regional and international journals devoted to pediatric surgery.

During the second half of the twentieth century the scope of pediatric surgery changed once again. The pioneers operated on all organ systems from cleft lip to club feet. At mid-century, as interest was drawn to cardiac and abdominal surgery, most North American pediatric surgeons gave up orthopedic work, leaving spina bifida and cleft lip to specialty surgeons. In Britain and continental Europe, by contrast, many surgeons continued to be real generalists.

The transition from mainly pediatric orthopedic work to general and cardiac surgery is best illustrated by the career of William T. Mustard (1914–1987). Dr. Mustard graduated from the University of Toronto in 1937, interned at the Toronto General Hospital and had a surgical internship at the Toronto Hospital for Sick Children. He then took a fellowship in orthopedics in New York and another six months in general surgery before he was caught up in World War II. During the war, he did neurosurgery at a hospital in England and then was given command of a front-line surgical field unit that went into Normandy two days after the first landing. There he made the first attempts during wartime to salvage legs in patients who had suffered vascular injuries. After the war, he took more training in orthopedics and was certified by the American Board of Orthopedic Surgery. He also spent one month with Alfred Blalock in Baltimore observing cardiac surgery. On Dr. Mustard's return to the Toronto Children's Hospital, he did orthopedics as well as the entire spectrum of abdominal and thoracic surgery. He helped develop the first heart-lung machine in Canada and carried out the first open heart operations in Toronto. He became Chief of Cardiovascular Surgery in 1957.

Dr. Mustard's name is attached to two operations; one is a transfer of the iliopsoas muscle for children with poliomyelitis, the other an ingenious creation of a new intra-atrial septum for "blue babies" who have transposition of the great vessels. Dr. Mustard was also one of the editors of a major textbook on pediatric surgery, published in 1962. He is remembered as one of the most versatile surgeons of the twentieth century.[41]

Some pediatric surgeons trained during the 1950s and '60s successfully performed general, cardiac and urologic surgery; most, however, found it difficult to do everything and gave up cardiac work. The scope of pediatric surgery changed once again when a few pediatric surgeons developed techniques to treat congenital abnormalities in the fetus. A tremendous amount of research exists on fetal surgery, but clinical work in this area is still confined to a few centers. Other pediatric surgeons took on kidney and liver transplantation, and still others did groundbreaking research in basic science.

General surgeons who treated adult patients were concerned about the splintering off of pediatric surgery, but the specialty surgeons were absolutely enraged when these new upstart surgeons invaded their territory. Urologists were especially upset when pediatric surgeons removed kidney tumors, operated on hypospadius and reimplanted ureters. The ear, nose and throat doctors who from the end of World War II had taken over all the tonsil and adenoid work were unwilling to give up endoscopy. The question of who removed foreign bodies from the bronchi or esophagus usually depended on who had the most training and could garner referrals. The advent of improved, flexible endoscopes allowed gastroenterologists and lung specialists to peer down the airways or esophagus.

When it became clear the adult subspecialists could not compete with pediatric surgeons, specialties created fellowships in pediatric urology, ENT, orthopedics, plastic and cardiac surgery. The result was improved care for children in all these specialties, and by the end of the century pediatric surgery in many places was almost limited to the abdomen and non-cardiac work in the chest. The ENT surgeons had transformed themselves into "head and neck" surgeons and looked longingly at cervical cysts and sinuses and even the thyroid gland. Others subspecialized in otology and developed cochlear implants for deaf children. Pediatric orthopedic surgeons took new and better techniques for straightening the spine and limb sparing operations for malignant bone and soft-tissue tumors. The Ilizarov technique, a Russian innovation for external fixation, opened up new opportunities for limb lengthening and better care for fractures. Plastic surgeons took on new and more complicated cranio-facial reconstructions and developed new and better techniques for cleft lip and palate repair. Pediatric neurosurgeons developed better methods for treating hydrocephalus. Enormous improvements occurred in the care of children, but the scope of general pediatric surgery was diminished. There was, however, more work to do in the abdomen and chest, partly because, by the 1980s most adult surgeons had given up even the most common pediatric operations.

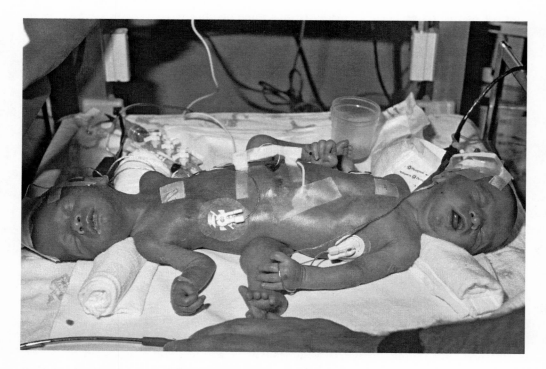

Conjoined twins represent one of the most difficult surgical and ethical problems in all of pediatric surgery. These twins were separated during a lengthy operation. The twin on the right has survived for more than 30 years. The weaker twin on the left died three years after surgery with congenital heart disease.

Advancements in Technology

The pioneer pediatric surgeons had to be first-rate clinicians because pediatric diseases were diagnosed by the parents' history, observation, palpation, listening with the stethoscope and plain X-rays. Surgeons often positioned infants and directed the technicians for special X-rays of the esophagus and imperforate anus. We then had to learn how to interpret exotic cardiac catheterizations, angiocardiography, ultrasounds, CT scans and magnetic resonance. "Old-timers" thought clinical examination was all that was necessary and grumbled about the cost and increased radiation associated with the new tests.

This author became an instant convert to ultrasound when a radiologist pointed out seven stones in a gallbladder. I scoffed at his diagnosis, but after counting seven stones in the removed specimen I humbly apologized. Before long, we were seeing patients whose diagnosis was made by prenatal ultrasonography before they were born, when the new techniques unearthed lesions we didn't know existed. There was a mini-epidemic of gastroesophageal reflux in vomiting babies that required a new operation, and the new techniques demonstrated lesions such as cysts of the bile ducts that had never been suspected. As CT scans became routine in patients with cancer, more metastases were found and operated on. In a way, the new means of making a diagnosis took some of the challenge from surgery.

There was once a saying "the bigger the incision, the bigger the surgeon." This was nonsense but accepted as gospel by young surgeons in the days when it was necessary to really open up the patient to expose the pathology. A few surgeons, like Dr. Orvar Swenson, carefully placed a small incision directly over the pathology. An example was his small flank incision for the removal of a spleen. His patients had less pain and recovered rapidly. For years, surgeons in Germany and France performed what become known as "keyhole," Band-Aid, or laparoscopic surgery. The Europeans peered inside the abdominal cavity with lighted telescopes attached to cameras for diagnosis and for removal of the appendix and ever more complex gynecologic operations. Dr. Stephen Gans introduced new endoscopic techniques and diagnostic laparoscopy to pediatric surgeons in the United States in the early 1970s, but at first there was little interest in diagnostic laparoscopy.[42] In the United States, the profession was outraged when a few adult surgeons commenced removing the gallbladder through three or four one-centimeter incisions. It was regarded as a publicity stunt and reviled because there was insufficient anatomical exposure. There were reports of injuries to the bile ducts, difficulty in the control of bleeding and tissue injury due to the injudicious use of the electrocautery. Once these problems were overcome, the advantages of less postoperative pain and more rapid recovery became obvious. Patients loved not having a long incision.

Like many other older surgeons, I scoffed at the new technique but became a believer when my colleagues insisted that I take the "pig" course to learn laparoscopic surgery. The anatomical exposure with the laparoscope was perfect, and with very little change in technique, the surgery was easy. Within a few years even the most complex abdominal and thoracic operations were performed with minimally invasive techniques. Discussions were no longer about survival rates but about comparing the need for pain medication and the time from surgery to discharge between traditional and minimally invasive techniques. There was also increasing concern about the cost, but the initial expense was balanced by the patient's earlier discharge from the hospital. More and more operations could be done on an outpatient basis.

In the latest advance in minimally invasive surgery, robots may do the actual dissecting, cutting and stitching while the "surgeon" sits at a computer manipulating levers and knobs while watching a television-like screen that demonstrates the patient's anatomy. The announcement of the World Robotic Symposium for June 2011 described all phases of robotic surgery, including operations on the kidney, ureters and adrenal gland.

Pediatric surgery had become kinder and gentler as a result of these techniques and better methods of pain control. This increased concern for gentle care of the pediatric surgical patient may also be the result of the increasing numbers of women who have joined the profession.

By the end of the twentieth century, pediatric surgery had made great strides in developing countries. Chinese pediatric surgeons developed training programs and rapidly adopted new technology such as organ transplantation and laparoscopy. The Chinese had considerable experience with biliary anomalies and contributed new methods to the treatment of choledochal duct cysts. Opportunities for training at institutions such as the 750-bed Beijing Children's Hospital attracted trainees from other countries. In the year 2000, Dr. Jin-zhe Zhang was awarded the Denis Browne Gold Medal for his efforts to improve the care of children in China. The workload and academic output of surgeons in India, as well as the rising survival rate of children with birth defects, indicate the "coming of age" of pediatric surgeons in India. The work of these surgeons is a worthy tribute to the *Sushruta Samhita* and the beginnings of children's surgery, centuries ago.[43] Cuba is an excellent example of a small country with severe economic problems that has made a major effort to improve child care. During a visit to children's hospitals in Havana, the author saw excellent surgical care that included splendid units for cardiac surgery and transplantation. Sub-Saharan Africa, that poor dark continent, is now the only place in the world that is underserved by pediatric surgeons. This huge area, with a high incidence of pediatric trauma and tumors, has only ten trained pediatric surgeons, poor or non-existent facilities and a high birthrate.[44] In this region and elsewhere around the globe, pediatric surgeons are challenged with overcoming poverty and apathy to bring optimum care to all children.

PART II

Specific Conditions and Treatments

CHAPTER 20

Robert E. Gross (1905–1988) and Patent Ductus Arteriosus

W. Hardy Hendren, M.D.

Robert E. Gross appeared on the international stage of surgery on August 26, 1938, when he successfully ligated a patent ductus arteriosus in a seven-year-old child.[1] Gross was then age 33 years and was Chief Surgical Resident at the Boston Children's Hospital under William E. Ladd. Gross chose that time when Dr. Ladd was away on a summer vacation because he was certain Ladd would not allow him to do this daring venture. Dr. Thomas Lanman, the most senior of the surgical staff, assisted Gross. After Ladd learned of this surgical success, for the next decade interactions between mentor and pupil were cool.

Gross was well aware that a patent ductus carried risk of cardiac failure, poor growth and streptococcus viridans bacterial endocarditis, which was usually fatal in pre-antibiotic days. He practiced the surgical approach in cadavers and living, anesthetized dogs.[2] He sought advice from Dr. Paul Dudley White, celebrated cardiologist at the Massachusetts General Hospital, and Dr. John Hubbard, who was coauthor of the paper about the first case. Previously, Dr. John Strieder in Boston had operated on an adult with patent ductus complicated by bacterial endocarditis, but that patient died.[3] Gross published papers on his success in the *New England Journal of Medicine*, the *Journal of the American Medical Association* and the *American Journal of Diseases of Childhood*. At the 1939 meeting of the American Surgical Association at Hot Springs, Virginia, by invitation Gross presented the leadoff paper, "Surgical Management of the Patent Ductus Arteriosus, with Summary of Four Surgically Treated Cases," from the Children's Hospital, the Peter Bent Brigham Hospital, and Harvard Medical School.[4] Although cardiologists felt many children with a patent ductus were healthy, Maude Abbott had reported 92 patients, with death from bacterial endocarditis in 28, slow cardiac failure in 24, abrupt cardiac failure in 16, acute ductile rupture in 2 and death at an average age of 24 years. Discussion of the paper was spirited and complimentary. It included mention of a paper by John E. Munro, who in 1907 had considered the feasibility of ductus ligation but who died in 1910 at age 58, having not had a chance to ligate a ductus![5]

Lorraine Sweeney (Nicoli), Dr. Gross' first patient, is alive and well today (June 2011). We met 32 years ago and she is now age 80 years old, a wife, mother, grandmother, and

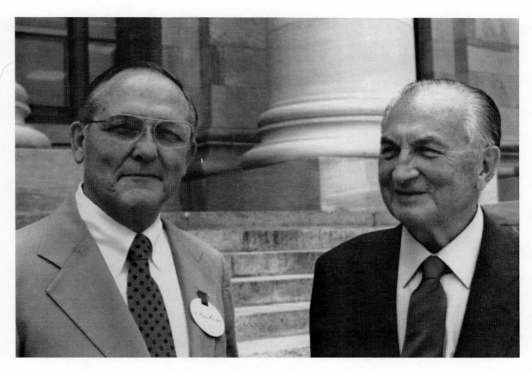

W. Hardy Hendren, left, with Robert E. Gross at the eightieth birthday celebration for Dr. Gross in 1985, when Dean Tosteson of the Harvard Medical School announced the appointment of Dr. Hendren as the Robert E. Gross Distinguished Professor of Surgery (courtesy W. Hardy Hendren, M.D.).

great-grandmother, Lorraine is living a normal and productive life. Her memory is sharp, as demonstrated in a two-hour oral history given by her to us as an important archive for Children's. She visited Dr. Gross in his retirement in Vermont and spoke at his memorial service in 1988 in Plymouth, Massachusetts. Lorraine illustrated poignantly the mission of pediatric surgery — to save a child's entire life. Lorraine had cardiomegaly, poor exercise tolerance, and failure to thrive at the time of her surgery, with predictable early demise were it not for Dr. Gross. The operative note he dictated in her case is a classic, in contrast to his usual short and terse notes for most cases. The culmination of his study of the anatomy in the autopsy room and the dog laboratory, it explains the physiology at hand by listening to and palpating the great vessels. It is reproduced, here, unabridged, with typos and misspellings, because of its historical importance.

   OPERATION RECORD
      Date: August 26, 1938
      Pre-Operative Diagnosis: Patent Ductus Arteriosis
      Post-Operative Diagnosis: "   "   "
      Operating Surgeon: Dr. Gross
      Assistants: Dr. Lanman, Dr. Tanner.
      Type of Operation: Ligation of patent ductus arteriosis
      Description of Operation:
      Anesthesia: Cyclopropane.
      Skin preparation: Iodine.

Prior to the beginning of the anesthesia, a constant intravenous was put in the right ankle vein and 10% glucose was run in slow drip during the operation, giving a total of 250cc. With the patient turned slightly towards the right, and the left arm drawn up toward the head, the skin of the chest in line of incision was infiltrated with 10 cc. of ½% novocain. A curved linear incision was now made beneath the left breast, running from the sternal margin downward beneath the breast tissue and then upward outside the beast along the anterior axillary fold. Incision was carried down through the subcutaneous tissue and the pectoralis major muscle was divided and reflected upward. Incision was now made in the third intercostal space, running from the internal mammary vessels backward to the anter-ior axillary line. The lung collapsed away in the lower portion of the chest. The third costal cartilage was now cut obliquely and the third rib displaced upward with self-retaining retrac-tion. This gave a beautiful exposure of the base of the heart, the aortic arch and superior part of the lung root. The lung was now held downward with a moist sponge. Palpating finger placed on the heart disclosed an astounding coarse and very strong thrill which was felt over the entire cardiac musculature. A finger running along the aortic arach and the thoracic aorta disclosed that there was practically no thrill over this vessel but when the finger was put on the pulmonary artery there was a thrill of extreme magnety. A longitudinal incision was now made in the parietal pleura for a length of about 5 cm., just posterior to the phrenic nerve, so as to expose the aortic arch and pulmonary artery. As the posterior flap of this pleura was now pealed backward, the recurrent laryngeal nerve was readily brought into view. This was followed along its course inferiorly and led directly to a large and patent ductus arteriosis.

This ductus was approximately ¼ inch in length and was about ⅜ inch in diameter. Its walls were readily collapsable by digital pressure. The walls seemed to me to be quite thin and more pliable than I had expected they would be. Pressure on the ductus with one finger completely removed the thirill which had previously been felt over the pulmonary artery and the heart. It was interesting to note that the ductus was like the aorta in that it had no palp-able thrill but that all of the thrill was on the pulmonary artery side of this abnormal arterial communication. One must assume, therefore, that the murmur and thrill are not caused by a rushing of blood against the orifice or walls of the ductus, but rather that they are caused by an eddying of cur-rents within the pulmonic artery or else are caused by a forcefull stream of blood directed against the pulmonic artery wall opposite to the ductus opening.

An aneurysm needle was now carefully brought around the ductus and a number 8 braided silk thread passed around the ductus and hitched to a hilar pulmonary clamp. This clamp was now drawn up tightly so as to obliterate the ductus. Just before this was done the stethoscope was placed on the heart and there was an extremely loud continuous murmur which was greatest during systole. When the stethoscope was placed on the pulmonic artery there was an almost deafening continuous sound like rushing steam, which was accentuated during systole. When the ductus was obliterated, all of these murmurs disappeared. This ligature was left on the duc-tus for a period of three minutes in order to see what effect obliteration might have on the patient's general condition. There was no cyanosis of any degree. Blood pressure taken at inter-vals showed some rise of diastolic pressure and a slight slowing of the pulse as shown on the accompanying anesthesia chart. Therefore, believing that the ductus has not stayed open as a compensary mechanism for some other cardiac defect, it was decided to ligate it permanently.

The clamp was taken off and the ductus was ligated with a single #8 braided silk circum-ambiant suture. An attempt was made to place another silk suture around the ductus but it was impossible because after the first suture had been tightened up the aorta and pulmonic artery were lying directly against one another. After this tie had been put in place it seemed as if every-thing was still in the operative field because previously there had been a continual buzz and thrill imparted to the finger through the instruments while working in the area, but now that the tie had been placed all of this buzz had completely disappeared.

Closure was now started, bringing together the separated edges of the mediastinal pleura was 4–5 "C" Deknatel silk sutures. About 5 cc. of eucupin solution were injected into the 2nd, 3rd, and 4th intercostal nerves in the posterior portion of the thorax in the hope of relieving discomfort from the operative wound. The two cut ends of the costal cartilage were now drilled and the ends brought together with #2 chromic catgut suture. The ribs were brought together with 4 interrupted sutures of #2 chromic catgut. The intercostal muscles were approximated with continuous #1 chromic catgut, and as the last of these stitches was being placed, the lung was re-expanded with positive pressure anesthesia. The pectoralis major muscle was now sutured down to the fourth rib with continuous #1 chromic catgut. The subcutaneous tissue was brought together with continuous triple 0 plain catgut and the skin approximated with continuous "C" Deknatel. A small dry sterile dressing was applied.

The patient stood the procedure exceedingly well and showed no evidence of shock. It was decided not to give a transfusion. She was warm, and the pulse was good. When returned to the ward there was a marked flushing of the right side of the face as contrasted with pallor of the left side of the face, which I assumed must be due to an irritative effect of eucupin on the left sympathetic chain, which I assume will wear off in a few weeks' time.

Dr. Gross' twelfth patient died during a party several weeks after the surgery following a massive hemorrhage. At autopsy, the ligature had cut through, causing a false aneurysm that had eroded into the adjacent esophagus or trachea. After this sad incident, Gross no longer ligated the ductus but changed to clamping, dividing and suture closure of each end of the ductus. Gross was reluctant to use the available vascular clamps (including the clamp used by Willis Potts of Chicago), for fear of crushing the sometimes fragile ductus. Instead he used four small hemostats, holding them gently closed with a rubber band encircling each clamp near the ratchet mechanism. The ductus was then transected between the two central clamps. The pulmonary site was sewn closed first, with a continuous fine silk suture in the cuff exposed by removal of the second clamp. The remaining clamp on the PA was slowly opened and observed for bleeding. A small sponge was placed over it and it was then gently retracted medially with a narrow ribbon retractor, to then concentrate on the more dangerous aortic wall closure. (A small piece of pectoral muscle was traumatized with a mallet and placed by Dr. Gross between the sutured ductus ends and covered with a flap of adjacent pleura when I worked with him in the 1950s.)

Gross used an anterior thoracic incision unless the ductus was very short or had high pressure. Then, he used a lateral thoracotomy that afforded more generous exposure. He also, in these cases applied a Potts-Smith excluding clamp on the aorta to provide the safest access for closing the aortic end of the ductus.

Gross was born in Baltimore in July 1905. His father was a piano maker. There were eight children, of whom he was seventh. His five sisters would include one physician and one college president, two brothers attended M.I.T., one worked as an engineer and the other was a college president. An academically accomplished family!

Gross discovered that he lacked vision in one eye when as a boy, he squinted at a lighthouse near Atlantic City, with first the good eye and then the other. Because he lacked good depth perception his father gave him clocks to take apart and then reassemble. This was repeated with timepieces of smaller size to hone his visual skills. None of his surgical residents in later life knew of his problem until, after retirement, he revealed his problem to a former resident who had lost an eye to melanoma. Gross urged him to continue on and learn to compensate as he did for an entire career. After retirement Gross sought consultation from Dr. Trygve Gundersen, an ophthalmology colleague at Children's. Gundersen removed the congenital cataract, giving Gross binocular vision for his remaining years. Gundersen related that to me at a Christmas party in the house of John Enders many years ago.

Robert Gross graduated from Baltimore Polytechnic High School and chose Carleton College in Minnesota to study chemistry. He was elected to Phi Beta Kappa and won a scholarship for doctoral training at the University of Wisconsin. His plans abruptly changed in his senior year when he was given Harvey Cushing's two-volume *Life of Sir William Osler*. While at Carleton, Gross met Mary Lou, a surgeon's daughter, who became his wife. As a medical student on Gross' service in 1951, I recall Mrs. Gross coming to the hospital for an emergency case and watching the surgery from the gallery. She had been their means of support during medical school and eight years of surgical training. Mrs. Gross was very nice to the wives of the surgical house staff, having herself been in that role for many years. My wife remembers her genuine interest expressed in the activities and families of the wives of the surgical residents, who were all males in those days.

Having redirected his goal toward medicine, Gross went to Harvard Medical School in 1928. Soon after arriving in Boston he found his way to the gallery of the operating room of Surgeon in Chief Harvey Cushing, whose book about Osler had catalyzed Gross' own interest in medicine. When Cushing asked who he was, Gross said he was a medical student. Cushing sternly told him to depart and return when he was a full-fledged doctor. Gross never forgot that humiliating experience. Throughout his own career he was always cordial to students and visitors (although on one occasion when a visiting surgeon shuffled a morning newspaper audibly he was summarily escorted from the gallery by the circulating nurse, who then locked the door!).

In January of 1931, when Gross was a fourth-year Harvard medical student he received a letter of recommendation from Dr. Charles F. McKhann, a professor of pediatrics, at Children's, to be sent to Dr. William Ladd, then Surgeon in Chief.

My dear Dr. Ladd,

Mr. R. E. Gross, a member of the fourth year class at the Harvard Medical School, has asked me to write you concerning his qualifications for the position of house officer in the Children's Hospital.

Mr. Gross is an interested, eager and accurate student, somewhat above average, has a pleasant personality and a good appearance. He should make a satisfactory house officer.

Very sincerely yours,

Charles F. McKhann, M.D.

Gross graduated with honors and was elected to Alpha Omega Alpha. Evidently, Dr. Gross was not selected for a surgical internship, for his first residency slot was six months (July–December 1931) in Pathology at Children's. Dr. S. Burt Wolbach was Chief of Pathology at both Children's and the Peter Bent Brigham Hospital. This was fortuitous, because Wolbach became a lifelong mentor and supporter for Gross. The next job was in surgery at Children's with Dr. Ladd from January 1932 to March 1933. Gross then returned as Chief Resident in Pathology from May 1933 to August 1934 at the Peter Bent Brigham. From November 1935 to March 1937 he had surgery with Dr. Elliot Cutler at Brigham, and he had a Peters Traveling Fellowship from March 1937 to August 1937, when Germany was on the eve of World War II. He visited Professor Ferdinand Sauerbruch in Berlin. Dr. Gross described that visit one day over lunch when I was his cardiac surgical resident in 1956: "There was a long operating room in which there were six OR tables for patients undergoing various operations by multiple assistants. Sauerbruch observed all of the proceedings, scrubbing in as he chose. Although he was world famous as a pioneer of surgery in the thorax, Sauerbruch was a facile general surgeon." Gross related that Sauerbruch's demeanor toward the patient was cold and authoritative, typical for the German professorial *Geheimrat*. One unhappy female patient was subjected to multiple pelvic examinations by medical students before being anesthetized for surgery by Herr Professor. A book about that great German surgeon describing his life and those years after Gross visited him would interest those who appreciate surgical history.[6] During his visit in Edinburgh, Scotland, Gross worked on a laboratory project regarding the vagus nerve. After his travel time, Dr. Gross spent September 1937–August 1939 as Chief Resident in Surgery at Children's and overlapping September 1938–August 1939 as Chief Resident at Brigham.

Gross was a keen observer and meticulous dissector. He performed many autopsies. In some the cause of death was a surgically repairable problem, such as the patent ductus arteriosus (PDA). Another was the double aortic arch forming a vascular ring obstructing the trachea and esophagus. The postmortem to Gross was not an onerous task but a primer for the imaginative surgeon.

"Seek and ye shall find; knock, and it will be opened unto you" (King James Bible: Matthew 7:7). Gross found more than most! His first paper in 1933 described 2 cases of Idiopathic Dilatation of the Common Bile Duct in children.[7] His 15th paper was about the first PDA.[8] There followed papers on ano-rectal malformation, carcinoma of the stomach, subdural hematoma, intussusception, aberrant pancreatic tissue, gallbladder anomalies, nerve tumors, neuroblastomas, lung abscess, myxoma of fingers, branchogenic anomalies, plasma cell myeloma, and use of vinyl ether in children.[9] Gross told his residents that an academic surgeon should "pull a new rabbit out of the hat" periodically and that meant "burning the midnight oil." He surely led by his own example throughout his career, during which he published more than 240 papers and three books.

In 1941 Ladd and Gross published a landmark book, *Abdominal Surgery of Infancy and Childhood.*[10] In addition to beautiful medical illustrations by Miss Etta Piotti, the book included a statistical portrayal of experiences at Boston Children's during the preceding 25 years. That encompassed Ladd's time at Children's, which began in 1910, plus the decade with Dr. Gross. The book's writing is very similar to Gross' subsequent writing throughout his career. Most of the case material was Ladd's work but I think Gross penned most of the book. The first copy of the book was discovered in a barn in New Hampshire several years ago and presented to me as a gift. I was astonished to open the cover and read a handwritten inscription from Dr. Gross to Dr. S. Burt Wolbach, saying that the book arose from "your admonitions, precepts and constant help." Dr. Wolbach was a mentor and avid supporter of Dr. Gross.

Dr. Wolbach had two sons, the elder died and in his memory his father often wore a carnation. Some felt that Wolbach regarded Gross as a son. Wolbach's other son, William, was long the head of the board of trustees at Children's. How the book was found in a barn remains a mystery, because all principals who might know are now deceased.

Another book accompanied the copy of the Ladd and Gross work, namely *The Surgery of the Infancy and Childhood* by Robert E. Gross, published in 1953 by W. B. Saunders.[11] Again, I was taken aback to read Dr. Gross's handwritten inscription to Wolbach, expressing "deepest thanks for all you have done in so many ways." Two pages later is a formal dedication of the book to Dr. S. Burt Wolbach. These personal notes and the dedication indicate the enormous influence that Dr. Wolbach, the pathologist, had on Dr. Gross.

We referred to Gross's one-author book as "The Green Bible." It was reprinted multiple times, including in foreign languages. In 1953 it sold for about $20. Today a good used copy fetches $400 at old book stalls at the American College of Surgeons. The book had exactly one thousand pages. To his dismay, Gross had a telephone call from a surgeon seeking advice on the management of a newborn with a sacrococcygeal teratoma. When told to "look in my book," the caller said, "There is no chapter on that subject!" Gross found the manuscript of the missing chapter had fallen off the top of a radiator and disappeared from view! Late in his career Gross published an atlas of pediatric surgical operations illustrated in part by Mr. Janis Cirulis after the death of Miss Etta Piotti.[12]

Dr. Gross made seminal contributions to the treatment of coarctation of the aorta, although the Swedish surgeon Clarence Crafoord who operated on two adults in 1944 is credited with being the first to succeed in the correction of coarctation. He published those two cases in the Swedish literature. Dr. Charles A. Hufnagel, a Brigham surgical resident dropped out of the clinical grind with pulmonary tuberculosis to spend time in Gross' lab doing experimental studies on aortic resection in dogs. Their paper on experimental aortic resection was in press for publication in the *New England Journal of Medicine*[13] simultaneously with a paper being sent by Crafoord for publication in the American literature and allegedly reviewed by Robert Gross.[14] He immediately brought in two children with coarctation for resection. The first died when the aortic clamps were opened quickly. Undaunted, Gross did a second case a few days later with success. This time, he removed the clamps very slowly to avoid an abrupt pressure change. Those two pediatric cases were added as addenda in small print to the galley proof of the dog aorta laboratory paper in press to be published in September 1945. The Crafoord paper appeared in print a month later. Priority of publication sometimes results in unpredictable events! Later, Dr. Hufnagel became professor of surgery at Georgetown University and developed a caged plastic ball for insertion in the descending aorta to treat patients with aortic regurgitation. This operation was soon replaced by open heart surgery and direct repair of the aortic valve. Dr. Hufnagel related these events to me shortly before his death at age 72 in May 1989.

In 1970 Dr. Gross was awarded the Henry Jacob Bigelow Medal of the Boston Surgical Society for contributions to the advancement of surgery. To my great surprise, Dr. Gross had called me the previous week to ask if I would project his slides. I had finished as his chief resident a decade before and was then working full-time at the Massachusetts General Hospital. The equipment included a long electrical cord, a spare bulb, a new projector, a hemostat to extract a jammed slide, a coin to release the carousel projector tray, and a spare projector for backup. Gross always arrived early to rehearse his talk and to be sure all was in order, leaving nothing to chance. He gave a superb talk on surgery for congenital heart disease. Clarence Crafoord came from Sweden to pay homage to Gross. It was a memorable black-tie evening. I relived it again three decades later when receiving the Bigelow medal in 2001 and spoke of John Hunter (1728–1793), the Father of Scientific Surgery.

Gross pioneered vascular grafting using freeze dried, radiation sterilized human aortic homographs for coarctation cases with a long segment in which the ends could not be brought together.[15] The arterial grafts, procured by surgical residents from cadavers, were used until Michael DeBakey developed Dacron grafts in 1958. My wife and I were Sunday luncheon guests of Dr. and Mrs. Edward Churchill, then Chief of Surgery at the Massachusetts General Hospital. A third guest was Dr. DeBakey, who pulled a knitted graft from his vest pocket and with a small scissor on a pocketknife showed how a side hole could be made to which to anastomose another branch onto the graft.

The importance of arterial grafting was illustrated by the use of reversed venous autografts to replace injured blood vessels during the Korean War (1950–1953). Until then, the official military protocol for an arterial segmental loss was ligation to control hemorrhage, observation for circulatory demarcation of viability, and amputation when indicated. In addition, before arterial grafting was possible the treatment for aortic aneurysms was the insertion of long lengths of silver wire into the aneurysm to prevent rupture.

Many felt that Dr. Gross should have received a Nobel Prize for introducing a practical means to replace vessels. He did receive *two* Lasker Awards, the only person to be honored twice.

In 1945 Gross reported on the surgical relief for tracheal obstruction from vascular ring, and later he with E. B. D. Neuhauser reported 40 cases of vascular ring.[16] Gross' chapter on vascular rings in his 1953 book describes these malformations with greater clarity than anywhere else in the literature.

Gross was first to describe many pediatric surgical problems, including closure of the large omphaloceles with skin only, a procedure in use until Dr. Samuel R. Schuster used silastic membranes subsequently removed in stages to close the defect.[17] He also wrote on congenital diaphragmatic hernia, annular pancreas with duodenal obstruction, thoracic diverticula that originate from the intestine, and sacrococcygeal teratomas.[18] His first involvement with intracardiac surgery was the closure of atrial septal defects by suturing a rubber well at the right atrium. When blood filled the well to a depth that equaled the atrial pressure a finger reached inside the right atrium to palpate the defect and guide the placement of sutures through the edges of the septal defect. The sutures were tied "under blood" and cut. A patch was fashioned from polyvinyl sheet material to close large defects.[19] Other techniques used at that time included plicating the atrial wall onto the edges of the ASD while palpating the defect with a finger in the atrial appendage, and cooling the patient to 90 degrees, opening the atrium and sewing the defect closed. With hypothermia, the surgeon had to move rapidly and be certain that there were no anomalous pulmonary veins entering the right atrium. This method was still in use at the Hospital for Sick Children at Great Ormond Street in London, where I worked for a summer with Mr. David Waterston in 1962. The child was placed under anesthesia in a bathtub filled with ice and cooled; the surgeon had about eight minutes to sew the defect and close the atrium without cerebral damage.

These techniques faded from use when Dr. C. Walton Lillehei in 1953, successfully closed an interventricular septal defect by supporting the patient with cross circulation from his father.[20] Before that success, two patients at the University of Minnesotta had died following closure of ventricular septal defects using hypothermia. Lillehei's patient Gregory Glidden was scheduled for open heart surgery on March 26, 1953, but the Chief of Medicine tried to derail the plan by requesting that the Director of the University Hospital intervene. Owen Wangensteen, Chief of Surgery, held fast in support of Lillehei. Gregory's father was the "pseudo pump oxygenator." Blue blood from Gregory was routed by a tube to his father's femoral vein, and then returned bright red with oxygen from his father's lungs into Gregory. Dr. Lillehei and Richard Varco closed the ventricular septal defect in 19 minutes. The child's recovery was uneventful until April 2, when asthmatic breathing appeared and antibiotics were started. Death came four days later and a postmortem study showed the VSD closure had healed, but the boy had severe pneumonia. Dr. Lillehei successfully repaired ventricular septal defects in two more children. There was great interest in the method, but Dr. Gross offered no praise, perhaps because Dr. Lillehei had been critical of his atrial well technique.

The need for cross circulation ended when Richard DeWall, working in Lillehei's laboratory invented the bubble oxygenator and inaugurated the saga of open heart surgery. Dr. Gross, who had ruled supreme for the decade of the 1940s, was overtaken by many younger surgeons in the fifties, sixties, and seventies. In no way does that detract from his being the first to disprove that the heart is not sacrosanct.

Gross frequently related a story about a visit from Dr. Helen Taussig, a cardiologist at John Hopkins, after his success with ligating a patent ductus. She suggested that the creation of an artificial ductus arteriosus would be beneficial for a blue baby with poor pulmonary artery blood flow. Gross rejected the idea. Dr. Taussig then made the same suggestion to Dr. Alfred Blalock, professor and Chief of Surgery at the Johns Hopkins Hospital, who with Vivian Thomas, a talented and dexterous laboratory technician, devised a shunt from the subclavian artery to the pulmonary artery. The procedure, known as the Blalock-Taussig shunt, made Johns Hopkins the "blue baby" capital of the world.[21] Soon Willis J. Potts described a shunt between the left pulmonary artery and the adjacent descending aorta.[22] Gross frequently described those events as proof of the greatest judgmental error of his career. It is amazing to consider subsequent progress in cardiac surgery so that today tetralogy of Fallot is repaired completely in neonates with a 97–98 percent success rate and once inoperable conditions like transposition of the great vessels are repaired by switching the aorta and pulmonary arteries in neonates with 2–3 percent mortality!

After the retirement of his teacher Dr. Ladd, Dr. Gross was appointed to be the William E. Ladd Professor of Child Surgery at Harvard Medical School and Surgeon in Chief at Children's Hospital despite great opposition of his mentor. Twenty years later, in 1967, he was made Cardiovascular Surgeon-in-Chief. William Wolbach was Chairman of the Trustees at Children's at that time. Gross retired in September 1972, after a 41-year career at Children's and moved to Brattleboro, Vermont, with his longtime companion Ms. Jean Lootz.

Gross was succeeded in 1967 as Surgeon in Chief by Dr. Judah Folkman, who headed the Department of Surgery until 1982, when he resigned in order to manage full-time the enormous research laboratory effort he organized and directed involving angiogenesis. Dr. Folkman was succeeded by Dr. W. Hardy Hendren as Chief of the Department of Surgery from 1982 to 1998. Hendren had been previously head of pediatric surgery at Massachusetts General Hospital from 1960 to 1982. The Robert E. Gross chair in surgery at Harvard Medical School was activated in 1985 to coincide with the eightieth birthday of Dr. Gross. A daylong festschrift was held in his honor. At a dinner that evening Dean Daniel Tosteson named Hendren as the first incumbent of the chair.

Gross had in his operating room a sign:

> IF AN OPERATION IS DIFFICULT,
> YOU ARE NOT DOING IT PROPERLY.

When I succeeded Dr. Judah Folkman he gave that sign to me. It hung on the wall of OR 7 until I did my last case there in August 2004. The greatest blow of my own professional life was the premature and sudden death of Dr. Folkman on January 14, 2008. He had those talents and qualities that Gross possessed and was destined to win a Nobel Prize for his great discoveries. We all mourn Dr. Folkman's departure. Dr. Moritz Ziegler of Philadelphia followed Hendren from 1998 to 2002. Dr. Robert Shamberger became Chief of Surgery after Ziegler and continues to serve. He is also the current Robert Gross Professor.

During his long tenure Gross inspired many to enter the field of pediatric surgery. I can remember clearly his entering the lecture amphitheater at the Peter Bent Brigham Hospital in a stiffly starched white coat, collar upturned, and wearing a red bow tie to give a lecture about pediatric surgery to my medical school class. Having expected previously to practice general surgery in Kansas City, I soon changed course. Curiously in the class year book of 1931 Gross had listed general surgery in Minnesota as his future plan. His first Chief Resident at Children's had been H. William Clatworthy, Jr., who established the specialty at Children's Hospital in Columbus, Ohio. Of the 25 training programs extant when Dr. Gross died, 7 were headed by surgeons he trained and 13 by a "second generation Gross trainee" (trained by one of his pupils). That remarkable academic legacy, with 20 of 25 programs reflected his continuing influence in child surgery.

He was the President of the American Pediatric Surgical Association in 1970 and President of the American Thoracic Surgical Association in 1964 and had honorary degrees from Carleton College, Louvain University in Belgium, Turin University in Italy, Sheffield University in England, and Harvard University in Boston. He received 26 medals to honor his contributions to surgery. These included: the American Surgical Association Medallion for Scientific Achievement in 1973, The Denis Browne Gold Medal of the British Association of Pediatric Surgery, the Bigelow medal, and the Sheen Award of the American Medical Association. Gross modestly attributed his success to being at the right place at the right time.

The late Robert Allen of Memphis, one of his former residents, wrote of Gross: "Genius is a gift." Dr. Gross was given that gift. Greatness, however, had to be achieved by hard work. Through his technical surgical advancements, his publications, his residency training program, the genius and greatness of Robert Gross contributed more to pediatric surgery than any other surgeon of his time."[23] Enough said!

Dr. Gross developed Alzheimer's disease in his last three years and died quietly in his sleep on October 11, 1988, at age 83 years in Plymouth, Massachusetts. Children the world over benefited, and will continue to benefit, from the legacy of this great surgeon, scholar and teacher, and friend.

Mrs. Mary Lou Gross predeceased Dr. Gross; he was survived by two daughters Edith Smith of Laguna Beach, California, and Marcie Moore, of La Jolla, California.

CHAPTER 21

Hypertrophic Pyloric Stenosis

The earliest known reports of babies suffering with what seemed to be hypertrophic pyloric stenosis appeared as early as the eighteenth century. These were infants who vomited, survived for months or even years and at autopsy were found to have a hard, cartilage-like obstruction at the outlet of their stomachs. Dr. Harold C. Mack compiled these early reports in a comprehensive history of this common disease in 1942.[1]

Dr. Mark Ravitch, a colorful Hopkins-trained surgeon and a founding member of the American Pediatric Surgical Association, published another extensive review of the history of pyloric stenosis in 1960. Dr. Ravitch republished a report by Dr. Hezekiah Beardsley, "Cases and Observations by the Medical Society of New Haven," that appeared in one of the earliest American medical journals. The date was 1788:

> A child of Mr. Joel Grannis, a respectable farmer in the town of Southington, in the first week of its infancy, was attacked with a puking or ejection of the milk, and of every other substance it received into its stomach almost instantaneously, and very little changed. The feces were small in quantity and of an ash color, which continued with little variation till its death.... The child, notwithstanding it continued to eject whatever was received into the stomach, yet seemed otherwise pretty well, and increased in stature nearly in the same proportion as is common to that state of infancy, but more lean, with a pale countenance and a loose and wrinkled skin like that of old people.... It did not appear that he was attended with nausea or sickness at his stomach, but he often complained that he was choked, and of his own accord would introduce his finger or the probing, so as to excite the heaving of the stomach and an ejection of its contents.

The child died at five years of age despite many medical consultations and a variety of medicines. Dr. Beardsley performed an autopsy, but because of the intolerable stench of the body and the impatience of the people who had gathered for the funeral he was unable to do as complete an examination as he would have liked:

> On opening the thorax, the esophagus was found greatly distended beyond its usual dimensions in such young subjects; from one end to the other of this tube, between the circular fibers which compose the middle coat were small vesicles, some of which contained a tablespoonful of a thin fluid like water, and seemed capable of holding much more. I next examined the stomach, which was unusually large, the coats were about the thickness of a hog's bladder when freshly distended with air; it contained about a pint of fluid exactly resembling that found in the vesicles before mentioned, and which I supposed to have been received just before his death. The pylorus was invested with a hard compact substance or schirrosity, which so completely obstructed the passage into the duodenum, as to admit with the greatest difficulty the finest fluid; whether this was the original disorder, or only a consequence, may perhaps be a question.[2]

This baby certainly suffered with pyloric stenosis. The child was male, and the vomiting of unchanged milk without bile began in the first week of life. The "schirrosity" of the pylorus found at autopsy exactly describes the operative findings. It is amazing that the child lived for five years.

The first definitive description of pyloric stenosis did not appear until 1888, when Harald Hirschsprung, head physician of the Queen Louise Children's Hospital in Copenhagen, described the clinical course and pathology of two babies who died with hypertrophy of the pyloric muscle. In view of the eventual surgical treatment, he made an important observation: "the mucosa showed six ledge-like parallel columnae protruding along the entire length of the canal. These ledges form a rosette which projected into the cavity."[3] This description makes clear that pyloric muscle hypertrophy caused the obstruction.

Many physicians attributed pyloric hypertrophy to spasm and treated these babies with gastric lavage, electrical stimulation, diet and drugs. There was intense resistance to any consideration of surgical treatment despite the fact that Theodore Billroth in Vienna had successfully performed a gastric resection for a carcinoma of the stomach and his student Anton Wolfler performed the first gastroenterostomy for an inoperable carcinoma that obstructed the pylorus in 1881.[4] Arguments over medical versus surgical treatment between pediatricians and surgeons occurred as least as late as the 1950s, when I was a surgical resident hungry for cases.

A New York pathologist who had performed an autopsy on a three-month-old girl with pyloric stenosis was one of the first to suggest surgical treatment with this statement: "The diagnosis being once established, surgical interference alone will be of any avail or benefit to the patient."[5]

Carl Stern, a Düsseldorf surgeon, performed the first gastroenterostomy in 1897 in a two-month-old baby who stopped breathing, eviscerated and died.[6] Within a few months, Willy Meyer of New York did the second gastroenterostomy, using a Murphy button to make the anastomosis. The button was too large and this infant also died.[7] Both of these operations failed, primarily because delay had resulted in the infants becoming severely malnourished. Unfortunately, these early deaths reinforced the opinions of those who favored conservative treatment.

According to both Dr. Mack and Dr. Ravitch, who was fluent in German, a German surgeon named Lobker performed the first successful gastroenterostomy on a ten-week-old infant in 1898.[8] At the time of Lobker's report, given to a congress of German surgeons in Berlin during April of 1900, the child was alive and well at two years of age. We should credit Lobker not only for his surgical success but also for recognizing the importance of keeping infants warm during surgery. He said, "Such children should be handled as are the prematurely born. I admit the mother to the hospital with the child. Even during the operation, the mother must lie in bed with the lower part of her body uncovered and her knees drawn up so that her lap provides an artificial brooder."

At the same congress, H. Kehr presented a paper titled "Gastroenterostomie an Einem Halbjahrigen Kinde mit Pylorusstenose." The infant described in this paper was eight weeks old when operated on in 1899 and at the time of the report was eight months old and well.

During this same period, surgeons from various centers devised operations directly on the obstructed pylorus. In 1887, Loretta of Bologna passed instruments through the stomach to divulse the pylorus in three adult patients.[9] In 1900, the Scottish surgeon James Nicoll first considered resecting the pylorus, but because of the infant's enfeebled condition modified Loretta's operation: "I opened the stomach by the incision and passed in a pair of dressing forceps, forced this with a screwing motion down through the constriction into the free intestine below, and then expanded its blades until the peritoneal coats ruptured, thus widely dilating the thickened and practically completely stenosed pylorus.... The infant made a perfect recovery from the operation."[10]

The next direct attempts to cure pyloric obstruction in adults were developed independently by Walter von Heineke in 1886 and Johann von Mikulicz-Radecki in 1887. These surgeons cut across all layers of the pylorus longitudinally and sutured the wound transversely. The operation is still known as the Heineke-Mikulicz pyloroplasty.[11] In 1902, Clinton Dent, a London surgeon, successfully applied this technique in two infants. Surprisingly, he had little difficulty in suturing the firm, hypertrophied pyloric muscle.[12] Though Dent was successful, other surgeons who attempted the Heineke-Mikulicz operation encountered peritonitis as a result of gastric spillage, infolding of the mucosa and an inability to suture the thickened pylorus. Thus far, surgeons had been applying operations that were successful in adults to infants. If they had studied the cross sections of the pylorus demonstrating the thickened muscle and infolded mucosa, they might have come to the idea of an extra-mucosal pyloromyotomy.

In 1905, James Nicoll introduced an extra-mucosal V-Y pyloroplasty to a meeting of the Glasgow Medico–Chirurgical Society. He reported only one death in six infants, the best results yet reported. He evidently didn't entirely trust the operation, because he also passed a forceps through the pylorus from an incision in the stomach wall, thus combining the Loretta operation with his pyloroplasty.[13]

The problem of treating infants with pyloric stenosis had thus far excited great interest among German, British and American surgeons. They were working under enormous handicaps because of delayed diagnosis, the problems of dealing with the delicate tissues of an infant and little understanding of fluid, electrolytes and nutritional therapy. Furthermore, this was the time of transition from Lister's antiseptic methods to modern aseptic operating conditions. It is a tribute to the safety of open drop ether and chloroform anesthesia that they encountered so few anesthetic complications.

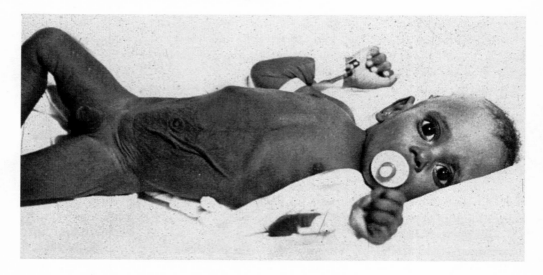

An infant with hypertrophic pyloric stenosis. The wrinkled abdominal skin and sunken eyes are evidence of severe dehydration due to vomiting and a neglected diagnosis.

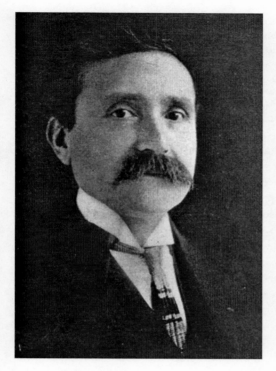

Pierre Fredet, the Paris surgeon who in 1907 first described an extra-mucosal pyloroplasty for congenital pyloric stenosis, one of the landmark operations in pediatric surgery.

On September 1, 1907, Paris surgeon Pierre Fredet performed a Heineke-Mikulicz pyloroplasty on a severely emaciated infant who had been vomiting for one month. The operation consisted of a longitudinal cut through both muscle and mucosa that was then sutured in a horizontal fashion. When his sutures cut through the mucosa, Fredet sutured the duodenal serosa to the pyloric antrum. The infant died the next day after "abundant hematemesis." A month later, a second infant with vomiting and an eight-hundred-gram weight loss was admitted to the Hôpital St. Louis-Enfants. The baby had a distended stomach, a palpable pyloric mass and scant urine, but "his face was good and he had a good cry." The attending physician, Henri Dufour, and Dr. Fredet decided to operate on the baby before he suffered further malnutrition. An intern gave chloroform and Dr. Fredet carried out a double extra-mucosal pyloroplasty. Two instructive intra-operative complications occurred. The hugely distended stomach had to be emptied with a trocar and the small intestine eviscerated because of "insufficient anesthesia," but the infant survived. From this experience Dr. Fredet learned to empty the stomach with a catheter prior to surgery and refined the anesthetic technique. A month later, Dr. Fredet operated on another infant who also survived.

On November 15, 1907, Dufour and Fredet presented their work to the Société Medicale des Hôpitaux de Paris: "We have the honor to present to you an infant, now three months of age, diagnosed with hypertrophic pyloric stenosis, upon which Monsieur P. Fredet, surgeon of the hospitals, at the age of two months performed a double submucous pyloroplasty, and who is now well." Dr. Fredet described the operation as follows:

> With the stomach emptied the pylorus is immediately recognized beneath the liver and grasped by the operator between the index finger and thumb. It gives the impression of a little tumor about the size of a cherry, and extraordinarily hard. One considers a pyloroplasty, an operation which seems a priori, the easiest and least dangerous — incision about 2 cm. long on the axis of the pylorus in the middle of the superior aspect. This longitudinal incision carries through the peritoneum and the muscularis to the exclusion of the mucosa. The bistoury cuts a white tissue, edematous and very hard, creaking under the instrument, having every appearance of certain uterine myomas. The incision cuts entirely through the sphincter to a depth of several millimeters, and the lips of the wound are gently spread. A series of sutures of linen, placed according to the method of Heineke and Mikulicz, transform a longitudinal wound into a transverse wound, a plastic procedure which manifestly enlarges the pylorus. The sutures, to the number of six or seven, take the entire thickness of the muscle mass and are tied successively to avoid their cutting through

... then to attempt to obtain a still greater enlargement of the pylorus, one attempts to repeat the same plastic procedure lower down on the anterior aspect. But the suture offers very great difficulties, and it is necessary to leave a little lozenge-like space without coverage. The threads cut as one attempts to approximate the two ends of the longitudinal incision.[14]

These two successes reflect the wisdom of an early operation and Dr. Fredet's extra-mucosal pyloromyotomy that avoided spillage of gastric contents and bleeding from the mucosa. He had learned from his earlier experience.

Pierre Fredet was born in Clermont-Ferrand, where his father was a professor of medicine. At medical school in Paris Pierre won competitive examinations to become an extern and then an intern. After a year of military service, he returned to Paris to pursue a career in surgery as an intern to Felix Terrier. Fredet learned asepsis with "inflexible rigor" and became a prosector in anatomy in 1898. His doctoral thesis was on the anatomy of and surgical approaches to the uterine artery. For 25 years he was an associate and then head of a department of surgery at the Charité and the Pitié hospitals. A true general surgeon, Dr. Fredet performed abdominal, thoracic and orthopedic surgery. He was an exacting educator who said of interns, "There are two categories of interns, the pests and the useless. Try to be only useless help." When an intern demonstrated improvement, Fredet would smile and say, "Well! Not bad progress!"[15] At a meeting of the Society of Surgery in 1926, fellow surgeon Victor Veau said of him, "In pediatric surgery Fredet is the greatest benefactor of our generation."[16]

In 1908, Fredet and Dufour published a meticulous statistical analysis of 72 reports describing the 135 operations performed for pyloric stenosis prior to December 1907.[17] The authors differentiated congenital pyloric atresia from stenosis by the asymptomatic period after birth and stressed the importance of forceful vomiting, using the term "projectile." They noted the absence of bile in the vomitus, visible gastric peristalsis and a palpable pyloric tumor. Dufour and Fredet were among the first to recommend an early operation to avoid severe malnutrition. They also analyzed gastric contents to demonstrate the elevated chloride levels that later explained the metabolic alkalosis in babies with pyloric obstruction. In 1910, Fredet and Louis Guillemot carried out a remarkable review of the world's literature on pyloric stenosis, even to finding Beardsley's 1788 report.[18] They noted the increased incidence in males, forceful vomiting, weight loss, oliguria, gastric hyperperistalsis and the pyloric tumor. They also advocated gastric lavage to rule out the presence of bile and to determine hyper-chlorhidria and hyperacidity. The authors illustrated the gross and microscopic appearance of the pyloric muscle and the infolded mucosa. They advocated reduced feedings, gastric lavage and atropine, but if there wasn't a prompt response, surgery was indicated. Fredet again reviewed the various operations, including his own extra-mucosal pyloroplasty.

In 1912, Dr. Fredet reported that the extra-mucosal pyloroplasty couldn't be done if the pyloric muscle was too large. He said, "Gastroenterostomy has the great advantage of being applicable in all cases, indistinctly." This may have been because in one case he was unable to suture the muscle horizontally and performed a gastroenterostomy. The baby died.[19] Dr. Fredet evidently was still concerned about leaving the muscle open. During the First World War Dr. Fredet served as a military surgeon, and he didn't address pyloric stenosis again until 1921, when he reported 11 cases, 9 of whom had gastroenterostomies. His report referred to Conrad Ramstedt's success with a pyloromyotomy. Though Dr. Fredet expressed confidence in his extra-mucosal pyloroplasty, he didn't think it could be done when the pyloric mass was large and he would not leave the mucosa exposed.[20] Dr. Fredet's reluctance to perform his pyloroplasty on all patients is a mystery, though his ambivalence may have stemmed from his recognition of the difficulties in suturing the thickened muscle and his reluctance to leave the mucosa exposed.

In 1927, Dr. Fredet made another major contribution to the treatment of infants with pyloric stenosis.[21] This time, he clearly preferred the simple, Ramstedt-type pyloromyotomy: "Hypertrophic stenosis is easily curable by a simple operation. In the section of the sphincter muscle, or longitudinal extramucosal pyloromyotomy." Dr. Fredet had abandoned horizontal suturing of the muscle and left the mucosa exposed. In this paper he points out, possibly for the first time in the surgical literature, how to avoid perforation of the duodenal mucosa while at the same time sectioning all the muscular fibers. He illustrated the protrusion of the pyloric muscle beneath the duodenal mucosa and acknowledged the inevitability of death following an unrecognized duodenal perforation. He used subcutaneous fluids and preoperative gastric lavage and emphasized the importance of keeping the infant warm during surgery. Though many surgeons used a local anesthetic, Fredet preferred chloroform in "infinite doses" while incising the skin, replacing the stomach within the abdomen and closing the incision. The anesthetic was "suspended" at other times. After surgery, the infant was placed in a warm chamber and given more subcutaneous saline injections; oral glucose was started two hours after surgery.

In this series of 25 pyloromyotomies, one baby with extreme cachexia died immediately after surgery. Another died with an intercurrent infection at eight days. In his last papers on pyloric stenosis, Dr. Fredet reported that his two original patients had normal gastrointestinal function and normal radiographs. He also showed slides demonstrating how the pyloric muscle returned to normal following pyloromyotomy.[22]

In 1908, without knowing of Fredet's work, Wilhelm Weber of Dresden did an extra-mucosal pyloroplasty in two babies, both of whom survived. He reported his work in 1910.[23] The surgeons thus far who had been zealously working to find a cure for hypertrophic pyloric stenosis finally understood that section of the muscle was sufficient to overcome the obstruction. They were, however, reluctant to leave the mucosa uncovered. After all, approximation of the sero-muscular layers was and still is a tenet of gastrointestinal surgery. Then came one of those truly historic moments in surgery. In 1911,

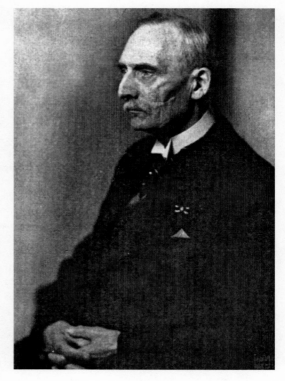

Conrad Ramstedt of Münster, Germany, who modified the extra-mucosal pyloroplasty. The Ramstedt pyloromyotomy is still performed with the same technique as first performed in 1911. No other operation has withstood the test of time for one hundred years.

Conrad Ramstedt of Munster performed the operation that bears his name and remains the standard operation for hypertrophic pyloric stenosis after one hundred years.[24]

The son of a physician, Conrad Ramstedt was born on February 1, 1867. He was educated in Heidelberg, Berlin and Halle, where he was an assistant to Professor Dr. von Bramam in the surgical clinic. Ramstedt worked as a military surgeon in Münster and, after serving in the German army during World War I, became Chief Surgeon in the Raphael Clinic in that same city.[25] When Dr. Mark Ravitch requested a photograph of Professor Ramstedt for his 1960 article, Ramstedt himself sent the photo. At the time, he was a stern-looking gentleman with a scarred face and a generous mustache.[28] Here are his descriptions of his first two operations for hypertrophic pyloric stenosis. Note that he attributes the pyloroplasty to Weber, because at that time he was unaware of Fredet's work:

> When in September 1911 ... I was first confronted with an operation for pyloric stenosis, I decided to perform the partial pyloroplasty according to Weber. During the operation I noticed, after section of the firmly contracted, almost bloodless and hypertrophied muscular ring, that the wound edges gaped markedly; I had the impression that the stenosis was already overcome. Nevertheless, I sutured the edges transversely in order to complete the Weber pyloroplasty. The tension of the wound edges was, however, very great and the sutures cut through so that the union of the wound edges in the opposite direction was incomplete. I therefore covered the sutured area with a tag of omentum for protection.
>
> The child is cured. Today, about one year after the operation, he is developed as well as any child of his age.
>
> The convalescence, however, was not without concern and was quite protracted. During the first eight days, vomiting continued at times, despite feedings of minimal amounts of breast milk. One gained the impression that the stenosis had not entirely been overcome and that the mucosa, perhaps as a result of the transverse closure, was folded in the pylorus, causing additional obstruction. At this time I decided not to carry out the transverse closure of the incised muscle in the next case, but merely to leave the incision gaping and unsutured.
>
> Based on these considerations I operated on a second young boy.... June eighteenth of this year in the manner I had planned. The result was a complete cure; the child never vomited again and under careful dietary management made a rapid recovery.
>
> Several objections might be raised against this operation. First of all, that the mucosa, uncovered by muscle and serosa, might become gangrenous. I believe that this need not be feared because the exposed area of mucosa is very small, ½ millimeters wide; nutritional disturbances are therefore not to be feared. Dufour and Fredet, who in 1908 recommended pyloroplasty without opening the mucous membrane, in one case had to leave a portion of the mucosa uncovered because the tension on the transverse suture was so great; they noted no ill effects. In order to be safe [as I did in my first transverse closure] one may cover the cleft with a tag of omentum. This brings up the question: Cannot the edges reunite, giving rise to recurrences? I believe I can answer that in the negative. When the circular muscle is cut down to the mucosa it gapes to such an extent that reunion of the separated muscle fibers [except by connective tissue] seems unlikely for a long period of time.[27]

Professor Ramstedt continued to write about pyloric stenosis, pleading for earlier operations, even suggesting exploratory laparotomy when the diagnosis was in doubt. In 1939, he refers to the "USA, where my operation is better known than in Germany herself."[28]

Either because of slow communications in those days or more likely because American surgeons didn't know French, news of the Fredet operation never seemed to reach surgeons in the United States. In 1911, Arthur Dean Bevan, Chief of Surgery at the Rush Medical School in Chicago and a founding member of the American College of Surgeons, reported four gastroenterostomies with three survivors. "The children I have operated upon have developed in every way as healthy normal children. I pray you to give these poor little chaps, who are born with this defective plumbing, the benefit of a good job of plumbing done early under the best aseptic and operative technique."[29] Dean Lewis, who left Chicago to become professor of surgery at Johns Hopkins, was also a proponent of gastroenterostomy: "Gastroenterostomy is well stood by infants if performed rapidly and without much trauma. We have had five cases with no deaths. In all cases the children have developed normally."[30]

In 1914, H. M. Richter, an assistant professor of surgery at Northwestern University, reported on 22 operations for pyloric stenosis with three operative deaths.[31] This was the largest series of operations for pyloric stenosis in North America and one of the world's best survival rates. In 19 patients he had performed a posterior gastroenterostomy with two deaths. In two babies he did a submucous pyloroplasty, and in one he divulsed the pylorus. Dr. Richter's paper marks the end of enthusiasm for gastroenterostomy. Though surgeons at the time claimed there were no sequelae, in later years it became evident that jejunal ulcer with bleeding often followed gastroenterostomy.

In 1914 W. A. Downes introduced the Ramstedt operation to the Babies' Hospital in New York, and by 1920 165 operations had been performed, with a 17.1 percent mortality rate. In infants operated on within four weeks of the onset of symptoms, mortality was less than 8 percent.[32] Downe's numerous publications and the fact that many American doctors took postgraduate courses in Germany prior to the First World War led to the rapid acceptance of the Ramstedt operation in the United States.

In 1936, William E. Ladd reported on 620 cases; in his most recent 160 patients, there were no deaths. Dr. Ladd repeated the cardinal signs of hypertrophic pyloric stenosis and said that X-rays were neither necessary nor desirable.[33] Over the next 20 years, centers devoted to the care of children continued to report mortality rates of less than 1 percent. The only deaths were in premature infants.[36, 37] These amazing results were obtained prior to an understanding of fluid and electrolyte abnormalities, and at a time when open drop ether and novocaine injected locally were the anesthetics of choice.

We are indebted to those gifted clinicians, such as Hirschsprung, Fredet, Ramstedt, Downes and Ladd, who demonstrated that superior results could be obtained by surgeons who took a particular interest in children.

Today, diagnosis is often made by ultrasonography within a day or two of the onset of symptoms and surgery is performed by video-assisted laparoscopy. The essential step in the procedure remains the extra-mucosal separation of the pyloric muscle described over a hundred years ago. I would hope that pediatric surgeons continue to take students on rounds to see the peristaltic waves marching across the abdomen from left to right and to see the expression of joyous discovery when the student first palpates the pyloric "olive."

CHAPTER 22

Ano-Rectal Anomalies

EDWARD DOOLIN, M.D.

A closed, or imperforate, anus is an easily observed birth defect, well known to ancient physicians. Anomalies of the anus, like those of the genitalia and face, aroused fear and shame. Alois F. Scharli, professor of pediatric surgery in Lucerne, Switzerland, captured these emotions in his excellent history of imperforate anus. In a quote from an Egyptian papyrus dated 1600 B.C.E., a mother prayed to the evil daughter of Osiris "not to attack the anus of her child, since even the gods are seized by loathing by this." Scharli also used the following quotation from a stone slab in the library of King Assurbanipal of Nineveh (650 B.C.E.): "When a woman bears a child whose anus is closed, then the whole world will suffer."[1]

Anomalies of the anus, with its complex function and contribution to health, remained the subject of myth, lore and obsession for many years.[2] It was not only the superstitious and ignorant who held these ideas, so strange to us today. Cotton Mather, a prominent seventeenth-century Puritan and Harvard graduate, believed witches and demons caused disease. Mather was involved with the Salem witch trials and suspected witchcraft when his own son was born with an imperforate anus: "Witchcraft and its mysteries called for investigation of deaths related to suspected conjuring by a witch. In these incidences, surgeons were enjoined by authoritative governing bodies to look for evidence of witchcraft in the bodies examined. Cotton Mather suspected witchcraft on noting the findings in the autopsy of his son. The child died at four days of age and had an imperforate anus."[3]

No systematic approach existed for cataloging congenital anomalies, which were seen as inexplicable and unmanageable, until the nineteenth century. Even then, speculation about the etiology of congenital defects focused more on the mother than on intrinsic errors of embryogenesis. The following quotation sums up the prevailing attitude in earlier times: "Might not the result of power acting upon the fetus in utero through the imagination or feelings of the mother be the cause of malformation?"[4]

In the seventh century, Paul of Aegina opened the occluding membrane of an imperforate anus with a scalpel and then irrigated the wound with wine. Other Greek and Arab surgeons recommended puncturing the imperforate anus with a finger or scalpel. This treatment was satisfactory when the anus was covered with a thin membrane, but too often the rectum ended well above the skin. Early attempts to cut through the skin and tissue to reach the blind-ending rectum usually ended in death. If the child lived, the raw wound was kept open until it healed with scar tissue. When the obstruction could not be relieved, the infant's abdomen became greatly distended and the child vomited and died within a few days. The wide variability in these lesions must have confounded ancient surgeons.

During the Middle Ages, there were more efforts to treat a "closed anus" by incision and dilatations. Male infants sometimes had a minute opening on the perineum with a tract that led to the rectum. The end of the tract can be identified when a small spot of green meconium appears under the skin. This could have been the type of lesion that Johann Scultetus treated in 1640. The parents refused an operation, so Scultetus gradually dilated the tract with gentian roots. Scultetus had learned the technique from a midwife who first incised the anus, then inserted a gentian root that absorbed moisture and swelled, gradually dilating the anus.[5]

In boys, the rectum most often ends well above the skin and is connected with the urinary tract. Medical writings from the Middle Ages include reports of male infants who expelled feces and gas in their urine. Some of these patients lived for several months before succumbing to urinary tract infections.[6] Postmortem dissections gradually revealed the complexities of these lesions, but there were still vain attempts to treat babies with imperforate anus and "high" lesions with blind thrusts of a knife or trocar. These efforts often damaged the bladder or peritoneum. Rarely the incision reached the blind rectal pouch releasing meconium, but death was the usual result.

The early difficulties of treating these infants were documented in Nuremberg in 1718, as shown by the following quote:

> Children are sometimes born with a grown-together or closed bottom, which people then usually notice when no filth passes from the children in the first few days, and those children are called atreti; in some, the bottom is only closed by the skin, in others by flesh. In such children it is necessary to make an opening, in order that the filth can pass from the body, otherwise they have mighty colics in the body, spasms, vomiting and finally must die.
>
> When the bottom is covered only by thin stuff, one probes this either with a large lancet or with a two-edged scalpel up into the bowel-cavity. When the incision has been accomplished, one inserts a large pack bound to a strong cord into the bottom, so that it may not grow back together.
>
> "When a thick stuff is present, one should seek signs of a cavity of the bowel and mark the spot with ink, then at the designated place make a fingers-breadth-long incision and feel with a finger for the bowel cavity. When the surgeon at last enters the bowel cavity, he should then cut through whatever further tissue is necessary and attempt to enlarge the bottom as has been instructed above.[7]

In girls, the rectum usually connects with the lower portion of the vagina, so a physician could determine the location of the rectum by probing: "Mr. Mantal operated in September 1786 on a female child with imperforate anus. A small opening existed between the rectum and vagina. In the spring of 1788, he had to repeat the operation in consequence of the closure of the artificial anus. Another surgeon previously performed the operation for the second time."[8] This case illustrates the problem of scar and stricture as a result of leaving a raw area, uncovered by epithelium, between the rectal mucosa and the perineal skin.

During the eighteenth century and for some time afterward, lesions that were too high to reach from the perineum were often regarded as untreatable. Alexis Littré, a French anatomist and surgeon who had studied in Mount Pilliar and Paris, was present at an anatomy demonstration of an infant who had died with an imperforate anus in 1710. Littré proposed opening the abdomen and bringing the colon to the exterior as an "artificial anus" for babies with ano-rectal atresia: "Unfortunately, in the case where the operation is most needed, those in which the rectal pouch is furthest from the skin, the operation is not always practicable; and in other cases, adhesions of the rectum, the bladder or vagina may be an insuperable obstacle. In cases of failure to establish a new anus in the anal region, colostomy should be performed at once."[9] By 1776 there were 29 published cases of colostomy, 21 for imperforate anus. Only four of the patients survived.[10]

Eighteenth- and nineteenth-century physicians and surgeons who cared for these patients struggled with the operations and postoperative care. Surviving patients were committed to multiple perineal dilatations and chronic difficult wounds. Death often occurred through sepsis. Those with an artificial anus had difficulties with hygiene. Several physicians at the time felt that technology would improve and that these children could lead meaningful lives. However, as the nineteenth century began most concluded that all but the simplest anoplasties resulted in painful, difficult and highly morbid conditions. A French surgeon named Martin in Lyon presented another option to the Société de Santé de Lyons. He proposed that an anterior incision be made in the left lower quadrant and through a small incision in the colon one could pass a probe distally to make the perineal exploration much more efficient. Martin's technique met with mixed reviews, though a fellow French surgeon, Velpeau, and others embraced it with success.

Many repairs ended fatally or with poor, painful function, making life difficult for the patient. By 1835, of all the known cases, only three children, all born with high ano-rectal agenesis, were known to be alive.[11] We can visualize the scene when the operation was carried out, prior to anesthesia and in poor light. An assistant held a screaming, struggling infant with its legs wide apart. The baby would move as the surgeon thrust his knife into the perineum, hoping to find the rectal pouch. He then blindly probed deeper until he encountered a gush of green meconium that flowed from the raw wound.

Jean-Zuidema Amussat, a Parisian who studied under Dupuytren, had no doubt seen the ill-fated results of surgery for imperforate anus. In 1835, Amussat operated on a two-day-old girl with a fistula to her upper vagina. He opened the perineum anterior to the coccyx, dissected up to the rectal pouch, divided the fistula, then mobilized the rectum and sutured it to the perineal skin. The anus, lined with endothelium, healed quickly without scar tissue and allowed for better passage of stool with fewer septic complications. The operation was a success, and the patient was well 19 years later.[12] Nonetheless, problems continued because of the difficult location of the surgery and the complications of stool passage. In addition to improving on the perineal repair of imperforate anus, Amussat published a series of articles describing an extra-peritoneal colostomy placed in the lumbar region.[13]

Despite Amussat's success, many nineteenth-century surgeons were reluctant to treat babies with imperforate anus because of the bad prognosis and miserable lives led by the survivors. W. W. Keen, a versatile and prolific surgeon from Philadelphia, tried to dispel this notion: "Some surgeons when the bowel cannot be reached through an anal incision advocated leaving the case alone, saying the child is better off dead than with a false anus in the groin, but the fact remains that individuals have grown to full maturity in comfort with such openings and have even married and lived to advanced age."[14]

Commencing in the Middle Ages, postmortem dissections and the accumulation of specimens of ano-rectal anomalies led to a greater understanding of this difficult problem. As early as 1736, A. Keith, M.D., in England grouped these patients according to sex and the relationship of the rectum to the genitourinary tract: "My classification differs from that of others in that sex and relationship of the rectum to the sexual organs are made the basis of grouping. In the male, the abnormality where the rectum opens into the urethra is made the central form round which the others are grouped; in the female, the type where the rectum opens in the vulva is made the central form."[15]

Anecdotal case reports and demonstrations of children with imperforate anus accumulated over the years. This information led to fairly comprehensive observations of the variety of anomalies. William Bodenhamer, a nineteenth-century American proctologist born in Pennsylvania in 1808, studied at the Worthington Medical College of Ohio and by mid-century was practicing in New York. In 1860, Bodenhamer published *A Practical Treatise on the Etiology, Pathology and Treatment of Congenital Malformations of the Rectum and Anus.* This 368-page masterpiece combines clinical observation and theory with an extensive review of the literature to that time. Bodenhamer classified nine types, or species, of ano-rectal anomalies according to anatomy and embryology and proposed treatment based on the severity of the lesion.[16] He treated anal stenosis and membranous atresia (species 1 and 2) with dilatation or puncture. More severe varieties, such as absence of the anus, rectal atresia with a deep anus and anal atresia with a fistula (species 3–6), were treated with perineal operations. He described the details of dissecting in the midline with reconstruction of the sphincter muscles: "...the perineal artificial anus should always he explored exactly in its mesial line of the sphincter of ani muscle..." He sutured rectal mucosa to the skin, as Amussat suggested. When the rectum was absent, Bodenhamer recommended a colostomy. His species 7 appeared to be a persistent cloaca in which the rectum, genital tract and bladder emptied into a common channel. Bodenhamer offered no treatment for this severe lesion.

As the years passed, improved instruments and anesthesia made possible much more detailed operations, such as sphincter dissection. The ability to refine the operation necessitated a more discriminating classification system in order to choose the correct procedure, whether a simple anoplasty, a more extensive perineal reconstruction or an abdominal perineal repair. Bodenhamer's classification system stood until well into the twentieth century. In the meantime, improvements in colon and rectal surgery came from a different direction.

Pediatric surgeons are indebted to the German and English surgeons who during the nineteenth century worked out techniques for excision of rectal carcinomas.[17] The first attempts to excise the rectum with a perineal approach resulted in hemorrhage and sepsis. Theodore Kocher excised the coccyx to improve exposure, a method used by Verneuil of France in babies with imperforate anus. In 1876, the prize essay of the Royal College of Surgeons on treatment of rectal cancer was won by Harrison Cripps, a demonstrator of anatomy at St. Bartholomew's Hospital. Cripps' essay was based on 53 cases of rectal carcinoma treated surgically between 1826 and 1875. The immediate mortality rate was 20 percent. Paul Kraske (1851–1930), a student of Volkman and later the Director of Surgery at Freiberg, read a paper on a posterior approach to the rectum at the Fourteenth Congress of the German Society of Surgeons in 1885. His paper was published in 1886 in the *Archives of Clinical Surgery* (German), Volume 33.[18] Kraske improved exposure of the rectum by resecting not only the coccyx but a portion of the sacrum as well. Other surgeons rapidly adopted and modified Kraske's classic approach to the mid-rectum. The procedure was abandoned for a time but then readopted to repair ano-rectal anomalies nearly one hundred years later.

According to Mark Ravitch, credit for the first combined abdomino-perineal pull-through in the United States goes to John Wheelock Elliot, a surgeon at Harvard and the Massachusetts General Hospital.[19] In his report to the 1896 meeting of the American Surgical Society, Elliot described being unable to find the rectum through the posterior Kraske incision in a two-day-old infant. Elliot then opened the abdomen and found a hugely distended colon, which he emptied with a trocar. When the bowel collapsed, he was able to push it down in front of the sacrum and suture it to the skin. The child went home on the twenty-seventh day following surgery, gaining weight with his wounds healed.

In 1897, Rudolph Matas of New Orleans presented a hundred-page paper titled "The Surgical Treatment of Congenital Ano-Rectal Imperforation Considered in Light of Modern Operative Procedures [Stromayer's suggestion: "Kraske's Operation and Its Modifications — Etc."] to the American Surgical Association. In his lengthy treatise, he reflected on all the variations, procedures and implications used to deal with imperforate anus.[20] His article is replete with procedures attempted over the years, including detailed tabulations and descriptions of complications along with the sometimes fatal outcomes. He took his extensive literature review largely from Bodenhamer. Matas reviewed the results of the Kraske operation, which allowed better visualization and mobilization of the pelvic structures. Matas used the Kraske operation and insisted on keeping the dissection in the midline to avoid damage to the sphincter muscles. He said: "The perineal-sacral anus, if properly performed, is almost certainly to be voluntarily controlled in the course of time." This optimistic prognosis would be made time and again by advocates of new operations. Matas also mentioned rectal mucosal prolapse, a complication that would plague future surgeons who extensively mobilized the rectum.

During the early part of the twentieth century, studies of embryology brought about a better understanding of the pathogenesis of ano-rectal anomalies.[21] By comparing the anatomy of a particular defect with the embryology, a surgeon could visualize the arrested development and the communications with the uro-genital tracts. More important, by predicting locations of fistulas between the rectum and bladder in boys and in the vagina in girls surgeons could devise a plan of treatment.

The next step in planning optimum treatment came from Owen H. Wangensteen, Chairman of Surgery at the University of Minnesota from 1930 until 1967. Dr. Wangensteen and his associates devised an ingenious technique for determining the level of the blind rectum.[22] The baby was held upside down so that gas could percolate to the end of the bowel, and a radio-opaque marker was placed in the anal dimple. An X-ray then demonstrated the distance between the air and the marker. It was necessary to wait until the baby was 15 to 20 hours old to give the air time to reach the rectum. Errors occurred when there was a proximal intestinal atresia or if the baby was not held upside down long enough. When the gas was within two and a half centimeters of the marker, a perineal operation was indicated.

Between 1908 and 1939, 214 patients with ano-rectal anomalies were admitted to the Boston Children's Hospital.[23] Dr. William Ladd and Dr. Robert Gross documented a 28 percent incidence of associated congenital defects in this group of patients. The most common defects were in the genitourinary tract, heart and esophagus, but anomalies turned up in almost every organ system. These associated defects contributed to the 26 percent mortality rate in these patients. In their 1941 book, Ladd and Gross advised a long midline incision, extending from the tip of the coccyx to the vagina or the scrotal raphe in boys. This incision was deepened through the sphincter muscles to reach the rectal pouch. According to Ladd and Gross, "it is impossible to be dogmatic about how much one should attempt in perineal exploration. Certainly a rectal pouch which is 1 or 2 cm. above the anal plate can be easily reached and brought down to the peri-anal skin. If the pouch is 3 cm. or more above the anal pit, the operator may experience great difficulty in mobilizing it in the tiny pelvis." They recommended a colostomy when the baby was in poor condition or when the rectal pouch was too high to reach easily.[24] They also admitted to great difficulty in closing recto-urinary fistulas in males through the perineal approach. Their main emphasis in 1941 was preservation of the baby's life; future continence was hardly mentioned. This volume by Ladd and Gross represented the end of an era in which surgeons attempted to reach a high rectal pouch through a perineal incision.

Up until 1944, surgeons had made sporadic attempts to combine a perineal or sacral operation with an abdominal incision; this approach was not widely accepted until Dr. Jonathan E. Rhoads and his associates at the University of Pennsylvania published their results with the abdomino-perineal pull-through operation.[25] Dr. Rhoads applied his experience in the treatment of rectal cancer in adults to children with high rectal atresia; he emphasized meticulous dissection in the pelvis with protection of the surrounding anatomy. Dr. Rhoads and Dr. Koop later provided a template for the organized approach to infants with anal atresia.[26] In 1948, Dr. Gross in Boston began using the abdomino-perineal pull-through operation as a primary treatment for babies with high rectal atresia. By 1953, surgeons at the Boston Children's Hospital had performed 507 operations for imperforate anus and had used the abdomino-perineal pull-through operation in 77 cases.[27]

Based on this experience, Dr. Gross issued a warning: "It is apt to be followed in a few cases by loss of urinary or rectal control, because of injury to nerves during the extensive pelvic dissection; just how frequent these complications are must be determined by future study. On the favorable side is the fact that the operation makes it possible to mobilize any blind rectum or sigmoid — regardless of its level — and has solved completely the problem of treating any existing fistulas."[28] With Dr. Gross' seal of approval, the abdomino-perineal pull-through became the standard of treatment for babies with high rectal atresia.

Willis Potts of Chicago, in his usual empathetic, philosophical manner, ended his chapter on atresia of the rectum in *The Surgeon and the Child* with the following observation: "This conclusion is inescapable: In general, atresia of the rectum is more poorly handled than any other congenital anomaly of the newborn. A properly functioning rectum is an unappreciated gift of greatest price. The child who is so unfortunate as to be born with an imperforate anus may be saved a lifetime of misery and social seclusion by the surgeon, who with skill, diligence and judgment performs the first operation on the malformed rectum."[29] Dr. Potts improved the perineal anoplasty for girls with a low vaginal fistula. He delayed the operation until the child was several months old and then he made two small incisions rather than one long midline cut. He dissected directly around the fistula and freed the rectum from the vagina; next, he made a small incision over the anal dimple and, without cutting the sphincter muscles, transplanted the rectum to its proper position. He advocated the Rhoads abdomino-perineal pull-through in the neonatal period for high lesions and performed a colostomy only for weak, debilitated babies. Dr. Potts was also one of the first writers to openly discuss the problems of incontinence, especially in boys. He recommended a program for toilet training to avoid accidents and ridicule by classmates. "These boys are put on such constipating diets that their stools are constantly firm. They may have accidents, but not offensive ones. From time to time just a little hard ball rolls out of their pants leg." Dr. Potts also recommended a daily enema when these boys started kindergarten and said that hopefully, they would develop bowel control by the time they were five or six years old.

For many years, considerable prejudice existed against colostomies in newborn infants with anal atresia. Most surgeons wanted to correct the defect as early as possible, and colostomies had their own complications. When performed in the adult manner by simply bringing a loop of bowel up to the skin and holding it in place with a glass rod, there was a substantial risk that loops of small intestine would herniate between the colon and the abdominal wall. Also, a colostomy did nothing to prevent urinary tract infections due to the intact recto-urinary tract fistula. Furthermore, when placed low in the abdomen, the colostomy could interfere with eventual repair. These complications were largely eliminated by placing the colostomy in the left upper quadrant of the abdomen and suturing the layers of the intestine to the abdominal wall. Complete division of the colostomy prevented spillover of stool into the urinary tract.

Despite prejudice against a temporary colostomy, there were drawbacks to complete correction of high lesions in the neonatal period. The abdomino-perineal pull-through operation was extremely difficult because the pelvis of a newborn boy is small and it is difficult to see the anatomy. The lower end of the operation was done under direct vision by blunt dissection through the center of the external sphincter. The upper end, the dissection of the rectum and the fistula, could also be done under direct vision. Unfortunately, connecting the two ends was done blindly by passing a long instrument from the perineum to the abdomen. Surgeons often dissected in a posterior direction to avoid injury to the urethra; some instructions said: "...dissect in the hollow of the sacrum." This plan led surgeons to miss the puborectalis muscle, of vital importance to continence. Finally, when the operation was carried out in the newborn period, surgeons might well overlook associated congenital anomalies, such as an esophageal atresia.

The increasing realization of less than satisfactory results after the pull-through for high lesions came out in the open when William B. Kiesewetter — a suave, distinguished, silver-haired gentleman surgeon from Pittsburgh — presented a paper to the Section on Surgery of the American Academy of Pediatrics. Dr. Kiesewetter truthfully disclosed the problems he had encountered with the abdomino-perineal pull-through performed on newborn infants.[30] Dr. Kiesewetter's paper, delivered in 1966, introduced his American audience to the work of F. Douglas Stephens, who since 1953 had advocated for a preliminary colostomy and later a sacral-perineal operation.[31]

Frank Douglas Stephens' father was a distinguished pediatric surgeon to the Melbourne Children's Hospital for 50 years. The younger Dr. Stephens trained at the Royal Melbourne and the Children's hospitals and in 1939 joined the Australian army medical service. He spent six years in the army, mostly in Africa. Dr. Stephens was operating when his hospital was struck by an artillery shell, but he went right back to operating after he was pulled from the rubble. After the war, he underwent further training at the Melbourne Children's Hospital and then at the Great Ormond Street Hospital in London with Sir Denis Browne. During Dr. Stephens' training in London, he spent a good deal of time with Martin Bodian in the pathology laboratory dissecting post-mortem specimens in order to better understand ano-rectal anomalies. Dr. Stephens later became Director of Research and a full-time surgeon to the Children's Hospital in Melbourne, where he continued his postmortem studies of infants with pelvic abnormalities. In his own words, he described his career this way:

> I was also appointed Consultant Pediatric Surgeon to the Royal Women's Hospital. I was able to work there with the pathologist. It was an absolute golden opportunity for special studies of any abnormality, because I had the opportunity to study abortuses, stillborns, and newborn babies with birth defects. That is where a tremendous amount of material came from for a study by myself, E. Durham Smith, Robert Fowler and Justin H. Kelly. While the wonderful specimens that I was able to obtain and study there and hand on to various members of my unit [sic]. All of this work was done on post-mortem studies.[32]

He continued his work after he became a visiting research fellow at the Children's Memorial Hospital in Chicago during the 1970s. Dr. Stephens was truly an international pediatric surgeon, well known throughout the world. After Australia awarded him the OBE, we referred to him as Sir Douglas. He made keen observations on the causal relationship between the in-uterine position of the fetus and pelvic anomalies.[33] On rounds, he would examine a baby with an imperforate anus and demonstrate how, in utero, the baby's foot had been jammed against his perineum, causing the defect. Dr. Stephens' first book, *Congenital Malformations of Rectum, Anus and Genitourinary Tract*, was published in 1963. In 1971, Dr. Stephens and his colleague Durham Smith published the classic *Ano-Rectal Malformations in Children*. Aside from the timeliness, several other characteristics of this landmark book are apparent. It included chapters on history, comparative anatomy and embryology, with an extensive cataloging of a variety of specimens; the authors included a broad group of investigators listing the many techniques, classifications and outcome studies performed up to that time; and finally, the personal touch — the authors' clear dedication to their subject, along with unique illustrations and artwork — all added up to an iconic publication.[34]

Attention to anatomic detail was the signature of Dr. Stephens' work. In addition to surgical dissections, he amassed a collection of neonatal specimens available due to fatal comorbidities. Using whole mount histology, in-depth detailed analysis of the pelvic anatomy and abnormal relationships of the organs added a great deal of insight into the understanding of how this disease could be approached.[35]

Dr. Stephens' most vital contribution was his realization of the importance of the puborectalis, a "sling" of muscle that normally encircled the rectum but in cases of high atresia in males hugged the urethra. A preliminary colostomy with delay of the posterior-sacral operation enabled the pelvis to grow. This allowed the surgeon to dissect the puborectalis away from the urethra under direct vision. Dr. Stephens then drew the rectum through this sling and the internal and external sphincters to the perineum. He, Durham Smith and John Huston published another book on congenital anomalies of the uro-genital tract in 1996, which was revised in 2002.

Dr. Stephens also wrestled with the problem of classification of ano-rectal anomalies in an effort to correlate the various lesions with the position of the continence muscles. In cooperation with many of his colleagues, he created a classification system focused on the level of the atresia and the presence or absence of different types of rectal fistulae.[36] This classification system allowed surgeons in various centers to compare their results. Stephens tried to explain how his system made sense as an anatomic method and how it related to classifications used in the past:

> (Wood Jones, 1904) Abnormalities of development of the proctodeal pit and membrane constitute the anal group, which is more common and more easily treated (Denis Browne, 1951) and which provides the greatest number of satisfactory surgical cures. The rectal group consists of those abnormalities in which the terminal end of the hind-gut ends at the level of the verumontanum or higher in the male, and in the female lies at a corresponding level in the pelvis or opens into the posterior wall of the vagina. These are referred to as imperforated rectum, with or without a communicating fistula to the urinary tract or vagina. It is this group of visceral deformities of the spine, sphincters and levator ani, with which this paper is concerned.

In order to standardize a system of classification, Dr. Stephens brought together an international group of pediatric surgeons at Wingspread, a retreat sponsored by the Johnson

Wax Corporation in Racine, Wisconsin.[37] The result was a highly workable classification system that differentiated between high, intermediate and low lesions in males and females and a separate group, the cloaca, in females. One of the most important contributions of this system was the intermediate group, which fell in a sort of no-man's-land between the high and low lesions. Dr. Stephens created an illustration in poster form that was invaluable in determining the proper treatment for various lesions.

The detection and treatment of associated anomalies improved care and increased the survival rate of these infants during the 1960s and '70s. There was a 41.6 percent incidence of other defects, mainly in the uro-genital tract, among 1,420 patients.[38] There was also recognition of VACTERL syndrome, an acronym for associated anomalies of vertebra, anus, cardiac, trachea, esophagus, the renal system and limbs. Defects of the sacrum and spinal cord made it much more difficult for children to become continent of feces.

The sacral pull-through did not solve all the anatomical problems. The distal, bulbous rectum, if left behind, became a reservoir for feces and caused severe constipation. There was also concern that dissecting out the distal rectum deep in the pelvis could damage the pelvic nerves. Furthermore, if the distal bowel or fistula had penetrated a portion of the levator sling, dissection could damage the muscle. Among others, Professor Fritz Rehbein of Bremen — a pioneer pediatric surgeon with a wide breadth of experience — solved this problem by dissecting out the rectal mucosa and leaving the muscle wall with its plexus of nerves.[39]

Surgeons and their patients remained dissatisfied with the available operations for high rectal atresia. Part of the problem was that no one surgeon did enough of these operations to become skillful and follow-up of patients, especially in a clinic setting, was often inadequate. There was always the vain hope that a particular operation would be the panacea. In 1982, Alberto P. Peña and Peter A. DeVries presented a "new" technique — the posterior sagittal anorectoplasty or PSARP — to the American Pediatric Surgical Association.[40] Dr. Peña had trained in general surgery and medical pediatrics in Mexico City and then went to the Boston Children's Hospital for three years' additional training in pediatric surgery. He then became Surgeon in Chief at the National Institute of Pediatrics in Mexico City. His remarkable presentation, complete with a movie, demonstrated Dr. Peña's superior technical skill and convinced many pediatric surgeons that this was the procedure of choice.

The definitive operation, preceded by a colostomy, was a variation of the century-old Kraske operation. Peña and DeVries made a midsagital incision from the sacrum to the anal dimple on the perineum. They identified the muscles with an electric nerve stimulator, then divided and retracted each muscle laterally until the rectal pouch, the fistula and the back of the vagina in the female or the urethra in the male was identified. They then divided the fistula, narrowed the dilated distal rectum, brought it to the skin and sutured the muscles over the bowel. The appeal of the operation was the ability to dissect each structure under direct vision. Dr. Peña also identified errors in original operations that caused incontinence, such as failure to center the bowel within the muscle complex, which could be corrected with the PSARP.[41] Dr. Alberto Peña tells the story of how he came to this new operation in his book *Monologues of a Pediatric Surgeon*, published by Atlas Books in June 2011, just as this book was going to press. Early in his practice, Dr. Pena was influenced by the work of Douglas Stephens, but in his own operations on a large number of patients with ano-rectal malformations he was unable in the living child to identify the puborectalis muscle that Dr. Stephens had found in cadaver dissections. Dr. Peña was not alone in this difficulty, since it was really impossible to identify specific muscles during the usual operations. He extended his incision and religiously identified sphincter muscles with an electric nerve stimulator that were different from those shown in the usual illustrations. Even more important that his developing concepts concerning anatomy, Dr. Peña kept meticulous records on his patients and worked hard to follow each and every one of his patients.

Peña and DeVries forced everyone to restudy the muscles involved in continence. Many pediatric surgeons adopted the new operation, but reports soon arose of complications including refistulization between the bowel and genitourinary tracts.[42] Dr. Peña amassed a large number of patients and continued reporting on his work after moving to the United States in 1985.[43] Despite the complications with the PSARP, any surgeon who proposed a new or different operation had to measure his results against Dr. Peña's.

The electric nerve stimulator, with the aid of magnification and bright, focused headlights, enabled surgeons to see and define the sphincter muscles with great precision, regardless of their approach. Surgeons in several centers continued to use the abdominal pull-through operation but took great pains to dissect anteriorly within the puborectalis muscle and more distal sphincter muscles.[44] The results of these operations were reportedly little different than those obtained with the PSARP.

Dr. Keith E. Georgeson, a proponent of minimally invasive surgery, introduced the laparoscopically assisted ano-rectal pull-through in 2000.[45] The operation was carried out in seven infants who had a previous colostomy and in four newborn infants. This appears to be a reversion to the abandoned abdomino-perineal pull-through, but with the laparoscope the operation was performed under direct vision, except for the "middle" part when the surgeon directed a small needle through the sphincter complex toward the lighted laparoscope. The bowel was then guided through the levator and exterior sphincter muscles that were first identified with an electric nerve stimulator. A Japanese study in 2010 comparing a small series of patients found no difference in fecal continence between patients operated on with the laparoscope and Dr. Peña's PSARP operation.[46]

It is difficult to compare results among the different operations. An individual surgeon's assessment of his own patients is often clouded with optimism. In addition, we have only recently attempted to deal with the emotional distress brought about by the birth of an infant with a defect that may cause incontinence of stool, with all the shame and distress that entails. After all, every mother likes to brag about how quickly her child became toilet-trained. Some parents may deny that their child has "accidents," yet on examination fecal soiling is visible in the child's underwear. One of the first efforts to measure fecal incontinence by clinical examination was a continence "score" from zero to three: zero being totally normal and three being continuously incontinent.[47] Unfortunately, any scoring system obtained by clinical examination is subjective; in order to compare the results of various operations on eventual continence, it was preferable to have objective criteria for ano-rectal function.

While at Johns Hopkins University in the late 1960s, Dr. Louise Schnaufer used meticulous, reproducible measurements of pressures and myo-electric evaluations to identify the functional defect in children with ano-rectal atresias. She and her colleagues felt that electromyography would help avoid mal-placement of the rectum through the perineal sphincter.[48] Other investigators used imaging studies, such as CT scans, ultrasound and MRI, to determine if the bowel was accurately placed within the sphincter complex in postoperative patients.[49] More dynamic studies, such as defacograms and manometry, were used to evaluate muscle function. These tools may not have statistical significance, but they play a key role in answering questions about an individual's deficiency.[50]

From these studies, concerns about constipation, incontinence, urinary infections and poor growth were monitored. In addition, the effect of such a handicap on the child and his family was considered and recorded in a "quality of life" score.[51] Though no number can rate an individual's life, this was an important step beyond simple survival and surgical complications. Lifestyle, impact on families and access to mainstream school and work all became important aspects of the problem.

As more surgeons adhered to the principles of surgical treatment, patients achieved a marginal improvement in function. However, despite the low surgical complication rates and more uniform approach, all children did not enjoy a normal lifestyle. As these children grew older, the insoluble shortcomings of the anal reconstruction became obvious. Defective innervation of the rectum and associated muscles caused by associated anomalies of the vertebra or sacrum could not be remedied by any operation. The majority of patients could have a voluntary bowel movement, but fecal soiling and constipation were concerns.

Clearly, more tools were needed to afford these patients a normal life. Many were challenging the decades of work up to this point and considering different operations. However, the procedures had to be complemented with adjuvant therapy to optimize the results. Dr. Durham Smith of Australia offered this insight: "My purpose has been to endeavor to select from the mass of material what we have learned that is new and productive, and what we dare not discard in the excitement of the new. We certainly need to change the bath water and put in new water, but don't let the baby slip out the plug hole."[52]

Secondary operations to improve the situation occasionally helped an individual patient. The removal of a dysfunctional, aperistaltic segment of colon sometimes improved constipation unresponsive to laxatives or enemas.[53] As early as 1952, K. L. Pickrell — a plastic surgeon — wrapped the gracilis muscle around the anus in an attempt to create an artificial sphincter with skeletal muscle.[54] The operation was successful in about half of older, highly motivated patients who felt the sensation of "fullness" and could learn to relax the muscle voluntarily or with the aid of an enema have a bowel movement.[55] In 2000, R. D. Maydoff reviewed anal sphincter replacement with muscle wraps, stimulated muscle transplants and sacral nerve stimulation. Most of this work was done in adults and may not apply to children.[56] Others have proposed artificial bowel sphincters and transanal muscle electrostimulation and have claimed some good results.[57] These "sphincters," whether of skeletal muscle or some sort of balloon, do nothing more than provide an obstruction. They don't improve sensation or motility. Other treatments, such as physiotherapy and biofeedback, have their proponents but so far have not enjoyed universal success.[58]

In the 30 years since he introduced his operation, Dr. Alberto Peña has operated on twenty-four hundred patients with ano-rectal problems; 75 percent of his patients have voluntary bowel movements without further treatment. In addition to this vast experience, Dr. Peña created an international referral center for the management of fecal incontinence and has developed a passion for the care of his patients: "The authors consider a moral obligation the management and long term follow-up of patients that receive an operation. This includes treatment for those that suffer from fecal incontinence."[59]

Dr. Peña instituted a bowel management program for incontinent children that depends not on new operations or magic remedies but on personal attention together with an ancient remedy, the enema. Dr. Peña's team of physicians, nurses and nutritionists evaluates each patient to devise a tailor-made therapy plan. The evaluation includes a contrast enema to determine the degree of motility in the child's colon. Based on this information, together with close observation, the team prescribes the type and amount of enema fluid. Their most difficult task is to overcome the parents' reluctance to embark on a program of enema therapy. The team accomplishes this with individual teaching and demonstrations until the child and his parents accept the treatment. In addition, the patient may be given a special diet or medications to slow motility of the bowel. The goal, a most worthy one, is to keep the patient completely clean 24 hours a day, so that he can function as a normal child. When the management program works — or if it appears that a patient with a poor prognosis will require lifelong management — Dr. Peña offers an operation, the Malone continent appendicostomy.[60] The patient may then self-administer a so-called ante-grade enema with greater ease than a rectal administration. This program to manage fecal incontinence has a 95 percent success rate.

The earliest writers of medical literature mentioned infants with a closed anus. There followed the observation, dissection, investigation and analysis required for surgeons to understand the problems. During the second half of the twentieth century, dissatisfaction with simple survival and a desire to restore all aspects of a patient's life drove a few doctors to constantly improve treatment. The quest to restore function remains elusive, however, as the relationship between structure and function is not obvious. This reality has given us an intriguing history of investigation, which is a metaphor for all scientific inquiry.

CHAPTER 23

Clubfoot Through the Ages

NORRIS CARROLL, M.D.

Idiopathic clubfoot is one of the most common problems in pediatric orthopedics. A true idiopathic clubfoot is characterized by a complex three-dimensional conformity of the foot. From a historical perspective it is often difficult to know if the description is of clubfoot, equinus due to poliomyelitis, or the result of cerebral palsy.

From time immemorial the fate of a child with a deformity depended on the attitude of society. When ancient man led a nomadic life, a frail child or one with a deformity could be a burden on the family in the struggle for existence and hence was unlikely to survive very long. Deformed children in ancient Sparta were "laid out" to die of exposure. In ancient Indian society, they became outcasts. An exception to this attitude is found in the Ajur-Veda of the tenth century B.C.E., where clubfoot is described and massage is recommend as treatment.[1]

In their studies of Egyptian mummies, G. Elliot Smith and Warren R. Dawson found that Pharaoh Siptah of the XIX Dynasty had a deformity they referred to as clubfoot.[2] Smith's drawing depicts a foot in extreme equinus, which was more likely the result of poliomyelitis or cerebral palsy rather than congenital clubfoot. In Greek mythology Hephaestus, the blacksmith of Olympus, had twisted feet and a stumbling gait. The work of ancient Greek artists demonstrates that he had bilateral clubfeet.

About 460 B.C.E., an Aesclepiad family on the island of Cos had a son, Hippocrates. It was he who gave Greek medicine its scientific spirit and ethical ideals. Hippocrates (circa 400 B.C.E.) described clubfoot and its treatment in the luminous work begun by him and continued over the next four centuries and eventually collected as the *Corpus Hippocraticum*. He believed the deformity was caused by mechanical pressure and advised beginning treatment as soon after birth as possible.

His treatment consisted of gentle manipulation to correct the deformity and bandages to maintain the correction. He advocated overcorrection and used special footwear to prevent a recurrence of clubfoot.[3]

The next contributor to ancient orthopedic surgery was Galen (second century C.E.), who studied muscles, nerves and blood vessels and wrote about the treatment of deformities.[4] Anthyllus (third century C.E.) recommended tenotomy in the treatment of joint contractures.[5]

The Middle Ages (fifth through fifteenth centuries) saw very little progress in surgery and the light of Hippocrates was all but extinguished. During this time medicine and surgery

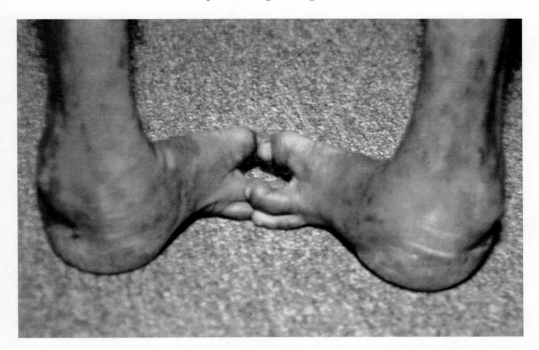

Untreated clubfeet in an adult. The photograph was taken with the knees pointed forward. The soles of his feet are pointed backward. This man was forced to tie pieces of motorbike tires to his feet in place of shoes. This severe deformity can be prevented by treatment during the newborn period or early childhood. This congenital defect was well known to ancient surgeons. Hippocrates treated clubfeet with bandaging and special shoes.

were influenced by mysticism stemming from Asia Minor and by Arabic culture that abhorred dissection. Cripples and dwarfs were subject to scorn and derision. Hunchbacks with crooked limbs and deformed feet were depicted as devils. It became fashionable to have cripples and dwarfs as court jesters, and there is some evidence to suggest that children were deliberately maimed so that they could become jesters.

About a thousand years, ago foot binding became fashionable in China. The so-called lotus blossom foot became a symbol of feminine beauty and resulted in a slow, graceful gait. In foot binding, manipulation and bandages were used to produce rather than correct deformity. This custom waned in the late nineteenth century and became illegal in the first half of the twentieth century.[6]

The birth of the great universities in the Western world in the fourteenth and fifteenth centuries marked a reawakening of medical sciences. The Renaissance (fifteenth and sixteenth centuries) brought with it the acceptance of scientific methods and anatomical studies. Leonardo da Vinci began describing human anatomy and the function of muscles.[7] Vesalius added physiology to the medical sciences.[8] And in 1575, Ambroise Paré described clubfoot and his method of treatment — manipulation, bandaging and special boots.[9] In the sixteenth century, it is reported that Dr. Haerdael of Holland treated the clubfoot of the infant Duke of Braunschweig by restraining him in an instrument and by repeated forcible manipulation of his foot with another instrument. The resulting correction greatly improved the young duke's gait.[10]

With the passage of the Poor Relief Act of 1601, derision toward the unfortunate gave way to sympathy and the crippled began to receive care. Painters began demonstrating empathy in their works. In *Le Pied-bot*, which hangs in the Louvre, José Ribera depicts a crippled Neapolitan beggar holding a paper authorizing him to beg that reads in Latin: "Give me alms for the love of God."

In 1658, Arcaeus gave us a description of clubfoot. He made a mechanical device for correction of the deformity.[11] About this same time, William Fabry described a device with a turnbuckle for gradual correction of clubfoot.[12] Isacius Minnius, a Dutch surgeon, established the principle of dividing tight tendons to correct joint contracture, and in 1685 he performed the first tenotomy for wry neck.[13]

In the eighteenth century, orthopedic surgery became established with the appearance of the first book devoted to orthopedics and the creation of the first orthopedic hospital. At age 83 in 1741, Nicolas André produced his treatise and gave us the word "orthopedic" from the Greek *orthos*, meaning "straight," and *pais*, a "child." He stressed the role of muscle imbalance in the creation of deformities. He illustrated the effect of molding and bandaging with his drawing of a crooked tree tied to a straight pole. He described clubfoot and recommended soaking the limb to soften the ligaments, followed by manipulation and splitting with wood or a small plate of iron held on by a carefully applied bandage.[14] Not quite forty years later, in 1780, Geneva physician Jean André Venel established the first orthopedic hospital in Orbe. He developed braces for clubfoot and designed a clubfoot shoe.[15]

The eighteenth century was the golden age for the bonesetter. There was no anesthesia and no antisepsis, and surgery was relegated to the barber. In England, William Cheseldon fractured his elbow when he was a boy. The fracture was set by Mr. Cowper, a bonesetter at Leicester, who wrapped the arm in rags dipped in egg whites mixed with a little flour. When they dried, the rags grew stiff, thus holding the limb in a good position. When he grew up, Cheseldon became a surgeon and anatomist and he developed an interest in clubfoot. He referred his cases to Mr. Presgrove, a professional bonesetter, who manipulated the feet to a neutral position and maintained the correction with bandages. Cheseldon modified the technique and, remembering the experience with his own arm, began using bandages in the treatment of clubfoot.

For 40 years Cheseldon used this technique with great success. Le Dran, a surgeon in Paris, described Cheseldon's technique with illustrations in his textbook *Operations in Surgery*.

In 1782, Lorenz in Frankfurt performed the first Achilles tenotomy for clubfoot. August Brückner stimulated interest in clubfoot in the German-speaking world with the publication of his monograph in 1796.[16] He deviated from Hippocrates' teaching in recommending forcible manipulation followed by corrective footwear.

The Nineteenth Century

The nineteenth century saw the gradual development of orthopedic surgery and the introduction of more surgical procedures to supplement conservative manipulation treatment. In 1798, Timothy Sheldrake, trussmaker to Westminster Hospital, published his *Essay on Club Foot*.[17] He had a good knowledge of anatomy and pathology and emphasized defective muscle action in the pathogenesis of the deformity. He designed an appliance with a spring to replace defective muscle action. Sheldrake reported considerable success, but one of his failures was the case of Lord Byron. He attributed this failure to the "unwillingness of the noble patient to submit to restraint and confinement." Sheldrake was, however, able to improve Lord Byron's gait with a "walking instrument." Lord Byron and Sir Walter Scott, two of the greatest poets of the nineteenth century, both had clubbed feet that were not cured. Sir Walter Scott reportedly was not self-conscious of his gait, but Lord Byron was very sensitive about his deformity.

Antonio Scarpa published his work on clubfoot in 1803, thereby marking a turning point in interest on the subject.[18] He felt there was a dislocation of the forefoot on a normal talus due to a derangement of the soft tissues. His manipulations were forceful, followed by the application of a complicated apparatus that we would now refer to as an orthosis.

Delpech of Montpellier began using tenotomy in the treatment of clubfoot.[19] When I visited the ancient medical school in Montpellier, I discovered that I was not the first to use nautical terms in the description of clubfoot. Delpech likened the bones of the hind foot complex to the hull of a boat.

Tenotomy was unfortunately associated with a high infection rate. To avoid infection, George Frederick Lewis Stromeyer of Hanover developed the technique of subcutaneous tendo Achillis tenotomy.[20] Stromeyer was chagrined to see people whom he felt he could help with untreated deformity on the streets of the great cities he visited. He abhorred the term "congenital" and insisted that the adjective did not imply that clubfoot was untreatable. In 1831, he first performed his new procedure on a 14-year-old schoolboy whose conservative treatment had been unsuccessful. Stromeyer's enthusiasm for the technique stimulated other surgeons to adopt his method, and two years later four hundred cases were reported. In New York in 1885, D. L. Rogers and his assistant, Lewis A. Sayre, performed the first tenotomy for clubfoot done in North America.[21]

William John Little, who was born in the East End of London in 1810, became Stromeyer's most famous patient. Little developed a deformed foot following a fever in infancy. Through the study of French literature, he learned of the French surgeon Delpech of Montpellier, who advised against Little having surgery for fear of infection. Little's study of comparative anatomy enabled him to become a member of the Royal College of Surgeons at the tender age of 22. Being unsuccessful in obtaining a position at the London Hospital, Little went to the University of Berlin. There he continued his dissections of deformed feet and concluded that there was a soft tissue problem (with muscles and tendons) that should be amenable to surgery. He therefore went to Hanover to see Stromeyer and had an operation, which was a great success. Little then stayed in Hanover to learn the technique. When he returned to Berlin, his colleagues Muller and Dieffenbach were amazed by the results. Dieffenbach learned the technique and within the year operated on 140 clubfeet. *The Nature and Treatment of Clubfoot* was the title of Little's doctoral thesis at the University of Berlin.

After receiving his doctorate, Little returned to London and set up a clubfoot practice, performing his first surgery on February 20, 1837. He divided the tendo Achillis and the tibialis posterior and flexor hallucis tendons. With the help of friends and relatives, he founded the Orthopaedic Institution in 1838, which later became the Royal Orthopaedic Hospital. Following in their father's footsteps, his sons Louis Stromeyer Little and Muirhead Little became surgeons.

In 1839, Little published his *Treatise on the Nature of Club-foot and Analogous Distortions.*[22] He described various types of clubfeet and recognized that pes cavus was a different entity. Little was determined to become a physician, but his busy surgical practice delayed his election to fellowship in the Royal College of Surgeons until he was 67 years old. He continued to study deformities and muscle action and gave us the first description of spastic diplegia, which became known as Little's disease.[23]

Tendo Achillis tenotomy was often unsuccessful in correcting a clubfoot deformity, and with the advent of the anesthesia in 1846 and Lister's antiseptic technique in 1862 surgeons became more aggressive in clubfoot surgery.[24] In 1867 Streckeisen performed the first medial release, and Phelps in 1884 added elongation of the tibialis posterior and flexor hallucis longus tendons and the division of the medial ligament to the procedure.[25]

For the more resistant forms of clubfeet, surgeons began performing operations on the bones. In 1875, Little advised Solly to remove the cuboid for a severe deformity, but the procedure was not successful.[26] The first record of the excision of the talus was by Lund in Manchester in1872, and in 1875 Davies Colley performed a wedge resection on the lateral side of the foot. In Liverpool in 1883 Pughe removed the head of the talus, and in the same year Phelps added osteotomy of the neck of the talus and a wedge resection of the calcaneus to medial release.

Plaster of Paris was first developed by J. R. Guerin in 1836, and 20 years later it came into use as a means of maintaining the correction obtained by manipulation of a clubfoot.[27] Plaster of Paris was a big advance for those opposed to radical surgical treatment of clubfoot.

Some surgeons adhered to Hippocrates' teaching that treatment should begin as soon after birth as possible, but often toward the end of the nineteenth century treatment was deliberately delayed until early childhood. Little started treatment when the child was old enough to walk; but Dieffenbach and William Adams recommended starting treatment as early as possible. The fundamental research done in the dissecting room by Little and Adams led to the theory that muscle action caused the deformity in clubfoot. Further observation and research enabled clinicians to classify clubfeet and to recognize, as separate entities, deformities due to poliomyelitis, cerebral palsy and other disorders. Scarpa and Paré, for their part, agreed with Hippocrates that the deformity was caused by mechanical pressure in utero, a theory revived by R. W. Parker and S. G. Shattock in 1884.[28] Like Tubby, they believed that early in pregnancy fetal feet are inverted and that increased pressure could lead to muscle damage and clubfoot deformity.[29] A study of human fetuses led Fritz Bessel-Hagen to the same conclusion.[30]

In Liverpool at the Robert Jones Clinic, it was found that manual correction as a daily routine was often sufficient to correct clubfoot. Manual correction and immobilization in a plaster of Paris cast or by strapping was used at the Hospital for the Ruptured and Crippled in New York. This procedure was performed once a week.

Hugh Owen Thomas, an enthusiastic manipulator of clubfeet, devised a wrench "to aid in the treatment of clubfeet of every variety."[31] He maintained that the foot became instantly more pliable after stretching and "the use of the wrench very materially shortened the period of treatment." The Thomas wrench was adopted by Grattan of Cork, Bradford of Boston and Lorenz of Vienna. Later, Lorenz used a padded pyramid as a fulcrum to "break" the deformity. In his novel *Madame Bovary*, the French writer Gustave Flaubert gives a vivid description of the attempted forceful correction of severe clubfoot and all the tragic consequences.[32] On the other side of the spectrum, surgeons like Taylor and Freiburg in the United States believed in prolonged and gradual leverage to correct the deformity.

During the twentieth century, clubfoot continued to be one of the most common congenital deformities of the musculoskeletal system. Epidemiological studies reported that the incidence of clubfoot varied from one to four per thousand live births. In some races the incidence is as low as 0.6 per thousand; in others, as high as 6.8 per thousand (Polynesia). This means that there must be a hereditary factor in the causation of clubfoot. This became obvious to me when on their third visit to my clinic in Toronto two mothers who each had a male child with a right clubfoot discovered that they were married to the same truck driver, who also had a right clubfoot. There is a higher incidence in males two to two and a half years old; 30 to 50 percent of cases have one side only involved, while the rest have bilateral involvement.[33]

Classification, Pathogenesis and Treatment of Idiopathic Clubfoot

Clubfeet can be divided into four general classes based on their cause and response to treatment:

1. Postural — benign, resolves completely with stretching and casts.
2. Idiopathic — true congenital clubfoot of variable severity.
3. Neurogenic — as seen in spina bifida.
4. Syndromic — associated with other anomalies. These feet are often quite rigid.

The following have been implicated in the pathogenesis of clubfoot: early developmental arrest of the foot, primary germ plasm defect in the talus, muscle imbalance due to a developmental neurological insufficiency, medial retraction fibrosis, mechanical factors such as intrauterine molding and oligohydramnios, and vascular insufficiency.

Throughout the twentieth century, most orthopedic surgeons agreed that treatment should be started as soon as possible after birth. At the turn of the century, forceful correction of the deformity as espoused by Hugh Owen Thomas was in vogue. R. C. Elmslie used the Thomas method in a modified form, in which he corrected the forefoot adductus and varus before correcting the equinus.[34] Denis Browne popularized the use of his splint after an initial forceful correction.[35] J. H. Kite is credited for recognizing the harmful effects of forceful manipulation that led to damage of the articular cartilage and resulting joint stiffness.[36] He recommended repeated gentle manipulations and serial plaster casts.

In a clubfoot, the soft tissues are more resistant to pressure than the bones. With this concept in mind, soft tissue procedures were developed in which the capsules and ligaments were released surgically, on the theory that the scalpel was much less damaging than the pressure of forceful manipulation on the articular cartilage of a deformed clubfoot. After it became clear that the simple elongation of the tendo Achillis was not sufficient to correct an equinovarus deformity, I. Zadek and E. Barnett released the posterior capsule of the ankle at the time of tendo Achillis lengthening.[37] A. Codivilla added elongation of the tibialis posterior, flexor digitorum longus and flexor hallucis longus at the time of tendo Achillis lengthening.[38]

I. V. Ponseti in Iowa developed his technique in the late 1940s and first published his method in 1963. He manipulated the feet weekly and applied above-knee casts. The cavus was corrected by supination of the forefoot and then the whole foot was abducted over the fulcrum of the thumb against the lateral aspect of the head of the talus. Once heel varus and forefoot supination was corrected by full abduction with maximal external rotation under the talus, attention was directed to the equinus. In most cases, subcutaneous tenotomy of the tendo Achillis was used to speed up correction of the equinus. Ponseti reported that the average cast treatment lasted two to three months, following which he used long-term abduction splinting to avoid relapse.[39]

Parallel with what was happening in Iowa and Ponseti's clinic, more aggressive surgery was practiced in many centers. In Connecticut, V. J. Turco popularized a one-stage posteromedial release through a medial incision.[40] J. Leonard Goldner at Duke University described a four-quadrant release in which the deltoid ligament was lengthened.[41] He developed this procedure on the premise that the primary deformity was internal rotation of the talus in the ankle mortise. In Washington, D.C., Douglas W. McKay developed a procedure designed to correct horizontal rotation and lateral displacement/equinus of the calcaneus.[42] He felt the talus was in neutral alignment in the ankle mortise. He found that sometimes it was necessary to do a complete release of the talocalcaneal interosseous ligament to achieve a full correction. In Milwaukee, George W. Simons developed a procedure for the treatment of clubfoot that produced an extensive circumferential release of the subtalar joint and a release of the talocalcaneal interosseous ligament.[43] Alvin Crawford in Cincinnati popularized the "Cincinnati incision," developed by Giannestras for extensive clubfoot surgery.

In Paris, Henri Bensahel was using physical therapy and taping as his initial treatment for clubfeet. For a clubfoot requiring surgery Bensahel described an à la carte approach: "Do only what is necessary to give a good correction of the foot."[44] In Montpellier, Alain Dimeglio was using continuous passive motion and splinting prior to any surgical intervention.[45] Meanwhile, north of the border in Toronto, I studied the pathoanatomy of clubfoot in embryological and fetal specimens.[46] My team and I then digitized sections of clubfeet and developed a computer graphic representation of the deformity. I described external rotation of the long axis of the body of the talus.[47] I agreed with Bensahel that each foot had slightly different pathology and thus needed slight modification of surgical technique. I also felt that all components of the deformity needed to be corrected at the time of surgery. For a severe clubfoot that required both a medial and posterior release, I used two incisions: one medial, one posterior lateral, as I felt that the tendon sheaths behind the medial malleolus were analogous to "no man's land in the hand."[48]

Unfortunately, human wounds heal by a patching-up process called repair. The losses are made good not with the original tissue but with a material that is biologically simple, cheap and handy—connective tissue scar. Over time and with longer follow-up studies, surgeons began to realize that scarring can lead to stiffness, residual and/or recurrent deformity and pain. For these reasons, the pendulum has taken a massive swing toward the Ponseti method, which many pediatric orthopedic surgeons now regard as the initial treatment of choice (surgery being reserved for the most severely deformed feet). Ponseti taught us that the treatment of clubfoot is not only a science but also an art and it is better to have some residual deformity and a mobile foot than a fully corrected stiff and painful foot. Some of the major players in the Ponseti Technique are Herzenberg, Mosca, Lehman, Pirani, Penny and Richards.[49]

CHAPTER 24

Appendicitis

STEPHEN DOLGIN, M.D.

The vermiform appendix lurked in obscurity through antiquity and the Middle Ages. Leonardo da Vinci depicted this seemingly innocent anatomic structure in 1492; it is not known to have been displayed before then.[1] Though people suffered from severe and often fatal inflammatory events emanating from the right lower quadrant, the devastating role of the appendix was not widely accepted by the medical world until the late decades of the nineteenth century. The cause of the serious inflammatory processes was thought to be from the cecum or the surrounding tissues (typhlitis or perityphlitis) or the psoas itself. How appendicitis came to be understood and how for so long the crises arising from the right lower quadrant were attributed to other causes is a story of considerable interest. Factors far removed from physiology influenced the slow advance of insight into the disease process. Isolated voices suggested that the appendix was at times responsible for this condition, but they were not influential because louder voices said otherwise. In addition, there was little incentive for understanding appendicitis prior to the introduction of general anesthesia in the mid-nineteenth century. Very little intra-abdominal surgery was possible before then.

In 1886, Reginald Heber Fitz convinced the clinical world of the appendix's essential role in causing inflammation in the right lower quadrant, often with widespread consequences. Fitz had authority as a respected pathologist and physician at the Massachusetts General Hospital and was a faculty leader and a beloved teacher at Harvard. He offered evidence with many carefully dissected cases, and his well-supported contention by then had a practical implication for physicians and patients.

A hundred and fifty years before Fitz's publication, Claudius Amyand, a London surgeon, performed the first recorded appendectomy in 1736. It was not an abdominal operation. The patient was an 11-year-old boy with a hernia and a fecal fistula exiting the wall of the scrotum. Through a scrotal incision, Amyand found the appendix, which had been perforated by a pin. He removed the appendix, fixed the hernia and cured the fistula.[2] It is not surprising that some of the earliest patients in the history of this condition were children. Nor is it surprising, given the absence of anesthesia, that this first known appendectomy was for an atypical form of appendicitis that did not require an abdominal operation.

Occasional reports attributing illness to the inflamed appendix appeared, but they did not substantially change the standard dogma that the appendix had no significant role in most cases of right lower quadrant inflammation. Parkinson in 1812 reported the death of a five-year-old boy whose autopsy revealed peritonitis. The patient's appendix contained a fecalith and was perforated distal to the obstruction.[3] In France, Louyer-Villermay in 1824 described two patients whose deaths he attributed to inflammation arising from the appendix.[4] Three years later, Melier, also in France, added six more fatal cases and attributed the condition and the outcome to inflammation arising from the appendix. These voices, however, were drowned out by the authoritative opinion setters in European medicine. The prominent French physician Dupuytren insisted that the cecum was the original site of inflammation, and his influence was overwhelming. Baron Guillaume Dupuytren (1777–1835) reigned as the Chief of Surgery at Hôtel-Dieu in Paris for more than 20 years. He lectured often and was forceful in his opinions and highly influential. He never doubted that inflammation arose from the cecum and surrounding tissues and not from the appendix. His pronouncements were generally accepted standard teaching and echoed by leading figures in European medicine.

Patients who developed peritonitis were often said to have typhlitis or perityphlitis. *Typhlo* is a Greek word for "cecum." These conditions were described and split into various forms, with detailed distinctions made between subtypes. The appendix was not generally identified as having a role in these often catastrophic processes.

It is unusual that the careful dissections of Rudolph Virchow in the mid-nineteenth century did not unearth the role of the appendix. It is possible that by the time the patients came to autopsy the appendix was in part autolyzed or highly disrupted and the chronic inflammation was widespread. Such dense uncontrolled inflammation may well have obscured the origin of the condition.[5] Virchow did not have the chance to see an appendix in the early stage of inflammation.

What was it about Reginald Heber Fitz that caused his advocacy of the appendix to be accepted quickly? Fitz had traveled to Europe after completing his studies at Harvard Medical School in 1868. He worked in the laboratories of leading figures in medicine in Vienna, Paris, and London and in Berlin under Rudolph Virchow. Fitz then returned to Boston and impressed the prominent establishment. A publication celebrating his sixty-fifth birthday described him as follows: "...his ability and attainments were at once recognized, especially by the older and powerful group of men at the Massachusetts General Hospital and the Harvard Medical School, so that in 1871 he was made microscopist to the former and at the latter Instructor in Pathological Anatomy.... He has, throughout his career, looked upon pathology and allied medical sciences as the handmaidens of clinical medicine rather than goddesses to be pursued for their own charms."[6]

Fitz took multiple leadership roles in the medical school, reflecting his ability as a teacher and clinician both as a pathologist and physician. It is noteworthy that the clinical world became convinced the appendix was the culprit and that a timely operation was appropriate for appendicitis not by a surgeon but by a respected, careful, insightful pathologist and physician.

Fitz had clarity, humor and humility. He was highly respected in the medical world, well established as an educator and clinical observer at Harvard.[7] His seminal paper, "Perforating Inflammation of the Vermiform Appendix; with Special Reference to its Early Diagnosis and Treatment," was originally presented at the first meeting of the Association of American Physicians on June 18, 1886.[8] William Osler and other medical dignitaries were present. Fitz was speaking from a central position in the burgeoning medical world of the United States.

This remarkably influential work details the contributions of others who identified the appendix as key in causing abdominal inflammation. It never suggests that the author himself is offering anything radical or exceptional. The paper is based on no fewer than 257 autopsies. The facts are recited with a matter-of-fact clarity, as if the conclusions simply flowed from the observations, making it clear that the appendix is responsible for the illness and that prompt appendectomy is necessary for a good outcome. Fitz also depicts local and widespread consequences of the disease when left to non-operative management. He describes liver abscesses, pylephlebitis, portal embolism, and diverse and widespread fistulas. His observations include commonly found foreign bodies, usually inspissated feces. For the conditions outlined in this remarkable discussion Dr. Fitz proposed the term "appendicitis."

An encomium written on the death of Reginald Heber Fitz summarized the personal traits that helped him convince the medical community of the validity of his claims. These are the words of the Philadelphian surgeon W. W. Keen: "...I need not dwell on his charming personality, his fine character, his diagnostic acumen, his painstaking, faithful examination, his sober, well considered judgment — the Man as well as the Doctor. His influence as a consultant, teacher and writer will long survive in his students and in turn in their students, his professional children and grandchildren. His name is writ large and high on the Roll of Honor of our Guild."[9]

Surgeons were quick to learn and teach appendectomy for appendicitis. The acceptance of Fitz's principles was so quick that just three years after Fitz's monumental paper the surgeon Charles McBurney in New York wrote: "The fact that inflammatory affections of the vermiform appendix give rise to a considerable number of the so-called pericaecal inflammations is now accepted in every part of the medical and surgical world, although one still reads of perityphlitis and paratyphlitis, and of intraperitoneal and extraperitoneal abscesses."

In this same presentation, McBurney described the clinical findings necessary to establish the diagnosis: "The exact locality of the greatest sensitiveness to pressure has seemed to me to be usually one of importance. And I believe that in every case the seat of greatest pain, determined by the pressure of one finger, has been very exactly between an inch and a half and two inches from the anterior spinous process on a straight line drawn from that process to the umbilicus."[10]

A particular historical event had substantial impact as well, though as a consequence of sociological rather than physiological factors. This event helped secure the role of the appendix and of the surgeon in treating appendicitis. About six months after Queen Victoria's death, Edward VII developed appendicitis just before his planned coronation. A team of illustrious physicians recognized the likelihood of appendicitis and asked the busiest surgeon in London, Sir Frederick Treves, to see the future king. Treves advocated an operation, though not an appendectomy; given the advanced state of the illness, the plan was to drain the patient's right lower quadrant abscess. Edward is alleged to have initially refused an operation because of his long-awaited coronation, saying he had to go serve his people. Treves reputedly told him, "Then, Sire, you will go as a corpse!" The coronation, scheduled for June 26, 1902, was delayed so the operation could be performed. The patient did well. Treves' fame increased and he earned part of his place in history for his bold response to a VIP. This was the most famous operation for appendicitis in history.[11]

Attention to appendicitis was dramatically enhanced when Edward VII, an older man, was afflicted by the condition that most often affects young people. Almost half (48 percent) of the patients studied by Fitz were between 20 months and 20 years of age. Only 9 percent were older than 40.[12] The presentation from which McBurney was quoted earlier reviews cases that include a ten-year-old boy and several teenagers.[13] It was not long before the medical establishment turned its focus to childhood appendicitis. In 1905, less than a decade after Fitz's paper, John Blair Deaver's text *Appendicitis* appeared in its third edition; that edition included a chapter titled "Appendicitis in Children."[14]

Deaver was a prolific and prominent surgeon in Philadelphia. He confirmed that the illness was rare in children younger than 2 years of age and most common between ages 5 and 15. He found a marked predominance of male patients, an observation also made by Fitz. Strikingly, Deaver notes that there were no deaths in the most recent 75 operations for appendicitis at the Children's Hospital of the Mary J. Drexel Home. This is a remarkable accomplishment in an era prior to the development of antibiotics and only half a century since ether was introduced as an anesthetic in Boston.

The section in Deaver's text on the history of appendicitis echoes the observation that the appendix lurked largely unappreciated until Fitz: "So many times does it appear that acute observers stumbled on the very threshold of the discovery that the original lesion in these conditions was in the appendix, that it seems scarcely credible that for less than twenty years have we had any adequate knowledge of appendicitis."[15]

Deaver, a busy surgeon writing before pediatric surgery was a recognized specialty, made the following insightful observation about childhood appendicitis: "As regards symptomatology, the main difficulties in connection with the subjective symptoms are referable to the inability of the patients to make themselves understood, or even to accurately analyze their own reactions."[16] He reviews the differential diagnosis and warns about the possibility of pneumonia masquerading as appendicitis in children. He advocates for an early appendectomy in the course of the illness.

In 1938, William E. Ladd, addressing a wide clinical audience from his specialized focus on the surgery of childhood, lamented that in recent decades it had seemed "the last word had been said for appendicitis and that the situation was well in hand about it," but that, sadly, the mortality rate from the condition was substantial in the United States. He quotes evidence that mortality from childhood appendicitis was increasing in Massachusetts. From 1926 through 1936, appendicitis was the third most common cause of death in Massachusetts after accidents and pneumonia.[17] In Dr. Ladd's department, with focused attention to pediatric surgical care, deaths from appendicitis were rare. Keen on helping clinicians make a prompt and safe intervention, Ladd reviews some epidemiology. He finds appendicitis "extremely rare" in the first year of life, infrequent in the second and then common. While confirming that the clinical history from sick children may be vague, he describes periumbical pain that migrates to the right lower quadrant. He offers a guide to the examination of the child that would seem quite familiar to a pediatric surgeon today and is worthy of quotation for the pediatric surgeon of tomorrow: "...the child's confidence must be gained before starting the examination. It often requires much patience and time to accomplish this, but it is time well spent."[18]

Ladd gives details for the physical exam and history that aid in the diagnosis. He argues against the interval appendectomy, favoring prompt operation. Only in the dehydrated child does he spend some hours for narcotics, gastric decompression and "intravenous glucose and saline solutions." He favored a right rectus incision, removing the appendix in advanced cases if it could be done safely and inserting two drains, one in the pelvis and one in the iliac fossa. It is interesting that the latter approach regarding the use of two drains was still advocated at the Children's Hospital in Boston 45 years later.[19] The source of that practice, advocated in 1983, is not mysterious. With his approach, Ladd reported a mortality rate of 3.5 percent in the most recent 632 cases, including children with severe peritonitis.

The mortality rate on that service continued to decline. In Robert Gross' first edition of the textbook *The Surgery of Infancy and Childhood* in 1953, he listed declining mortality with no deaths from 384 cases of acute, unruptured appendicitis and one death (.02 percent) in 345 cases of acute, ruptured appendicitis from July 1944 through 1950.[20] Dr. Gross emphasized the way to conduct a careful examination adapted to the frightened young patient. He also encouraged admission to the hospital for frequent observation in uncertain cases. By this time, antibiotics had become part of the armamentarium. The use of two Penrose drains remained standard; these were inched out and removed by about postoperative day six in cases of perforated appendicitis.

Today, with the cacophonous beat of drums from the imaging suites dominating the management of children who may have appendicitis, the wisdom of our clinical forefathers provides a still, quiet voice of common sense and inspiration. The path to our present understanding is not a direct consequence of accrued physiological insight. Instead, it reflects the unsteady progress of an all-too-human enterprise.

CHAPTER 25

Necrotizing Enterocolitis

Necrotizing enterocolitis was unknown until 50 years ago. The diagnosis did not appear in textbooks, and experienced clinicians were puzzled when premature infants suddenly developed abdominal distention, vomiting and sometimes bloody stools. When operating on these infants, surgeons found patchy areas of intestinal necrosis with bubbles of air in the wall of paper-thin intestine. No obvious cause existed for these findings; the disease was usually confined to the terminal ileum, but some patients had a patchy distribution through most of the bowel. In a few tragic cases, the entire intestine was necrotic. By the time an operation was performed, the patients were suffering from intestinal perforations and generalized peritonitis. Babies with similar but milder symptoms recovered with gastric drainage, intravenous fluids and antibiotics.

This puzzling, mysterious disease appeared during the 1960s and within a few years became the most common surgical emergency in newborn infants.[1] It was particularly distressing because at that time the care of neonates, especially premature infants, was improving as a result of better incubators for temperature control, antibiotics, sophisticated methods of respiratory support and what was thought to be better nutrition.

Isolated perforations of the gastrointestinal tract, especially in newborn infants attributed to stress ulcers, infection or Hirschsprung's disease, were seen during the 1950s and early '60s.[2] These perforations caused a striking X-ray sign: free air within the peritoneal cavity or pneumoperitoneum. The abdominal X-rays in this new disease also demonstrated bubbles of air in the wall of the bowel, termed "pneumotosis cystoides intestinalis." These air bubbles in the intestinal wall became the most significant radiologic feature that led to the diagnosis.[3]

A disease in newborn calves, well known to veterinarians as the "scours," had similar features, including bubbles of air in the intestinal wall.[4] The disease occurs in newborn animals that cannot obtain their mothers' milk during the first few hours after birth. This first flow of milk, colostrum, is rich in nutrients and contains antibodies necessary for intestinal immunity. When the animal could not obtain colostrum, bacteria were free to migrate through the intestinal wall, causing sepsis. Cold stress and exposure to infectious bacteria contributed to the disease in animals.

These same factors seemed to be involved in the premature infants who developed necrotizing enterocolitis, or NEC. These small infants, too weak to nurse, were given intravenous fluids and then fed with artificial formulas. Episodes of asphyxia, hypovolemia, congestive heart failure and hypothermia — problems common in premature infants — also seemed to be etiologic factors. The lack of oxygen and lowered blood flow was thought to induce a shift of circulation from the intestine and extremities to more vital organs, a phenomenon observed in diving mammals and known as the "seal diving reflex." This shift in blood flow was thought to cause localized areas of ischemia and necrosis in the intestinal wall.[5] This concept is logical, but recent evidence suggests that more is involved than ischemia.

No other disease, save possibly diaphragmatic hernia, resulted in so much research, clinical study and discussion at meetings. The earliest long series of patients and experimental work originated from Dr. Thomas V. Santulli and his colleagues at the Babies' Hospital in New York. This group demonstrated in animal models that breast milk did play a role in protecting newborn animals and that hypoxia and cold stress caused findings similar to NEC.[6] Umbilical artery catheterization to monitor blood pressure or for exchange transfusion also seemed to be associated with NEC. Evidence suggested that artificial feedings could cause direct mucosal damage and that such feeding was a substrate for the growth of bacteria. These bacteria produced the gas bubbles seen in the intestinal wall and even in mesenteric blood vessels.[7]

Intense research by a number of centers added little to our understanding of this complex disease that affected 5 to 10 percent of infants weighing less than fifteen hundred grams at birth. Efforts to prevent NEC by giving corticosteroids to the mother before birth, prophylactic antibiotics and delayed feedings did not reduce the incidence of NEC. As our experience with total intravenous nutrition developed, it became common practice to delay oral feedings and provide nutrition by the intravenous route. Technical difficulties arose with inserting intravenous catheters into tiny infants, however, and during the early years these babies suffered a high incidence of catheter sepsis. It was difficult to provide enough calories and protein for the baby to grow, and parenteral nutrition appeared to cause liver disease. Despite delayed feedings, the incidence of NEC remained high.

While the researchers attempted to discover the cause of NEC and the neonatologists worked to prevent the disease, surgeons were faced with the decision to operate or not and what to do at the time of surgery. The consultation to see a terribly sick infant would come late in the day. The poor wizened infant, often weighing a thousand grams or less, would be connected to monitors with multiple wires. He would have intravenous lines for the delivery of multiple medications and was attached to a mechanical ventilator. He may already have suffered from an intracerebral hemorrhage, retinopathy, and be in congestive heart failure. The findings of a distended abdomen with a bluish discoloration around the umbilicus indicated the presence of meconium free in the peritoneal cavity. When slight pressure was applied to the abdominal wall, the baby would lift his legs and sometimes grimace. It was his way of saying, "My stomach hurts." When the X-ray demonstrated free air in the peritoneal cavity, indicating intestinal perforation, the decision was made to perform surgery. There was usually no alternative, but sometimes we felt as if we were being asked to operate on a baby who was well past saving.

When the findings were not so definite, it was difficult to decide to operate. We did not want to perform unnecessary surgery on a desperately ill, tiny infant. Once, a neonatologist asked, "Why do you always wait until the intestine perforates?" I had no good answer, except that the presence of free air in the abdominal cavity indicating an intestinal perforation was about the only definite indication for an operation. Even this was not always true; a few babies with pneumoperitoneum did not appear to be sick, and their abdomens were not tender. These infants were on a ventilator, and the pressurized air had ruptured a part of the lung and dissected its way down to the abdomen.

Other signs, such as gastrointestinal bleeding, air in the portal vein, or refractory acidosis, likewise indicated the need for surgery. Surgeons searched for clues to an earlier diagnosis of intestinal gangrene. Needle aspiration of the abdomen demonstrating brown-stained fluid with bacteria was considered another indication for surgery.[8] There was, however, some reluctance to poke a needle into the abdomen of a tiny infant. No matter the diagnostic method, the decision to operate was agonizing. These babies were so fragile that we often would not move the baby to the operating room but would arrange a sterile field inside the infant's incubator and do the surgery in the nursery. At first this outraged the nursing service and the administrators, but it became common practice.

The usual treatment for intestinal gangrene or perforation is removal of the diseased segment, with either immediate reconnection of the bowel or exteriorization with a later anastomosis. This could be done in babies with NEC when the disease was localized, but too often there would be patchy areas of necrotic intestine with multiple perforations. This presented a terrible problem. Removal of all diseased tissue might leave the baby with insufficient bowel to absorb nutrients. Thus was born a new condition, "short bowel syndrome." In an attempt to save every possible fragment of intestine, we sutured suspicious areas, patched perforations and exteriorized proximal perforations in an attempt to heal the distal intestine.

Surgeons slavishly adhere to rules laid down by their mentors and professors as if Moses had written them in stone. It was considered absolutely essential to remove necrotic or perforated intestine, and drainage of the entire abdomen was thought to be impossible. The profession reacted with disbelief when Sigmund Ein and his associates at the Hospital for Sick Children in Toronto reported on the efficacy of simple drainage of the peritoneal cavity under local anesthesia in infants with intestinal perforation due to NEC.[9] Many surgeons showed deep reluctance to try this new method, but when they were faced late at night with a terribly ill, tiny baby unlikely to survive an operation simple drainage was a welcome alternative to doing nothing. At first, drainage was used to stabilize a sick infant; to our surprise, as many as 40 percent of these infants survived and needed no further surgery. This outcome was a mystery. Had the perforation and gangrenous intestine spontaneously healed? A partial answer came when infants treated with peritoneal drainage later required surgery for an intestinal obstruction. It appeared that the perforations had been sealed by dense adhesions between adjoining loops of intestine and scar that obliterated the lumen.

Between 1980 and 1987, Richard Ricketts in Atlanta, Georgia, operated on 91 infants with NEC. The overall survival rate was 72.5 percent, even though the entire intestine was gangrenous in 14 percent of his patients and all of those infants died. A quarter of his patients weighed less than one thousand grams, but even in this high-risk group the survival rate was 58 percent.[10]

R. L. Moss and his associates carried out a multi-institutional randomized study of 117 infants under fifteen hundred grams to determine if drainage or open operation was superior and found no statistical difference in mortality rates for either group.[11] Almost simultaneously with this study, a group of 31 neonatal units in 13 countries carried out another randomized study of infants under one thousand grams with NEC and found that laparotomy gave superior results over simple drainage. The difference was that in this second series drainage was usually followed by a laparatomy.[12] Both of these studies used the most sophisticated statistical analyses, and the patients were treated in the most modern neonatal units. The differing results may indicate the difficulties in applying science to complex clinical problems.

At the 2010 meeting of the American Pediatric Surgical Association, M. A. Hull and her colleagues presented data collected from 545 hospitals on 79,445 neonates who weighed less than fifteen hundred grams at birth.[13] Nearly 7,000 of these patients — 6,852, to be exact — developed NEC. A laparotomy was performed in 54 percent of these infants, while 26 percent had only peritoneal drainage. The overall survival rate was 67 percent, with a better survival rate in those treated with an open operation. Since the higher-risk, smaller infants were more likely to have had only peritoneal drainage, it is difficult to interpret this difference in survival rates.

Dr. Ekhard E. Zeigler and his colleagues at the University of Iowa have shed new light on the nutritional needs of very low birthweight babies.[14] For many years, neonatologists have delayed enteral feedings for fear of causing NEC. There was also reluctance to provide sufficient calories and protein for growth and neurologic development. Dr. Zeigler and others have demonstrated that it is possible to provide more parenteral amino acids and more calories in the form of lipids than was given in the past. More important, they have shown that withholding enteral feedings delays maturation of the gastrointestinal tract and increases the risk of NEC. Early "trophic" feedings of as little as two milliliters of human milk every four to six hours, started on the day of birth, provide nutrition to the intestine and stimulate growth. If fresh mother's milk is not available, banked donor human milk is almost as effective. These findings showing the beneficial effects of early feeding of human milk may spell the end of this plague that has affected premature infants during the past 40 years.

I was involved with necrotizing enterocolitis from the beginning and therefore may be permitted a few personal observations. The disease began at what might be termed the dawn of high technology as applied to the care of a newborn infant. Dedicated pediatricians could save ever smaller infants by the application of mechanical ventilation, antibiotics, better incubators, monitoring and parenteral nutrition. Surgeons contributed to this increased survival with improved techniques of vascular access and the early treatment of complications such as a persistent ductus arteriosus. At the same time, industry produced convenient infant formulas so that mothers no longer had to sterilize bottles and mix canned milk with sugar and water to feed their babies. Mothers were less interested in breast-feeding, and some doctors thought the new artificial formulas were as good as or better than human milk. We ignored the nutritional and immunologic benefits of human milk and forgot the lessons learned by veterinarians on the importance of colostrum to the well-being of newborn animals. We even ignored some of the earliest research on the benefits of milk in preventing NEC. When it became apparent that infants became ill coincident to enteral feedings, the solution for years was to delay feedings. All of this may indicate a certain arrogance about our reliance on technology rather than nature. Perhaps the doctor doesn't always know best.

CHAPTER 26

Esophageal Atresia and Tracheo-Esophageal Fistula

N. A. Meyers, surgeon to the Royal Children's Hospital in Melbourne, Australia, and two surgeons from Kansas City, USA — Tom M. Holder and Keith W. Ashcraft — have written extensive reviews of esophageal atresia and tracheo-esophageal fistula.[1] According to these and other authors, the first reported case of an esophageal atresia was by William Durston, an English physician. Durston delivered thoracopagus-conjoined twins in Plymouth on October 22, 1670. The twins died; the case was so remarkable, he obtained permission to perform an autopsy. The esophagus was open in one twin, but in the other it ended blindly; Durston also found multiple other anomalies.

Thomas Gibson, another English physician, in 1697 was the first to describe a baby with a classic esophageal atresia and tracheo-esophageal fistula. Holder and Ashcraft reproduced the pertinent parts of Gibson's *The Anatomy of the Humane Bodies Epitomized* in their excellent monograph published in 1966. Gibson wrote:

> About November 1696 I was sent for to an infant that would not swallow. The child seem'd very desirous of food, and took what was offered it in a spoon with greediness; but when it went to swallow it, it was like to be choked, and what should have gone down returned by the mouth and nose, and it fell into a struggling convulsive sort of fit upon it. It was very fleshy and large, and was two days old when I came to it, but the next day died. The parents being willing to have it opened, I took two physicians and a surgeon with me.... We blew a pipe down the gullet, but found no passage for the wind into the stomach. Then we made a slit in the stomach, and put a pipe into its upper orifice, and blowing, we found the wind had a vent, but not by the top of the gullet. Then we carefully slit open the back side of the gullet from the stomach upwards, and when we were gone a little above half way towards the pharynx, we found it hollow no further. Then we began to slit it open from the pharynx downward, and it was hollow till within an inch of the other slit, and in the imperforated part was narrower than in the hollowed. The isthmus (as it were) did not seem ever to have been hollow, for in the bottom of the upper and the top of the lower cavity, there was not the least print of any such thing, but the parts were here as smooth as the bottom of an acorn cup. Then searching what way the wind had passed when we blew from the stomach upwards, we found an oval hole (half an inch long) on the fore-side of the gullet opening into the aspera arteria [trachea] a little above its first division, just under the lower part of the isthmus above mentioned.[2]

There would never be a better description of the symptoms and pathology than that given by Thomas Gibson over three hundred years ago. Unfortunately, it would take almost as long before this distressing lesion could be successfully treated.

176

More reports cropped up throughout history of infants who were unable to swallow, choked on feedings and died within a few days. In at least two infants, physicians diagnosed an obstruction by passing a bougie into the esophagus.[3] In 1840, Thomas P. Hill, an American physician, saw an infant who salivated excessively, coughed, became cyanotic and regurgitated each feeding. Hill suspected that the symptoms were due to "flatulence" and ordered an enema. The nurse who attempted to give an enema couldn't find the anus. At autopsy, the baby had an esophageal atresia, a fistula from the trachea to the distal esophagus, and an imperforate anus with a recto-urinary fistula.[4] This common association of congenital anomalies almost defines the specialty of pediatric surgery — defects of separate organs that would normally require three different surgical specialties to correct.

Harald Hirschsprung, that remarkable Danish physician who described pyloric stenosis and his namesake disease, wrote his doctoral thesis on congenital occlusion of the esophagus. This report on 14 cases included four patients he had seen while on the obstetric service and seven from the literature.[5] In 1880, Morell Mackenzie (1839-1893) published "Malformations of the Esophagus," a review of 57 patients including those with atresia, fistula without atresia, fistulas to the bronchi, an adult with esophageal stenosis and what sounds like a duplication of the esophagus.[6] Like his predecessors, Mackenzie described the inability to swallow, "distressing" attacks of suffocation and death by exhaustion in infants with esophageal atresia. He also said that the passage of a bougie into the blind esophagus made the diagnosis. Five of the patients in his review were anencephalic monsters; others had spina bifida, an absent anus, a horseshoe kidney, deformed hands, and intersex anomalies.

Mackenzie also described the normal embryological development of the esophagus and trachea from a single tube. He concluded that malformations were the result of an arrest of separation of the primitive tube. At the time of Mackenzie's paper there had been no attempt at surgical treatment, but some had suggested a gastrostomy in cases of atresia without fistula. Mackenzie also correctly pointed out that food introduced into the stomach in the presence of a fistula would result in food regurgitating into the lung.

A pioneer laryngologist and one of the first physicians to use a laryngoscope, Mackenzie had an extensive Harley Street practice. He was called upon to treat the Crown Prince of Germany, who later became King Frederick III. German physicians had diagnosed throat cancer, but Mackenzie claimed the lesion was benign. He was proved wrong when the King died of throat cancer a year later.[7]

One of the first attempts to operate on the esophagus of a child was the removal of a foreign body from the cervical esophagus in 1833.[8] The 28-month-old child had swallowed a bone from a rib of mutton six days before the surgeon, James Arnott of London, was called in consultation. The child could swallow only small amounts of liquid and the bone was immovable. Arnott opened the esophagus through an incision in the right side of the neck and was able to feel the bone half an inch below his incision. He extracted the bone with a forceps, but the child died 56 hours later. This case demonstrated extraordinary courage on the part of the surgeon, not only to operate but also to report an unsuccessful case so that others could learn from his example.

One report from 1888 describes an attempt to cure a day-old infant with what turned out to be esophageal atresia without fistula. The infant had choking spells and became livid on attempts to swallow. The attending physician, unable to pass a sound beyond five inches from the baby's mouth, diagnosed an esophageal obstruction. Charles Steele, M.D., the surgeon in the case, thought there might be a membrane obstructing the lumen. The baby was sustained through the night with milk enemas. The next morning, when there was enough light and with the infant under chloroform, Steele made a midline abdominal incision and sutured the stomach to the skin. After opening the stomach, he proceeded as follows: "A bougie was passed down the oesophagus [sic] as before and another upward from the stomach for a short distance; but they did not approach each other by what we judged to be an inch and a half. I then cut a gum-elastic catheter in half, and passed it from below, introduced up it a long slender steel probe, and pressed it upwards as much as was justifiable, in case the lower part of the tube might be twisted or narrowed, and capable of being rendered pervious."[9]

The infant died after 24 hours. At autopsy, the proximal and distal ends of the esophagus were an inch and a half apart. This operation might have been successful had the obstruction been a simple membrane, but things are rarely so simple. The reasoning behind the operation was sound and was similar to our attempts at passing catheters and dilators retrograde from the stomach up through the esophagus in children with strictures.

Even with anesthesia and antisepsis/asepsis, there were many obstacles to direct repair of an esophageal anomaly. There were no suction devices to remove secretions from the proximal pouch or lung and no intravenous fluids or antibiotics. These poor infants rapidly develop aspiration pneumonia and soon become malnourished and exhausted. The most daunting surgical problem was maintaining lung ventilation while the chest was open. Surgeons had drained pus from the pleural cavity for centuries, but if the lung was not adherent to the chest wall the introduction of air caused the lung to collapse. This is a rapidly fatal complication in a small infant.

A few surgeons had removed foreign bodies from the intrathoracic esophagus through a posterior incision into the mediastinum without opening the pleural cavity.[10] This is essentially the same incision later used for the retropleural approach to esophageal atresia. However, even with this incision, a perforation of the thin, delicate pleura would have collapsed the lung. In later years, some surgeons made successful repairs of esophageal atresia and fistula with local anesthesia, but this is precarious, with a high risk of injury to the pleura in a moving infant. In practical terms, before operations on intrathoracic organs could be successful, there had to be a way to provide positive pressure to the lungs.

Tracheotomy had been since ancient times the only way to secure control of the airway. Armand Trousseau, a French physician in Paris, popularized the operation for children with diphtheria in 1831.[11] In 1853, while experimenting with the effects of chloroform on the heart, Joseph Lister performed a tracheotomy on a donkey, tied a tube into the trachea and connected the tube to a bellows. With this apparatus, he administered chloroform and inflated the lungs with positive pressure. The donkey died, but the experiment proved that with an endotracheal tube and positive pressure a surgeon could open the chest.[12]

Joseph O'Dwyer, working at Columbia Hospital in New York, in 1887 published his work on intubation of the trachea with a metal tube for children with croup. Any physician could learn to insert an O'Dwyer tube, but there was concern about damage to the larynx.[13] During the 1888 meeting of the American Surgical Association, Professor Thomas Annandale of Edinburgh told of a patient who stopped breathing during an operation for a thyroid tumor but was revived after the insertion of a gumelastic catheter into the trachea.[14] The addition of a bellows to the O'Dwyer tube provided for positive pressure, similar to Lister's apparatus. Rudolph Matas of New Orleans, a brilliant and innovative surgeon, devised a piston similar to a bicycle pump that on the backward stroke drew in air and on the forward stroke pumped air over a bottle of ether to an O'Dwyer tube in the trachea. A manometer controlled the inflation pressure. In his 1900 report, Matas had used his apparatus only on dogs and cadavers.[15]

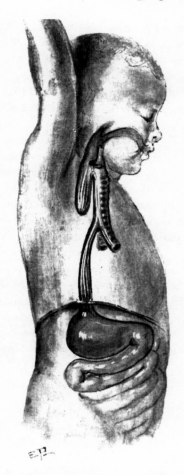

Esophageal atresia and tracheo-esophageal fistula, the most common esophageal defect. The proximal esophagus ends as a blind pouch, while the distal esophagus is connected to the trachea. The child can't swallow and his gastric secretions reflux into his lungs. This illustration from *The Surgery of Infancy and Childhood* by Dr. Robert Gross (W. B. Saunders 1955 is an example of the artistry of Etta Pioti, who illustrated Dr. Gross' book (courtesy Elseuier Limited).

There were many animal experiments with intra-tracheal intubation and artificial respiration, but William MacEwen of Glasgow in 1880 was the first to use endotracheal anesthesia in a human. The patient was an adult with an extensive cancer at the base of the tongue. MacEwen passed the tube through the patient's nostril into the larynx and the operation proceeded smoothly.[16] In 1909, Theodore Janeway of Columbia University used endotracheal, positive-pressure anesthesia to operate on a boy for empyema.[17] In 1911, Charles Elsberg of New York made a detailed report on 30 patients operated on using endotracheal intubation with an electric pump that delivered oxygen and ether vapor.[18]

Sad to say, most surgeons were comfortable with ether delivered by face mask and especially in children were concerned about postoperative laryngeal edema. In the United States, where poorly trained interns, nurses and even students were likely to be the anesthetist, this was a reasonable fear. The United Kingdom, where skilled physicians delivered most anesthetics, saw more rapid progress.

The real impetus to thoracic surgery came from a German, Ferdinand Sauerbruch, an assistant in the clinic of Professor von Mikulicz-Radecki who was interested in esophageal cancer. Sauerbruch built a low-pressure chamber large enough to accommodate the patient's body and the surgeons, while the patient's head protruded through a sealed aperture. In the chamber, the patient's airway was exposed to atmospheric pressure while his chest was opened. The device maintained inflation of the lung and allowed Sauerbruch to operate on the esophagus and tuberculous empyema. He established his reputation as a thoracic surgeon, but despite a lecture tour with demonstrations, his chamber never caught on in the United States. Sauerbruch led a sensational life and served as a medical officer in the German army during both world wars.[19]

In comparison with the great European and British medical centers and the well-established Eastern U.S. medical schools, Chicago was a medical backwater. However, the city did boast a group of well-trained, innovative surgeons at the end of the nineteenth century. Christian Fenger from Copenhagen had established a "school" of scientific surgery, based on pathology and bacteriology, at the Cook County Hospital. One of his students was the internationally known John B. Murphy, a general surgeon and a founder of the American College of Surgeons. Other Cook County graduates, such as Alan Kanavel, Dallas Phemister, Loyal Davis and Roswell Park, would head departments of surgery and serve as Presidents of the College of Surgeons.

Northwestern Medical School was scarcely 50 years old when, between 1910 and 1913, three Northwestern physicians — Joseph Brenneman, a pioneer pediatrician; Robert F. Zeit, a pathologist; and Harry M. Richter, a young surgeon — reported on five infants with congenital esophageal atresia and tracheo-esophageal fistula.[20] The papers discuss the same infants and, taken together, document the clinical symptoms, signs, pathology, embryology and treatment of esophageal atresia. The diagnosis was made in each infant without resort to X-ray by passing a catheter down the proximal esophagus and noting gastric distention, indicating the fistula. One infant was judged too ill for an operation and another died following a feeding jejunostomy. Dr. Richter did a gastrostomy on one and in the other two performed transthoracic ligations of the fistula. All three patients died, but his thoughtful paper pointed the way to ultimate success.

Dr. Richter had been an intern at the Cook County Hospital and was an assistant professor of surgery there. From his work with pyloric stenosis he knew of the need for gentleness and fine suture material and the importance of preventing heat loss by wrapping infants and using hot water bottles on the operating table.[21] Most important, in 1908 he had reported on his own apparatus to deliver positive-pressure intra-tracheal anesthesia, and he was the first to use this method in a newborn infant. Here is his description of the anesthesia machine:

> My apparatus consists of a motor and a pump, giving a free current of air at a pressure varied readily by a reostat, with a valve in the connecting tubing, through which excess air may be allowed to escape. The air passes over ether contained in a Wolff bottle, or is shunted directly to the tracheal tube as desired. A manometer and a mercury "blow off" as a safety valve are in the circuit. The whole is simply the type of apparatus of Meltzer and Auer. Just before beginning differential pressure, and not until the operator is ready to begin it, a pad should be firmly bandaged upon the abdomen; otherwise the stomach and intestine will be greatly distended by inflation through the tracheo-esophageal fistula.[22]

Richter had done a gastrostomy on his first patient and observed the regurgitation of fluid from the stomach to the lung that caused "drowning." He realized that a simple gastrostomy would suffice for an infant with pure esophageal atresia but that the "fatal factor" in the most common type of anomaly was the free regurgitation from the stomach to the lung. He observed the anatomy of the tracheo-esophageal fistula in the autopsy of his first patient and knew that separation of the fistula and a direct anastomosis of the esophagus was the only curative operation. He thought this would eventually be possible, but as a first step he planned on dividing the fistula so the infant could be fed by gastrostomy. He admitted his lack of familiarity with the anatomy of and the hazards of operating on a newborn infant.

In his first operation, performed on July 16, 1913, he did a gastrostomy and passed a flexible sound up the distal esophagus. Then he opened the infant's left chest through the seventh interspace, divided five ribs and ligated the esophagus at the trachea. Richter admitted that the incision was too low and in the wrong pleural cavity. The infant died two hours after the operation. An autopsy demonstrated that the lungs were inflated, indicating the success of Richter's anesthetic apparatus. The ligature was watertight and at the junction of the trachea and esophagus. We can wonder at his choice of a left thoracotomy; Richter may have been influenced by surgery for carcinoma of the esophagus. Only a few months before Richter's operation, Franz Torek of New York had performed the first successful resection of a carcinoma of the esophagus through an incision in the left, seventh intercostal space.[23]

Richter realized his mistake and used a right thoracotomy for his second operation, performed on August 14, 1913. The infant was three days old:

> Child had a marked purulent secretion in its mouth and gullet and showed marked respiratory retraction of ribs and abdomen. Preliminary intubation of gullet from below, as in previous case. Clamp placed on jejunum to prevent inflation of bowels. Temporary closure of abdominal incision. Change to intra-tracheal ether anaesthesia. Incision in right sixth intercostal space about two inches long, the posterior end carried upward and the sixth, fifth and fourth ribs cut across near their angles. Retraction of ribs gave perfect view of operation. A blunt hook passed around gullet at tracheal junction and ligature placed. Chest closed as before, raising the intrapulmonary tension sufficiently to bring the lung up to the chest wall. Gastrostomy of the E.J. Senn type. The child took approximately 8 ounces of fluid through the gastrostomy tube in the next twenty hours without showing any evidence of regurgitation into lungs. Its breathing lost the dyspneic type at once. No attacks recurred. Reaction rapid. Auscultation showed lung maintained in fully inflated condition. Death twenty hours later. No post-mortem examination permitted.

Richter realized that a primary anastomosis was possible, but with the danger of mediastinal infection it was safer to ligate the fistula and hope for some type of reconstruction in the future.

Dr. Richter was Surgeon in Chief at the Northwestern Medical School from 1929 to 1932. He was a founding member of the American College of Surgeons, published 40 articles and practiced surgery for 50 years. Long before it was accepted, Dr. Richter adopted early ambulation for his surgical patients. He was warmhearted, kind and so concerned about his patients' welfare that he advocated pre-paid medical care, even "socialized medicine" if it would help patients obtain care. He retired from practice at 74 years of age in 1946.[24] He never again operated on a baby with esophageal atresia.

Dr. Richter's concept of staged treatment, with endotracheal positive-pressure anesthesia, a right-sided incision and immediate division of the fistula, was largely ignored by future surgeons. During the next few years there were more reports, mostly with theories of etiology, discussions of embryology, confusing classifications and futile attempts at therapy. There were also suggestions that, since the prognosis was so poor, surgery should not be attempted. Two surgeons from Tulane University in New Orleans, M. Gage and A. Ochsner, attempted to prevent reflux of gastric juice into the lungs by ligating the esophagogastric junction through the abdomen in two babies. Their plan was to feed the infants by gastrostomy and eventually reconstruct the esophagus. Both their patients had attacks of cyanosis and respiratory failure and died of aspiration pneumonia. It is notable that one was treated with a Drinker respirator, a device used to support breathing in children with poliomyelitis.

The discussion of the Gage and Ochsner paper covers two important points. Dr. Blair of St. Louis said that if an operation were to succeed, it must take place immediately after birth. Another surgeon observed that at autopsy there were flecks of barium in all foci of pneumonia.[25]

In 1940, Thomas H. Lanman reported on what may be the longest series of patients operated on with a 100 percent mortality rate. The four surgeons who operated on these patients were Harvard professors and surgeons at the Boston Children's Hospital, located not far from Bunker Hill, where the first shots in the Revolutionary War were fired. Lanman's report gave detailed descriptions of operations performed on 31 patients with esophageal atresia and tracheo-esophageal fistula and one with atresia without fistula. All operations were carried out with local procaine anesthesia, supplemented with ether or cyclopropane given through a "tight mask". Endotracheal tubes and positive-pressure devices were not used. Two infants died without an operation; several others died during or immediately following surgery.

The first operation, performed by Dr. C. G. Mixter in September of 1929, was a gastrostomy, extra-pleural ligation of the fistula, and insertion of a catheter into the distal esophagus, which was then sutured to the skin. The infant died at the end of the procedure. This operation — a posterior mediastinal, extra-pleural approach with division of the fistula and exteriorization of the distal esophagus — was done in 11 more patients. One survived for 32 days.

The first of four attempts to make an esophageal anastomosis occurred in 1936. One infant lived nine days; its subsequent death resulted from overhydration with parenteral fluids. Discouraged by direct division of the fistula, surgeons made two attempts to ligate the cardio-esophageal junction and in two other patients the stomach was completely divided. Thomas Lanman operated on 16 of these babies; one can only imagine his terrible disappointment with the results, but he passed on important lessons. He favored the posterior mediastinal, extra-pleural approach because drainage was better than with a transpleural incision and he believed drainage was important. Dr. Lanman recommended giving patients intravenous fluids and transfusions but cautioned against overhydration. He warned against using contrast material in the proximal pouch because of an increased risk of aspiration pneumonia; the curled catheter in the proximal pouch made the diagnosis of atresia. Despite this important warning, radiologists persist in using contrast material to make a pretty picture.

Lanman's final comment was prophetic: "Given a suitable case in which the patient is seen early, I feel that, with greater experience, improved technique and good luck, the successful outcome of a direct anastomosis can and will be reported in the near future."[26]

After a review of the literature and his own failures, N. Logan Leven at the University of Minnesota became convinced that gastrostomy followed by obliteration of the fistula was necessary. In 1939, he achieved the triumphal success of operating on the first infant to survive treatment for esophageal atresia with fistula.[27] The baby, a full-term infant, was two days old when she was admitted to the hospital on November 28, 1939. The first operation, a gastrostomy with passage of a feeding tube into the jejunum, was done the next day. Surprisingly, the baby tolerated five milliliters of tube feeding every fifteen minutes, with only occasional cyanotic attacks. On December 6, Dr. Leven attempted to electo-coagulate the fistula through a bronchoscope. When this failed, he ligated the fistula through an extra-pleural approach on December 29. The baby thrived, and it wasn't until March 27 of 1940 that Dr. Leven did a cervical esophagostomy to drain saliva from the proximal pouch. In addition to Dr. Leven's surgical skill, this baby must have had a small fistula to survive for one month before the fistula was divided. When she was two years old, the infant had a three-stage, ante-thoracic jejunal interposition and was able to swallow.[28]

Also, on November 28, 1939, a one-day-old girl was admitted to the Boston Children's Hospital. Dr. William E. Ladd, discouraged with his attempts at direct anastomosis of the esophagus, did a gastrostomy and an extra-pleural ligation of the fistula.[29] Though Dr. Ladd carried out his operation almost simultaneously with that of Dr. Leven, Dr. Ladd graciously said: "It is interesting to note that Leven, at almost the identical time, came to the same conclusion about methods of attacking this problem and adopted principles identical with ours, with only minor variations of technic. So far as I know, he has the oldest living patient with esophageal atresia and tracheo-esophageal fistula, his patient being twenty-four hours older than our oldest living one."[29]

Dr. Ladd connected the proximal esophagus and the stomach with tubes constructed from skin flaps on the anterior chest wall in his patient. By the time she was four years old, she was eating a moderately varied diet and indulged in fairly normal activities for a child of her age.

Dr. Cameron Haight at the University of Michigan in Ann Arbor was the first surgeon to successfully anastomose the esophagus in a baby with esophageal atresia.[30] A pioneer thoracic surgeon, Dr. Haight had performed the second total pneumonectomy in the world and the first in the United States in 1932. The patient was a 13-year-old girl who had aspirated part of a rubber mouth gag during a dental procedure. The piece of rubber lodged in her left main bronchus, and she developed a septic lung, an empyema and bronchiectasis. Dr. Haight drained the empyema, later removed the left lung and did a thoracoplasty to obliterate the pleural cavity. The patient was well after this formidable series of operations.

The saga of the first baby to survive esophageal anastomosis — and it was indeed a saga — began in March of 1941 in Marquette, Michigan, a city on the shores of stormy Lake Superior. When a baby girl became cyanotic with feedings, the obstetrician passed a catheter into the esophagus and injected Lipiodol that outlined the atresia and was aspirated into the lungs. The X-ray also demonstrated copious amounts of air in the stomach. The baby was then transported from Michigan's Upper Peninsula to the hospital in Ann Arbor, a distance of five hundred miles that included a ferry trip across the Straits of Mackinac. The baby was 12 days old and weighed eight pounds, four ounces on admission to the hospital. Despite the long journey and having aspirated Lipiodol, the baby was robust and her lung fields were clear. She was given parenteral fluids to correct her dehydration and on March 14, 1941, Dr. Haight made a left extra-pleural incision under local anesthesia. He resected four centimeters of the second, third, fourth and fifth ribs and divided the intercostal muscles to gain exposure. Since his incision was on the left side, it was necessary to mobilize the subclavian artery and the aorta arch to expose the distal esophagus. One can imagine the difficulties encountered by the following excerpt: "Traction on the tension suture allowed the blind upper pouch to be drawn down to the level of the distal segment, but when the patient struggled or cried, the upper segment retracted up into the neck and out of sight. The tip of the upper segment was opened for a distance corresponding to the diameter of the distal segment and the interior of the two segments was cleansed with a 1:3000 solution of flavine. When an attempt was made to unite the two segments, the first suture pulled out when the child strained. When the upper segment again disappeared into the neck, open drop ether was then begun. The complete relaxation that was obtained allowed the segments to be approximated without tension."[31]

The postoperative course was complicated by bouts of cyanosis when mucus accumulated in the baby's throat and by edema, probably from excess amounts of subcutaneous saline solution. On the seventh postoperative day, saliva appeared at the drain site and a Lipiodol swallow demonstrated a large anastomotic leak. The baby was treated with oxygen–carbon dioxide inhalations to stimulate respiration, sulfadiazine and frequent transfusions of blood and plasma. On the tenth postoperative day, Dr. Ransome, a general surgeon, performed a feeding gastrostomy. The esophageal leak was so large that gastrostomy feedings escaped from the thoracic wound and a catheter inserted through the mouth emerged from the drainage site. Despite these serious complications, the leak healed and by the thirty-ninth day the baby took feedings by mouth. From then on, the baby thrived despite a stricture at the anastomosis that required one dilatation. She was discharged from the hospital in December 1941, after a 20-month hospitalization. According to a recent report from Dr. Arnold Coran, the former Surgeon in Chief of the C. S. Mott Children's Hospital at the University of Michigan, the patient was still alive at 69 years of age.

The survival of this remarkable patient, despite a delay in diagnosis, aspiration of Lipiodol, a difficult operation, bouts of cyanosis and a major anastomotic leak, was due to the skill and tenacity of her physicians. Also, she survived in no small part because of her high birth weight and strength. We should also note that the administration of sulfadiazine, one of the first antimicrobials, contributed to the success of this fortunate child.

At the time of his report in 1943, Dr. Haight switched to a right extra-pleural incision and had four more survivors. By 1986, 426 infants with esophageal atresia had been operated on at the University of Michigan Medical Center. By the end of that period, the survival rate of infants operated on was over 80 percent despite increased numbers of premature infants and babies with multiple associated anomalies.[32]

After Haight's report, direct anastomosis of the esophagus became the standard of treatment in the United States.[33] England was still suffering from the effects of the war when, in 1947, a London surgeon named F. H. Franklin successfully operated on two babies with atresia and fistula.[34] Both operations were performed with local anesthesia through a right retropleural incision and both babies were given penicillin. The first infant suffered a large anastomotic leak and a near-exanguinating hemorrhage from the incision. Perhaps as a result of wartime scarcity, the anastomosis was made with 0 silk!

W. E. Ladd, Orvar Swenson and Robert Gross operated on 76 patients at the Boston Children's Hospital from 1940 through 1946. The authors emphasized the importance of preoperative care, including supplemental oxygen, suction of the proximal pouch and the head-up position to minimize pulmonary aspiration. Cyclopropane administered with a closed system was the anesthetic of choice, and they had settled on using a right extrapleural incision. They closed the fistula in all cases and when possible did a primary anastomosis of the esophageal segments. When the two ends of the esophagus were widely separated, they divided the fistula and then performed a gastrostomy, a cervical esophagostomy and a later reconstruction using an ante-thoracic skin tube and a segment of jejunum. Forty-three patients had staged operations, with 16 survivors; 14 of 32 patients with direct anastomosis survived. The authors noted that lessons learned from earlier cases as well as the routine use of sulfadiazine and penicillin helped reduce the mortality rate. At the time of their report, they had performed a primary anastomosis in 14 patients with only two deaths. The survivors included premature infants and those with associated birth defects.

Here is Dr. Swenson's account of an infant who had an associated ileal atresia:

> Through a transthoracic approach the tracheo-esophageal fistula was ligated and divided. Although the upper esophageal segment was within 1.5 cm. of the fistula, a primary anastomosis was not done as the time consumed would have been prohibitive. A long abdominal incision was made and a malrotation and atresia of the ileum with a minute cecum and colon were found. The terminal ileum ended in a bulbous sac about five centimeters in diameter. The malrotation was corrected and the terminal bulbous ileum was resected with a Mikulicz spur between the terminal ileum and cecum. A gastrostomy was made. Nineteen days later the ileostomy was closed. Two weeks later a primary anastomosis of the esophagus was made through a retropleural approach. Ten days later feedings were well taken by mouth. The patient continued to do well and was discharged taking all feedings by mouth and gaining weight.[35]

This one baby with multiple anomalies, treated by Dr. Orvar Swenson, illustrates the burgeoning specialty of pediatric surgery. In 1970, when Dr. Swenson was Chief of Surgery at Children's Memorial Hospital in Chicago, I watched him operate on another baby with a tracheo-esophageal fistula. He exposed the atresia and fistula through a small right extrapleural incision and repaired the defect with deftly placed 6-0 silk sutures, tied with perfect square knots. The baby literally did not "turn a hair."

Dr. Robert Gross, in his landmark *Surgery of Infancy and Childhood* published in 1953, reviewed 259 infants with esophageal atresia and tracheo-esophageal fistula seen at the Boston Children's Hospital from 1929 to 1952. At that time, 109 patients had survived treatment, though nearly half weighed less than five pounds. Nine patients were not operated on because they were in extremis or had Mongolism or serious cardiac abnormalities. The oldest living patient was 14 years of age.

Dr. Gross stressed the importance of total care, including the administration of penicillin, streptomycin, oxygen, suction of the proximal esophagus and careful roentgen examination. He still advocated cyclopropane anesthesia given through a tight-fitting mask, explaining that an intra-tracheal tube caused irritation of the trachea. He used a right transpleural incision, a two-layer anastomosis and a temporary feeding gastrostomy in all patients. He reviewed the experience with staged reconstruction, using skin tubes and segments of jejunum, but said, "We now feel strongly that multiple-stage construction of an antethoracic esophagus is obsolete therapy; it is greatly inferior to esophageal anastomosis in the mediastinum or[primary esophago-gastrostomy within the mediastinum] as a one-stage repair of the esophageal malformation."[36]

In one patient, the stomach had been brought up into the right chest to allow an esophageal anastomosis. In the years since Dr. Haight's first success, little had changed in the diagnosis or surgical technique. The improved mortality partly stemmed from the use of antibiotics: first sulfadiazine, then penicillin, and by 1953 the combination of penicillin and streptomycin that was effective against a wide spectrum of bacteria. Another major factor was the presence of dedicated surgical house officers at the Boston Children's Hospital. Dr. Gross stressed the necessity for the surgeon to take control of all phases of care.

Other centers couldn't match the results obtained at the Boston Children's Hospital. Hospital mortality remained between 30 and 50 percent, mostly due to associated anomalies and prematurity. Dr. Willis Potts in Chicago, using a transpleural approach and a two-layer anastomosis, reported only two anastomotic leaks in 50 patients.[37] He also stressed the importance of meticulous postoperative care to aspirate mucus from the proximal pouch and feeding the baby with a medicine dropper in order to avoid aspiration of milk into the lungs. In the Chicago series, there were ten cases of atresia. An anastomosis could be made in only one case, and that child, with Down's syndrome, died the next day. Dr. Potts asserted that pulling up the stomach had failed and that staging the repair with a gastrostomy and a cervical esophagostomy was essential. He had abandoned subcutaneous reconstruction of the esophagus with jejunum for the ascending colon, placed behind the sternum.

Full-term infants without severe associated anomalies all survived a primary esophageal repair, but premature babies, especially those with associated defects, had only a 15 to 28 percent survival rate. The presence of aspiration pneumonia, primarily the result of regurgitation of gastric juice into the lungs via the fistula, added to the mortality rate. This led to a revival of staged procedures, consisting first of a gastrostomy performed under local anesthesia, and intensive support including frequent pharyngeal and tracheal suction and antibiotics. When the lungs improved, the fistula was divided through a retropleural approach under local anesthesia. Later, when the infant had gained weight and was vigorous, the esophagus was united. This program, reported in 1962, led to a survival rate of 10 infants out of 15. Deaths occurred in those infants who had severe associated cardiac disease.[38]

The members of the Section on Surgery of the American Academy of Pediatrics reviewed 1,058 patients with all types of esophageal atresia and tracheo-esophageal fistula, treated between January 1, 1958, and December 31, 1962.[39] Eighty-six percent had a proximal atresia with a distal fistula, 7 percent had an atresia without fistula and 4 percent had a fistula without atresia. The remainder had fistulas to either the proximal pouch or both proximal and distal segments. A little over half of the patients had an associated anomaly; the survival rate, as in previous studies, was related to the degree of prematurity and the severity of associated defects. The survival rate was somewhat better in patients operated on through a retropleural approach; infants with retropleural anastomotic leak had a 60 percent survival rate, while only 32 percent of infants with a leak into the pleural cavity lived. This study emphasized the importance of well-trained nurses, a competent house staff and expert anesthesia. Though several surgeons used local anesthesia for premature infants, the trend was toward general endotracheal anesthesia.

In 1962, David J. Waterston and his associates, in a study of 218 infants, published a risk classification based on the presence of prematurity, associated anomolies and the severity of lung complications.[40] This report clinched the need for early gastrostomy and a staged repair in high-risk patients.

During the next 40 years there were minimal changes in technique, but survival improved as a result of total intravenous nutrition, advances in anesthesia and respiratory support. A double lumen plastic sump tube to drain the upper pouch significantly reduced aspiration of saliva into the lungs.[41] Prenatal ultrasound made diagnosis possible prior to birth, and preoperative cardiac ultrasound identified infants who had a right aortic arch, an indication for a left-sided approach to the esophagus. The early recognition of cardiac defects also led to more aggressive treatment of associated anomalies. The survival rate in North America, Europe and Australia rose to well over 85 percent, with fewer anastomotic leaks and fewer delayed operations.[42] One of the most remarkable series, from the Medical College of Jaipur in India, reported on 25 years' experience, with an 85 percent survival rate in good-risk patients.[43] This increased survival rate of babies with esophageal and tracheo-esophageal atresia occurred over the lifetimes of a generation of surgeons trained by W. E. Ladd and Robert Gross at the Boston Children's Hospital. We owe these surgeons a debt of gratitude for their persistence, ingenuity and skill.

Increased recognition of the role of gastroesophageal reflux in stricture formation and respiratory complications led to the widespread use of antireflux operations in this group of patients during the 1970s.[44] There were also reports of a distressing incidence of respiratory infections, decreased respiratory function, chest wall muscular atrophy and thoracic scoliosus in long-term survivors of surgery. The respiratory problems could well be due to unrecognized gastroesophageal reflux and the chest wall deformities to the thoracotomy incision.

With the increasing enthusiasm for "minimally invasive" surgery, it was inevitable that the newest generation of pediatric surgeons would apply the latest technology to esophageal surgery. At the very end of the twentieth century, Tom E. Lobe and his associates in Memphis reported the first thoracoscopic repair of an esophageal atresia.[45] As usual, when faced with new technology, older surgeons claimed their methods gave excellent results and were critical of the new techniques. It quickly became evident that thoracoscopic repair not only was feasible, but also eliminated the muscular trauma associated with an open operation.[46]

Within five years, an international group of experienced thoracoscopic surgeons reported on a series of 104 newborn infants operated on for esophageal atresia and fistula.[47] The complication rates for anastomotic leak, stricture and the need for antireflux operations were essentially the same as with an open operation. Further series of patients have confirmed these excellent results.[48] There is no doubt that thoracoscopic repair of esophageal atresia, a product of the twenty-first century, is rapidly becoming the treatment of choice.

Isolated Esophageal Atresia — the Long Gap

Infants with esophageal atresia without fistula present an entirely different set of problems. There is no gastric regurgitation into the lungs, but the ends of the esophagus are too far apart for a primary anastomosis. As predicted by early authors, a simple feeding gastrostomy eventually allowed the survival of an infant with esophageal atresia without fistula. The first survivor was born in February 1935. James Donovan, a New York surgeon, performed a gastrostomy. Barium injected into the stomach demonstrated a distal blind esophagus. There was no fistula. The child thrived on gastrostomy feedings and when he was 11 years old Dr. George Humphries at the Babies' Hospital in New York brought up a long segment of jejunum through the left chest. The blind end of the jejunum was sutured to the mediastinal pleura. A month later, Dr. Humphries found that the end of the jejunum had necrosed and couldn't be anastomosed to the proximal esophagus. In 1951, when the patient was 16 years old, the jejunum was finally hooked to the proximal esophagus.[49] This was the first patient to survive with an esophageal atresia.

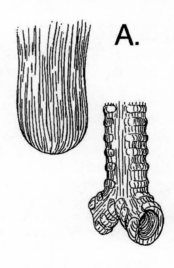

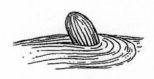

Unlike the near unanimity of opinion on the treatment of atresia with fistula, pediatric surgeons do not agree on the best treatment of babies with a long gap between the esophageal segments. The skin tube "esophagus" was quickly abandoned for small intestinal conduits of the type used in adults with lye strictures. At the height of the Second World War, in 1943, a group of American and English surgeons observed Dr. S. S. Yudin, a colonel in the Red Army, completing the second stage of a jejunal esophageal substitution by suturing the jejunum to the pharynx. At that time, Yudin had constructed 88 artificial esophagi with only two deaths. Twenty-one were with long segments of jejunum.[50]

The difficulty in maintaining the blood supply to the transplanted jejunum and widespread con-

Pure esophageal atresia, with the proximal esophagus ending blindly and the distal end near the diaphragm. The long-gap esophageal atresia is one of the most difficult problems in pediatric surgery (illustration from *Swenson's Pediatric Surgery*, 5th ed., ed. John Raffensperger, M.D., published by Appleton and Lange, 1990, and used by permission of the McGraw-Hill Companies).

cern about eventual jejunal ulceration at the gastric anastomosis led to a search for other methods of esophageal substitution.

In 1943, J. H. Garlock, M.D., brought up the entire stomach through the left chest after resecting a carcinoma of the middle third of the esophagus.[51] Unfortunately, the early results of pulling the stomach up through the chest in children were unsatisfactory because gastric distention compressed the lung.

In 1953, at the Surgical Forum of the American College of Surgeons, a general surgeon from Indianapolis named J. S. Battersby reported on using the right colon drawn up through the anterior mediastinum as an esophageal substitute in four patients with cancer of the esophagus.[52] This report led to widespread enthusiasm for the use of various segments of the colon connected to the cervical esophagus through a substernal tunnel.[53] It seemed for a while that the colon was a near-perfect substitute for the esophagus, especially when a long segment of terminal ileum was attached to the cervical esophagus and the ileocecael valve was left to control gastro-colic reflux.[54] Some surgeons reported difficulties with blood supply and leakage at the esophago-intestinal segment, and others reported growth delay in children with esophageal atresia following colon bypass.

Overall, the results of esophageal substitution appeared to be better in older children with strictures than in those with esophageal atresia, which may very well have been due to prematurity and associated anomalies.[55] Many surgeons thought that the long-term results justified the continued use of colon bypass.[56] Others preferred tubes made from the greater curvature of the stomach.[57] The iso-peristaltic gastric tube never became sacculated or tortuous, but the proximal esophago-gastric anastomosis was prone to leak and there was concern about connecting the squamous esophageal epithelium to a segment of acid-secreting stomach.

Louis Spitz and his colleagues at the Great Ormond Street Hospital in London overcame the problem of gastric distention in the pleural cavity by transposing the entire stomach through the posterior mediastinum to the cervical esophagus.[58] In this impressive series of 173 patients seen over a 21-year period, there were no graft failures, but there were nine deaths and a 20 percent incidence of anastomotic strictures.

In 1985, Arnold Coran at the Mott Children's Center in Michigan switched from using the colon conduit to gastric transposition through the posterior mediastinum. He cited conduit loss from poor blood supply and other complications with the colon. Twenty-six of his 41 patients with gastric transposition had esophageal atresia. He was satisfied with the operation despite a 36 percent incidence of anastomotic leak and feeding intolerance that required jejunal feeding in 20 percent of his patients. In response to concern about gastric reflux into the esophagus, as well as denervation of the stomach causing achlorhidria and possibly atrophic gastritis, Dr. Coran summed up the controversy this way: "There is no perfect substitute for the esophagus. We are not saying that the stomach is better than the colon, just that it works."[59]

Another option, laparoscopic-assisted gastric transposition, could be performed in small infants and allowed dissection of the posterior mediastinal tunnel under direct vision. This procedure offered a distinct advantage over blind dissection.[60]

Though a gastrostomy and the creation of a cervical esophagotomy preserve life and allow a later esophageal substitution, the delay itself can cause problems. Many of these infants develop "food aversion" despite sham feedings. Few surgeons have had the courage to perform any kind of esophageal bypass in the neonatal period, but D. K. Gupta and his associates of New Delhi performed gastric pull-up via the posterior mediastinum in 12 infants from 2 to 50 days of age with two deaths, one due to associated cardiac malformations and another due to septicemia at 41 days of age.[61] Other attempts at neonatal repair have included rare cases of colon substitution. C. Petterson of Göttenberg, Sweden, after reviewing all the current options for esophageal reconstruction, planned to do a colon bypass in a neonate when the opportunity occurred. His chance came on Christmas Eve 1959, when he was presented with a twenty-nine-hundred gram infant with a gap of four to five centimeters between the two ends of the atretic esophagus. Petterson immediately carried out a primary reconstruction with the transverse colon brought through the hiatus to the cervical esophagus, with an abdominal incision and a right thoracotomy. The distal end was hooked to the stomach. The colon was no larger than a lead pencil, but the fat-free mesentery allowed excellent visualization of the mesenteric vessels. When the child was one year of age, his mother said, "Now, he is just as normal as his brother."[62]

In 1965 at the Glasgow Children's Hospital, noting the "grave disadvantages" of a delayed operation, J. F. R. Bentley performed two colon bypass operations in neonates. One survived and was well at 18 months of age. The other died on the eighteenth postoperative day with tricuspid atresia and septal defects. Like Petterson, Bentley noted the advantages of easy visualization of the mesenteric vessels in the fat-free mesentery and the sterility of the neonatal colon.[63]

Colon bypass in the newborn never became popular, possibly because in the same issue of *Surgery* as Bentley's article P. W. Johnston of Los Angeles reported on stretching the esophagus with mercury bougies and subsequent anastomosis.[64] Various methods of elongating and saving the native esophagus by stretching the proximal esophagus with mercury bougies or with magnets placed in the proximal and distal pouches became popular.[65] In 1973, A. Livaditis was able to bring the esophagus together after a circular division of the muscular layer of the proximal pouch.[66] Many other surgeons devised ingenious techniques for lengthening the esophagus, but all required extensive mobilization of the distal pouch and the anastomosis was often under tension. They saved the native esophagus, but there were leaks, stricture, poor esophageal motility and a high incidence of gastro-esophageal reflux.[67]

The application of traction sutures to the two ends of the esophagus, by either an open operation or thoracoscopy, has also allowed direct esophageal anastomosis.[68] Spitz and Keily at the Great Ormond Street Hospital in London advocated primary anastomosis under "extreme" tension, with paralysis of the baby and ventilator support to save the native esophagus. Seventy-two percent of infants treated with this method developed strictures and 54 percent had gastroesophageal reflux.[69]

These and other results show that salvage of the native esophagus may not be completely desirable. V. Tomasselli and his associates in Milan studied esophageal function in 26 patients 8 to 28 years after surgery.[70] These patients had learned to cope with difficult swallowing, but all had disordered peristalsis, 50 percent had dysphagia and others had heartburn and aspiration pneumonia. The authors speculated that dissection of the distal pouch with denervation and traction contributed to a lack of peristalsis and poor clearing of acid from the distal esophagus.

The solution to the vexing and persistent problem of the long-gap esophageal atresia may well be an ingenious operation performed on a newborn infant by Craig T. Albanese and his associates in 1999.[71] The baby had a gap of 3.5 vertebrae between the two ends of the esophagus. The authors transposed a three-centimeter segment of transverse colon, based on the ascending branch of the left colic artery, through the esophageal hiatus into the posterior mediastinum. The segment was left open and four days later, through a right thoracotomy, the segment was found to have a good blood supply and was interposed

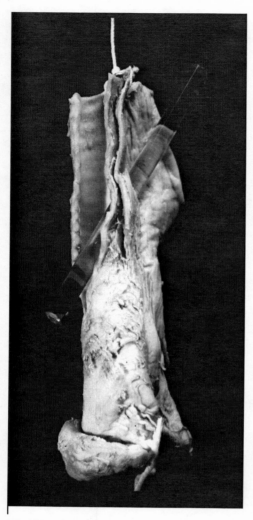

The first recorded case of congenital tracheo-esophageal fistula without atresia was not diagnosed until the autopsy. The child suffered coughing and choking spells until he died with pneumonia. Note the whalebone probe extending downward from the esophagus into the trachea (courtesy National Museum of Health and Medicine).

between the two ends of the esophagus with minimal mobilization of the esophageal segments. Ten years later, the child was swallowing normally and an esophagogram demonstrated minimal redundancy of the colon segment.

Dr. Albanese had done one more colonic interposition during the neonatal period with an 18-month follow-up.[72] This operation which avoids the disadvantages of a "spit fistula," long delay and anastomotic tension, may be the best solution to this problem. Some enterprising young surgeon should first clip the middle mesenteric artery with a laparoscope to increase collateral blood supply, then, a few days later, create a posterior mediastinal tunnel under direct vision and interpose the segment between the two ends of the esophagus. The challenge should be to create an esophagus so the baby can suckle at his mother's breast.

The "H"-Type Isolated Tracheo-Esophageal Fistula

The isolated, or "H"-type, tracheo-esophageal fistula is the rarest of esophageal anomalies, the most difficult to diagnose and the easiest to treat. The diagnosis is often delayed because the symptoms of chronic cough and frequent respiratory infections are usually attributed to other causes. One must think of this diagnosis when the cough immediately follows the ingestion of food and when there is intestinal distention from air forced into the fistula.

The first report of a patient with an isolated tracheo-esophageal fistula appeared in 1873. The infant had suffered with strangling and "lividity" at every attempt to nurse and also exhibited prominent flatulence. Death came at seven weeks of age. The autopsy revealed consolidation of the right lung, and a fistula was found between the trachea and esophagus half an inch below the cricoid cartilage. This unusual specimen was contributed to the Army Medical Museum.[73]

The first child to survive with an "H"-type fistula was born in 1931, but the diagnosis was not made until he was eight years old.[74] The surgeon was Charles J. Imperatori of New York, but the case history was written by the patient's father, a physician. The child had coughed and choked since birth and had difficulty with feedings. When X-rays demonstrated food retention in the stomach, a diagnosis of cardiospasm was made. At surgery, an adhesion across the pylorus was divided. Next, in conjunction with the diagnosis of cardiospasm, the patient underwent a series of esophageal dilatations. He also had a tonsillectomy at six years of age. When his symptoms continued, he swallowed a string to guide bougies for dilatation of "cardiospasm." The string passed through to his rectum, but his cough was aggravated and at bronchoscopy a part of the string was found in his right main bronchus. At this time, he was so desperately ill that a tracheotomy was necessary. Finally, at seven years of age, when he was acutely ill and coughing up a pint of sputum a day, another bronchoscopy revealed the tracheo-esophageal fistula. The position of the fistula was verified by passing a ureteral catheter from the trachea through the fistula into the esophagus. Two operations performed through the trachea were required to close the fistula. The prolonged course of this child is typical of early reported cases when the diagnosis was often made at an autopsy or via an exploratory thoracotomy.[75]

In 1965, D. A. Killen and H. B. Greenlee made the diagnosis in a six-and-a-half-year-old girl by passing a catheter through the fistula using a forward-viewing cystoscope. They repaired the fistula through a cervical incision. At that time, there were 115 cases in the literature; only 12 had been repaired through a cervical incision.[76] With improved radiological techniques, the correct preoperative diagnosis was made in 14 of 19 cases at the Toronto Children's Hospital.[77] The introduction of improved optics and ventilating bronchoscopes simplified the identification and localization of the fistula, so that a correct diagnosis could be made in every case.[78] Exact localization of the fistula allowed a transcervical repair in almost every instance.

CHAPTER 27

Wilms' Tumor

Childhood cancers, at the borderland between embryology and pathology, are totally different from adult cancers that mainly arise from endothelium in the breast, gastrointestinal tract and lung. In children, malignant tumors originate from connective, lymphoid or nervous tissue. Cancer in the adult, especially breast cancer, has been known since ancient times, but it wasn't until the eighteenth century that Percival Pott described cancer of the scrotum in chimney sweeps. There was little understanding of cancer until the nineteenth century, when researchers discovered abnormal cells in malignant tumors.

Physicians took no a real interest in childhood cancer until the middle of the twentieth century, when vaccines and antibiotics had subdued poliomyelitis, rheumatic fever and the most deadly infectious diseases. During the second half of the century, the incidence of cancer in all age groups rose, most notably in children. This increase may stem from environmental toxic chemicals such as the insecticide DDT and its by-products or generally increased exposure to all forms of radiation following the Second World War. As early as 1956, researchers in Britain observed an increased incidence of malignancy in children who had been exposed to diagnostic radiation while in utero.[1]

The history of Wilms' tumor of the kidney, from its early recognition through the first stumbling efforts at surgical treatment to the brilliant success of chemotherapy, is representative of all childhood cancers. Mark Ravitch and Bjorn Thomasson found scattered cases of kidney tumors in children starting in 1814, when Thomas Ranee of London reported on a 17-month-old child with an asymptomatic flank mass.[2] The tumor grew steadily; the child became febrile and late in the course developed hematuria. Another tumor appeared in the opposite flank and the child died 13 months after discovery of the lesion. At autopsy, the tumors occupied most of the abdomen and the larger mass was of a soft, medullary appearance. The diagnosis was "fungus hematoides of the kidneys." Most of these early reports of cancer involved children younger than two, but one concerned a seven-year-old boy. In this child, the enormous tumor weighed 31 pounds. This case, presented to the Pathological Society of London, was examined microscopically and said to be cancerous.

In 1880, while still at McGill University in Montreal, William Osler provided one of the best pathological descriptions of what we now call Wilms' tumor. In fact, one has to wonder why it isn't termed "Osler's tumor."[3] His first case was a 19-month-old boy, healthy until he was vaccinated, who subsequently developed severe gastrointestinal symptoms and died within 12 hours. The child's left kidney contained a grayish-white, spongy tumor, seven centimeters in diameter and composed of round cells the size of blood corpuscles, with a large nucleus, spindle cells and striped muscle cells. Osler commented: "I have rarely seen in any specimen the 'sarcous cells' so well marked."

His second case was a three-and-a-half-year-old girl with a soft tumor in her left hypochondrium. She suddenly collapsed and died with a "choking fit." At autopsy, Osler discovered a tumor measuring 15 by 7.5 centimeters in the right kidney. Soft, pulpy tumor tissue in the renal vein and metastases blocking the tricuspid and pulmonary valves in the heart explained her sudden death. Microscopically, the tumor was similar to his first case. Osler's diagnosis was striated myo-sarcoma of the kidney, although he described two types of cells and referred to it as a "mixed tumor." At the time of his report, Osler called these tumors "oncological curiosities" and had found six similar cases in the literature. The presence of tumor in the renal vein and in the heart illustrates the propensity of these tumors to metastasize via the bloodstream. These early cases are representative of the deadly, rapidly progressive natural history of childhood cancer.

Until the end of the nineteenth century, there was confusion about the cellular nature of renal tumors in children. Some were termed "sarcoma," others "carcinoma," "adeno-myosarcoma," "embryonal adenosarcoma" or "malignant embryoma." In 1894, F. V. Birsch-Hirschfeld pointed out that all these reports dealt with a mixed tumor with features of both carcinoma and sarcoma that developed in fetal life. The variations in ratios of the various elements accounted for the different terms.[4]

In 1899, Carl Max Wilhelm Wilms (1867–1918) published a monograph on various types of mixed tumors that included seven cases of kidney tumors in children.[5] Wilms graduated with a degree in medicine from the University of Bonn in 1890 and during the next four years studied pathology. During this time, he became interested in childhood cancers; he proposed that the cells in renal tumors found in children originated from embryonic tissue. His theory of a unified origin for these apparently diverse tumors led to the eponym "Wilms' tumor." Max Wilms worked with Frederich Trendelenburg in Leipzig, then became professor of surgery at Basel; in 1910, he was appointed to the chair of surgery in Heidelberg. He was also known for perineal prostatectomy and collapse therapy of pulmonary tuberculosis. In May 1918, Wilms performed a tracheotomy on a French prisoner of war who had diphtheria. Reportedly, the soldier lived, but Wilms died of diphtheria caught from his patient. Wilms was only 50 years old.[6]

Wilms' monograph was often quoted and his name became eponymous with all renal tumors in childhood, but there were still efforts to classify these tumors by their histolology. Edgar Garceau, a surgeon to St. Elizabeth's Hospital for Women in Boston, extensively reviewed embryonic tumors in a 1909 textbook devoted to kidney disease.[7] Garceau's extraordinary discussion differentiated the more benign rabdomyomas from the common malignant mixed tumors containing endothelial structures. Garceau argued that since these tumors were found in newborns and even fetuses and simultaneously in both kidneys, there was even more proof for their origin from early embryonic tissue. It would take another 60 years and the advent of multi-institutional studies before we realized that responses to treatment were related to the tumor's histology and that not all "Wilms'"tumors were the same.

The first successful nephrectomy for Wilms' tumor was performed by Mr. Thomas Richard Jessop (1837–1903) at the Leeds infirmary in England in 1877.[8] Mr. Jessop graduated from the Leeds School of Medicine in 1856 and became MRCS in 1859. He was the house surgeon at the Leeds infirmary in from 1860 until 1865 and five years later was appointed surgeon to the infirmary. Later, he served as Senior Vice President of the Royal College of Surgeons of England. The two-year-old boy who underwent the nephrectomy had hematuria and dysuria, suggesting bladder stones. Mr. Jessop "sounded" the bladder but found no stones. He diagnosed a malignant tumor of the kidney because the boy had a rapidly enlarging flank mass. At surgery, Mr. Jessop "peeled out" the tumor with finger dissection and ligated the ureter and renal vessels en masse. There was considerable venous hemorrhage. The kidney weighed 16 ounces and was "encephaloid" in appearance. The child died from recurrent tumor nine months later.

A year after Jessop's operation, Theodore Kocher of Bern, Switzerland — best known for surgery of the thyroid — removed the kidney from a child, who died two days later. In 1888, Czerny at Heidelberg reported on a nephrectomy for tumor in an 11-year-old child who died of septic peritonitis.[9]

Roswell Park, M.D., professor of surgery at the University of Buffalo, claimed to have performed the first successful nephrectomy in a child in 1885.[10] Born in Chicago, Park graduated from Northwestern University in 1876, interned at Cook County Hospital and became professor of surgery at the University of Buffalo in 1883. He is perhaps best known for operating on President William McKinley, who was shot and killed by an anarchist in 1901.[11]

Park's claim regarding the child nephrectomy was based on the survival of his patient for seven months at the time of his report in 1886 and the deaths of patients in previously reported cases. The child was perfectly well when a nurse noted an enlargement on his left side. Over a month later, Dr. Park examined the child under anesthesia and found a firm tumor the size of a child's head in the left flank. He aspirated 15 cc of a brownish liquid from the tumor. The liquid contained para-albumin and cells of the type found in renal cysts. A month later, the child was again examined under anesthesia and more fluid was aspirated from the mass. By that time, the child was deteriorating and the tumor had grown so large that he needed a suspensory belt to support it.

The operation was performed ten days later under "strict antiseptic conditions." The boy was first anesthetized with chloroform, but ether was substituted halfway through the operation. Dr. Park shelled out the tumor, then doubly ligated and seared the pedicle with thermocautery. The tumor weighed nearly four pounds and was a fibrocystic degeneration of the kidney. There was no mention of a microscopic examination, so we don't know if this was a Wilms' tumor. The entire operation lasted only 45 minutes and only 15 cc of blood was lost. After surgery, the boy's fever climbed to 106 degrees but was successfully treated with injections of aconite root and tincture of digitalis. Within two hours, his temperature fell to normal and the boy recovered. He was the "picture of health" seven months later.

At the end of his paper, Dr. Parks remarked that the abdominal incision wasn't his choice but that the tumor was so large it required a transperitoneal incision. This was prophetic, because in the future the transperitoneal incision proved superior to the usual flank approach to kidney tumors.

A report in 1892 by Robert Abbe, at the Babies' Hospital in New York, is of particular interest because Abbe gives us a glimpse of postoperative care during this period and the confusion surrounding the diagnosis of these tumors.[12] The tumor in the first child described in the report, a two-year-old, filled the entire right side of the abdomen. It was shelled out by finger dissection through a long transverse lumbar incision. The author stressed the need for swathing the child in cotton batting to retain heat during the operation and to keep the child in a steep, head-down Trendelenburg position to minimize blood loss. After surgery, the child was sustained with oral milk and lime water mixed with thirty drops of whisky every two hours. The microscopic diagnosis of "carcinoma sarcomatosum" illustrates the confusion of classifying kidney tumors in children. The child was well a year and a half later.

The second child, aged one year and two months, had a rapidly growing tumor that when removed weighed seven and a half pounds. Dr. Abbe noted huge veins over the surface of the tumor that almost precluded its removal, but with the patient in a steep Trendelenburg position he was able to bluntly dissect the tumor and control bleeding with gauze pressure. In this case the tumor was connected to the kidney by a pedicle and he was able to separate the tumor from the kidney. The operation appeared to have been a hemi-nephrectomy. The child was under ether for about an hour and a half but "suffered little shock." Postoperatively he was kept in the Trendelenburg position, swaddled in cotton batting and sustained with hypodermics of brandy and strychnine. The child "rallied beautifully" and returned home five weeks following the operation. The diagnosis was "rhabdo-myo-sarcoma" and the bit of attached kidney was free from tumor. It would be nearly 70 years before partial nephrectomy with salvage of renal tissue became an acceptable operation.

Early in the twentieth century radical nephrectomy was recognized as the treatment of choice, but in 1915 at the University of Freiburg there was a report of X-ray treatments given in the postoperative period to three children, two of whom had died by the time of the report. The author recommended X-ray treatments as useful if given early after nephrectomy and in high doses.[13]

In that same year, Arthur Friedlander at the Cincinati General Hospital treated a four-year-old boy with a "growth so large that no surgeon was willing to undertake its removal."[14] The boy was given 20 X-ray treatments a week apart over the course of five months. At first, the tumor shrank and the child gained weight. The tumor then increased in size and the boy died after a bout of measles complicated by bronchopneumonia. At autopsy, there were metastases in the liver and lungs, but a large portion of the tumor was necrotic, apparently as a result of the X-ray treatments.

In 1941, William E. Ladd, at that time Chief of Surgical Services at the Boston Children's Hospital, and Robert R. White published one of the most definitive articles ever written on Wilms' tumor.[15] The authors described the clinical course, diagnosis and pathology of children with Wilms' tumors. The article made mention for the first time of intravenous pyelography in the differential diagnosis of Wilms' tumor from neuroblastoma by the outward or downward displacement of the kidney caused by neuroblastomas. In their extensive review of the literature, the authors found 563 reported cases with only 26 cures. They specifically addressed the issue of pre-operative radiation: "From a statistical point of view, then it can be stated that the chance of survival for a patient with embryoma of the kidney is far greater if the policy of immediate operation is adopted rather than the policy of delayed operation following roentgen therapy." Dr. Ladd noted the friability of the tumor after radiation and suggested that the delay resulted in metastases.

At the time of the report, the authors had performed 23 nephrectomies for tumor with no hospital mortality. This excellent result was attributable to an immediate operation by a vertical transperitoneal incision with ligation of the renal vessels prior to mobilizing the tumor. This operative approach continues to be the choice of most surgeons. Dr. Ladd had no objection to postoperative radiation but doubted its benefit. In their reported series of 60 cases, 18 were still living and 14 children appeared to have been cured. In 16 patients under one year of age, 50 percent were cured. This indication that young children had a better prognosis was later confirmed by Wilms' tumor study groups.

Between 1940 and 1947, 38 children with Wilms' tumors were treated at the Boston Children's Hospital, with a survival rate of 47.3 percent. Dr. Gross stressed several details that may seem minor but that led to this improvement:

It is important to have as little trauma as possible in the handling of these patients, because repeated palpation of the mass or squeezing of the tumor may discharge malignant cells into the blood stream and give rise to distant metastases which vitiate any possibility of a permanent cure. Aspiration biopsy has been recommended by some for confirming the diagnosis by microscopic study. This procedure is a thoroughly unsound one, since puncture of the mass may seed the peritoneal cavity or the surrounding tissues with neoplasm and spoil the surgeon's opportunity for complete removal of a lesion, the prognosis of which otherwise might have been favorable. We abandoned this procedure more than twenty years ago.... It is firmly believed that these subjects should be operated upon very promptly. There is little excuse for having them lie in the hospital for several days or even weeks before surgery is undertaken. While we do not regard such operations in the category of emergencies, we have found that it is generally possible to admit the patient, gather the important data and surgically remove the neoplasm within four or five hours.

Dr. Gross was emphatic in his opposition to pre-operative radiation. He said: "We began in 1949 to give such irradiation to every other patient who entered our service. Two to three thousands roentgens were given over the presenting mass, in divided doses extending over a period of ten to fifteen days. Within a year it became so evident that the fatality rate was skyrocketing above former figures, that we felt completely sure that such irradiation before operation was very detrimental; we have therefore completely abandoned it." He went on to say, "During the last twenty years at the Children's Hospital, the large size of the tumor has never been considered a contraindication to operation."[16] He stressed the need for a long transperitoneal incision and immediate ligation of the renal vessels prior to mobilizing the kidney. Pediatric surgeons followed these principles for many years. Today, the issue of preoperative chemotherapy for "tumors too big to remove" and needle biopsy is again on the agenda. Some have asked, "Is the tumor too large or is the incision too small?"

At mid-century, the cure rate for Wilms' tumor remained constant at 30 to 40 percent. There were attempts to surgically remove or irradiate lung metastases, but there was little hope for children with recurrent or metastatic disease until a miracle happened. The miracle was actinomycin-D, an antibiotic derived from the bacteria *Streptomyces parvulus* by Dr. Selim A. Waksman in 1941.[17] Another cancer treatment, chemotherapy, commenced when nitrogen mustard — a poison gas used in the First World War — was found to temporarily reduce tumor mass in patients with Hodgkins' disease. Intravenous nitrogen mustard was tried in children with metastatic Wilms' tumor, with no success. Dr. Willis Potts, Surgeon in Chief at the Children's Memorial Hospital in Chicago, said: "The child who in spite of widespread metastases is happy and still has a good appetite, will, I believe, receive just as much benefit from a nice, juicy nitrogen-rich hot dog touched with mustard to taste and taken by mouth as from nitrogen mustard injected into a vein."[18]

Sidney Farber (1903–1973), the first full-time pathologist at the Boston Children's Hospital, reported the first real success with chemotherapy in childhood cancer.[19] The drug aminopterin, a folic acid antagonist, produced temporary remissions in ten children with leukemia. As a result of this initial success, Farber persuaded a charitable club to establish the Children's Cancer Research Foundation at the Boston Children's Hospital in 1948. This would become the Sidney Farber Cancer Institute.

In 1955, Farber's group discovered that actinomycin-D potentiated radiation therapy and was effective in treating Wilms' tumors.[20] Even prior to Farber's report in 1960, we were able to obtain actinomycin directly from the Eli Lilly Pharmaceutical Company. The drug, a yellow powder, was dissolved in alcohol and given intravenously over five days. We gave the first dose prior to surgery and the second during the operation and then one dose daily for three more days. The idea was to destroy any malignant cells that broke free from the tumor during surgery. We were amazed to see lung metastases melt away and children survive. Then came the hard lesson of drug toxicity. One of my patients was an older girl; I calculated the dose based on her body weight, rather than surface area. The toxic overdose depressed her bone marrow and she died. It became apparent that hematologists were better equipped to administer these toxic drugs and the specialty of hematology-oncology was born.

At the 1966 meeting of the American Surgical Association, Dr. Orvar Swenson, Chief Surgeon at the Children's Memorial Hospital in Chicago, reported on his spectacular success in treating metastatic Wilms' tumors with a combination of radiation, actinomycin and (when necessary) surgical resection. Five of his patients were alive and free from disease two to five years following pulmonary lobectomy or pneumonectomy. At the same meeting, C. E. Koop from the Philadelphia Children's Hospital and E. J. Beattie from Memorial Hospital in New York reported the successful treatment with actinomycin-D of children with bilateral Wilms' tumor and those with pulmonary metastases.[21]

The survival rate of children with Wilms' tumors dramatically improved, but some patients required multiple courses of therapy; drug and radiation toxicity became an increasing problem. No single institution had enough patients to determine optimum treatment. The National Wilms' Tumor Study Group (also known as NITWITS) was formed from a consortium of institutions to refine treatment schedules and if possible to reduce treatment in low-risk patients. In the trial, which commenced in 1969, 359 of 606 patients were randomized.[22] Completed in 1974, the study demonstrated that children under two years of age whose tumor was confined to the kidney and completely removed had a 90 percent survival rate without radiation. Children with more advanced tumors and metastases fared better with a combination of actinomycin and vincristine, a drug derived from the Madagascar periwinkle, *Cantharanulus roseus*. The study also demonstrated that Wilms' tumor was not a single entity but that there were different pathologic types. The degree of cellular anaplasia and the presence of sarcomatous tissue as well as lymph node involvement carried a poor prognosis.

As a result of the first study, we made a greater effort to remove all lymph nodes from the iliac fossa to the diaphragm. The second National Wilms' Tumor Study Group enlisted 755 children; and the third, 1,439 patients. These studies demonstrated a better than 90 percent two-year, relapse-free rate for children with favorable histology and no distant metastases when treated with a combination of surgery, vincristine and actinomycin. The relapse-free rate for children with "unfavorable" histology was less than 70 percent, even with the addition of more chemotherapy agents. The improved cure rates came with the additional hazard of pulmonary fungus infections, liver fibrosis and even death from drug toxicity. Doxorubicin combined with irradiation to the chest resulted in cardiac myopathy that on occasion led to a heart transplant.[23]

Bilateral Wilms' tumors presented the additional problem of salvaging renal tissue. With improved imaging techniques, ultrasonography and CT scans, more bilateral tumors were found at the time of initial diagnosis. Prior to chemotherapy, resection of the largest tumor combined with radiation to the opposite kidney resulted in a surprising number of cures, suggesting that these lesions had a lesser degree of malignancy. Swenson in the 1960s removed the kidney with the largest tumor and did a partial nephrectomy on the side with the smallest lesion. After Weiner's report of bilateral partial nephrectomy or "tumorectomy," many surgeons attempted to save both kidneys by shelling out the tumor from normal kidney.[24] After 1982, surgeons at the Great Ormond Street Hospital in London first did core biopsies of the tumors, then administered chemotherapy and later operated. Forty-three patients had tumors with "favorable" histology and three "unfavorable." In 20 kidneys, the tumor either progressed in size or shrank less than 50 percent. The survival rate of 74 percent in this series was only slightly better with preoperative chemotherapy.[25] Results from the most recent National Wilms Tumor Study Group again emphasized the poor prognosis in tumors with anaplastic histology.[26] There were 27 kidneys with anaplastic histology among 189 patients with synchronous bilateral tumors. These patients had a much worse prognosis, and the study also demonstrated that a core needle biopsy was not a reliable indicator of anaplasia. In a further attempt to define those children at increased risk for recurrence, the fifth NWTS study demonstrated that tumors in which there was a loss of heterozygozity for chromosomes 16q and 1p had a poor prognosis.[27]

The desire to preserve renal function led a group of surgeons in Rome to carry out partial nephrectomy or enucleation of the tumor in a select group of children with unilateral tumors that had favorable histology.[28] They treated their patients with actinomycin and vincristine preoperatively and removed the tumor with at least a half centimeter of normal kidney. Their results suggest that children with favorable histology fared as well with this renal sparing procedure as with more drastic surgery.

The controversy over treating Wilms' tumors assumed international proportions when in 1969 the European International Society of Pediatric Oncology commenced clinical trials with pre-operative chemotherapy and delayed surgery. In a 25-year, single-institution study, M. L. Capra saw little difference in the results of immediate versus delayed surgery and an overall survival rate of 90 percent. Others on the Continent believed that preoperative chemotherapy could potentially reduce tumor size and rupture with spillage.[29] A Japanese study group formed in 1982 used the U.S. protocol of surgery followed by chemotherapy and also reported an overall five-year survival rate of 87.8 percent.[30]

Few diseases in the history of medicine have had such intense, cooperative study as Wilms' tumor. At times, it appeared as if the decisions made by the study group were pragmatic and arbitrary, but the results speak for themselves. The improvement in survival while minimizing the side effects of treatment has been astounding and has led to a not-so-subtle change in the surgeon's role. Until about 1970, patients with tumors were referred directly to a surgeon, who with dispatch removed the tumor, initiated chemotherapy and ordered radiation. Now, oncologists see the patients first, order a prolonged workup, and rather grudgingly refer the patient for an operation. Oncologists still require a surgeon to perform biopsies, insert central venous lines and treat some of the more disastrous complications of chemotherapy, however. At one time, in a discussion of surgery versus more chemotherapy, referring to a child who suffered cardiac myopathy, I shouted at an oncologist, "No child ever had to have a heart transplant as a result of surgery." The oncology team approach also includes specially trained nurses and social workers to look after the physical and emotional well-being of the patient and his or her family.

Dr. Audrey Evans, who was involved in the very first work on actinomycin-D and serves as head of hematology-oncology at the Philadelphia Children's Hospital, became concerned about the families of children who spent weeks and even months in the hospital for cancer treatment. Her concern led in 1974 to the founding of the first Ronald McDonald House, a home, where families could live while their children were hospitalized. Dr. Edward Baum, a pediatric oncologist at Children's Memorial Hospital in Chicago, together with the father of one of his patients, founded a not-for-profit organization to open the second Ronald McDonald House. They then formed the National Advisory Board of Children's Oncology Services, Inc., which helped found Ronald MacDonald Houses for families of hospitalized children near almost every children's hospital. There are also summer camps and trips arranged just for children with cancer. All these activities have contributed to the well-being of cancer-stricken children and have raised the public's awareness of childhood cancer.

Sad to say, children whose Wilms' tumors have been "cured" continue to face long-term complications, including an increased risk for a secondary malignancy, decreased fertility, scoliosis, decreased bone growth, and liver and lung fibrosis.[31] Though we remember Drs. Jessop, Ladd and Gross for their pioneering efforts in surgery for Wilms' tumor, the real heroes are Selim Waksman, Sidney Farber and all those who worked on the protocols and painstakingly analyzed the data for the National Wilms' Tumor Study Groups. The story will not end until we can cure the tumor and spare the child.

CHAPTER 28

History of Intussusception

SIGMUND H. EIN, M.D., *AND* ARLENE EIN, R.N.

During Roman times (400 B.C.E.), the word "intussusception" was derived from the words *intus* (within) and *suscipere* (to receive).[1] According to Hippocrates, there were attempts to reduce an intussusception by the injection of air or oil into the rectum using a bronze bellow to "untangle the bowel," and Praxagoras of Cos even advised an operation to solve this problem. However, Littré claimed the rectal injection was really being done for an ileus and the latter operation for a mechanical obstruction. Apparently, during these times and for these medical incidents there was never any mention of intussusception (bowel invagination or involution, the passage of gross blood per rectum, or the fact that this type of bowel problem was peculiar to infants and children).[2]

In the early 1600s, in his six-volume textbook of surgery, Nang Ken-tung described an intussusception in a five-month-old baby with an egg-sized mass in the abdomen. He said this baby was so sick, with a dark face, staring eyes and cold lips, nose, hands and feet, that it was unable to eat, passed dark bloody stools and subsequently died.[3] In the mid-1600s, Paul Barbette of Amsterdam was the first to describe an intussusception as "intestinal invagination" (a most apt term). He also suggested that laparotomy and manual reduction was preferable to letting these patients die.[4] In 1677, J. C. Peyer was the first to clearly record the clinical differentiation between a small bowel volvulus and an intussusception. He also described the lymphoid follicles of the terminal ileum (now referred to as Peyer's patches) as the pathogenesis of an intussusception.[5]

In 1742, Cornelius Velse performed the first successful operative reduction of an intussusception in an adult.[6] In 1761, Morgagni published in his huge book cases of intussusception that he said were caused by worms; he even described an intussusception in a dog.[7] Twenty years later, G. Langstaff (in discussing Herrin's successful operative reduction of an intussusception in France) commented that both medicine and surgery did not help treat intussusception and therefore the best chance of cure was the spontaneous sloughing of the invaginated portion of bowel.[8] A most radical and rare solution for this problem!

At the end of the 1700s, Hunter was the first to describe in detail what he called an "introsusception," his word for intussusception. He said it happens most frequently in the first 15 years of life, is uncommon in older people, never occurs only in the colon and can be differentiated from a rectal prolapse if and when it presents at the anal margin. The suggested treatments at that time were bleeding and quicksilver, to which Hunter added emetics to reverse the peristalsis of the gut (which he considered important in the pathogenesis of intussusception), followed by purgatives if the former failed. Despite these ideas and attempted reductions from below with enemas, infant intussusception remained almost universally fatal into the early 1800s. Hunter reported a case of a classic ileocolic intussusception in a nine-month-old infant who subsequently died; the pathological specimen can be found in the Hunterian Museum at the Royal College of Surgeons of England.[9]

Within the first four decades of the 1800s, three separate authors — Blalock, Mitchell and Gorham — described the first pneumatic air enema (AE) reduction. However, these cases were not well documented; some involved adults, and many were doubted.[10] At about the same time, John R. Wilson reported the first successful operative reduction of an intussusception in an adult in the United States. Like Hunter, he called it "a case of introsusception." Samuel Mitchell in England reported the first successful AE reduction of a pediatric intussusception using an enema tube and "a common pair of bellows."[12] H. Hachmann reported that Gersonon performed the first laparotomy for an intussusception in a 12-week infant, but the gangrenous intussusception was perforated during the attempted manual reduction and the infant died. Both Hachmann and T. Spencer-Wells also separately attempted laparotomy for reduction and/or resection of an intussusception, but without success.[13]

In 1864, David Greig, a surgeon from Scotland, was the first to suggest strict criteria for the diagnosis of an intussusception. He also tried to persuade others that his use of the common fireplace hand bellows successfully reduced four out of five pediatric intussusceptions. He wrote: "Contrary to our expectations, the air passed readily into the bowel and seemed to give the child great relief." Other methods to treat intussusception at that time were belladonna, long bougies per rectum, cold-water effervescent powder, electricity, hypertonic saline and opium. Needless to say, these were not very successful, and intussusception remained fatal in most infants and children.[14] Several years later, English surgeon Jonathon Hutchinson performed the first successful operative reduction of an ileocolic intussusception in a two-year-old infant under chloroform anesthesia after a failed hydrostatic reduction; Hutchinson said the procedure was "an extremely simple one and had not taken more than two or three minutes." Nonetheless, operative intervention remained quite hazardous.[15]

In 1876, Harald Hirschsprung of Copenhagen started reporting his personal cases of hydrostatic reduction of intussusception, but unfortunately, mortality was also common with this method. Hilton Fagge and Henry Havse at Guy's Hospital in England clearly described the proper mechanism for manual reduction of an intussusception: "Pulling at the (proximal) end was quite ineffectual, though as much force as was considered justifiable was exerted in this way. Under a kind of kneading movement, however, combined with circular pressure upon the farthest (distal) intussuscepted part of the gut, it began to yield, and when once started, the process went on readily, until the last part of the intestine was reached."[16] Leichtenstern pointed out that the mortality in reported cases at that time was 88 percent in the first six months of life, 82 percent in the second six months and 72 percent from two to ten years.[17]

In 1885, Frederick Treves (whose sister died of an intussusception) advised no oral intake and the gradual administration of warm-water enemas in a relaxed child (by opium or chloroform anesthesia) as the initial treatment for an intussusception. Failure of enema reduction prompted him to proceed immediately to laparotomy under chloroform anesthesia using strict antiseptic precautions; this operative treatment remains almost unchanged to the present day. The mortality rate for his first 33 cases of intussusception was 73 percent. He found that those undergoing an easy manual reduction had a mortality of 30 percent compared with those who had a difficult reduction, where the mortality was 91 percent. He proposed that the resection of a gangrenous intussusception should have stomas rather than a primary anastomosis.

Treves described intussusception as responsible for 30 percent of all cases of intestinal obstruction, distinguished idiopathic intussusception (mostly seen in children) from that caused by a pathological lead point (PLP; that is, a polyp, Meckel's diverticulum or lymphoma), pointed out that intestinal obstruction and strangulation need not coexist, discussed chronic intussusception, and recognized transient small bowel intussusception, antegrade and retrograde intussusception, and the passage of a gangrenous intussusception per rectum. Moreover, he believed the treatment of intussusception should be prompt and active.[18] He certainly had a good understanding of the disease.

A popular area of investigation was the study of pressure tolerances of the human colon during intussusception reduction. W. E. Forest of New York questioned whether liquid, gas or both was the best agent to use for the hydrostatic and pneumatic methods of intussusception reduction; he later calculated that six pounds of pressure per square inch was acceptable in attempting to reduce an intussusception by these means. He advised "...laying the child in the hallway, inserting the enema tube and slowly ascending the stairs, enema bag in hand, exercising caution after ascending ten feet"; thus started the "battle of the pressures."[19] Mortimer in England and Nordentoft in Denmark injected colons of adult and newborn cadavers, obtaining perforations from five feet and upward. Nordentoft later reported treating 204 of 419 cases of intussusception by barium enema alone; he stated that the hydrostatic pressure used was generally one to two meters (six feet) and it should never exceed the latter.[20]

In 1893, Nicholas Senn in Chicago was one of the first to perform experimental studies on intussusception. He found that manually produced intussusceptions in cats would reduce spontaneously if not fixed by sutures. He reduced these experimental intussusceptions by insufflation of hydrogen gas into the rectum; he considered this safer than fluid and therefore the preferred method of therapy in patients. He said the reduction should never exceed two pounds per square inch, unlike Forest's six pounds. Senn's studies were the only ones at that time dealing specifically with the mechanism of reduction by gas or fluid pressure and aimed at establishing the utility and safety of this method. Furthermore, Senn's studies were the only ones before those of Ravitch and Robert M. McCune, Jr., 60 years later (in 1948), which concluded that "...the 3 or 3½ feet of pressure used in patients would appear to provide a safe margin."[21]

In 1897, in the first edition of his textbook *Diseases of Infancy and Childhood*, L. Emmet Holt said the treatment of intussusception was insufflation with the bellows and simultaneous manipulation through the abdominal wall. His method was to give an enema, holding the reservoir four to five feet above the patient and raising it if necessary as high as six to eight feet. If this failed, an operation was necessary. Holt reported only one bowel perforation in his 225 cases of using air or fluid.[22] Meanwhile, Clubbe reported the first successful resection of an intussusception in Australia.[23] As the 1800s came to an end, it was understood and accepted that successful reduction of an intussusception by the hydrostatic and pneumatic methods depended on the pressure exerted, and various devices were being developed to capitalize on the growing popularity of this form of treatment even though debate still existed over the exact amount of pressure exerted at how many feet above the patient.

By the beginning of the 1900s, hydrostatic reduction of an intussusception was widely accepted, though that did not prevent some enterprising and daring surgeons from still trying operative reduction. The debate about the merits of dry versus wet taxis in the reduction of intussusception continued; dry taxis meant the kneading of the intussusception out of the intussuscipiens, and wet taxis meant reduction with a water enema. Some felt these measures could be undertaken at home, and others felt they should be performed in a hospital.[24] In 1905, Hirschsprung had collected 107 cases of hydrostatic reduction (which at that time was fatal in over 80 percent of cases), with a reported mortality rate of only 35 percent. These results were so superior to those previously reported that his contemporaries doubted his conclusions. His technique was superior to operative treatment but still met with limited acceptance until the late 1900s. Meanwhile, the drift toward the surgical treatment of intussusception was under way, and as surgical techniques slowly improved, so did their results, particularly in the United States, Britain and Australia. At the same time, Scandinavian interest in hydrostatic pressure reduction continued.[25]

The first successful resection of an intussusception in the United States was reported by Peterson.[26] In 1909, Parry and Rutherford individually reported successes with an anastomosis around an irreducible intussusception, leaving the latter in situ. This method was revived by Montgomery and Musil in 1930 and has since been referred to as the Montgomery operation. At the same time, Lehman first used bismuth enemas for diagnostic imaging, but he did not report these findings until 1914, one year after William E. Ladd in Boston reported the same thing. In retrospect, many consider this the most important advancement in the diagnosis and non-operative treatment of intussusception.[27] However, Ladd was convinced that this procedure was only a good diagnostic device. In the same paper in which he reported the first use of X-ray in the diagnosis of intussusception, along with the first published roentgenologic photographs of an intussusception, he also reported that the "improved" operative mortality for intussusception from the Boston Children's Hospital was still 45 percent.[28]

In 1921, Perren observed that scattered lymphocytes in the jejunal wall became more concentrated Peyer's patches in the ileum and they formed a lymphatic ring as they approached the ileocecal valve. He focused his attention on this lymphatic tissue as an explanation for and possible cause of intussusception. It is unfortunate that his work was neglected for so long, because viral infections became implicated as the ultimate cause of lymphoid hyperplasia, causing the distal ileal circular lymphoid tissue to be the non-pathologic lead point of most ileocolic intussusceptions. Perren correctly observed that the large majority of intussusceptions were caused by viral illness that did not need a surgical correction.[29] Around this time, Australia was quite involved in the non-operative treatment of intussusception; Hipsley published a series of 100 cases, 62 of which were treated by hydrostatic saline enema with only one death. Ironically, S. Monrad (previously an assistant to Hirschsprung in Copenhagen) continued to advocate laparotomy and manual reduction of the intussusception as the primary mode of treatment.[30]

Meanwhile, the use of contrast barium enema (BE) to allow fluoroscopic control of the hydrostatic pressure reduction was the natural consequence of the introduction of X-rays, and it became popular in Scandinavia (Olsson and Pallin), South America, France (Pouliquen) and the United States (Retan and Stephens). Despite this newly described ability of the radiologist to not only diagnose an intussusception but also treat it by hydrostatic reduction (and watch the attempted reduction by fluoroscopy), surgery remained the primary mode of treatment in the United States. Even though G. M. Retan had used contrast BE and fluoroscopy in the hydrostatic reduction of intussusception, he also wrote: "The injection of gas into the bowel in the hope of relieving an intussusception is a dangerous procedure. First, it is difficult to control the pressure used. Secondly, the procedure is a blind one, and it is impossible to know what is occurring in the abdomen. This method is a relic of the pre-surgical age and should not be used."[31]

When Mark Ravitch was a junior resident in 1939, he became enthusiastic about investigating the hydrostatic pressure reduction technique of Clubbe, Hipsley and Hirschsprung (and his successors in Scandinavia).[32] Within ten years, Ravitch and McCune (who started as a medical student and contributed to Ravitch's laboratory experiments and clinical analyses) were still reporting a surgical mortality for intussusception of 32 percent. However, their laboratory research focused attention on non-operative fluoroscopic hydrostatic BE reduction as the primary mode of therapy for intussusception. They produced evidence from their animal experiments to repudiate criticisms that hydrostatic reduction of intussusceptions risked perforation or reduction of non-viable bowel, and even showed that these reductions were possible up to 36 hours after the intussusception started and were safer and the patients had shorter hospital stays and fewer complications.[33]

In spite of the research and publications of Ravitch and McCune in Boston, both William E. Ladd and his successor Robert Gross steadfastly maintained that operative reduction was the definitive treatment for intussusception. Operative reduction at that time was done by using two fingers through a small abdominal incision; if the intussusception was irreducible, enterostomy or a bypass was regarded as safer than resection. To prove their point, Gross reported 702 cases of intussusception over 40 years at the Boston Children's Hospital, showing a gradual decline in the mortality rate from 60 percent in 1900 to zero in 92 cases from 1948 to 1950.[34] Additional reports up to 1958 from Ravitch and McCune showed that hydrostatic BE reduction had reached success rates of up to 75 percent with a zero mortality. This non-operative method persisted and finally became the primary, safest and most successful means of treating intussusception.[35]

By the mid–1900s, Zachary Cope's text describing the symptoms and signs of intussusception remained unparalleled in its clarity and completeness.[36] In 1954, at the First Annual Congress of the British Association of Pediatric Surgeons in London, Robert B. Zachary presented a paper highlighting two serious problems that frequently confronted the pediatric surgeon at that time: "...the management of a gangrenous intussusception and the role of conservative treatment." He further suggested that "...a selective policy of conservative or operative management was appropriate ... [but] ... the procedure should be in responsible hands and the child must be under the direct care of the surgeon who may have to operate."[37] Radiologists like E. S. Fiorito in 1959 and J. Z. Guo in 1986 continued to be at the forefront of successful non-operative treatment of intussusception (reaching a 90 percent reduction rate), achieving further advances in technique with air used as the contrast medium (pneumatic reduction).[38]

At roughly the same time, during the 1970s, there was a shift in the operative practice of intussusception to resection and primary anastomosis.[39] In 1977, L. F. Burke and E. Clarke introduced ultrasonography in the United States for screening, diagnosis and monitoring the reduction of an intussusception. This combination of U.S. screening and pneumatic reduction (air enema, or AE) increased the success rate to 92 percent with a lower incidence of complications.[40] By the end of the 1970s, the mortality rate from intussusception in the United States was 6.4 (0.00064 percent) per 1 million live births.[41]

In 1986, Guo introduced the concept of delayed repeat enema attempts, which further increased the non-operative success rate for intussusception, finally making surgery a backup form of therapy to radiologic-guided reduction.[42] By the 1990s, laparoscopy was being used for diagnosis and, in some cases, treatment of intussusception, but this new mode of therapy after a failed enema reduction only achieved an overall reduction rate of 50 to 65 percent.[43] By the end of the 1990s, A. D. Sandler and the group from Toronto showed that repeated attempts at enema reduction increased the reduction rate of irreducible intussusceptions by 60 percent. The remaining irreducible intussusceptions, therefore, frequently required surgical resection.[44] The intussusception mortality rate in the United States dropped even more to 2.3 (0.00023 percent) per 1 million live births.[45] Now, after successful AE reduction, patients were being sent home after a short period of observation.[46]

Around the turn of the twentieth century, rotavirus vaccine was implicated as a direct causal link to intussusception and its routine use was therefore withdrawn. However, many studies throughout the world have since shown that there is no epidemiologic evidence for such an association.[47] The medical profession realized that pediatric intussusception will continue to occur unless viral illnesses are eliminated, as well as all of the PLP. Realistically, the best one can expect is the current 90 percent success rate for enema reduction (including repeated attempts), thus eliminating approximately 10 percent that are unsuccessfully reduced through this procedure but are found spontaneously reduced when operated on. That should only leave the following intussusceptions for operation: those that require difficult manual reduction; resection for ischemic, gangrenous, and necrotic bowel; repair of a perforation from the attempted BE or AE; and resection of a PLP.[48]

CHAPTER 29

A Historical Review
of Hirschsprung's Disease

SIGMUND H. EIN, M.D., *AND* ARLENE EIN, R.N.

The people involved in the discovery and clarification of Hirschsprung's disease (congenital, aganglionic megacolon) are some of the most famous and recognizable names in the world of medicine and surgery, especially pediatric surgery. By the year 2000, more than five hundred articles had been published to clarify Hirschsprung's disease, despite the fact that this bowel problem took a number of centuries to be properly understood, diagnosed and treated.[1] Generally speaking, since aganglionic megacolon was initially not differentiated from other types of megacolon (idiopathic and chronic constipation), the literature up to 1950 was muddled by the inclusion of inappropriate material.[2]

Probably the first known description of the clinical pathology of megacolon appears in the text *Observations Anatomico-Chirurgicarum Centuria*, published in 1691 by Frederick Ruysch, a Dutch professor of anatomy, botany and surgery.[3] Ruysch made mention of an extremely dilated colon in a number of patients.[4] However, later on T. Ehrenpreis felt the clinical and autopsy findings in some of these patients did not produce enough evidence to make the definitive diagnosis of Hirschsprung's disease.[5] Little appeared in the literature about this bowel problem until 1825, when Parry reported the earliest autopsy findings of a narrow rectosigmoid and a dilated proximal colon, indicators for Hirschsprung's disease. The autopsy subject was an adult with chronic constipation who died after an acute colonic obstruction.[6]

In 1830, Harald Hirschsprung was born in Copenhagen, where his German father owned a tobacco factory. Harald completed his medical studies at the University of Copenhagen in 1855 and interned at the Royal Maternity Hospital, where he began his lifelong concern with pediatrics.[7] His doctoral thesis dealt with esophageal and small bowel atresia. As a pediatrician, he was interested in, and wrote about, a wide range of neonatal problems that still posed difficulties for pediatric surgeons in the twentieth century.[8] These lesser-known writings were of equal or even greater importance than his description of the disease that now bears his name. As a matter of fact, more than 20 reports written before January of 1886 preceded his classic description of congenital megacolon.[9]

Despite a certain natural timidity, Hirschsprung was accorded deference when attending medical congresses, usually accompanied by his two pretty daughters. Everyone at the prestigious meeting of the Society of Pediatrics in Berlin listened intently when he presented his paper titled "Constipation in Newborns Due to Dilatation and Hypertrophy of the Colon." This paper concerned two infants who had suffered with constipation and abdominal distention from birth. The first child died at 11 months of age with what appeared to be enterocolitis. At autopsy, the sigmoid and transverse colon, but not the rectum, were enormously dilated and hypertrophied.[10] Hirschsprung offered no definite opinion as to the etiology or treatment of the disease in these two newborn cases, though the title of his talk indicated his attitude toward this problem.[11] He believed this was a new, rare, congenital condition in infants and children, because he thought it inconceivable that any other mechanism could produce a megacolon so soon after birth. This view, shared by many medical authors of his time, soon became known as the malformation theory.

Of more significance, though Hirschsprung noted the narrow rectosigmoid, he did not understand its significance and never pursued this observation.[12] Instead, he focused (as did subsequent authors) on the dilated

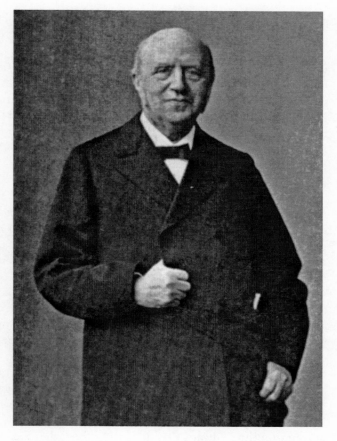

Harald Hirschsprung, the Danish pediatrician who described the clinical and pathologic findings in the disease that is named for him. Dr. Hirschsprung also described hypertrophic pyloric stenosis and contributed to the treatment of intussusception. He was a medical pediatrician but was intensely interested in what are now surgical diseases.

proximal colon and actually believed the entire colon was congenitally defective.[13] Though he failed to recognize that the cause of the proximal megacolon was in the distal, normal-appearing, aganglionic rectosigmoid (which contributed to the 60-year delay in eventual complete understanding of the pathogenesis of this disease), his presentation was the classic description of the disease that would eventually bear his name. His 1886 talk was finally published in 1887.

By the 1890s, in the United States the term "dilatation of the colon" was used more often than "Hirschsprung's disease."[14] At the same time, Sir William Osler treated two children with colon dilatation who undoubtedly had Hirschsprung's disease.[15] One was a ten-year-old boy with long-standing constipation and a huge distended abdomen. For many months Osler treated him with rectal irrigations at Johns Hopkins University Hospital. Finally, on April 10, 1892, William Halsted operated on the boy. Through a midline incision, he opened the massively distended sigmoid colon, and while Osler did a rectal examination Halsted put his hand down the colon to touch Osler's finger. The "handshake" of these two great surgeons ruled out an intrinsic anatomic obstruction. Halsted then performed a sigmoid colostomy. The boy recovered from the operation and was eventually discharged home.

A second child, also constipated from birth, who suffered from episodes of acute obstruction, was treated by enemas with a long catheter. Osler advised the following treatment: "Regulation of the diet and in very young children, relieving the distention by irrigation several times a day so as to prevent the accumulation of liquids." Thus, Osler and Halsted at John Hopkins Medical School clearly described the disease and suggested rational medical and surgical treatments that are still in use. Osler thought there was a defect in the innervation and contraction of the colon; he also said, "One finger in the throat and one in the rectum makes a good diagnostician."[16]

In 1894, G. Mya introduced the term "congenital megacolon" to go along with the name Hirschsprung's disease as well as the original name, megacolon congenitum.[17] About the same time, A. Marfan said a long, redundant sigmoid caused obstruction, producing dilation and hypertrophy of the proximal colon, and this obstruction could be relieved by passage of a rectal tube.[18] These early reports of massive colon distention in children and adults could well have been descriptions of patients suffering from Hirschsprung's disease who survived infancy. One such case was described in 1897 by William Lewitt, a demonstrator in anatomy at Rush Medical College in Chicago.[19] The patient was a 21-year-old man with a long history of constipation and episodic fecal vomiting who died after the administration of powerful cathartics and enemas. The autopsy demonstrated huge dilatation of the colon, which had perforated, causing generalized peritonitis. The rectum was empty despite a proximal fecal impaction. Other authors writing about congenital megacolon said that symptomatic relief of the colonic obstruction could be obtained by colonic irrigations and/or by colostomy. Ironically, both of these treatments still play an important role in today's preoperative and occasional postoperative management.

In 1898, the English surgeon Frederick Treves (most famous for performing an appendectomy on King Edward VII and writing about the "Elephant Man") had a valuable insight into the cause and treatment of Hirschsprung's disease. Treves not only accurately described the gross pathology of Hirschsprung's disease but also surmised that there was a congenital defect in the rectum: "I have ventured to think that there is strong evidence to support the suggestion that all cases of 'idiopathic dilalation of the colon' in young children are due to congenital defects in the terminal part of the bowel; that there is in these cases an actual mechanical obstruction and that the dilalation is not idiopathic."[20] Treves proved his theory in a five-year-old girl whose gigantically distended sigmoid tapered to her rectum, which was only the size of a forefinger. In spite of this, on January 13, 1897, Treves performed a sigmoid colostomy on the child. This relieved her symptoms and signs, though he failed to appreciate the functional rectosigmoid obstruction as the real cause.[21] On October 29 of the same year, he resected all the proximal dilated colon and the narrow rectosigmoid and pulled the splenic flexure through to the anus, where he sutured it in place. This created an incontinent perineal colostomy. Treves considered the anus to be at fault.[22] The child survived the operation, but had a minor infection between her new anus and the vagina. In 1957, 60 years after her operation, this patient was seen with an adhesive bowel obstruction. Her colon was free and without dilatation; she was continent and had regular stools twice daily.[23] For whatever reason, the physicians of his day paid no attention to Treves' observation about a congenital defect in the rectum.

At the beginning of the twentieth century, the name Hirschsprung's disease was commonly used, but it was restricted to dilatation and hypertrophy of the colon. All efforts to explain Hirschsprung's disease continued to be focused on the dilated colon. Case reports of the absence of ganglion cells being found in this disease started to appear but were considered rare medical curiosities. These reports were refuted by as many reports of normal ganglion cells in similar cases, possibly from the normal, dilated, proximal colon in cases of congenital and idiopathic megacolon. At the same time, W. M. Bayliss and E. H. Starling published a study showing how peristalsis carried material through the colon and described its autonomic nerve supply.[24]

During the first quarter century of the 1900s, there were three concepts of the pathogenesis and many different treatments, procedures and operations for this disease. The first was congenital megacolon and malformation (Hirschsprung and Mya); resection of the dilated proximal colon was the accepted treatment for this cause. M. Wilms and W. S. Fenwick identified as a second cause spastic (neuromuscular) obstruction, similar to hypertrophic pyloric stenosis.[25] Wilms considered long-term anal spasm as the main cause of the secondary megacolon. Parasymphathomimetic drugs, electric enemas, spinal anesthesia and lumbar sympathectomy were the accepted treatments for this apparent cause. A perfect example of the confusion and debate about these differing theories was Perthes' resection of a dilated colon along with a low colorectal anastomosis; he believed he had thereby removed the "vent mechanism" that caused the Hirschsprung's disease. Wilms, on the other hand, believed Perthes had interfered with the anal sphincter, which accounted for his successful treatment.[26] Fenwick also made a strong case for the abnormally tight anal sphincter resulting from a spastic rectal contraction acting as a mechanical obstruction and causing the proximal colon to dilate.[27] However, his therapy did not lead to any improvement in the treatment of megacolon.

Marfan and Perthes identified a third pathogenesis: mechanical obstruction and vent mechanisms caused by an unusually long sigmoid bending, folding and twisting.[28] Rectal tubes, enemas and irrigations, anal dilatation, rectosigmoid myotomy and occasional resection were the accepted treatments for this apparent cause. Though many of these treatments temporarily succeeded, recurrences were almost inevitable after a short period of time, especially if the diagnosis was really Hirschsprung's disease.

In 1904, two milestones occurred in the world of Hirschsprung's disease. K. Tittel published the case of a 15-month-old infant with abdominal distention that started eight days after birth, and Hirschsprung wrote the first textbook chapter on congenital dilation of the colon. In Tittel's case, the infant was developing fairly well while breast-feeding but developed a chronic bowel obstruction after switching to cow's milk, culminating in death.[29] The autopsy revealed megacolon, and as Tittel noted, "It was interesting that the ganglia of myenteric plexus could hardly be found. Normal findings were found in ileum." He thought a probable cause of the impaired peristalsis was a disorder of intramural innervation — an insight very close to the truth. Hirschsprung's chapter on congenital dilation of the colon was based on his own series of patients, along with his observations of other contemporary publications.[30] He retired from practice in the same year. Despite some clarity given by Hirschsprung's chapter to the disease, Kredel still said: "It is astonishing that it should be possible to put forward so many different opinions on one and the same thing."[31]

In the United States, J. M. T. Finney performed a colostomy on a boy with a huge colon; he later resected the colon and did a colon anastomosis protected by another colostomy. This was eventually closed under "cocaine anesthesia." The resected colon was extensively studied microscopically and ganglion cells were found in the dilated and hypertrophied colon. Two years later, in 1908, Finney wrote "Congenital Idiopathic Dilatation of the Colon," the most comprehensive paper to date on Hirschsprung's disease. In it, Finney reviewed 207 references in the world's literature (including papers by Osler and Treves). However, like all the others of Finney's time, he arrived at the wrong conclusion by focusing on the obviously dilated bowel.[32] At the same time, H. P. Hawkins stated: "The origin of the disease is mysterious." He believed a neuromuscular defect caused a rectal spasm, producing an obstruction; he treated this condition with enemas, a rectal tube and resection. Unfortunately, his resection was not distal enough and ultimately resulted in failure.[33]

Hirschsprung died in 1916, at age 86. Amazingly, his contributions to pediatric knowledge over his very productive academic lifetime go far beyond the disease named after him. Aside from his many publications, his clinical observations on biliary and intestinal atresia, hiatus hernia and spina bifida established for him a rare and unusual reputation as a pediatrician who became a pioneer in pediatric surgery.

Between 1918 and 1927, Wilms tried anal sphincter dilatation and E. Martin and V. G. Burden reported rectosigmoid myotomy as treatments for Hirschsprung's disease.[34] Starting in the 1920s and continuing for 20 years, the spastic (neuromuscular) theory became popular, giving rise to easier operative procedures than bowel resection (such as spinal anesthesia and lumbar sympathectomy) with lower morbidity and mortality. R. B. Wade and N. D. Royle believed normal colonic function could be restored by dividing the sympathetic nerve supply of the colon; they based this conclusion on the observations of W. J. M. Scott and J. J. Morton, who described the colonic evacuation of a patient with Hirschsprung's disease after receiving a spinal anesthesia.[35] These results were initially successful but ultimately failed with longer follow-ups.[36] Others, like V. P. Ross in 1935, reported that this procedure was of questionable value for congenital megacolon.[37] No wonder Bolling wrote at that time: "The outlook is poor whatever the treatment."

In spite of all the preceding efforts, in 1920 A. DallaValle was the first to report a total absence of ganglion cells from the rectosigmoid and normal ganglion cells in the dilated proximal colon in two brothers with typical symptoms and signs of Hirschsprung's disease.[38] Unfortunately, these correct observations fell on deaf ears. Almost 20 years later, H. E. Robertson and J. V. W. Kernohan from the Mayo Clinic again reported the absence of ganglion cells in the rectosigmoid and correctly correlated it with the proximal colonic obstruction of infancy.[39] In spite of these insightful reports, W. A. D. Adamson and I. Aird still concluded that the rectosigmoid aganglionosis was a rare, secondary change caused by chronic stasis and dilatation of the proximal colon.[40] K. S. L. Grimson, L. Vandergrift, and H. M. Datz later proposed subtotal colectomy and ileosigmoidostomy as the best treatment after they observed failures of segmental resection, but their procedure also failed because they did not go low enough with their resection.[41] By 1945, F. Whitehouse echoed the thinking of the past few decades: "The literature related to the therapy of congenital megacolon is rather chaotic and difficult to evaluate."[42] Despite all these findings, observations, opinions and theories, most doctors still saw Hirschsprung's disease, with its hypertrophic and dilated colon, as a congenital disorder. By the middle of the 1900s, the continuing poor outlook for infants and children with definite Hirschsprung's disease was reflected in contemporary pediatric surgery textbooks. At the same time, William E. Ladd and Robert Gross of Boston stated, "It is axiomatic to say that no one has been permanently cured of this condition."

T. Ehrenpreis' doctoral thesis was considered a pioneer work in the history of Hirschsprung's disease.[43] He summed up the prevailing opinions regarding ganglion cells, or the lack thereof, in the colon: Tittel in 1901, Brentano in 1904 and Cameron in 1928 showed that the aganglionic changes in Auerbach's plexus in the rectosigmoid had pathologic significance. However, Smith in 1908, Retzlaff in 1920 and Passler in 1938 could never confirm these findings and therefore considered them as probable secondary changes.[44] Ehrenpreis was the first to appreciate that the proximal colon became dilated because of a distal malfunction (obstruction) of the narrow rectosigmoid. He based these conclusions on his clinical observations and repeated contrast enema examinations of 110 patients with Hirschsprung's disease. The unfortunate aspect of this clinical work was that he never mentioned the narrow rectosigmoid as the cause of the disease. In fact, he tried to prove through his clinical investigations that Hirschsprung's original theory (the congenital nature of megacolon) was incorrect; instead, Ehrenpreis pointed out that this problem developed shortly after birth, could be diagnosed in a neonate, and did not involve the entire colon. He said: "A critical review of the evidence offered previously as support for the different theories on pathogenesis satisfied us that none of this material was conclusive." Consequently, he defined Hirschsprung's disease as "a dysfunction of evacuation of the colon of as yet unknown origin, occurring in the absence of morphological and mechanical causations and giving rise secondarily to a characteristic dilation of the colon."

From Hirschsprung's first report in 1886 until Orvar Swenson and his colleagues in Boston entered the picture, there had been about two hundred case reports of megacolon, with an equal amount of speculation about the etiology. As Swenson said, "At the time we began our work ... there was no consensus regarding the absence of Auerbach's plexus in congenital megacolon ... and no new therapy had evolved from these findings."[45] Confusion about the cause of this disorder continued because some children with idiopathic megacolon were included in the mix with those who indeed had congenital megacolon.[46] At the same time, at the Boston Children's Hospital there was continuing confusion about different treatments, especially when the disease recurred and these patients "had not been helped." Initially, Swenson and A. H. Bill proved the cause of Hirschsprung's disease by careful clinical observation, without concern about the ongoing debate over ganglion cells.[47] They established for the first time that the narrow rectosigmoid was the cause of the disease. Swenson subsequently felt that the lack of ganglion cells in this narrow rectosigmoid in pediatric patients of all ages with congenital megacolon supported the concept that resection of this aganglionic segment was the treatment of choice for Hirschsprung's disease.[48] He proposed resection of the rectosigmoid with preservation of the sphincters and an extra-

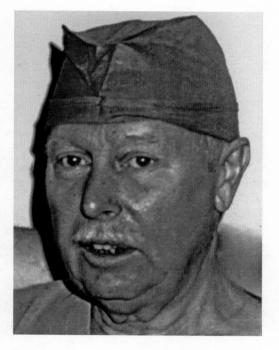

Dr. Orvar Swenson in 1973 at the Children's Memorial Hospital in Chicago after his last pull-through operation for Hirschsprung's disease. Dr. Swenson was a meticulous, highly skilled technical surgeon who followed his patients for many years (courtesy Juda E. Jona, M.D.).

corporeal (outside the anus) anastomosis of the small residual distal aganglionic rectum to the proximal ganglionic colon (which came to be called the Swenson pull-through procedure).

Swenson and Bill's conclusions were verified by comparing the clinical picture, colonic motility studies, contrast barium enema results and observation during surgery. From all these findings, Swenson deduced that only the surgical treatment of Hirschsprung's disease could be successful and definitive.[49] Swenson's surgery brought for the first time a realistic hope that children with Hirschsprung's disease could be cured. In January 1948, Swenson and Bill presented their work to the Society of University Surgeons. They reported that radiographic and balloon manometry demonstrated an area of spasm and lack of peristalsis in the rectosigmoid. It was "the first absolute concrete evidence that the etiology of the disease was the defective narrow distal segment," and it explained why removal of the dilated proximal colon did not cure the disease. They presented a successful operative technique (plus a temporary colostomy). Before this, they had developed an operation experimentally on dogs whereby the entire rectum and appropriate lengths of dilated, proximal bowel were removed, preserving the internal anal sphincter for continence. This anal pull-through procedure was then used successfully in a child with Hirschsprung's disease.[50] The patient, Joseph Murphy, was alive and well with normal bowel function as of December 1986: a 40-year follow-up. Swenson, who was born in Sweden not far from Hirschsprung, "provided the genius and scientific curiosity to correlate the physiology and pathology of Hirschsprung's disease and to devise a curative operation."[51]

In 1948, W. W. Zuelzer and J. L. Wilson reported on a series of 11 infants who had the classic clinical, roentgenological and pathological findings typical of Hirschsprung's disease. No mechanical cause for the obstruction was found, but microscopic examination of the myenteric plexus of the narrow rectosigmoid showed no ganglion cells. All 11 infants died. Zuelzer and Wilson initially suggested that their patients be treated by temporary enterostomy "at the lowest level of normal intestinal motility ... to decide whether resection of part or all of the non-mobile portion of the intestine is a desirable and practical procedure." The authors thought this bowel obstruction was functional and due to a congenital neurogenic cause, but they did not call it congenital megacolon. Nonetheless, they had made the correct diagnosis.[52] Swenson, H. F. Rheinlander and I. Diamond showed that the narrow rectosigmoid had no peristalsis, had abnormally high intraluminal pressure, and was aganglionic. All of these findings combined to form a physiological functional obstruction resulting in a dilated, proximal megacolon. They felt this was due to the fact that smooth muscle contracts when denervated (Cannon's Law, 1934) and concluded that patients with Hirschsprung's disease could be cured by removal of this defective rectosigmoid.[53]

M. Bodian, F. D. Stephens and B. L. H. Ward analyzed 73 cases of megacolon and distinguished between congenital and idiopathic, based on the presence or absence of a narrow, spastic, aganglionic rectosigmoid. Fifty percent of their cases belonged to each group and the prognosis was very different between them: Hirschsprung's disease carried a high mortality rate, while no children with idiopathic megacolon died.[54] In 1951, R. B. Hiatt also showed by manometric studies that the rectum (and maybe some proximal sigmoid and colon) was the pathological site of Hirschsprung's disease. This segment of bowel was narrow, spastic, contracted and devoid of peristalsis but still able to have a mass contraction. Hiatt also noted a lack of the normal, reflex relaxation of the internal anal sphincter. He described very short segments of aganglionosis and demonstrated that an incomplete resection of the distal, aganglionic rectosigmoid initially had an excellent result, but in time the same functional, distal obstruction returned.[55] This was shown to be a correct observation when D. State described a low, anterior resection as his answer to the treatment of Hirschsprung's disease. However, after a long follow-up it became obvious that leaving more than a few centimeters of aganglionic rectum cured no patients.[56] At this time, the mortality in newborn Hirschsprung's was 70 percent.

In 1955, Swenson, J. H. Fisher and H. E. MacMahon introduced the rectal biopsy as a precise, almost complication-free test to establish the diagnosis of Hirschsprung's disease; they reported it as superior to the barium enema. Their biopsy was done under general anesthesia and consisted of removing a 0.5 × 1 centimeter, full-thickness section of the posterior, rectal wall three centimeters from the mucocutaneous junction (pectinate line); the procedure needed a two-layered closure. The specimen required a histopathological search for ganglion cells in the intramuscular nerve plexuses; the presence of ganglion cells absolutely ruled out the diagnosis of Hirschsprung's disease.[57]

After the Swenson pull-through procedure was introduced, all pediatric surgeons had finally agreed that the defective rectosigmoid was the cause of the disease, but many objected to the deep pelvic dissection required by this operation. The objections led to the development of other procedures by B. Duhamel, F. Rehbein and F. Soave.[58] Essentially, these new operations modified the Swenson anastomotic method, following removal (or bypass) of the aganglionic rectosigmoid. Duhamel described the first of these new operations in1956: a posterior colorectal side-to-side anastomosis just above the internal sphincter, with crushing of the colorectal septum using two Kocher clamps (with their points touching at the top of the septum in the shape of an inverted V and their handles sticking out of the rectum). The clamps were left in place to cut through the septum and fall out in 10 to 14 days. This Duhamel procedure was done to leave anterior rectal mucosa (believed to be important in sensation) and to decrease injury to the pelvic nerves from the perirectal dissection.

These newer operations underwent further modifications by others. In 1958, Rehbein adopted State's anterior resection technique but improved it significantly by doing a lower resection and anastomosis within three to four centimeters of the mucocutaneous line. Because this operation was done entirely from an abdominal (pelvic) approach, his modification was limited to patients about three months of age and was really a low anterior resection. Duhamel originally incised the posterior ano-rectal wall less than one centimeter above the mucocutaneous line for his posterior anastomosis. However, he either destroyed or bypassed the internal (anal) sphincter, resulting in partial continence or incontinence for gas and liquids. M. Grob, N. Genton and V. von Tobel raised this posterior anastomotic incision to between 2 and 2.5 centimeters above the mucocutaneous line, preserving the entire internal sphincter, but the patients suffered constipation, often with fecaloma formation in the residual blind anterior rectal pouch.[59] Eventually, R. Pagès and Duhamel placed the retrorectal incision in the middle of the internal sphincter 1 to 1.5 centimeters above the mucocutaneous line; this preserved some of the posterior internal sphincter, and with it normal fecal continence.[60] Swenson reported exactly this result in 1964.[61] Grob again modified the Duhamel operation, this time by shortening the anterior rectal pouch, in hopes of minimizing the common occurrence of a postoperative fecaloma.[62] However, the fecaloma problem did not go away, so in 1968 R. T. Soper and F. E. Miller again modified the Duhamel procedure by trying to eliminate the all-too-common colorectal septum, which was the cause of the anterior rectal pouch fecaloma. They accomplished this by opening the top of the residual anterior rectum from the abdomen to make sure that the two Kocher clamps had completely eliminated the colorectal septum. This rectal opening was then closed and placed below the peritoneal reflection.[63]

Steichen, Talbert and Ravitch again modified the original Duhamel operation by using staples instead of Kocher clamps to crush and divide the colorectal septum. These staple cartridges were long enough to be placed in one or two bites only from below and not leave any septum at the top of the pouch, which no longer had to be opened from above. This variant came to be known as the Soper modification.[64] In 1964, F. Soave also modified the original Swenson procedure by doing a submucosal dissection from below and removing only the mucosa of the aganglionic rectosigmoid starting eight centimeters above the muco-cutaneous line. Then he performed an endorectal pull-through of the proximal ganglionic colon, via the residual aganglionic rectosigmoid muscular cuff, and left the proximal bowel protruding five to ten centimeters out of the anus so that adhesions developed between the pulled-through colon and the muscular cuff, after which the prolapsed bowel was amputated by cautery in 15 to 20 days. The severed proximal end then spontaneously withdrew into the anal canal. The principal advantages of the Soave endorectal pull-through were technical ease, minimal pelvic dissection, and no anal anastomosis.[65] S. J. Boley then modified Soave's original endorectal pull-through by trimming the prolapsed proximal colon at the original operation and performing a primary ano-rectal anastomosis.[66]

In 1971, M. Kasai, H. Suzur and K. Watanabe modified the original Soave procedure by doing a longitudinal myotomy of the aganglionic rectosigmoid muscular cuff and a higher ano-rectal anastomosis to eliminate some common postoperative cuff stenosis problems.[67] Even Swenson modified his own original pull-through procedure. In 1964, he published his first few hundred cases and reported significant postoperative enterocolitis in a number of his patients, requiring an internal sphincterotomy. He blamed this frequent postoperative enterocolitis on the amount of distal rectum left by his original pull-through procedure, leaving the patient with the equivalent of a rare case of ultrashort Hirschsprung's disease. When he began leaving an anterior distal rectal cuff of two centimeters and a posterior cuff at one-half to one centimeter (removing a portion of the posterior internal sphincter), the incidence of postoperative enterocolitis requiring a sphincterotomy virtually disappeared while continence was maintained.[68]

About five years after Swenson reported his first rather extensive full-thickness rectal biopsy, M. Bodian attempted to make the diagnosis of Hirschsprung's disease easier by a smaller rectal biopsy including only mucosa and submucosa, searching for ganglion cells in Meissner's submucosal nerve plexus.[69] In 1961, B. Shandling improved this small rectal biopsy technique by using a laryngeal biopsy forceps and doing only a submucosal (punch) biopsy from the low posterior rectal wall. This procedure required no anesthesia in newborns, infants and some older children, and closure of the biopsy site was not required.[70] A further refinement of the rectal biopsy came along in 1965 when W. O. Dobbins and A. H. Bill, Jr., reported that suction biopsy of the rectal mucosa and submucosa was just as reliable as other smaller biopsy techniques, especially when the absence of ganglion cells was combined with histochemical staining for excess acetylcholinesterase associated with the increased number of hypertrophied nerve trunks that were also being found with the lack of ganglion cells.[71]

By the 1970s, medical professionals had begun to focus on the aganglionic internal sphincter of the Hirschsprung's patient. L. Schnaufer and her coauthors reported that the absence of aganglionic internal sphincter relaxation was the most important finding in the manometric diagnosis of Hirschsprung's disease.[72] This was a relatively non-invasive way to make that diagnosis, with the risk of a false positive or false negative reading arising only in the newborn.[73] Ehrenpreis reported that the principal complication of all the operative procedures for Hirschsprung's disease was related to the aganglionic internal sphincter. If too much sphincter was damaged or bypassed, incontinence resulted; if more than the sphincter remained, constipation and other obstructive symptoms and signs (often with enterocolitis) returned.[74] By the end of the 1970s, S. Kleinhaus and coauthors surveyed the members of the American Academy of Pediatrics' Section on Surgery and found that satisfactory results could be obtained with all of the pull-through procedures and their modifications; the key was performing the procedure correctly.[75] Nonetheless, in 1982 A. M. Holschneider reported that all of these procedures and their modifications still had their own peculiar postoperative problems.[76] At the same time, using special stains, W. Meier-Ruge described pathognomonic criteria for a "strange" disease (intestinal neuronal dysplasia) that mimicked Hirschsprung's disease.[77] This diagnosis continues to be hotly debated throughout the world.

Beginning in the 1980s, a new approach to the operative repair of Hirschsprung's disease appeared. Throughout this decade, several case reports focused on a small series of successful one-stage pull-throughs. Except in infants with enterocolitis, none of the patients with these one-stage procedures received a colostomy. Newborns also benefited from this approach, which quickly gained favor as its efficacy and safety were proven, with long-term results yet to be determined.[78]

The 1980s also saw a focus on the pathogenesis and genetic influence of the disease. Physicians developed two theories of the former, both of which focused on the neural crest stem cell. The first theory hypothesized that stem cells fail to migrate effectively from their neural crest niche.[79] The second theory postulated that the stem cells either involute or fail to differentiate once they arrive at their terminal location.[80] After development of the first animal models of aganglionosis in 1966 and the initial report of genetic rat mutations involved in Hirschsprung's disease in 1967, this area of research went dormant until the 1980s, when there was a flurry of genetic research. G. Martucciello and colleagues identified the first Hirschsprung's-specific genetic defect for a sporadic case of the disease. They reported an interstitial deletion in the long arm of Chromosome 10 in a child with total colonic aganglionosis and no family history. These investigators, along with others, narrowed the location of this mutation to the region between 10q11.2 and 10q21.2.[81] In 1996, a mutation in the endothelin receptor type B (EDNRB) causing myenteric aganglionosis and coat color spotting was described in rats.[82] These rats exhibited congenital intestinal aganglionosis, resulting from failure of the neural crest-derived enteric nervous system stem cells to effectively colonize the intestine. Toward the end of the decade, C. E. Gariepy and colleagues demonstrated that a single gene mutation may be responsible for Hirschsprung's disease.[83] Investigators found a link between dental pigmentation and intestinal aganglionosis, while others reported a role for EDNRB in Lethal White Foal Syndrome. The latter syndrome, a disease of horses, produces foals that are nearly all white and have total colonic aganglionosis, mimicking human Hirschsprung's disease.[84]

At the end of the 1990s, two simultaneous papers described a novel and completely transanal approach to existing pull-through procedures.[85] This unusual modification of existing techniques used an anal approach through which the rectal mucosecetomy, distal aganglionic colon resection, and actual pull-through procedure were all performed. The apparent benefits of staying out of the peritoneum had the potential advantages of less damage to pelvic structures, less bleeding and fewer adhesions, as well as no large abdominal scars. However, the long-term results remained to be determined. Since their original reports, Langer, Durrant and De la Torre, along with other investigators, have presented a multicenter review of 141 patients undergoing this transanal pull-through operation.[86] They reported comparable morbidity to the open approaches but less postoperative pain and shorter time to feeding and discharge. Nonetheless, some concerns have been reported about the transanal operation: increased anal anastomotic stricture formation, postoperative enterocolitis and possibly increased incontinence. These may result from the intra-operative anal opening retraction when doing all of the above through the anus of an infant. Meanwhile, K. E. Georgeson and his colleagues modified the Soave pull-through by a laparoscopic approach, making it easier to identify the transition zone and perform the mesenteric dissection, thus improving postoperative complications and recovery time.[87]

By the turn of the twenty-first century, the American Pediatric Surgical Association reported that newborn mortality in Hirschsprung's disease had declined from 70 percent in 1954 to 1 percent. They attributed this improvement to earlier and more precise diagnosis, as well as more effective and aggressive surgical management. However, long-segment aganglionosis remained a problem. In 2003, M. L. Proctor and colleagues reported that in 10 percent of patients with long-segment Hirschsprung's disease the preoperative barium enema did not correctly predict the level of aganglionosis.[88] Two years later, in spite of the increasingly favored transanal pull-through, some surgeons believed this approach was relatively contraindicated for patients with long-segment Hirschsprung's disease, mainly because of the difficulty in diagnosing the transition zone. Instead, some of these surgeons used laparoscopy to confirm the transition zone. Others suggested an umbilical incision for both the diagnostic laparoscopy and a colostomy, if needed.[89] Most surgeons continued to believe that the Duhamel procedure gave better functional results when long-segment disease existed.[90]

By 2004, at least ten genes and mutations were identified as having a possible link to Hirschsprung's disease, as reviewed by P. Puri and T. Shinkai.[91] However, it remains unclear what role they play in the development of this disease.[92] T. Iwashita and colleagues provided the strongest evidence that Hirschsprung's disease is linked to dysfunctional neural crest stem cells, and the likely candidate gene was thought to be necessary for neural crest stem cell migration.[93] However, the focus of scientific research remains on the loss of bowel function due to RET mutations. The research goes on.

CHAPTER 30

Abdominal Wall Defects

RICHARD RICKETTS, M.D.

This chapter explores the evolution in our understanding and treatment of patients with abdominal wall defects: omphalocele (also known as exomphalos) and gastroschisis. Infants with abdominal wall defects were originally called monsters and they had no chance for survival. Not until the late 1700s were omphaloceles successfully repaired, and gastroschises were not successfully repaired until the early 1900s, though the mortality rate for each remained exceedingly high. With the persistence of surgeons in developing novel operative and non-operative techniques and with the availability of antibiotics, anesthesia, and parenteral nutrition, all of these infants are now salvageable unless they have life-limiting associated congenital anomalies.

Omphalocele (Exomphalos)

Though probably known in ancient times, the first "modern" description of an abdominal wall defect, probably an omphalocele, is credited to the sixteenth-century French surgeon Ambroise Paré in his chapter titled "Of the Relaxation of the Navel in Children." He wrote:

> Often times in children newly born, the navel swelleth as big as an egg, because it hath not been well cut or bound, or because the wayith [sic] humors are flowed thither, or because that part hath extended itself too much by crying, by reason of the pains of the fretting of the child's guts, many times the child bringeth that tumor joined with an abscess with him from his mother's womb: but let not the surgeon assay [sic] to open that abscess, for if it be opened, the guts come out through the incision, as I have seen in many, and especially in a child of my Lord Martigues; for when Peter of the Rocke, the surgeon, opened an abscess that was in it, the bowels ran out at the incision, and the infant died; and it wanted but little that the gentlemen of my lord's that were there, had strangled the surgeon. Therefore when John Gromontius the carver desired me, and requested me of late that I would do the like in his son, I refused to do it, because it was in danger of its life by it already, and in three days after the abscess broke, and the bowels gushed out, and the child died.[1]

Here Dr. Paré sought to explain the etiology behind an omphalocele by blaming the infant for excess crying, or he blamed those who delivered the infant and cut and "bound" the umbilical cord. He also warned surgeons not to operate on these, lest the surgeon be strangled! He pointed out the futility of surgery in these patients since they were all destined to die anyway.[Editor's note: See "Some New Birth Defects" in part 1 for the work of Johannes Fatio and others who during the sixteenth century saw and treated infants with abdominal wall defects.]

Giovanni Battista Morgagni, professor of anatomy and President of the University of Padua, described several abdominal wall defects in "Of Diseases of the Belly" in his book *The Seats and Causes of Diseases Investigated by Anatomy* (published in 1769). He presented the case of a 41-year-old "mother of many children ... who brought forth a monstrous infant" in 1735: "The abdomen was open in the middle; and the intestines were pushed out from thence. And the exit of the intestines from the abdomen; the blame of which is often thrown upon the rough and violent handling, and pressure of the midwives, when they deliver the infants; in this case, where there could be nothing of that kind, certainly must be attributed to the abdomen itself of the fetus never having been shut up; or at least not sufficiently shut up."[2]

Morgagni described this condition as a congenital anomaly, not the result of mishandling of infants by midwives. This could be a description of a ruptured omphalocele or gastroschisis. He then attempted to describe the embryological error as incomplete abdominal wall closure, indicating that this was probably an omphalocele: "For from the original formation ... it[the abdominal wall] is open. And afterwards, unless the peritoneum, the muscles and the common integuments firmly and closely shut it up, it must, without doubt, either remain open,[gastroschisis?] as many have found it; ... or must be relaxed into a purse of the same kind; ... and if the covering is very thin and slender, it may easily be broken through by the very weight of the viscera. For when it is made up of peritoneum only, it is so thin, as even to suffer the peristaltic motion of the intestine to be seen through it[omphalocele]."

Morgagni also describes an infant who probably had an omphalocele and a sacrococcygeal teratoma, or a meningo-myelocele: "...[The child] was deformed with two tumors in particular, the one at the os sacrum, and the other under the navel, where the intestines, and other viscera, coming out through the hiatus of the abdomen, greatly raised up the peritoneum, in which they alone were contained."[3]

The prevailing attitude in the eighteenth century seems to have been that congenital anomalies stemmed from maternal imagination or the mother's life experiences. Morgagni credited several other authors of the time with accounts of "monsters" being born to mothers who seemed to have déjà vu experiences: "But if you examine the greater part of those authors, from whom these examples are produced, you will see how readily they are accounted for from the imagination of pregnant women; and that when even they could be very fairly deduced from some external violence, a part is nevertheless assigned to the imagination likewise."[4]

Morgagni threw doubt on this theory, but with some reservations: "Though I cannot approve these things, yet, on the other hand, there are cases where it seems to me to be very hard to depart from that opinion, which is common to the greatest men, totally and altogether. What Boerhaave, what Van Swieten, what other grave authors of undoubted credit assert to have been seen by them that relates to this question, no one will doubt the truth of."

He described several cases in support of maternal imagination or experiences as a cause of congenital anomalies, such as an infant with a "mulberry protuberance" on its nose from a mother who had a mulberry fall on her nose; a female infant born to a woman who had a caterpillar fall on her neck, subsequent to which the child had "...on the skin of[her] neck, the form of a caterpillar, ... being various colors, and having upright hairs..."; an infant born with a "hair-lip" after the mother had seen a beggar with a "hair-lip"; and an infant with anencephaly born to a woman who had seen two drowned children taken out of a lake "without any skull" and who had "excruciated herself with that fixed and obstinate imagination, and with personal rumination on the past evil."[5]

However, Morgagni did not believe maternal imagination accounted for the abdominal wall defect he described.

The congenital theory was soon accepted, and by the early 1800s what we now call omphalocele was termed "hernia congenita umbilicus" or "exomphalos." William Hey, senior surgeon of the General Infirmary at Leeds in England, is credited with the first successful repair of an omphalocele in 1772 (reported in 1803):

> I found the funis umbilicus distended to the bulk of a hen's egg ... its external coat so transparent, that I could already discern through it the folds of the small intestine, which had been protruded through the navel before the child was born. I immediately reduced the intestine.... I procured some plaster spread upon leather, cut into circular pieces, and laid upon one another in a conical form. This compress I placed upon the navel, after I had brought the skin on each side of the aperture into contact, and had laid one of the lips a little over the other. I then put round the child's abdomen a linen belt, and placed upon the navel a thick, circular, quilted part, formed about two inches from one extremity of the belt ... and at the expiration of a fortnight from that time the aperture at the navel was so far contracted, that the crying of the child, when the bandage was removed, did not cause the least protrusion.[6]

The repair, then, was skin closure followed by a pressure dressing, wound contracture and cicatrixation. Hey later had "an ingenous mechanic in Leeds" construct a truss to be used in treating exomphalos (figure 1). Unfortunately, Hey's truss method for treating omphaloceles did not work well with another infant, who in 1791 had a large omphalocele that was "difficult to reduce ... but by gentle pressure I made them (intestines) all return to the abdomen in the space of about a half an hour." He placed his truss and "the hernia did not return but the child became uneasy after the reduction; and, although it had two natural stools, yet it died about 48 hours after the operation."[7]

The first American report of an omphalocele came from A. C. Robinson, lecturer of anatomy at the University of Maryland. He reported in 1841 on a female infant he cared for, non-operatively, in 1839:

> When the infant was exposed, I discovered a large umbilical hernia, caused by incomplete development in the abdominal parietes. The viscera were not entirely covered, however, for the sheath of the cord had been expanded to complete the abdominal walls, and confine them within some limits. Although thus partially confined, the abdominal contents were not concealed from view by their pellucid covering, but were as distinctly perceptible as if viewed through a thick moist watch glass.... This was quite large, measuring 10 inches around its base, and 5 inches and three quarters of an inch from side to side, over its most prominent point ... while crying the tumor became so tense, as to induce the fear, that its frail walls might yield, and the intestines be at once rolled out.[8]

He describes what amounts to the natural history of untreated omphaloceles in the era prior to antibiotics: The sac became dry and withered and began to separate on the ninth day, "exposing the peritoneal membrane, overlaid by a delicate web of cellular tissue, which soon became covered with granulations, as if nature was struggling to complete her work by filling up the breach in the abdominal walls." The infant developed peritonitis on the nineteenth day and died 48 hours later. Up until that time, "the child lived ... with all the functions of its systems in an apparently healthy state." The baby had been eating and stooling normally.

C. Visick reported the first successful repair of a ruptured omphalocele or perhaps a gastroschisis in 1873:

> ...I found the cord had been divided in the usual place; but that the part next to the skin had been developed into a hernia sac the size of a hen's egg, very thin and transparent and lined with peritoneum, much congested, and communicating with the abdomen by an orifice of the diameter of a cedar pencil. This sac had either ruptured during labor or had been opened by the midwife.... The greatest possible difficulty was experienced in returning the large mass, from the minute size of the orifice[hence possible gastroschisis] and the violent expulsive efforts of the child: but after more than an hour's patient coaxing, the whole was returned.[9]

He closed the defect with wire and the baby survived. Visick commented that perhaps he should have further opened the abdominal wall gap to facilitate easier reduction.

William Fear of Kent published the first report of successful treatment of a ruptured omphalocele using the sac as a silo in 1878. This patient was a full-term female infant whose "...cord was very large through its abdominal half and oedematous, especially so at its attachment to the umbilical ring, where it presented also a funnel-shaped condition. The viscera were found to escape through an umbilical ring an inch and a half in diameter, to enter the expanded base of the cord, and then emerge from its split side."

Dr. Fear inspected the eviscerated small bowel and stomach and felt meconium in the colon, "which could be recognized and passed along by the finger" in the abdominal cavity. He then reports using the sac as a "natural" silo: "With caution and difficulty, I slowly restored the entire contents from the last to the first, being embarrassed by the threat made upon the bowels when the infant cried. Then, lifting by the cord the umbilical region came into a cone; I encircled it with a skein of thread, strangulating a narrow ring of skin, and with it as much abdominal wall as I could around the umbilicus....Within 6 weeks, cicatrisation was completed."[10] The baby made an uneventful recovery.

In 1887, R. Z. Olshausen reported the case of a newborn with probable Beckwith–Widemann syndrome (unknown at the time), where he repaired an omphalocele with a novel technique: "She weighed 4,280 gm and her length was 57 cm. She demonstrated, besides a large umbilical cord hernia, significant macroglossia. The by all dimensions overly large tongue resided at 6 months still between the upper and lower jaw but could be retracted within the jaws."

Shortly after the baby was born, Olshausen incised a thin rim of skin around the defect and "with pick-ups ... the amniotic layer was peeled off the peritoneum, which covered the inside of the hernia sac." Having separated the sac into its two components, he then closed the wound in layers over the peritoneal surface. Olhausen felt it was important to preserve the peritoneum, "which secures healing in the likely event of a wound dehiscence because peritoneum-derived tissue will quickly fill the base of the wound..." The wound partially dehisced but closed by secondary intention, leaving a "broad scar." The baby lived for six months. Olhausen wrote: "In cases where the hernia contents are non-reducible, this surgical approach is of course not feasible..."[11]

In 1888, D'Arcy Power made two observations in "a case of congenital umbilical hernia." First, that it may be necessary to enlarge the umbilical ring in order to reduce the viscera in cases where the umbilical ring is small, and second that "the external surface (of

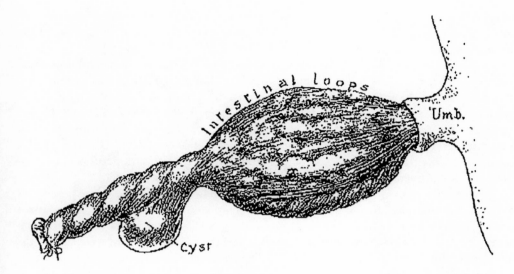

A case of "congenital umbilical hernia," which is actually an omphalocele. D'Arcy Power reported this case in 1888. The illustration in his original article was reproduced on page 460 in *Embryology Anatomy and Diseases of the Umbilicus* by Thomas Cullen, published in 1916. Coils of intestines were contained in a translucent sac of the umbilical cord. The umbilical ring was enlarged to permit reduction of the intestine into the abdomen and the defect was closed with silver wire sutures. The baby died with peritonitis three days later. Today, this would be considered a small omphalocele and would be easy to repair.

the sac) was polished, and closely resembled the outer surface of the cord, whilst internally the sac is covered with a smooth layer, which is apparently derived from the peritoneum."[12] A little over a decade later, in 1899, F. Ahlfeld proposed for the first time painting the sac with a disinfectant and sclerosing agent (alcohol) in cases of giant "inoperable" omphalocele: The mature boy demonstrated an umbilical hernia with approximately 8 cm. diastosis at the base. The structure stood over the abdominal wall like a huge apple ... through the wall we saw liver and intestines.... We rubbed the skin with 96 percent alcohol ... and covered the hernia with cotton soaked with 96 percent alcohol, then a broad binder was placed. The same process was repeated after a few days.... The big sac was not only entirely covered with skin but also retracted in a way that one could only see when the child was crying how the small palm-sized anterior part of the abdomen consisted of a thin wall and protruded."[13]

In 1916 Thomas Stephen Cullen, associate professor of gynecology at Johns Hopkins University, published *Embryology, Anatomy, and Diseases of the Umbilicus Together with Diseases of the Urachus*: the first and most complete treatise on umbilical disorders up until that time. It took Cullen more than three years to review the literature up to 1912. "Such an extensive survey of the literature as was here undertaken would have been absolutely impossible had it not been for that gold mine of medical information — the Surgeon-General's Library in Washington[now the National Library of Medicine], where the curators took infinite pains to see that every article in any way dealing with the umbilicus was brought to me."[14]

The book includes a detailed, illustrated account of the embryology of the umbilicus. Cullen noted: "...In our study of the embryology of the umbilical region we have seen that in the early months a large part of the small bowel lies out in the umbilical cord. Later

4-12 wks

the intestine recedes into the abdomen. The cavity in the cord becomes obliterated and the umbilical ring closes." The embryological basis for omphalocele was thus recognized at the beginning of the twentieth century.

Cullen divides his chapter on umbilical hernia into "Hernia of the Umbilical Cord," "Amniotic Hernia," "Congenital Nipping Off of an Umbilical Hernial Protrusion," and other sections. In the first section, concerning what we would now term "umbilical cord hernia" or "small omphalocele," he describes three cases as illustrated in figure 2. Cullen points out that the sac consists "for the most part of the amnion and the peritoneum." In these cases he recommends "radical operation at once," since with delay or non-operative management "the thin-walled sac ... consisting mainly of amnion and peritoneum ... [is] likely to tear and there will then be great danger of peritonitis."

In the section on amniotic hernia (or amniotic umbilicus), Cullen describes seven cases of what we would now term "omphalocele" or "exomphalos" of various sizes. One patient with a giant omphalocele, which Cullen termed "total hernia," underwent an operation on the second day of life. Half the liver was resected and the muscle and skin were closed; the baby died within 24 hours. Because of this, Cullen states that "the time to operate is immediately after birth, before there is any drying out of the (sac) and before the hernial protrusion has been increased in size by the accumulation of fluid in the stomach." With respect to another patient with a giant omphalocele (14 × 17 cm), who died with non-operative treatment, Cullen again states: "It is obvious that in such cases the only chance of saving the child is by operation immediately after birth." This became the prevailing attitude toward the treatment of omphaloceles at that time.

Cullen describes two cases of congenital nipping-off of an umbilical hernial protrusion, which we would now term "closed gastroschisis" (but might really be a closed omphalocele). Meckel observed one such case in a four-month-old fetus. Ahlfeld probably described the first case in 1782 of a child who "at the navel [had] an irregular tumor the size of an apple. The tumor was attached to the umbilicus by a very thin pedicle. It was clearly evident that the tumor consisted of a nipping-off of intestinal convolutions." The "tumor" was removed and an attempt was made to do an "artificial anus" above the umbilicus, but the child died.[15] At autopsy, the proximal jejunum and the ascending colon ended blindly at the umbilical ring. Cullen states that "should such a condition be noted at birth, immediate operation is indicated. After the umbilical growth has been cut off, the abdomen should be opened and the upper and lower portions of the bowel united by lateral or end to end anastomosis."

E. J. Klopp in 1921 was the first to report stage one of a staged closure of a giant ruptured omphalocele. The defect occupied "the greater part of the abdominal wall" and contained liver, small bowel and colon. Klopp removed a portion of the ruptured sac after replacing the bowel and closed only the skin after raising wide flaps: "No attempt was made to bring the muscles together. The skin was incised around the margin of the hernia and extensively undermined in all directions, then sutured vertically over the amnion."[16]

The baby survived and did well until the age of five months (figure 3), when he died of otitis media even though both tympanic membranes were incised and "there was copious discharge of pus from both ears." Klopp summarized: "...It is questionable whether one should attempt ... to bring the muscles together when there is a large defect in the abdominal wall."

In 1928, A. F. Herbert reported a personal series of three cases of "hernia funiculi umbilicalis" and reviewed the literature up until that time. He found 18 cases with 16 survivors up until 1890, which "were all of the small variety, with the intestines the only contents of the sac."[17] He summarized the reports of sixteen infants between 1890 and 1928, including his own three patients. By reviewing the records of several large metropolitan areas, he concluded that the condition occurs in about one in ten thousand live births. He cites different opinions as to the etiology of "congenital umbilical hernia"; various authors attributed it to pressure on the fetal abdomen due to faulty position traction on the cord "because of winding about the fetal body," "pulling of the vitelline duct on the intestine in the root of the umbilical," or adhesive bands holding the viscera out of the abdomen.[18]

Dr. Carrington Williams was the first to describe closure of a giant omphalocele with skin only, leaving the sac intact: "It appeared impossible to dissect the skin away from the membrane without opening the abdominal cavity, so an incision was made about ¼ inch from the skin edge, leaving the small circle of skin attached. The skin was undermined for about 2 inches around the whole defect without disturbing the muscles, the excess strings of the umbilical cord were removed and the skin easily closed down the midline with interrupted sutures."[19]

The baby died 12 hours afterward. The autopsy revealed pus between the membrane and the skin, a potential problem identified by Gross many years later.[20]

Norman M. Dott in 1932 provided a colorful description of the etiology of omphalocele (exomphalos) and umbilical hernia:

> Hence the abdominal viscera protrude into the umbilical cord, which is probably an integral part of the abdominal wall in early embryonic life. Later, when the developing embryo has decided to use the tissue of his cord for another purpose, he hurriedly withdraws the viscera into the abdomen proper and seals up the umbilical orifice. As is so often the case with after thoughts, his plans may miscarry into lesser or greater degree, and he fails to abolish his umbilical hernia. The least degree of error consists in the persistence of a little pouch of umbilical coelom in the thickness of the abdominal wall, which is later expanded into an ordinary skin-covered umbilical hernia. The greatest degree of error consists in the larger part of the abdominal viscera remaining in the umbilical cord.[21]

Dott proposes two types of exomphalos: the "embryonic" type, containing liver adherent to the upper portion of the sac (which we now call "giant" omphalocele), and the "foetal" type, in which the liver is not in the sac or adherent to it and in which "surgical reduction and repair is relatively easy." He accurately describes the problems facing surgeons in dealing with the "embryonic" type of exomphalos: "Here one is faced with an enormous gap to close, and with an abdomen of small capacity which has never held its allotted contents, a huge protrusion, including the solid liver, which is awkward to manipulate through an aperture without rupture, and above all which is intimately adherent to the sac wall over a large surface."

Dott describes his primary repair of a giant omphalocele ("embryonic" type), illustrated in figure 4. He excised the sac off of the liver "with the greatest care and patience, to avoid tearing and bleeding," and then he had to "pack these bulky viscera into a little abdomen which had never known them.... After about an hour's careful packing and adjustment, linen sutures were placed in the musculature on each side and the abdominal wall gradually stretched and brought together over the viscera. The packing had been done very tight and it seemed impossible that the viscera should function under such tension. However, so adaptable is Nature that the abdominal wall rapidly stretched, the suture line held, and on the second day vomiting ceased and feedings commenced." At the time of that report, the baby was one year old and thriving.

In the 1930s and 1940s, several case reports appeared of omphalocele, variously titled

"Hernia into the Umbilical Cord, Containing the Entire Liver and Gallbladder," "Eventra-tion," "Exomphalos" and "Umbilical Hernia."[22] In one case of a giant omphalocele, primarily repaired, the author makes a remarkable statement: "Lastly, a severe manhandling type of operation was easily weathered by a newborn child.... No doubt at this early age the child is adapted to the trauma of birth and is well able to accommodate itself to what may be described as merely an extension of this trauma in the form of a major abdominal operation ... we may say that surgical obliteration of the extra-embryonic coelom in a newly born infant is merely a greatly accelerated physiologic event brought about artificially by surgery, to which the developing child is already adapted and to which therefore it presents little reaction."[23]

Charles O'Leary presented a comprehensive literature review of congenital umbilical hernia in 1941. He reviewed 7 cases from the University Hospital of Oklahoma City along with 84 cases from the literature (91 cases total). He made the following observations:

- the ratio of male to female incidence was 2:1
- one-third had associated anomalies
- about 3 percent were ruptured at birth
- about one-third had a diameter more than five centimeters
- mortality was related to the time of repair: 21 percent mortality up to twelve hours after birth, 44 percent 12 to 24 hours after birth and 62 percent more than 24 hours after birth
- in patients with delayed surgery or with conservative treatment, mortality was due to peritonitis
- sac adherent to the liver should not be removed because of the danger of profuse bleeding
- the incidence was about one in five thousand deliveries[24]

In 1948, Robert E. Gross made some cogent observations concerning giant omphaloceles and recommended a new method for repair. From a series of 60 babies at the Boston Children's Hospital, Gross noted that the mortality rate was directly related to the size of the defect. If it was less than seven centimeters in diameter, the mortality rate was 25 percent; from seven to nine centimeters, 70 percent; and greater than nine centimeters, 85 percent. He attributed this to three problems arising from increased intra-abdominal pressure: respiratory distress from upward displacement of the diaphragm; impaired venous return from compression of the IVC; and intestinal obstruction from compression of the stomach and small bowel.

In order to avoid increased abdominal pressure, Gross supported a two-stage procedure (skin closure followed later by fascial closure) for treating giant omphaloceles, as first attempted by Klopp. Gross was concerned about potential weakness of the skin closure and the development of dense adhesions between the bowel/liver and the overlying skin. He described a "new technique" to avoid these potential problems: leave the omphalocele sac intact and bring the widely mobilized skin flaps over it. Gross did not credit Dr. Carrington Williams with first attempting this technique in 1929 (reported in 1930) but did report the successful use of this two-stage procedure in two infants. The subsequent fascial closure was delayed ten months and six months, respectively. A third infant had the first-stage procedure but had not yet undergone the second operation at the age of ten months because Gross felt the abdominal cavity was still too small to accommodate the viscera. Gross noted that there was no problem with infection of the buried sac, seroma formation between the sac and the overlying skin, or necrosis of the widely mobilzed skin flaps.[25]

In his landmark textbook *The Surgery of Infancy and Childhood* (1953), Gross beautifully illustrates his two-stage operation for giant omphaloceles ("umbilical eventration"). He described 88 infants, 10 of whom were not operated on because they were in extremis and/or had other life-threatening anomalies; all of these babies died. Of the 78 surgically treated infants, 48 survived (a 38 percent mortality rate). There is no breakdown between those primarily repaired and those having a staged procedure.

Interestingly, in this landmark textbook there is no mention of gastroschisis. However, Gross describes 17 infants seen between 1940 and 1950 with "rupture of an omphalocele sac," with some of these occurring in utero and some after delivery. He points out that those occurring in utero have intestines that are "thickened, edematous, and matted together."[26] The picture in the textbook (figure 5) certainly could be a patient with gastroschisis, and many of the so-called ruptured omphaloceles in this chapter and in the literature probably are patients with gastroschisis. Gross notes that prior to 1940, all of these cases were fatal from peritonitis. After the advent of antibiotics, Gross reported that six of his seventeen patients survived and that those who ruptured after delivery did better than those who ruptured in utero (gastroschisis).

The standard of care for omphaloceles, ruptured or intact, was immediate surgery, in either one or two stages as outlined by Gross. He says: "...There is no hope that the skin will grow over the sac or that the contents may be returned to the peritoneal cavity by simple taxis. The clinical progress is invariably towards rupture of the sac as it dries out, infection ensues, and death is inevitable and not long delayed. There is therefore no warrant for attempts at conservative therapy."[27]

A. A. Cunningham first challenged this belief in 1956 when he reported treating two infants in 1948 and 1949 with absolute alcohol dressings applied to the sac twice daily. (Cunningham credited Ahlfeld with first using this method in 1899.) Cunningham also used parenteral and/or oral penicillin, which was available by then. He described and illustrated in detail the escharization, sloughing, contraction, and gradual epithelialization of the defect with the "conservative therapy" for large omphaloceles.[28] M. Grob from Switzerland also used and popularized the conservative treatment of large omphaloceles, pointing out: "...The principle of treatment lies in the fact that the omphalocele will be covered spontaneously by normal skin growth starting from the border of the sac."[29] He used a 2 percent aqueous solution of mercurochrome to prevent infection and dry up the sac. Epithelialization occurred in six to eight weeks. Of his 16 patients treated conservatively, 13 survived (a less than 20 percent mortality rate). Two died of midgut volvulus and one from pneumonia.

The next major advancement in the treatment of large omphaloceles was introduced by S. R. Schuster in 1967.[30] He first used his technique in 1959 for secondary repair of large omphaloceles that had initially been managed with skin closure only, and then he applied his technique to newborns. In infants undergoing the secondary repair, the skin is opened in the midline, a sheet of Teflon mesh is sutured to the edge of each rectus muscle, a piece of polyethylene film is placed inside the Teflon mesh to keep bowel from adhering to it, the two sheets of Teflon mesh are sewn together in the midline while applying moderate downward pressure to the viscera, the excess Teflon is excised and the skin is closed over the mesh, excising the excess skin. This process is then repeated every week or so until the mesh can be removed and the recti brought together and covered with skin.

In newborns with large omphaloceles, the management is the same after extending the opening from the xiphoid to the pubis, except that the skin is not closed over the mesh but attached to it as high as possible. The mesh is covered with sterile dressings and then seri-

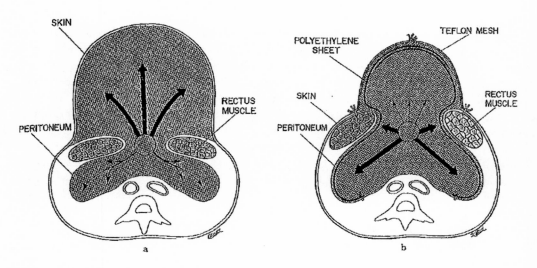

The image on the left illustrates the problem of large omphaloceles. A small amount of viscera is confined to a space between the muscles and the posterior abdominal wall. The remainder of the intestine and liver are outside the abdominal cavity. Forcing the viscera back into the abdomen causes respiratory distress and kinking of blood vessels. Suturing plastic membrane to the fascia surrounding the sac allows the surgeon to gently push the viscera into its proper location while gradually enlarging the abdominal cavity. It is also possible to reduce the viscera by treating the antiseptics to allow a gradual shrinkage of the sac (from S. R. Schuster, "A New Method for the Staged Repair of Large Omphaloceles," *Surgery, Gynecology and Obstetrics*, Vol. 125 [1967]: 837–850).

ally excised until the fascia can be reapproximated. Of 11 newborns treated by this method, 9 survived, 6 of whom had complete repair during the initial hospital stay of 24 to 63 days. Three had partial repair with planned secondary repair at a later hospitalization. There were two episodes of sepsis, one necessitating removal of the mesh and one resulting in a death.[31]

The theory supporting the effectiveness of this method is well illustrated in Schuster's figure 6. The inelastic mesh directs the intra-abdominal pressure laterally and posterolaterally to expand the abdominal wall, rather than anteriorly to expand only the skin. Schuster points out that the success of this technique derives from the avoidance of respiratory and vascular compromise by a series of gradual reduction of the viscera into the slowly enlarging abdominal cavity. At the time of this writing, Schuster was developing a single sheet of material consisting of teflon mesh lined on either side by silastic material, with a cuff of unlined mesh to sew to the rectus muscles.

In 1969, R. C. Allen and E. L. Wrenn introduced the next major advance in treating large omphaloceles and gastroschisis.[32] They used Silon®, which consisted of a sheet of Dacron mesh lined with silastic except for an uncovered cuff to be used for suturing to the fascia (as Schuster was developing). They also used reinforced Silastic® sheeting in some patients. This material was sutured circumferentially to the full thickness of the abdominal wall and the two edges were sewn together along the side and over the top of the viscera. This "chimney" was then covered with an antibiotic- (or silver nitrate–) soaked dressing to help prevent infection. Using sterile gloves, the size of the chimney was reduced every one to three days by pushing the viscera down and applying a tie around the sac. Two newborns with gastroschisis and three with ruptured omphaloceles were treated by this method. The first infant died from sepsis (antibiotic dressings were not used until after this incident); one developed a fecal fistula, which was closed but then recurred and eventually closed spontaneously; and three survived without significant complications. The authors proposed the use of steroids (to help prevent sclerema), gammaglobulin, local and systemic antibiotics, and strict sterile techniques to help prevent infection.

Realizing that the application of Silon(r) carried a serious risk of infection and that application of tincture of iodine (or mercurochrome) carries the risk of toxicity from absorption, S. H. Ein and B. Shandling introduced another non-operative method for initial management of "huge" omphaloceles in 1978.[33] Two newborns with large omphaloceles, one ruptured, were treated by covering the sac with Op-Site(r) and applying a dry sterile dressing over that. The underlying sac liquefied and was replaced with granulation tissue by three and six weeks, respectively, at which time the Op-Site(r) was removed. Skin eventually covered the sac, leaving a large ventral hernia, which was closed at 13 months in one baby and was awaiting closure in the second baby at the time of the paper.[34]

S. H. Kim nicely summarized the "modern" treatment of omphaloceles in 1976.[35] Initial resuscitative measures, non-operative management, and operative management including primary repair, staged repair, and repair using silastic chimneys are thoroughly discussed. Other methods, including use of tissue expanders, component separation and a combination of these techniques, are used in selective cases.[36] Using these modern methods, the survival rate for infants with omphaloceles is now approximately 75 percent, with most deaths due to severe associated anomalies.[37]

One of the syndromes associated with omphaloceles is now termed "Pentalogy of Cantrell." The first description of this syndrome found by this author came from D. J. Thompson in 1944. She described a full-term South Indian baby boy with microcephaly and "...a large omphalocele, with an opening in the abdominal wall 3 inches in diameter. Parts of the intestine, the liver, and spleen were prolapsed, and the heart was also lying outside the chest wall, enclosed in the pericardiaum."[38] The "monster" lived for three-quarters of an hour.

In 1958, J. R. Cantrell, J. A. Haller, and M. M. Ravitch described 5 personal cases and referenced 16 others with a syndrome consisting of the following features: a midline supra-umbilical abdominal wall defect, a lower sternal defect, an anterior diaphragmatic hernia, an absent diaphragmatic pericardium and a congenital cardiac defect (figure 7). The 21 cases demonstrated a wide spectrum of severity for each of the five anomalies, but in only one case was true ectopia cordis present and in only three were the anomalies severe enough to preclude successful correction. The presentation is so variable that no specific management plan can be formulated; each must be individualized depending on the findings in the patient. Immediate treatment of the omphalocele by either primary or skin closure, with concomitant repair of the diaphragmatic defect, is recommended. Repair of other defects should be individualized, but the authors recommend that they be managed in the newborn period, except for the intracardiac defects, for which treatment can be delayed.[39]

Another syndrome associated with omphalocele, known as cloacal exstrophy or vesico-intestinal fissure, was first described in 1908 by Arthur Keith, professor and conservator of the Hunterian Museum. In presenting "Malformations of the Hind End of the Body," he describes a newborn female with a defect from the umbilicus to the perineum:

> Near the middle of the exposed area of mucous membranes there is a depression; into the upper part of the depression opens the ileum; into the lower part opens the cecum together with a diverticulum representing the colon and rectum.... The median depression

has on each side of it an area of vesical mucous membrane, the two areas representing a divided upper vesical area of the usual type of ectopic bladder.... The vulvar cleft is widely open, the halves of the clitoris, prepuce, and labia minora being represented by tags on the margin of the exposed mucous area. In the male, there is a corresponding condition, the halves of the penis and scrotum being un-united. The exposed mucous surface usually reaches up as far as the umbilicus ... the rectum is imperforate and usually forms merely a cecal process ... the appendix is occasionally bifid ... spina bifida is present without exception ... the testicles are undescended in the male..."[40]

At the time there were eight such specimens in the Hunterian Museum, five females and three males, and Keith knew of four other males and two other female specimens in other museums.

The term "vesico-intestinal fissure" was introduced by Schwalbe in 1909 to describe this condition, but the term was popularized and the syndrome codified by P. P. Rickham in 1960.[41] According to him, Meckel described the first case in 1812. However, according to K. J. Welch, Littré reported the first patient in 1709.[42] Rickham presented four patients, three of whom died, one with non-treatment, one from malnutrition, and one from multiple intestinal obstructions. The surviving patient was incontinent of stool via a perineal ostomy (he had a primary pull-through) and drained his solitary kidney with a cutaneous uretero-ileostomy after his exstrophied bladder had been excised.

Kenneth Welch summarized the world's experience of 157 patients, including 23 from the Boston Children's Hospital, in 1979, and established the management principles still used today. These principles include: individualizing each case; immediate management of the omphalocele by either primary closure, skin closure, silastic membrane staged closure, or non-operative treatment with antibiotic/antiseptic dressings; salvage of all existing intestine, including the diminutive hindgut, and bringing that out as end ostomy in the left lower quadrant; delaying abdomino-perineal pull-through; delaying closure of the exstrophied bladder in most cases; consideration for urinary diversion, especially in cases of upper urinary tract damage; delayed genital reconstruction and cystectomy (if necessary); and consideration for female gender assignment in males with no hope for phallic reconstruction. Of Welch's 23 patients, only 6 survived and these were treated late in his series. The survival rate for cloacal exstrophy in the 1970s was about 50 percent; it is now 90 percent.[43]

While it is now possible to treat these patients with excellent survival rates, the functional outcome has been a concern. Several groups have demonstrated very good outcomes with respect to continence of urine and stool, though intermittent catheterization and/or bowel management programs are frequently necessary; few patients develop voluntary continence of both urine and stool.[44]

Gastroschisis (Belly Separation)

Early descriptions of specimens that may have been infants with gastroschisis were recorded by N. Steno in 1673 and L. Schroeck in 1677.[45] J. Calder, a Glasgow surgeon, wrote the first clear description of a baby with a gastroschisis in 1733. Calder was called to see a baby with the intestines "...lying without teguments of the abdomen; I at first imagined the containing part had been torn in the birth, but upon examination found the navel entire, and a perforation half an inch above it, thro' which the guts had fallen out, with the skin closely united to them.... The guts were inflated, and had no peristaltic motion that I could observe, gradually inflamed, and before the child died, were become perfectly black."[46]

Calder also comments that the mother could not remember being surprised, hurt, or frightened during the pregnancy. This comment is another example of the feeling that maternal experiences during pregnancy caused deformities in the newborn.

Among the collections of the Hunterian Museum, amassed by John Hunter in the eighteenth century, is a specimen of a fetus with what appears to be gastroschisis (figure 8). In 1769, Morgagni described a baby he saw in 1736 with a probable gastroschisis: "This child, if you looked at it, had one disorder, which was a tumor equal to the size of a man's fist, in that part of the abdominal region, on the right side, which is called umbilical, and a little above the navel itself."[47] This appears to be the first time gastroschisis was described as being to the right of the umbilicus.

William Hey from Leeds not only described the first successful repair of an omphalocele but also described the first repair of a gastroschisis, though the baby died: "In the year 1775, I was called to see a newborn child, whose intestines had escaped at the navel out of the cavity of the abdomen. I found the whole of the small intestines lying upon the belly, not enclosed in any sac ... the intestines had an inflamed appearance ... I reduced the intestines immediately, and as carefully as I could; but the baby died within a few hours after the reduction."[48]

Taruffi in 1894 proposed a classification system for gastroschisis:

- epigastro-schisis: epistric region [gastroschisis]
- epi-omphalo-schisis: epigastric region [probably omphalocele]
- thoraco-omphalo-schisis: umbilical aperature continuous with the sternum [probably Pentalogy of Cantrell]
- hypogastro-schisis: Aperature in hypogastrium [probably exstrophy of the bladder]
- hypogastro-etro-schisis: aperature in hypogastrium including the pubis[probably exstrophy of the cloaca]
- pleurosomata-schisis: lateral trunk aperature
- hologastro-etro-schisis: entire abdominal wall aperature extending to the pubis symphisis [probably giant omphalocele or exstrophy of the cloaca]

The first American report of a baby with gastroschisis appeared in 1913, from E. N. Reed of Clifton, Arizona: "...the whole intestines, both small and large, [were] outside the abdominal cavity. Examination showed that the bowels had passed along inside the cord for about two inches, at which point the walls of the cord had ruptured, allowing the bowels to escape laterally ... the bed was filthily dirty and the mass of intestines was thickly sprinkled with bits of straw, feathers, crumbs of food and fecal matter from the mother."[49]

He took the baby to the Arizona Copper Company's hospital, and when the infant was two hours old the bowels "...were cleaned gently with sponges and warm salt-solution, but this cleaning was not very thorough, of course. The appendix ... was removed. The umbilical opening ... was enlarged half an inch upward and downward and the cord-bearing edges were trimmed off. The intestines were then replaced..." and the abdominal wall closed. The child made an uneventful recovery. Reed described enlarging the opening as needed and freshening up the edges of the defect prior to closure, techniques that are still employed today.

P. Bernstein in 1940 was the first to really draw attention to the differences between gastroschisis and "umbilical hernia" (omphalocele): "Gastroschisis differs from true umbilical hernia ... in that the latter is covered by a peritoneal sac, whereas in the former the extruded organs develop extracorporeally, immersed in the surrounding amniotic fluid, containing vernix caseosa, debris, and meconium."[50] In his patient, the defect was to the left of the

umbilicus and consisted of a "...cyanotic and injected cluster of bowel loops, matted insep-
arably together by transudative adhesions into a firm mass, which was larger than the chest
and abdomen combined."

The viscera could not be reduced and the baby died. Not knowing of Reed's 1913
report, Bernstein stated: "...Surgical treatment of gastroschisis, unlike umbilical hernia,
does not yield any success, according to reports in the recent literature. Undoubtedly the
incompatibility between the size of the herniated viscera ... and the underdevelopment of
the empty abdominal cavity, cannot be satisfactorily altered surgically for the normal resump-
tion of physiologic function." Here Bernstein brings attention to the abnormal function of
the herniated bowel, a fact that led to the demise of many babies before the availability of
parenteral nutrition.

Up until 1943, except for Reed's case in 1913, there were no reports of survivors following treatment of gastroschisis, probably because gastroschisis was not recognized as a
separate entity from omphalocele until 1940. D. E. Watkins points out that before 1943
babies with gastroschisis did not survive because of the disproportion between the size of
the eviscerated viscera and the abdominal cavity; abnormal function of the intestines; peritonitis; dehydration; and, as he states, "the viscera are generally found to be thickened and
leathery, cyanotic and injected, with adhesions matting the loops into clusters..."

In his case, "...it was found that there was a slit about one inch long, just to the left
of the base of the umbilical cord. There was no torn peritoneum or evidence of a sac. The
edges of the opening were smooth and thickened."[51] Watkins opened the ring, replaced the
viscera with some difficulty, then "sprinkled into the peritoneal cavity" some sulfonilamide
crystals and closed the wound with full-thickness interrupted sutures. Interestingly, the
umbilical cord was not removed. The baby was supported with normal saline given by
hypodermoclysis each day, small doses of atropine and prostigmine to stimulate peristalsis
of the bowel, and "lactic milk" as tolerated. The baby was discharged on the sixteenth hospital day, tolerating P.O. feedings.

T. C. Moore and G. E. Stokes provided a clinical classification system to differentiate
omphalocele, intussusception of the ileum through a persistent omphalomesenteric duct,
and gastroschisis in 1953. They also treated two patients, both of whom died, modifying
the Gross method for treating omphaloceles by mobilizing skin flaps to cover the bowel,
creating a large ventral hernia. Thomas Moore, Gross' thirteenth trainee, was the first to
report using this modification of the "Gross technique" for treating babies with gastroschisis.
Gross utilized this procedure in 17 patients with "rupture of the omphalocele sac" between
1940 and 1950. Some of these were probably babies with what we would now term "gastroschisis." Six of these babies survived, and according to Gross in *The Surgery of Infancy
and Childhood*, "...If the rupture and evisceration had taken place after birth, the outlook
was far brighter than in those cases where rupture had occurred during intra-uterine life
and the intestines had become edematous, swollen, and matted together."

Both of Moore's patients had defects to the right of the umbilicus (figure 9). Both had
malrotation. One baby had multiple intestinal atresias, which were not repaired during the
first operation (skin closure only). By this time, babies could be supported with intravenous
fluids and blood and penicillin was available. Peristalsis was noted on the eighteenth postoperative day, so the baby was returned to the OR for repair of the atresias. Moore noted:
"...The gelatinous matrix in which the intestines had been embedded had disappeared....
Furthermore, the formerly discolored and thickened intestine had become normal both in
color and consistency."

The atresias were bypassed, gastric suction and parenteral fluids were maintained post-operatively, but the baby died from respiratory failure three days after the procedure. The authors bring attention to the functional impairment of the intestines in babies with gastroschisis, which "...might have been due to the thickness of the bowel wall from the profuse serosal granulation tissue and to the dense gelatinous matrix in which the intestines were embedded."[52] They stress the need for gastric suction and parenteral fluid until the physiological abnormalities subside.

From that time on, the treatment of gastroschisis paralleled that of omphalocele. Patients were either repaired primarily (rarely), or had skin closure only, or were repaired utilizing the Schuster "silo" technique, depending upon the condition of the baby and the herniated viscera.[53] Having these three techniques available, plus neonatal total parenteral nutrition, S. R. Luck and others reviewed a series of 106 consecutive newborns with gastroschisis treated between 1970 and 1985.[54] They achieved primary (skin and fascia) closure in 28 percent and skin closure with a very small ventral hernia (subcutaneous fasciotomy and minimal skin mobilization) in another 55 percent; only 17 percent required a prosthetic silo. Principles of this technique include:

- decompression of the upper gastrointestinal tract with an orogastric tube
- decompression of the lower gastrointestinal tract with a rectal tube and rectal irrigations
- mobilizing a one-centimeter skin flap circumferentially
- manual stretching of the abdominal wall, particularly in the flanks as described by R. J. Izant, Jr.[55]
- subcutaneous fasciotomy if necessary
- fascial and/or skin closure under only "moderate" tension (otherwise use of a prosthetic silo)
- long Steri-strips(r) dressing to distribute tension away from the midline

D. W. Shermeta and J. A. Haller, Jr., advanced the Shuster technique by introducing a "pre-formed transparent silo" for treating babies with gastroschisis in 1975. A compressible silicone polymer ring fit inside the abdomen and was held in place with four internal sutures. The transparent bag allowed visual inspection of the bowel during the reduction process, which generally took 9 to 12 days. Eight of nine newborns with gastroschisis were treated successfully with this technique; one infant died of aspiration pneumonia at the age of three months.[55]

The next advance was the spring-loaded Silastic(r) silo (manufactured by Dow Corning of Midland, Michigan) introduced by J. D. Fischer in 1995.[57] This silo has the advantage of not requiring sutures to hold it in place. It comes in various sizes and can be placed in the nursery without the need for anesthesia. Use of this silo has become standard practice for treating babies with gastroschisis when primary repair is not feasible.[58]

Probably the most significant advance in the management of infants with abdominal wall defects, particularly gastroschisis, was the development and introduction of total parenteral nutrition by S. J. Dudrick and D. W. Wilmore in 1967. Six beagle puppies were fed intravenously for 72 to 255 days. Compared to their litter mates, they all surpassed the controls in weight gain (figure 10) and matched them in skeletal growth, development, and activity.[59] The story of this remarkable achievement is best told by Dr. Stanley Dudrick himself:

> We originally were going to try to infuse them by peripheral vein, because Dr. Rhoads felt very strongly that clinicians would never accept central venous feeding. So I tried to feed the dogs peripherally by hindpaw or forepaw veins, but that was difficult. I added steroids to reduce inflammation.

I started to feel stymied, and so I just decided that I was going to go central and see what happens. So I bought a couple of dogs from the pound. They were a couple bucks apiece, and as a trial I put a central (venous) catheter in through the jugular vein.

I asked Dr. Rhoads if he would come by and take a look at something I had in the laboratory, so he walked down to my lab, and I showed him these puppies, and I had my graphs and my work all lined out there for him to see, and he said, "That's very impressive, Stanley." He said, "Good for you," he said, "and what peripheral vein are you using?"

And I thought, "Oh, my god! I'm gonna get fired right here tonight." I said, "Well, Dr. Rhoads, I'm using the external jugular as access, but I actually run the catheter down into the superior vena cava." He said, "Oh, so you're infusing them by central vein." I said, "Yes, sir." I said, "The solution is about 25 to 30 percent solute, and there's no way you can give it by peripheral vein. It burns like liquid fire, Dr. Rhoads." And I said, "I've calculated that, judging from blood flow and judging the rate at which we're giving this [formulation], that the solution is really dissolved, like, 200 or 300 to one per minute." And I said, "If you'll excuse the expression, sir, it's like whizzing in the ocean." I said, "Everybody does it, but everybody still goes in the ocean." It just gets diluted.

We originally tried to feed puppies from birth, and I actually had pregnant dogs brought to the Harrison Department near whelping, a couple days before they were going to deliver. I didn't want anything by mouth for these puppies. And they were little puppies. They were 200

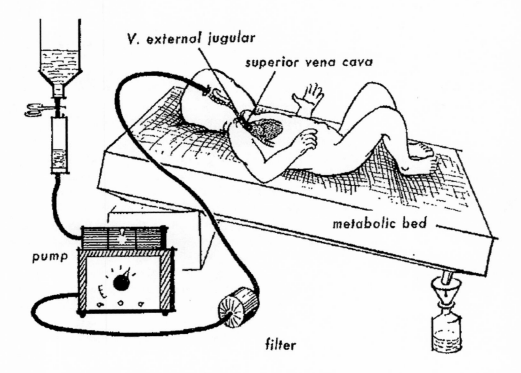

Parenteral nutrition or TPN is perhaps the most important factor in the survival of babies born with abdominal wall defects or major intestinal problems. The original technique involved passing a plastic catheter from the external jugular vein into the superior vena cava. At first, the catheter was tunneled to the scalp. Now, the catheter exits through the skin of the chest wall (from W. D. Wilmore, and S. J. Dudrick, "Growth and Development of an Infant Receiving All Nutrients Exclusively by Vein," *Journal of the American Medical Association*, Vol. 203 [1968]: 149–144).

to 250 grams, which would be about the size of a big rat. I miniaturized the technology for them and the delivery apparatus, and I began to try to grow the puppy from birth.

But then I had problems because I had—first of all, to get the puppies I literally would sleep in the animal quarters with them. I'd set the alarm to wake me up every hour to see if the mother-to-be was okay, and when I'd wake up I'd have roaches and mice and rats running around my body because they came out at night, and that was kind of fun. And I actually then suspended an Army cot from the ceiling with four piano wires so that I could lie on this cot away from the vermin, but they would crawl [down the cords]—[chuckles]. I don't know how they did it, but somehow they'd get on me anyway. So I lived through that a month or two. But it was "fun."

The baby was a direct application or translation of fundamental basic science and practical basic science in the laboratory to the clinical situation, and although I was motivated by adults requiring the nutrition, when the baby came along after we had already done six adults.[60]

The six adults had supplemental parenteral nutrition. The first human fed exclusively parenterally was an infant who had suffered massive bowel loss as a result of a Type III–b intestinal atresia. The baby was supported for 44 days with TPN and showed normal weight gain associated with increases in length, chest circumference, and head circumference. Balance studies proved positive nitrogen balance during the 44 days of total parenteral nutrition (figure 11). The baby eventually died one month after the Ethics Committee discontinued TPN, because it was deemed "experimental."[61]

The story of how this baby came to Dudrick's attention is also noteworthy, as colorfully described by him:

> Diller Groff called me up, and he said, "Stan," he said, "I've heard about your work with the beagle puppies. Would you mind coming down here to Children's Hospital of Philadelphia and giving us a talk on that tomorrow morning?" I said, "Yes, I'll be happy to." I was flattered. So I went down and they had this grand rounds, jam-packed, and I'm showing them my puppy data that I had, which was not complete at this time, but it was enough to be impressive. At the end of it, people had a lot of questions, and Dick asked, "Could you play your puppy trick on a baby that we have here?" That's how he said it. I'll never forget: "Can you play your puppy trick on a baby that we have?" And we got the baby to start growing. I knew that we had accomplished something.[62]

S. J. Dudrick, D. B. Groff and D. W. Wilmore described the technique for central venous cannulation in 1969.[63] In that same year, the first large series of "infants with catastrophic gastrointestinal anomalies" supported with TPN was presented. There were 18 neonates, 4 with abdominal wall defects, supported with TPN for seven to four hundred days. Normal growth and development, weight gain, wound healing, and increased activity were demonstrated. Complications of TPN were few and included glucosuria (cleared with diluting the TPN) and cannula sepsis (cleared with removal of the line). Adherence to strict aseptic technique in handling the lines and solutions was emphasized.[64]

In an interesting phenomenon regarding abdominal wall defects, the incidence of gastroschisis has increased over the past two decades, without a corresponding rise in the incidence of omphalocele.[65] The increase in incidence is most marked in mothers less than 20 years old, who have an 11-fold increased risk of having a baby with gastroschisis than older mothers.[66] In addition to lower maternal age, other risk factors include use of illicit drugs (Ecstasy), methamphetamines, cocaine, pseudo-ephedrine, alcohol, and smoking (nicotine).[67]

CHAPTER 31

Diaphragmatic Hernia

Early authors like Hippocrates, Galen and Paré mentioned diaphragmatic hernias, usually due to trauma in adults. In 1701, the English physician Sir Charles Holt described an infant who had difficulty breathing from birth until his death at two months of age. At autopsy, the viscera from the stomach to the colon had passed through a foramen in the diaphragm into the chest.[1]

Giovanni Battista Morgagni, the venerable sixteenth-century pathologist, did not use the term "diaphragmatic hernia" but noted a variety of defects in the diaphragm that allowed the passage of viscera into the thorax.[2] Morgagni told of a young man wounded with a sword slash that entered his abdomen, penetrated the diaphragm and nicked the lung. The man died 13 hours after the injury; at autopsy, his stomach and omentum had passed into the left thoracic cavity via a hole in the diaphragm. There were other similar cases found at autopsy, either immediately or several months after the injury. Fighting with swords and daggers must have been a common way to settle disputes in those days. Morgagni also noted an anterior passage beneath the xiphoid, the diameter of two thumbs, that allowed the colon to herniate into the chest. The patient had died in "decrepit old age" without any symptoms. Today, a hernia through this opening, named the foramen of Morgagni, is often asymptomatic.

Morgagni quotes previous authors in the cases of children aged two months and four years, respectively, who at autopsy were found to have the stomach, spleen, omentum, duodenum and intestine "carried up into the left cavity of the thorax." The infant who died at two months had been in ill health since birth, and the other child had been sick during the last two years of life.[3] Morgagni had seen similar cases in fetuses with abdominal viscera in the left chest and the left lung was one-third the size of the right lung. He said these cases were due to "nature herself" and that the fetuses were "quite monsters in their formation." It is unclear from the text whether Morgagni used the term "fetuses" in reference to a newborn infant or a stillbirth or if the "monsters" had associated defects. These cases, described by Morgagni but attributed to others, are examples of hernias through the pleuro-peritoneal hiatus or canal, a posterior-lateral opening in the diaphragm that normally is closed by the eighth week of fetal life. This hernia is now named the Bochdalek hernia.

One of the best clinical and anatomical descriptions of a newborn infant with diaphragmatic hernia appeared in the *Philosophical Transactions of the Royal College of Physicians*, London, in 1754: "The child started, shuddered and breathed easily for a while, but soon relapsed and died in a few hours. With my ingenious friend, Dr. Hunter, I laid open the abdomen and only the colon was in the cavity. When the sternum was raised, the intestines, spleen and pancreas were in the left thorax having protruded through and aperture in the

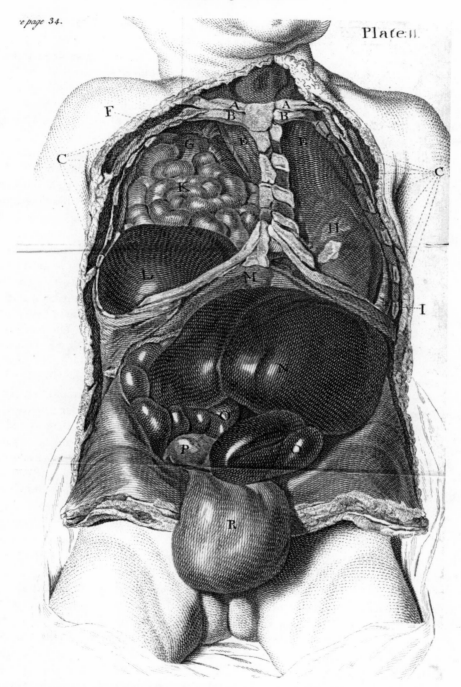

An autopsy performed with John Hunter in 1754 on a baby who died at a few hours of age with a right-sided congenital diaphragmatic hernia. The intestine and a portion of the liver are in the right chest and the heart is shifted to the left. Most of the liver, the colon, and the bladder are in the abdomen. Usually congenital diaphragmatic hernias are on the left side (from G. Mccauley, "An Account of Visceral Herniation," *Philosophical Transactions of the Royal College of Physicians*, [1754]: 6, 25 courtesy Dr. Charles Stollar).

diaphragm. The structures of the mediastinum were forced to the right side. The diminished size of the lungs resulted from the bulk of the abdominal viscera in the thorax."[4]

Sir Astley P. Cooper (1768–1841), surgeon to kings and consulting surgeon to Guy's Hospital in London, described in his book *Anatomy and Surgical Treatment of Abdominal Hernia* apertures through the diaphragm for the esophagus and blood vessels as well as defects in the muscle, or "unnatural openings," that allow abdominal viscera passage into the chest. He described two newborn infants who died as a result of such a hernia. In one, the left lung was no larger than a "small nutmeg."[5]

In 1846, Henry I. Bowditch (1808–1892), a physician at the Massachusetts General Hospital, examined a 17-year-old laborer paralyzed from the waist down after a falling derrick fractured his spine. Dr. Bowditch found the laborer's heart in the right chest, and instead of respiratory sounds on the left he heard "gurgling, whistling and blowing sounds like those heard over the abdomen and produced by flatus and intestinal motion." Dr. Bowditch diagnosed a traumatic rupture of the diaphragm with intestine in the left chest. The patient, however, had been aware that his heart was in his right chest from early childhood and he had been troubled all his life by palpitations. He died as a result of his fractured spine. At autopsy, the stomach, the major portion of the colon and several folds of small intestine were in the left thoracic cavity. The spleen and liver were in their normal positions; the right diaphragm was normal, but the left consisted of a band of muscle between the sternum and spine with a semi-lunar portion of muscle over the spleen. The peritoneum and pleura were continuous, forming a large cavity. Dr. Bowditch said: "It was evidently a foetal arrest of development." The account seems to describe a congenital hernia with a sac, but we cannot say for certain that the hernia was through the posterior-lateral pleuro-peritoneal canal.[6] Subsequently, Dr. Bowditch found 88 similar cases scattered through the medical literature from 1610 to 1846. In 41 cases, the hernia was on the left, in 18 on the right. The remainder involved both sides of the mediastinum. Bowditch determined that 26 cases were congenital, while 44 resulted from various types of trauma or unknown causes.

Dr. Bowditch was the son of Nathaniel Bowditch, a self-educated mathematician who in 1802 brought out the first edition of the *American Practical Navigator*, a guide to navigation of ships at sea. Dr. Bowditch graduated from Harvard Medical School and with his friend Oliver Wendell Holmes went to Paris for advanced medical training. There Bowditch became skilled in physical examination of the chest. He was also an ardent abolitionist who helped runaway slaves before the Civil War.[7] His interest in lung disease and his skill with a stethoscope resulted from his studies in Paris. His numerical analysis of the literature on diaphragmatic hernia also reflected his training in Paris.[8]

Vincenz Alexander Bochdalek (1801–1883), an anatomist and pathologist, studied and worked at the Charles-Ferdinand University in Prague. In 1845 he was appointed to be the head of the department of anatomy, and for the rest of his life worked in the laboratory.[9] In 1848, Professor Bochdalek published a paper whose title translates into English as "Some Observations About the Origin of Congenital Diaphragmatic Rupture as a Contribution to the Pathological Anatomy of Hernias."[10] This long, detailed and scholarly paper reads like an oral dissertation. Bochdalek commented that several other authors had written about the defect, but not in great detail, probably because there was little hope for treatment. The hernia, he postulated, is not as uncommon as previously believed and occurs in otherwise normal children. Typical of the era, he gives no bibliography. Bochdalek does not mention the number of specimens he has seen but refers to two examples, "which I have in front of me." Considering his detailed analyses of the posterior lateral diaphragmatic hernia, he must have examined many specimens. He described the defect as a split or separation of the fibers of the diaphragm where they insert in the structures of the posterior body wall. "This opening which I will call the posterior diaphragmatic gap [opening] is situated between the outer or third fascicle of the loin portion of the last fleshy point of its rib portion and the floating rib. It has mostly the form of a triangle, rarely it is arched, and even more rarely transversely oval." He also described a membrane devoid of muscle, indicating that he was aware that some hernias have sac. In the newborn, the defect measured five "linein" (about a centimeter) in length and three to four in width. He also knew that left-sided hernias were more common than right and that the liver may have had a protective effect on the right side. Bochdalek had also studied diaphragmatic hernias in adults and animals and speculated that if muscle fibers were missing, the pressure of abdominal viscera would stretch the sac (pleuro-peritoneal membrane) into the chest, where it could rupture. The membrane would then be absorbed. He even mentioned a specimen exhibiting this phenomena. He would leave treatment to "practical surgery," but suggested the possibility of making a cut below the last rib, one and a half inches away from the vertebral spine, and inserting a finger to press down the viscera into the abdomen. He thought that the expanding lung would hold the intestines in the abdominal cavity. In ending, he said he planned to continue his studies of the origins and development of the posterior portion of the diaphragm. An opportunity arose in 1867 when a coal miner suffered a fractured lumbar vertebra and had progressive difficulty with breathing after he had been crushed in a mine cave-in. The physical findings progressed, with the breath sounds becoming mucous rattling noises with a loss of the normal tympanic note on percussion of the chest. At autopsy, Bochdalek found an uneven fringed defect in the diaphragm as if it had been freshly torn, with the stomach and transverse colon in the left chest.[11] This was a traumatic, not a congenital, hernia. Professor Bochalek's name is also associated with a ganglion in the maxillary nerve plexus and valves in the lachrymal duct. Given his extensive work on the subject, it is totally fitting that the posterior-lateral diaphragmatic hernia should be named for Bochdalek. On rounds, the professor who may know little about the latest developments can always prove his superiority with questions concerning disease eponyms. The student who knows the difference between a Morgagni and a Bochdalek hernia goes to the head of the class.

Scattered case reports of diaphragmatic hernia found at autopsy appear during the remainder of the nineteenth century, but the authors were not as astute as Dr. Bowditch. J. O'Dwyer, a New York surgeon, operated on a three-and-a-half-year old child with the mistaken diagnosis of empyema. When O'Dwyer opened the chest, loops of small intestine emerged. He attempted to replace the bowel in the abdomen and suture the diaphragm, but the child died six hours later. At autopsy, the edges of the diaphragm had separated, presumably from intra-abdominal pressure.[12] O'Dwyer's observation of the "loss of domain" of the intestines in a small abdominal cavity would be important to the eventual repair of hernias in infants.

Some of the earliest successful repairs occurred in patients with traumatic hernias. In 1900, Cincinnati surgeon E. W. Walker reported the case of a "woodchopper" struck by a fallen tree. Twenty hours later, the man was in shock with a pulse of 145, dyspneic, and suffering agonizing pain in his left chest. The apex beat of the heart was displaced to the right, and a succession splash was heard in the left chest. Dr. Walker made a midline abdominal incision and found that the small bowel had passed through a rent in the left diaphragm. The bowel was viable; he sutured the diaphragm with four interrupted catgut sutures. The man survived to work as a carpenter.[13]

The wider use of the new roentgen ray resulted in increasing numbers of patients with traumatic diaphragmatic hernias who came to operation, though most congenital hernias in children were not discovered until after death. X-rays were often misinterpreted, as in a case of a six-year-old boy who died following a thoracentecis for a suspected pneumothorax. At autopsy, there was a posterior-lateral defect in the diaphragm with the stomach, colon and small intestine in the left chest.[14]

Dr. Lothar Heidenhain (1860–1940), a surgeon at the municipal hospital in Worms, Germany, performed what is likely the first successful operation for a congenital diaphragmatic hernia in 1905. His report was titled, "History of a Case of Chronic Incarceration of the Stomach in a Congenital Diaphragmatic Hernia, Which Was Cured by Laparotomy with Ensuing Comments Concerning the Possibility of Resection of the Carcinoma of the Esophageal Cardia."[15] The patient was a nine-year-old boy who had suffered two bouts of bronchopneumonia and in 1901 developed an empyema. A family doctor resected five to six centimeters of the left seventh rib and drained one liter of pus. The lung expanded down to the diaphragm, but six months later the boy commenced to vomit and had left shoulder pain. On physical examination, there was dullness to percussion over the left chest and the examiners heard gastric sounds. The removal of three liters of fluid from the stomach relieved the shoulder pain. At operation, Professor Heidenhain made an abdominal incision and found that the entire stomach had herniated through the diaphragm into the left chest. Only the pylorus was in the abdomen; adhesions between the omentum and the diaphragm had to be divided to free the stomach. The diaphragmatic defect was described as a two-and-a-half-centimeter slit extending horizontally from medially to the posterior axillary line.

Professor Heidenhain sutured the lateral portion of the defect. Medially, there were large blood vessels, and so rather than suturing the diaphragm, he packed the area above the liver with iodoform gauze to create firm adhesions. The boy recovered and later served at the front during the First World War. He was well 18 years later.[16] An assistant to Dr. Heidenhain, O. Aue, wrote a paper that recounted the first case as well as that of a "highly emaciated, cachetic" five-year-old boy who had vomited since birth. Roentgenograms demonstrated that his entire stomach was in the right thoracic cavity. From the description of the operation, the child appeared to have a hiatus hernia with the stomach in the right chest. Attempts were made to bring the stomach into the abdomen and repair the defect, but the hernia recurred and the child died after two weeks. The author speculated that the same approach could be used to resect a carcinoma at the esophago-gastric junction. There are some unusual aspects to Professor Heidenhain's first patient. The boy's symptoms appeared several months after drainage of an empyema. Was there a hernia sac separating the abdomen from the empyema or was the operation for the empyema somehow responsible for the hernia through the diaphragm? It is possible that the incision through the low inter-space may have injured the diaphragm, however, this was a bold, successful operation. I agree that Professor Heidenhain deserves credit for being the first to cure a congenital diaphragmatic hernia.

In 1925, Carl A. Hedblom — a surgeon from Madison, Wisconsin — collected from the English and continental European literature descriptions of 375 diaphragmatic hernias of all types where the patients had undergone an operation. Forty-four of these cases were thought to be congenital in origin.

Hedblom made little distinction between hernias through the esophageal hiatus and other parts of the diaphragm. Older children had suffered with difficult breathing, attacks of cyanosis and vomiting due to partial intestinal obstruction. There were 22 operations for all types of diaphragmatic hernia in children under 12 years of age, with nine deaths. The article is unclear as to the location of these hernias and none appear to have been operated on during infancy[17] The survival rate in these early cases was better with a thoracic rather than an abdominal approach, possibly because the older patients had dense adhesions between the abdominal viscera and the lung and pleura.

An extensive world literature review of diaphragmatic hernia in infants and children in 1929 painted a grim picture, especially for newborn infants.[18] The authors differentiated the symptoms of vomiting in babies with esophageal hiatal hernias from the weak cry, respiratory distress and cyanosis in those with posterolateral or Bochdalek hernias. They observed the absent breath sounds, dullness on percussion and dextrocardia in babies with left-sided hernias but noted that a roentgen examination was essential for a pre-mortem diagnosis. In older children, the X-ray was often misdiagnosed as a pleural effusion. All infants in whom the diagnosis was made during the first 36 hours of life died. This experience, and the fact that a few children with diaphragmatic hernia survived, led to the belief that even when a diagnosis was made during the early months of life, an operation should be delayed until the baby was older and stronger. Unfortunately, those sad children who survived with a Bochdalek hernia beyond infancy were chronically ill, malnourished and often misdiagnosed as having tuberculosis or some other more common disease.

This brings us to one of those unsung surgical heroes whose honesty and perseverance proved that children with diaphragmatic hernias could be cured. In 1921, Philomon E. Truesdale (1874–1945) — a surgeon from Fall River, Massachusetts — reported to the American Surgical Association on a child who developed a diaphragmatic hernia after being crushed under the wheel of an automobile.[19] X-rays demonstrated viscera in the chest. Dr. Truesdale operated through the seventh intercostal space and reduced the stomach, small intestine and colon into the abdomen; he closed the rent in the dome of the diaphragm with catgut sutures. Ten months later, the patient developed an intestinal obstruction due to a knuckle of colon caught in a small, recurrent hernia. This was again repaired through the chest, but when the child developed another intestinal obstruction Dr. Truesdale operated through the abdomen and released adhesions. The boy remained well after this third operation.

This case prompted Truesdale to study the effects of incisions on diaphragmatic function in dogs. His interest and writing on the subject led to referrals of more children who had been given up as "hopeless" by other surgeons. In 1935, he reported his experiences with operations in ten children, from 1 to 13 years of age, with both congenital and traumatic diaphragmatic hernia. This was the longest personal series of operations for diaphragmatic hernia in the world.[20] The only death was a nine-year-old boy who had suffered with cyanotic spells since birth. He also had a pectus excavatum and rheumatic heart disease. There were dense adhesions between the bowel and chest wall, and the boy died as a result of postoperative hemorrhage into his left chest. In all, Dr. Truesdale found only 36 children with a congenital diaphragmatic hernia who had survived an operation.

Dr. Truesdale graduated with honors from Harvard Medical School and founded in 1905 a hospital and later a clinic in Fall River. He served in World War II and was a founder of the American College of Surgeons and the New England Surgical Society. He was the first surgeon to use motion pictures as a tool to teach surgical technique. His work with children cast him into the national spotlight when the citizens of Omaha raised money to send a ten-year-old girl with an "upside-down stomach" in her left chest to him. The *New*

York Times described Dr. Truesdale as one of the few surgeons in the country qualified to do the operation.[21] The publicity from this patient led to a second child — a boy named Jimmy — traveling from California to Fall River to have his diaphragmatic hernia repaired. The headline from the March 18, 1935, edition of the *New York Times* read: "Soma Boy's Stomach Misplaced: Alyce McHenry's Surgeon Offers Services to Californian."

On April 7, 1935, the *New York Times* reported that the two-hour operation to relocate organs from Jimmy's left chest to his abdomen was successful. More than "forty prominent surgeons witnessed the operation."[22]

The first successful repair of a Bochdalek hernia in a newborn infant appears to have taken place in Glendale, California, in 1931.[23] The infant seemed strong and normal at birth, but when laid in the crib he developed dyspnea and cyanosis. Nothing was found on physical examination, but an X-ray taken the next morning demonstrated an "enlarged thymus" and shadows suggestive of gas. Barium introduced into the rectum and stomach showed the stomach and intestine to be in the left chest. When the infant was 40 hours old, Henry Johnson, the surgeon, opened the baby's abdomen under ether anesthesia. The viscera were reduced from the chest and the defect in the diaphragm was closed with chromic catgut. Breast-feedings were started four hours after the operation; the infant recovered and at nine months of age was perfectly normal. This terse, two-page case report from a surgeon practicing in a small community hospital is a landmark in children's surgery.

By 1939, two more infants — one 13 days and another three and a half months old — were successfully operated on for Bochdalek hernias in Chicago.[24] Both papers about these cases dwelled on the symptoms, physical signs and radiographic appearance of the hernia.

In their 1941 book, *Abdominal Surgery of Infancy and Childhood*, W. E. Ladd and Robert Gross reported 12 cures in children aged two days to ten years; two of these patients had esophageal hiatal hernias and the rest left postero-lateral hernias.[25] In the chapter on diaphragmatic hernias, Ladd and Gross stressed the importance of a vertical abdominal incision for reduction of the viscera and encouraged surgeons to search for anomalies of intestinal rotation. They "unrolled" the edges of the diaphragmatic opening and closed the hernia with interrupted silk sutures. They noted that since the viscera had been in the chest, the abdomen was poorly developed and complete closure would result in abdominal pressure on the diaphragm. They solved this problem by undermining the subcutaneous tissue and closing only skin, leaving a ventral hernia that could be closed later. They did not use a chest tube to drain air from the thoracic cavity. The air slowly absorbed as the small lung reexpanded and the mediastinum gradually returned to the midline. In later years, surgeons learned to their sorrow that a chest tube connected to a water seal rapidly withdrew air from the chest, but the hypoplastic left lung did not expand. Instead, the mediastinum came to the left and overexpanded the right lung.

Between 1950 and 1966, no deaths occurred among 36 infants more than 24 hours old who were operated on at the Boston Children's Hospital. Paradoxically, the mortality rate in babies younger than 24 hours of age increased.[27] Other centers reported similar results. The Denver Children's Hospital saw a 44 percent mortality rate in babies operated on during the first 24 hours after birth.[28] M. R. Harrison and his associates in Norway reported a "hidden" mortality rate because severely ill infants died in local hospitals and were not included in mortality statistics.[29] This "hidden mortality" was thought to explain the increasing incidence and severity of diaphragmatic hernia seen when better and faster neonatal transport brought sicker infants to pediatric surgical centers. In retrospect, this increased incidence may have been real, the result of environmental teratogens.

Several doctors noted a curious postoperative phenomenon, the "honeymoon" period. Some infants would appear to dramatically improve following an operation, then develop increasing respiratory distress and die. This decreased survival rate was associated with several changes in treatment. In many centers, a chest tube connected to a water seal was used routinely to rapidly remove air from the affected chest; few surgeons heeded Dr. Ladd's advice to create a ventral hernia to relieve intra-abdominal pressure. The rapid removal of air from the affected pleural cavity with overexpansion of the contra-lateral lung, together with pressure on the diaphragm from increased intra-abdominal pressure, may have contributed to some deaths. At about the same time, endotracheal intubation and mechanical ventilation were becoming more common in the treatment of infants with respiratory distress. This treatment did not seem beneficial in babies with diaphragmatic hernia. In fact, R. C. Raphaely and J. J. Downes, Jr., at the Philadelphia Children's Hospital observed a decreased survival rate in babies who were ventilated.[29] Our early, overzealous attempts at mechanical ventilation with endotracheal tubes resulted in barotrauma to the contra-lateral lung and, in some cases, pneumothorax.

Intense research involving fetal and neonatal lambs and cardiac catheterization suggested that the problem was one of persistent fetal circulation, with increased pulmonary vascular resistance and a right-to-left shunt through the ductus arteriosus and foramen ovale.[30] As a result of these and other studies, there were greater efforts to monitor pre- and postductal arterial gases and the administration of drugs to dilate the pulmonary vascular bed.[31] Survival rates increased, but some of the vasodilating drugs caused gastrointestinal hemorrhage, and mechanical ventilation damaged already tenuous lungs. Prolonged muscle paralysis resulted in atrophy of respiratory muscles. Some surviving infants were ventilator dependent for prolonged periods of time. The treatment of high-risk infants with diaphragmatic hernia was at an impasse, and there was little agreement among various centers about the best form of treatment.

In 1977, there was an amazing report of a baby with diaphragmatic hernia who survived when treated with extra-corporeal membrane oxygenation (ECMO).[32] ECMO provided near-complete cardiopulmonary support and no barotrauma to the hypoplastic lung. Survival rates climbed to over 70 percent.[33] Enthusiasm for ECMO continues, but its use decreased between 1997 and 2006, perhaps because of improved conventional therapy. ECMO requires a large team of technicians and constant attention from special-duty nurses and surgeons. In the United States, the cost is $250,000 per patient.[34] Despite concern about ligating and canulating the carotid artery, the early survivors appeared normal.

By 2009, the Extra Corporeal Support Organization's database included 4,115 infants who had been treated with ECMO during a 15-year period.[35] The survival rate in these highest-risk patients was 51 percent, but some infants had suffered seizures or brain infarcts, presumably due to asphyxia prior to going on ECMO but possibly due to carotid artery ligation. The evidence suggested that fewer neurological complications arose from veno-venous ECMO that did not require canulation of the carotid artery. However, as a group these patients were not as ill, so the impact of carotid artery ligation remains unclear.

Fetal surgery, starting with the creation of congenital anomalies in fetal animals during the 1960s, is one of the most spectacular features of twentieth-century medicine. The development of this field is a story of intense cooperation among obstetricians, pediatricians, ultrasonographers and surgeons to treat the earliest stages of birth defects. As a surgical intern in Boston, Dr. Michael Harrison envisioned treating fetuses with diaphragmatic hernia in utero.[36] During the 1980s, Dr. Harrison and his colleagues at the University of California Fetal Treatment Center in San Francisco operated on two thousand fetal lambs and five hundred fetal monkeys. Harrison succeeded in creating and then repairing diaphragmatic defects in fetal lambs, and in 1986 he reported success in treating diaphragmatic hernias in the human fetus. Unfortunately, in the highest-risk cases when the liver was herniated it was impossible to repair the defect without kinking the umbilical vessels. The results in cases where the liver had not herniated differed little in the neonate from standard treatment.[37] Encountering such tremendous difficulties, Dr. Harrison and his group ultimately abandoned fetal repair of the hernia. However, by the end of the twentieth century many centers throughout the world had begun carrying out fetal therapy, especially fetal endoscopic techniques.

The next attempt at fetal treatment of diaphragmatic hernia resulted from the observation that tracheal occlusion in the fetus resulted in lung growth.[38] A few trials of fetal tracheal occlusion have shown some promise in the treatment of human fetuses with diaphragmatic hernias. It is difficult to establish criteria for fetal treatment, and the results of tracheal occlusion among various centers vary widely.[39]

In 2000, Christopher S. Muratore and Jay M. Wilson — two surgeons at the Boston Children's Hospital, successors to Ladd and Gross — neatly summarized the changes in treatment of diaphragmatic hernia that had taken place during the last half of the twentieth century.[40] Surgeons slowly came to realize that a newborn infant with a diaphragmatic hernia need not be operated on as an emergency but should be stabilized with gentle, low-pressure ventilation, cardiac support, and if necessary ECMO prior to surgery. These authors also discussed the latest modes of treatment with nitric oxide to relax vascular endothelium and the intrabronchial installation of perfluorocarbon, a liquid with an extraordinary capacity to carry oxygen. They recommended the creation of a national registry to better coordinate the treatment of infants with diaphragmatic hernias.

The widespread use of ultrasonography in pregnant women has resulted in the fetal diagnosis of almost all diaphragmatic hernias.[41] There may be some difficulty with the differential diagnosis of congenital lung anomalies, but high-resolution ultrasound and fetal magnetic resonance imaging allows doctors to make the diagnosis and to estimate the severity of the hernia. The most important result of prenatal diagnosis has been the recommendation that afflicted babies be delivered in centers fully equipped to care for high-risk infants. Treatment may include placing the highest-risk infants on ECMO in the delivery room.

Babies with diaphragmatic hernia who have no need for ECMO or prolonged ventilation can now be operated on using minimally invasive techniques with less morbidity than an open operation.[42] It seems incredible that one can push neonatal intestine into the abdomen with thoracoscopic instruments. In his book *The Surgeon and the Child*, Willis Potts said: "The only time I tried a thoracic approach on the left side, it was impossible to push the loops of intestine into the unacommodating abdomen faster than they slid out; it was like trying to stuff foam into a bottle with a tweezer. In despair the chest wound was closed, the abdomen opened and the hernia satisfactorily repaired."[43] Apparently, air introduced into the chest to facilitate a thoracoscopic repair helps reduce the viscera. It is surprising that in thoracoscopic repair the small abdomen presented no difficulty and there is no concern about the accompanying intestinal malrotation.

Unlike less complex birth defects, pediatric surgeons have not adopted a uniform approach to babies with diaphragmatic hernias. As of 2011, surgeons at the King Abdulazis Medical Center in Saudi Arabia reported a 71.4 percent survival rate in 49 patients treated with high-frequency ventilation, nitric oxide and surfactant.[44] These results are comparable to those centers using ECMO and may indicate the way to future treatment.

By the end of the twentieth century, the incidence of diaphragmatic hernia was approximately one in twenty-five hundred to thirty-five hundred live births, a significant increase during the 70 years since Ladd and Gross described the definitive surgical treatment. Is this increased incidence simply the result of improved diagnosis? I doubt it, because postmortem examinations were routine in almost every hospital death and the coroner was required to perform autopsies on unexplained deaths, even in newborn infants. Perhaps the answer lies in research on the role of toxic chemicals in the production of diaphragmatic defects, pulmonary hypoplasia and pulmonary vascular anomalies in fetal rodents.[45] Nitrofen (2.4-dichlorophenyl-p-nitrophenyl ether), a potent herbicide, interferes at the molecular level with several genetic pathways leading to lung development. Following World War II, a variety of potent insecticides and herbicides such as DDT were applied to food crops all over the world. Some of these chemicals remain in soil, water and air for prolonged periods of time and are transmitted from the mother to the fetus and have even been found in mother's milk. This may be modern humankind's most dubious achievement during the twentieth century.

CHAPTER 32

Hydrocephalus and Spina Bifida

JOHN RUGE, M.D.

The rich, colorful story of hydrocephalus began with ancient descriptions of children with enlarged heads and a cast of characters who wore highly decorated gowns and wielded stone knives or bronze trephines to make holes in the skull. Today's neurosurgeons dress in crisp gowns and probe with sparkling, sophisticated, pencil-thin neuro-endoscopes to release spinal fluid trapped in the ventricles of the brain. The understanding of hydrocephalus could not begin until society allowed human postmortem dissections. Safe, effective treatment of hydrocephalus had to await the development of anesthesia, sterile techniques, and finally the parent of an affected child with no medical training who worked out a method of draining fluid from the brain.

The word "hydrocephalus" is a combination of the Greek word for head (*cephale*) with the word for water or fluid (*hydro*). Any enlarged head was termed a "hydrocephalus." Hippocrates thought that the fluid accumulated externally to the brain, but he knew the brain was the organ of thought and understanding.[1]

The Greek writer Celsus (first century B.C.E.) thought the enlarged head resulted from "a humor inflating the scalp, so that it swells up and yields to the pressure of the fingers."[2] The first treatments involved massaging a paste made with the herbs marshmallow or aristolochia, combined with wine, wax and olive oil, into the shaven scalps of infants with enlarged heads. This paste was thought to draw out the fluid and shrink the head.[3] Infants treated in this fashion may well have been suffering from edema or hemorrhage of the scalp resulting from a difficult birth.

Galen recognized the ventricles of the brain but believed they contained a psychic pneuma, the soul or animal spirit. He thought this pneuma underwent putrefaction and the pituitary gland cleansed the waste products out of the cerebrospinal fluid. This waste was then discharged out the nose as the "pituita." Galen also thought that the fluid accumulated externally to the brain.

No clear description of what we now term "hydrocephalus" appeared until Vesalius at Padua performed autopsies on children with excess cerebrospinal fluid [CSF] in the ventricles of the brain. He dissected a two-year-old child whose head was as large as a man's, and the brain weighed almost nine pounds. The volume of water in the brain was as much as three Augsburg measures of wine. The cerebellum and the whole base of the brain were normal.[4]

During the seventeenth century Franciscus Sylvius described the cerebral aqueduct that is named for him, and the Italian anatomist Antonio Pacchioni described "granular

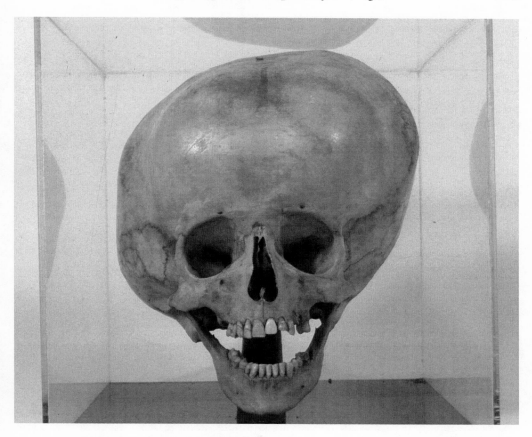

This specimen of neglected hydrocephalus shows the asymmetrical, enlarged skull of a 25-year-old man. This is a relatively mild example of hydrocephalus. Most untreated children died at a very young age (courtesy and © Hunterian Museum at the Royal College of Surgeons).

bodies" in the dura mater that were later found to be involved in the reabsorption of CSF.[5] Alexander Monro (Secundus), a professor of anatomy at Edinburgh, described the interventricular foramen; eventually, these ducts and foramina were recognized as sites of stenosis leading to obstruction of spinal fluid circulation.

Giovanni Battista Morgagni (1682–1771), the father of anatomical pathology, knew that the fluid originated in the ventricular system and described aqueductal stenosis as a cause for obstruction of CSF flow in children with hydrocephalus. Francois Magendie (1783–1855) thought spinal fluid formed in the subarachnoid space and flowed backward through the midline foramen, which is named for him. Lushka confirmed that the choroid plexus produced cerebrospinal fluid.

In the nineteenth century, Swedish anatomist Magnus Gustav Retzius (1842–1919) wrote *Das Menschenhirn* (The human brain), a book that brought together all aspects of brain anatomy and the pathology of hydrocephalus. In 1876, Ernst Axel Henrik Key — who worked with Retzius at the Karolinska Institutet — published *Studien in der Anatomie des Nerven Systems und des Bindegewebes*, a beautifully written treatise on the brain and cerebrospinal fluid circulation. This book detailed the passage of fluid through the ventricles and its reabsorption though the arachnoid (Pachioni) granulations. For the first time the circulation of cerebrospinal fluid was understood; the various anatomic locations where blockage of that circulation could occur and cause hydrocephalus were no longer a mystery[6]. Not until the twentieth century, however, did W. E. Dandy and I. Blackfan at Johns Hopkins devise a method of distinguishing communicating from non-communicating hydrocephalus by injecting a dye into the ventricles and then sampling lumbar spinal fluid. If the dye (phenolsuphonphthalein) appeared in the lumbar fluid, the hydrocephalus was caused by an obstruction.[7]

Early attempts to treat hydrocephalus with diuretics, head bandaging and irradiation by the sun were all unsuccessful; puncture of the ventricles through the scalp resulted in infection, leakage of spinal fluid and death. In 1751, Claude-Nicolas Le Cat reported the first device for repeated ventricular taps in a five-week-old baby with severe congenital hydrocephalus.[8] The family persuaded Le Cat to treat their child, though he believed the infant was incurable and that repeated punctures of the skull were dangerous because the integuments of the head were thin. The opening would never close sufficiently to stop the drainage when the cannula was removed. Le Cat made a trocar with a cuff and a screw top that could be "plastered" to stop the leak and left in place. He thrust the trocar and cannula into the brain and fastened a plaster made of linen cloths around the trocar. He then drew out four or five ounces of a liquid, the color of white wine and somewhat foul. He stoppered the cannula until the next day, when he withdrew more liquid. The infant at first worsened but improved a day later when Le Cat withdrew five more ounces of fluid. He also bound the head tightly, but the infant died five days after the start of his treatment. Le Cat concluded that the baby's hydrocephalus was the incurable sort.

In 1891, Heinrich Quinke eased the effects of hydrocephalus with intermittent lumbar punctures to drain tiny amounts of spinal fluid through a small cannula passed into the subarachnoid space.[9] W. W. Keen, a professor of surgery at the Woman's Medical College of Pennsylvania, gave precise directions for continuous drainage of the ventricles: "Choose a point one inch above the upper margin of the external auditory meatus and the same distance behind the meatus. Open the skull at this point with a three-inch trephine. On the opposite side of the head choose the point H two to three inches above the meatus auditorius. Through the trephine opening pass a groove director or a fine cannula towards the point H. The cannula should reach the ventricle at a depth of two to three inches. If drainage is required, introduce some threads of horsehair or a fine tube of rubber." All three of Keen's patients died, but he defended his priority as the first to perform the operation.[10] The site of his incision became known as Keen's point.

That same year, D. Hayes Agnew — another professor at Philadelphia — said: "...tapping the ventricles in cases of hydrocephalus is an old operation. The modern procedure consists in approaching the ventricles not through the fontanelles, but through a more dependent point, and by the use of subsequent drainage." He also said that most cases of hydrocephalus stemmed from tuberculosis. All five cases that Agnew reviewed, in children aged 2 to 14 years, died.[11]

Charles Balance of London and Harold Stiles of Edinburgh both ligated the carotid arteries in an attempt to reduce the production of spinal fluid from the choroid plexus.[12] Stiles pointed out the differences between communicating and non-communicating hydrocephalus and said he had tried all kinds of drainage into the subdural space and the abdomen, but with only temporary benefit. In 1896, J. Miculicz drained fluid from the ventricles to a space beneath a bone flap. He also tried various tubes made of glass or gold to drain fluid to the subarachnoid and subdural spaces, but without success.[13] In 1898, the English surgeon

G. A. Sutherland said it was important to operate early, before the mental powers were reduced. He and his associates drained fluid from the ventricles of the brain through the skull into the subcutaneous scalp tissues with tubes or strands of catgut and noted that it might be necessary to operate on both sides of the brain.[14]

Several German surgeons attempted to drain CSF through the corpus callosum into the lateral ventricle or into lymphatic and vascular channels using transplanted blood vessels. All of these ingenious techniques failed.[15] E. Payr of Leipzig used calf arteries to drain spinal fluid into the jugular vein; 8 of his 15 patients survived and 4 were "improved."[16] Forty years later, shunts to the vascular system were revived using plastic valved tubes.

The first installation of a ventriculo-peritoneal shunt with a rubber tube was performed in Germany by W. Kausch in 1905.[17] In 1910, Hartwell ran a silver wire from the ventricles to the peritoneum; his patient survived for two years but died from progression of a brain tumor. The shunt appeared to function, and at autopsy there was a tube of scar tissue connecting the ventricle and peritoneum.

Harvey Cushing, best known for his work with brain tumors, treated a child with hydrocephalus by modifying the German operations with a vein taken from the father to shunt fluid from the subarachnoid space to the jugular vein. Cushing's patient died two hours after surgery.[18] Cushing and Ferguson each attempted to drain CSF from the lumbar area to the peritoneum with silver wires or a cannula, but without success.[19]

Cushing's greatest contribution to pediatric neurosurgery came through two of his students, Walter E. Dandy and Franc Douglas Ingraham. Dandy, who graduated from the Johns Hopkins Medical School in 1910, worked in the Hunterian Laboratory and then became Cushing's Assistant Resident. Dandy became Halstead's Chief resident in 1916 and joined the Johns Hopkins staff in 1918. In the course of Dandy's career, he carried out extensive research on hydrocephalus and defined the obstructive versus non-obstructive forms of the deformity. Because he was a general surgeon, Dandy understood the significance of pneumoperitoneum, or free air, in the abdomen as a sign of a perforated viscus. This led him in 1918 to introduce air into the lumbar subarachnoid space. With the patient in the upright position, the air rose to outline the ventricles of the brain. Ventriculography was the most important diagnostic tool for brain disorders until the advent of the computerized tomography.

In 1921, Dandy reported a case of hydrocephalus caused by an obstruction of the outflow of CSF from the fourth ventricle of the brain.[20] This came to be known as the Dandy-Walker cyst. In 1918, Dandy treated non-communicating hydrocephalus by opening the third ventricle through either a sub-frontal or a lateral sub-temporal craniotomy and coagulating the choroid plexus.[21] Walter Dandy died in 1946 after spending his entire professional life at Johns Hopkins.

Franc Douglas Ingraham graduated from Harvard Medical School and in 1925 started his surgical training at the Peter Bent Brigham Hospital with Harvey Cushing. In 1929, after Ingraham spent a year on a traveling fellowship, Cushing sent him to the Boston Children's Hospital, where he established a pediatric neurosurgical unit. Ingraham helped develop the discipline of pediatric neurosurgery and, like William Ladd in general pediatric surgery, insisted that his staff direct all phases of patient care. Dr. Ingraham died in 1965, but in 1969 his associate Donald W. Matson published the second edition of *Neurosurgery of Infancy and Childhood*, in which he summarized the treatment of hydrocephalus.[22] In considering the indications for treatment, Matson wrote that there was little purpose in operating on a child with irreversible brain damage that would make acceptable development unlikely. He also recommended observation for children whose hydrocephalus was spontaneously arrested.[23] For older children with obstruction at the aqueduct of Sylvius, he recommended ventriculo-cisterostomy with a tube from the ventricle to the cysterna magna, as described in 1937 by Norwegian neurosurgeon Arne Torkildsen.[24] The Torkildson ventriculo-cisterostomy shunt was most often performed for benign stenosis of the aqueduct of Sylvius or for tumors involving the fourth ventricle and was popular until the advent of valved shunts.[25]

Matson also modified B. Heile's technique for shunting from the lumbar subarachnoid space to the ureter with a plastic catheter in babies with communicating hydrocephalus.[26] This operation successfully drained the spinal fluid but sacrificed a kidney, and the children suffered from fluid and electrolyte losses. Despite these complications, Matson had no immediate postoperative mortality and 41 of his 172 patients were free of symptoms for more than ten years. From 1952 until 1966, Matson also performed 98 ventriculo-ureteral shunts with plastic tubing.[27]

During the years immediately following the Second World War, there were many attempts to drain spinal fluid into the peritoneal cavity, chest, gallbladder, stomach, loops of intestine and bone marrow.[28] All of these techniques had complications, such as infection, kinking of the tube, abdominal adhesions and blood clots. In an effort to avoid adhesions related to the plastic tube in the peritoneum, Griffin R. Harsh III in 1954 published reports on a series of 12 children in whom he made a shunt from either the lumbar cistern or the ventricle to the fallopian tube and thence to the peritoneal cavity. He thought that the fimbriated end of the fallopian tube, serving as a natural entrance into the peritoneum, would avoid adhesions and allow for the natural absorption of CSF. Two of his patients died, and like all the others before it, the procedure was abandoned.[29]

These early results were so discouraging that many untreated children lived in institutions with heads too heavy to lift off the bed. The treatment of hydrocephalus languished until the development of a valved shunt that prevented backflow into the ventricles of the brain. In 1949, F. E. Nulsen and E. B. Spitz invented a shunt containing a platinum spring and two stainless-steel ball valves. It was placed in an 18-month-old child who did well, but the valve was difficult to make and expensive, and ultimately was deemed impractical.[30]

On November 7, 1955, Casey Holter — born with myelomeningocele and a Chiari malformation — developed meningitis and subsequently hydrocephalus. Two attempts at shunting him with polyethelene tubing failed. His father, John Holter, a machinist, believed his son's condition was a solvable mechanical problem. Working tirelessly in his garage and at the kitchen table, within three weeks John developed a new valve tube about the size of a pencil in diameter and three inches long. It was made of polyvinyl chloride and contained a slit valve at each end. Unfortunately, polyvinyl chloride was heat labile and could not be sterilized without affecting the valve pressure setting. Determined to find a better biomaterial, John Holter went to the Lee Tire and Rubber Company in Pennsylvania and found silicone that was being used as a grease to seal gaskets in high-altitude bombers. John Holter's silicone valve was first placed into a child in 1956; his son Casey received the second valve as a ventriculo-atrial shunt that was later changed to a ventriculo-peritoneal shunt. The shunt lasted until Casey died at age five from pneumonia related to his seizures.[31] John Holter's breakthrough invention eventually led to the development of biologically inert medical-grade silicone, used in later patients.

Simultaneously, Robert H. Pudenz also developed a valve system using silicone. These two valves and the ventriculo-atrial shunt were successfully used in the 1950s and 1960s.[32] However, the ventriculo-atrial shunts had to be lengthened as the child grew. Infections occurred in the shunts, and blood clots that formed on the catheter tips embolized. Glomeru-lonephritis was also associated with ventriculo-atrial shunts. Attention then turned to the peritoneum in hopes of finding a better terminus for the distal end of the shunt.

In 1966, Anthony J. Raimondi of Chicago used silicone tubing coupled with a distal Pudenz-Heyer slit valve to successfully perform ventriculo-peritoneal shunting.[33] His tech-nique, using the unified simple silicone shunt, became the world's most widely used shunt operation during the 1970s. However, continued problems with infection and peritoneal adhe-sions caused the shunt to malfunction. This led to more refinements in technique and even to drainage of the CSF into the gallbladder. Antibiotic-impregnated catheters have been devel-oped in an attempt to reduce shunt infection. These and other refinements, such as valves that can be programmed non-invasively to adjust fluid pressures, continue to be developed.[34]

Though the placement of plastic tubes to shunt fluid from the ventricles to the peri-toneal cavity remains the most common method of treating children with hydrocephalus, there have been attempts in recent years to cure the disease by endoscopic destruction of the choroid plexus, thereby reducing the production of CSF. This method eliminated the need to introduce foreign bodies such as shunt tubing into the brain.[35] For many years, sur-geons had attempted to coagulate the choroid plexus with a cystoscope introduced into the ventricles of the brain. The first instruments were bulky and difficult to use. Walter Dandy successfully performed the first endoscopic choroid plexectomy in 1922 but subsequently abandoned the procedure. Later, he described a one-year-old child whose head measured 54 centimeters in circumference, with a large, open anterior fontanelle. The cerebral cortex was about three-quarters of a centimeter thick and the dye test showed free communication between the spinal canal and the ventricular system. From April until June of 1936, Dandy operated on the child four times, removing first the glomus from the right lateral ventricle, then the glomus from the left lateral ventricle. Finally, Dandy cauterized the choroids plexus in the fourth ventricle and the body of the lateral ventricles. One year later, the baby could hold up his head and his mother thought he understood when she talked to him.[36]

In 1945, Dandy reported on 52 cases of open choroids plexectomy with an operative mortality of 17 percent. The hydrocephalus was arrested in 50 percent of his patients.[37] J. E. Scarf also used a ventriculoscope for cauterizing the choroid plexus in 1935, with limited success.[38] However, it wasn't until the British scientist Hopkins developed slender fiber-optic endoscopes with an "air-in-glass" lens that neuro-endoscopy became really feasible. M. P. Sayers and E. J. Kosnik reported on 40 cases of neuro-endoscopic third ventricu-lostomy, mainly in patients who had a functional shunt.[39] Others used neuro-endoscopy techniques in patients who already had a shunt.[40] The success rate of endoscopic surgery continued to improve, and by 1990 there were reports of children treated for obstructive hydrocephalus with endoscopic third ventriculostomy who did not require a shunt.

Surgical treatment of hydrocephalus has come a long way from binding the head or direct ventricular puncture, but even with the most modern methods these children often exhibit developmental delays and require care for prolonged periods of time.

Spina Bifida

Spina bifida, also known as myelomeningocele, is often associated with hydrocephalus. The lesion ranges in severity from spina bifida oculta, a minor lack of fusion of the vertebral bones, to an open spinal cord with lower extremity paralysis and incontinence of stool and urine. Spina bifida may well be the most complex treatable congenital anomaly consistent with life.[41]

Spina bifida has been found in skeletal remains from as early as 3000 B.C.E. and was depicted on ancient pottery and sculpture, suggesting the survival of individuals beyond infancy.[42] Both Hippocrates and Aristotle discussed this obvious abnormality but had no recommendations for treatment.[43]

A Dutch physician, Peter van Forest, ligated a cervical spina bifida in a child in 1587. The child subsequently died from infection.[44] Nicholas Tulp, another Dutch physician, used the term "spina bifida" in 1641 and stated: "...let the surgeon not imprudently open such a swelling, but force them to see the shame this would undoubtedly bring upon themselves."[45] Nicholas Tulp was the subject of one of Rembrandt's famous paintings, *The Anatomy Lesson of Dr. Tulp*, created in 1632.

Morgagni understood the common association of hydrocephalus with spina bifida and recommended against surgical treatment.[46] Friedrich von Recklinghausen (1833–1910) summarized the information available on spina bifida in 1886; his article titled "Untersuchungen uber die Spina Bifida" laid the foundation for the later treatment of the lesion.[47] Sepsis was the most significant impediment to treatment of these children, whether by aspiration, ligation or excision of the sac. When left untreated, spinal fluid could leak from the open lesions, causing infection. During the nineteenth century, many surgeons attempted to sterilize and sclerose the sac by the injection of iodine, potassium iodide or glycerine.[48] Daniel Brainard, the founder of Rush Medical School in Chicago, presented a paper in 1853 to the Society of Surgery in Paris titled "On the Injection of Iodine into the Tissues and Cavities of the Body for the Cure of Spina Bifida, Chronic Hydrocephalus, Oedema, Fibrous Effusions, Oedematous Ersipelas, Etc." On the basis of his paper, Brainard was elected to the society.[49] The iodine injection caused scarring and shrinkage of the sac, and the author claimed "cures."[50]

Carl Bayer introduced the modern technique for repair of spina bifida with a musculofascial flap in 1872. His layer-by-layer closure of the muscle, fascia and skin resulted in a near-anatomic repair. Here is an account of Dr. Bayer's technique:

> He [Dr. Bayer] rejects the use of the seton, the injection of iodine, and the excision of a portion of the sac, as being at the same time unsatisfactory and dangerous. He urges that the condition[spina bifida] is one analogous to hernia, and should be treated in a somewhat similar manner, that the danger of meningitis in the one case is no greater than the danger of peritonitis in the other, and that, as compared with the operation above mentioned, it is both safer and more radical. In a child 10 days old, in which there was a large meningocele the size of an apple, and who had already developed bed sores, he performed the following operation: the child was chloroformed, and the region of the bed sores cleaned and rendered aseptic. Two lateral flaps were made from the skin covering the tumor and were dissected down to its pedicle. The child was turned on its belly in order to avoid excessive loss of cerebrospinal fluid, and the sac of the meningocele was opened. The cauda equina was seen flattened out upon the posterior wall of the sac. It was loosened after dilatation of the incision, although in effecting this a slight laceration occurred on account of inflammatory adhesions. Two small arteries were ligated at the end of the cauda. No alteration of pupils and no spasm of the extremities were noticed. The cauda was replaced in the spinal canal, and the sac of meningocele was removed, leaving only two lateral flaps of dura, which was sewed together after thorough antiseptic cleansing of the wound. The muscles and skin were afterwards brought together separately.

The child recovered completely. Bayer suggests that in the future, through a greater development of the technique, a bony roof over the sewn sac may be produced by forming two lateral periosteal flaps from the canal of the sacrum.[51] Bayer's basic multilayered closure was widely accepted with only minor modifications and improvements during the twentieth century. The main problem lay in deciding who and when to treat, because closure of the spina bifida almost always led to a worsening of the associated hydrocephalus.

The father of modern neurosurgery, Harvey Cushing, attempted to control hydrocephalus in a newborn child by running a silver wire from the myelomeningocele sac through the lumbar vertebrae to drain spinal fluid. Within a week the child died from sepsis. In another seven-month-old child, Cushing closed the sac with the multilayered Bayer method; the child went on to do well and his macrocephaly stabilized without further intervention.[52]

Timing of an operation was often tied to the question of operating on a child born with crippling defects. In 1905, James E. Moore, professor of surgery at the University of Minnesota, analyzed 385 cases of operated spina bifida from the files of the Library of the Surgeon General's Office. The series began with the first known case operated on in the United States, in 1813 by H. H. Sherwood. Moore concluded that the operation should not be done at a "tender age" because of the high mortality and failure to cure the associated hydrocephalus or stop the progress of lower extremity paralysis. He thought a child should not be operated on until at least the age of five years.[53] By waiting, the children whose hydrocephalus spontaneously stabilized would survive.

James H. Nicoll of Glasgow took an entirely different approach and operated on all patients with spina bifida regardless of age or severity of symptoms. He said, "I have made it a rule to refuse to operate on no case sent to me."[54] By the end of May 1898, Nicoll had operated on 32 patients; 7 died within one month of the operation. Several of his patients had extreme hydrocephalus and may have died as a result of chloroform anesthesia. On child died of chicken pox a week after the operation. Here is Nicoll's report on one patient:

> Baby C., sent to me in November 1897 by Dr. J. Turnbull Smith. Spina bifida tumor, the size of an orange in lumbar region. Extreme hydrocephalus, the cranial bones of the vault rocking freely on the contents. On November 28, I excised the sac, and before suturing and closing the neck, I elevated the child and allowed a considerable quantity of cerebrospinal fluid to drain away. At the end of a week, the wound having healed by first intention and the health being perfect, we allowed the child who during the first week had been kept horizontal to sit up. The result was disastrous. In two hours the head had caved in like a cracked nut, and in a few hours more the child had expired in convulsions.

Nicoll also described a paraplegic and incontinent five-year-old boy who regained function after the operation. Nicoll's operating method consisted of excision of the sac and closure with flaps of fascia and muscle, with attempts to preserve the nerves. Nicoll also experimented with different means of treating the associated hydrocephalus by diverting the spinal fluid into the peritoneal cavity with tubes or by resecting portions of the lumbar vertebrae to allow suturing the omentum to the meninges.[55]

In 1944, Dr. Franc Ingraham published a monograph that reviewed 462 children seen at the Boston Children's Hospital over a 20-year period.[56] This splendid volume also extensively reviewed the literature on spina bifida and cranium bifidum going back to the sixteenth century. The outlook for children with spina bifida had changed very little since the turn of the twentieth century. Ingraham classified the lesions according to the presence of nerve tissue and the location and documented the presence of associated defects such as hydrocephalus, clubfoot, dislocated hip and urinary incontinence. He struggled with the question of who should be operated on. On the one hand, progressive hydrocephalus with neurologic disability was an indication to withhold treatment. Ingraham advised waiting until the child was 12 to

18 months of age to allow the neurologic condition to stabilize and for the sac to become epithelialized. On the other hand, if the hydrocephalus had stabilized, progressive deterioration in older children was an indication for surgery. In these cases, he thought progression of lower limb paralysis was due to tethering of the spinal cord as a result of growth. At the time of his writing, 46 of his patients were normal, 42 had mild neurologic disability and 60 had severe disability. We must remember that this group was treated prior to the advent of antibiotics, which would have controlled at least some of the complications seen in Ingraham's patients.

The situation did not improve until the mid-twentieth century, when valve-regulated shunts allowed children with spina bifida to live longer, with improved intelligence.[57] The intellectual outcome is also related to complications such as infections on the shunt that require revisions.[58]

An international ethical debate occurred in the 1970s when more children were surviving as antibiotics and shunting procedures improved. This led to a need for extensive services for the often multiple medical needs of the child with spina bifida. Many of these children would have serious urinary, orthopedic and cardiopulmonary issues in addition to neurologic impairments. Many physicians questioned the quality of life of children with severe spina bifida, and some suggested selecting for treatment those children with a better prognosis. J. Lorber's report from England on a series of patients selected for treatment based on their expected quality of life fueled the debate.[59] David G. McLone, a colleague of Dr. Raimondi in Chicago, analyzed multiple studies and provided a strong case against selection, as many of the most needy children led meaningful lives.[60]

McLone advocated closure of the meningomyelocele during the newborn period to avoid drying and further trauma to the nervous tissue. With micro-neurosurgical technique, using magnification, he preserved all neural tissue, reconstructed the spinal cord and closed the dura so the neural tube floated freely in cerebrospinal fluid. Ninety percent of his patients had a shunt operation for hydrocephalus, and all are followed closely with ultrasound or CT scans to determine changes in ventricular size. The presence of hydrocepalus and infection reduces motor function and hand-eye coordination and causes increased learning disabilities in children with meningomyelocele. Community ambulation was achieved in all of McClone's patients who had sacral or lower lumbar lesions. Children with higher lesions did not fare as well, even with orthopedic bracing.[61]

Surgeons operating in utero are currently writing the latest chapter in the treatment of spina bifida. In 1997, T. P. Bruner and N. E. Tulipan performed the first successful in utero repair of a child with an endoscope.[62] S. N. Adzick and his colleagues at the Philadelphia Children's Hospital further refined the technique and in 2011 compared the results of prenatal versus postnatal repair in a randomized trial of 158 patients.[63] The fetal surgery is performed between 19 and 25 weeks of gestation. A fetal surgeon opens the mother's abdomen and her uterus. The baby is rotated so that his back is uppermost, at which point a neurosurgeon removes the sac and closes the skin over the defect. The postnatal repairs were carried out in the usual manner. Only 40 percent of those operated on prenatally required a shunt, versus 82 percent of those operated on after birth. Babies operated on in utero also saw improvement in their mental and motor functions.

There is still no cure for infants born with spina bifida and hydrocephalus. The number of children disabled with this deformity has replaced the thousands of children with crippling poliomyelitis a half century ago. Some of the world's most brilliant surgeons have worked tirelessly against enormous odds so that today many children who would have died or lived with severe disability may now enjoy productive lives.

CHAPTER 33

Abdominal Trauma

For centuries children broke their bones by falling from trees or being thrown from a horse, wild animal attacks caused lacerations, and a mule kick or a thrown rock might fracture a skull. A boy who didn't have at least one broken bone or a laceration requiring stitches probably led a sheltered life. During the colonial wars, Native American children as well as adults were killed or injured by heavily armed Europeans and Americans. During the bloody wars of the twentieth century, children mangled by falling bombs were considered unavoidable collateral damage. Children's trauma escalated when boys as young as 12 were used as soldiers in Africa and Asia; their natural curiosity made children more susceptible to injuries by concealed landmines.

Doctors and even laypeople could diagnose and treat most fractured bones or lacerations, but a knife or bullet that penetrated the abdomen caused severe concealed damage. In earlier chapters, we saw instances when surgeons repaired and then replaced perforated intestines that had prolapsed through the abdominal wound. This procedure would have been more likely with a slash or stab wound; gunshot wounds make a small entrance hole but may perforate the intestine and damage the liver, spleen or major blood vessels. Prior to anesthesia and antisepsis, most victims of abdominal gunshot wounds died in agonizing pain from peritonitis or hemorrhage.

Very rarely, an intestinal perforation would fistulize or drain to the outside through the bullet hole and the patient would survive. Alexis St. Martin, a French-Canadian trapper shot at close range by a musket in 1822, became one of the most celebrated patients in the history of surgery.[1] The ball struck his ribs and penetrated his abdomen. William Beaumont, an army surgeon stationed on Mackinac Island in the Great Lakes between Canada and the United States, thought his patient would die. Instead, the stomach adhered to the abdominal wall and drained to the outside. Beaumont put bits of meat attached to a string in St. Martin's stomach to perform the first experiments on gastric digestion.[2] William Beaumont died in 1853; Alexis St. Martin outlived his surgeon, dying in 1880.

As recently as the American Civil War, a penetrating wound of the abdomen meant almost certain death. However, Dr. Samuel D. Gross reported on his experiments treating wounds of the intestines in dogs between 1841 and 1843.[3] His paper, published in 1843, was lost in a fire, but Dr. Gross reported his experience with a stab wound of the abdomen to the American Surgical Association 40 years later: "When faced with a stab wound of the abdomen, it will not do for the surgeon to fold his arms and look upon the scene as an idle and disinterested spectator. Far otherwise, he has a duty to perform, and that duty consists in dilating the external wound, if it not be already sufficiently large, in hooking up the injured bowel, and in closing the solution of continuity with the requisite number of stitches, at the same time the effused matter is carefully removed with tepid water and a soft sponge. All wiping must of course be carefully avoided as this would add much to the risk of peritonitis." Dr. Gross' report was advanced even for 1884, though he did not mention the outcome of his operation.

Samuel Gross was considered the father of American surgery and was the founder and first President of the American Surgical Association. He served for many years as professor of surgery at the Jefferson Medical School in Philadelphia.

According to Dr. Mark Ravitch, Dr. R. A. Kinloch of Charleston, South Carolina, was the first to perform a laparotomy for a gunshot wound of the abdomen. It was not, however, an acute operation.[4] Dr. Beiman Otherson, also of Charleston, reviewed Dr. Kinloch's original report and noted that the patient, a lieutenant, wounded at the battle of Bees Creek developed a fecal fistula and purulent drainage from his wound. Several months later, Dr. Kinloch opened the abdomen, resected and anastomosed the damaged intestine.

During the 1880s there were further animal experiments on intestinal suture and heated arguments about surgery for gunshot wounds. On the one hand, doctors were concerned about the legal implications if the patient died after surgery. Was the death due to the gunshot or to the operation? On surgeon expressed the opinion that all wounds of the abdomen should be operated on, with repair of stomach or intestinal wounds, suture of the liver and removal of a damaged spleen or kidney. The peritoneum was to be irrigated with bichloride of mercury and peritonitis treated with morphine, stimulants, cupping and leaching. During an 1887 meeting where the subject was discussed, W. W. Keen of Philadelphia reported on a woman wounded with a pistol bullet. He closed perforations of her stomach and intestine with silk and removed a "badly lacerated kidney." The patient died two weeks later; at autopsy, there was a short segment of intestinal gangrene due to an injured mesenteric vessel.[5]

Nicholas Senn, M.D., of Chicago, a city well known for gunplay, wrote in 1889, "...the operative treatment of penetrating wounds of the abdomen complicated by visceral injury of the gastrointestinal tract is now sanctioned by the best surgical authorities."[6] He differentiated wounds of the abdominal wall from those that penetrated and injured the viscera. If there was no visceral injury, there was no need for an operation, but if one waited for peritoneal signs, it might be too late to operate. Worried about the legal implications of an unnecessary operation, Senn thought of a test for visceral perforations similar to that used by plumbers to discover leaks in gas pipes. Senn experimented first on dogs and then healthy medical students to prove that gas instilled into the rectum could reach the stomach. In his final animal experiments, Senn fired a pistol bullet into a dog's abdomen and then insufflated hydrogen gas into the rectum: "On applying a lighted taper to the wound of entrance, and compressing on the abdomen, hydrogen gas escaped and was ignited. The gas burned with a continuous flame at the entrance wound." On opening the abdomen, he found two perforations of the stomach.

Senn used this technique not only to detect the escape of gas from the abdominal wound but also as an aid to discover all perforations at the time of surgery. There were no reports of exploding patients. In 1890, Senn attempted to demonstrate his technique for detecting visceral perforations before the Berlin International Medical Congress. He shot an anesthetized dog, a female, and an assistant commenced insufflating the gas. The abdomen did not distend and there was no escape of gas. The experiment was abandoned after an hour. The assistant had placed the catheter in the wrong orifice.[7]

The mortality rate and incidence of infection in wounds during the Spanish-American

War was dramatically reduced by the application of antiseptic dressings on the battlefield. Controversy remained about surgery for abdominal wounds, but one surgeon claimed that five of his nine patients recovered after surgery.[8] Despite this remarkable result, others still thought surgery was not indicated.

There were plenty of civilian gunshot wounds in the United States, and surgeons of the late nineteenth century — often operating on kitchen tables or even in the back of a saloon — established the principles of treating these injuries. They learned to close or exteriorize gastrointestinal perforations and to remove injured organs such as the spleen or kidney. During the latter part of World War I, when these principles were put into use, the mortality rate for penetrating abdominal wounds varied from 60 to 70 percent, depending on how soon the operation was performed. In civilian practice, this high mortality rate declined with improved resuscitation, especially when blood transfusions became available. Unfortunately, during the latter part of the century larger and more powerful weapons produced much more dreadful wounds.

Except for the occasional hunting accident or shooting in an urban gang war, penetrating injuries of the abdomen are rare in children. They are far more likely to suffer from blunt trauma as a result of falls, auto accidents or even falling on the handlebar of a bicycle. Morgagni, in his *Seats and Causes of Diseases* published in 1769, described a boy who at autopsy had a ruptured liver. His clinical description is classic for the signs of shock caused by intra-peritoneal hemorrhage: "...yet the pulse was barely perceived; the extremities were very cold."[9]

The fragile, vascular spleen, tucked up under the ribs on the left side of the abdomen, is the most common organ injured by blunt trauma in children. Ancient surgeons treated splenomegaly by thrusting red-hot cautery irons through the abdominal wall into the spleen. It was thought that splenectomy, or at least reducing the size of the spleen, increased an athlete's endurance. This is not entirely unreasonable, since an enlarged spleen is associated with certain forms of anemia and splenectomy cures the anemia.

The 1928 meeting of the American Surgical Association commenced with a symposium on surgery of the spleen.[10] The most common indications for splenectomy were the various forms of hemolytic disease associated with splenomegaly. William Mayo reported on five hundred splenectomies performed at the Mayo clinic between 1904 and 1928, with a 10 percent mortality rate. Arthur Dean Bevan of Rush Medical School in Chicago described the individual ligation of the splenic vessels, a technique for splenectomy still in use today. There was a report on 32 patients with splenic trauma from the Harlem Hospital in New York. Seven patients died without surgery and ten of the operated-on patients died as well. In 1933, Dean Lewis, who followed William Halstead at Johns Hopkins, reported that the mortality rate for blunt abdominal trauma had dropped from 70 percent between 1885 and 1890 to 22 percent in 1925.[11] This paper established the principles for treating blunt abdominal injuries that remained in place for the next 50 years. The indications for surgery were a history of trauma: abdominal tenderness, especially on the left side; a rising pulse rate; and a falling red blood cell count. The Hopkins surgeons recommended suture or packing of liver lacerations, removal of lacerated spleens, repair of intestinal wounds and conservative treatment for an injured kidney unless there was severe renal hemorrhage. There was a 28 percent mortality rate for ruptured spleens, but all deaths were due to associated injuries. The value of blood transfusions in the treatment of abdominal trauma was discussed, but at that time few hospitals were equipped to provide emergency transfusions.

These early discussions of abdominal trauma did not differentiate between adults and children, and it is quite likely that prior to widespread automobile use severe abdominal injuries in children were rare. Early textbooks on pediatric surgery discussed fractures, head injuries and burns but said little about abdominal trauma. The landmark 1941 text *Abdominal Surgery of Infancy and Childhood* by William E. Ladd and Robert Gross mentions two boys who suffered lacerated spleens.[12] The authors reiterated the signs that surgery was needed: abdominal tenderness, a rising pulse, a falling red blood cell count and the specific sign of left shoulder pain suggesting splenic injury. They also recommended removal rather than repair of the spleen. In his 1953 textbook, Dr. Robert Gross barely mentioned abdominal trauma. There were two patients with injuries to the extra-hepatic bile ducts, one as a result of the child being crushed between the bumpers of automobiles and the other from a fall. Gross also described 18 children operated on for ruptured spleens, of whom all survived. He recommended splenectomy in all cases but did say that in two patients with small tears in the capsule there was little bleeding.[13]

Societal changes following the Second World War may have influenced the incidence and type of childhood trauma. The movement of poor people into high-rise public housing resulted in children falling from unprotected windows onto concrete pavement. The increased use of automobiles led to more children who suffered multiple severe injuries. In the United States, the lack of firearms regulation led to the use of high-powered rifles and pistols in place of fists and slingshots in settling gang disputes. This urban warfare often involved children, who suffered the sort of high-powered bullet wounds once seen only on battlefields.

Family instability may have led to more child abuse during mid-century, but it was not until 1962 that pediatricians exposed one of mankind's darkest secrets.[14] Whipping and beating children as a disciplinary measure, as in "spare the rod and spoil the child," was common in many societies, but either the abuse became more common or physicians got better at recognizing a syndrome of old fractures, bruises, cigarette-type burns and retinal hemorrhages as indications of child abuse. In a particularly vicious form of blunt trauma, physicians sometimes saw infants with ruptured livers and a peculiar stomach laceration that we finally realized was due to a kick or punch to the abdomen while the stomach was full. It was as if someone had popped a paper bag filled with air. Often, a delay in bringing the child to medical attention resulted in a high mortality rate for abdominal injuries due to child abuse.[15] Society often turned a blind eye to these injuries or claimed that parents had a right to discipline their children. It took a great deal of effort on the part of pediatricians to change this attitude.

For many years, trauma victims were transported to the nearest hospital in police "paddy wagons" that also carried criminals, drunks and lost dogs. The victim was fortunate if he was taken to a large city-county hospital where the surgical staff was experienced in the trauma care. Local hospitals had neither the equipment nor personnel to care for seriously injured children. When it became evident that trauma was the most common cause of death in children aged 1 to 14, pediatric surgeons, previously interested mainly in birth defects and tumors, became concerned about trauma. Haller at Johns Hopkins proposed criteria for the pediatric trauma centers and a trauma registry.[16] Dr. Peter Kottmeier started the first pediatric trauma center at the Kings County Hospital in Brooklyn, New York, in 1962.[17] A few years later, trauma centers were instituted at the Cook County Hospital in Chicago and at the University of Maryland, both urban hospitals that treated large numbers of trauma victims of all ages. The American College of Surgeons Committee on Trauma established guidelines and training programs for personnel involved in trauma care. These efforts led to a system of treatment in the field by emergency medical technicians, transportation, triage and regional pediatric trauma centers. The program was similar to systems for trauma care that were common in Austria and Switzerland. Trauma centers were staffed by pediatric and specialty surgeons who were "on call" 24 hours a day, as well as special nurses and technicians. This system led to increasingly sophisticated, coordinated care for the child with multiple injuries.

One difference between abdominal trauma in children and adults is the incidence of preexisting congenital defects such as hydronephrosis or abdominal tumors that come to light after trauma.[18] The difficulties in the early diagnosis of intra-peritoneal injuries in very young children and in those obtunded by a head injury led to a search for improved diagnostic tools. Hospitalization with close observation of abdominal tenderness, the vital signs and serial blood counts was helpful. The majority of children with insignificant injuries improved dramatically within 12 to 18 hours, and the policy of continued observation resulted in no increase in morbidity or mortality.[19] Roentgenograms of the chest and abdomen were useful in detecting lung and mediastinal injuries, as well as free air in the abdomen indicating a perforated viscus. Early catheterization of the bladder was useful for monitoring urine output as well as discovering hematuria that indicated cystography with contrast material and an intravenous pyelogram. Tests for serum amylase and lipase helped detect pancreatic injuries. In experienced hands, these clinical and simple roentgen tests were sufficient in most cases.

Abdominal paracentesis with a syringe and needle was first used in adults to determine the presence of intra-peritoneal blood or fluid. The Tulane surgical group found a positive "tap" in all but 2 of 31 children who came to surgery for blunt trauma. There was only one negative "tap" in a child who was later discovered to have splenic trauma.[20] Unfortunately, a paracentesis or the even more invasive peritoneal lavage is not easy in a small, apprehensive child. There were also false positive taps that led to needless surgery.

Splenectomy for a lacerated spleen was the gold standard of treatment for over 50 years. A typical question for candidates for the American Board of Surgery was, "What would you do for a ruptured spleen?" The candidate would say, "Splenectomy"; the examiner would smile. Then the examiner would ask, "Suppose it was only a tiny laceration?" The correct answer was still "splenectomy." For many years, the spleen was regarded as a useless appendage, like the appendix, until reports arose of children developing fatal sepsis following splenectomy.[21] For several years, it was thought that splenectomy for trauma in older children did not result in postoperative sepsis, but this proved false.[22] There was absolute disbelief, even outrage, when Sigmund Ein and his colleagues reported that 35 of 56 children at the Toronto Children's Hospital recovered from splenic lacerations without surgery. The Toronto surgeons had observed a boy who had been suspected of a splenic injury but who was not operated upon. Later, after the boy died from an unrelated problem, at autopsy the spleen was found to be in two pieces, but healed. [23] This report coincided with the widespread use of computerized tomography that clearly demonstrated lacerations of the liver, spleen, pancreas and kidney and, with the addition of oral contrast aided in the diagnosis of duodenal injuries.[24]

Splenectomy for trauma was one of the most thrilling and satisfying operations in surgery. We regarded the operation as lifesaving but reluctantly abandoned surgery in favor of observation and non-operative management for most children with liver and spleen injuries seen on the CT scan. The argument then became how long the child should remain at bed rest and when to administer a blood transfusion. It probably didn't matter, because once the child felt well he was up and away. Continued hemorrhage as indicated by instability of vital signs and the need for transfusion became the only indication for surgery. Increased experience with interventional radiology and embolization led the non-operative management of some cases of intra-abdominal bleeding, such as liver lacerations with bleeding into the biliary tract.[25] Total intravenous nutrition also allowed conservative treatment for traumatic duodenal hematomas that had once required surgery.[26]

By the end of the twentieth century, many physicians became concerned about the cancer risk in children who had multiple CT scans.[27] A child with multiple injuries might have several brain scans and at least one scan of his abdomen and spine. Since fewer than 5 percent of children with abnormal scans required abdominal exploration, these concerns led to a plea for fewer CT scans.[28] Clinical examination with abdominal ultrasound was equally effective in evaluating children with abdominal trauma, without the risks of radiation.[29]

The concern over trauma during the past 50 years has led to an almost fanatic preoccupation with safety. Children are required to wear a helmet to ride a bike, and infants are restrained in special car seats. Children are warned not to go near the water or climb trees; all play is supervised for "safety." Despite uncounted committee meetings, educational efforts by medical and lay organizations, and sophisticated surgical technology, thousands of children in the United States still die as a result of injuries and more are disabled for life. Other countries, such as Britain, Sweden, Italy and Holland, have much lower death rates due to injury.[30] The high injury rate among children in the United States is not surprising when one considers our lax attitudes toward guns and automobiles. The public is outraged when a deranged student guns down his classmates, but politicians are too timid to limit access to high-powered automatic weapons. A drunk driver can kill half a dozen children, but a judge will rule that it was an accident and the driver may not even lose his driver's license. Automobile accidents are a leading cause of death among teenage drivers, but the idea of making driving contingent on high school graduation is not politically feasible. The reality of high death and disability rates for trauma appears to be a permanent feature of American life, at least in the near future.

CHAPTER 34

Inguinal Hernia

CATHERINE M. COSENTINO, M.D.

"No age, sex, rank, or condition of life, is exempted from it; the rich, the poor, the lazy, and, the laborious, are equal liable to it; it produces certain inconvenience to all who are afflicted by it; it sometimes puts the life of the patient in such hazard as to require one of the most delicate operations in surgery.
— Percival Pott, from *Treatise on Ruptures* in 1756[1]

The *Corpus Hippocraticum* consisted of 72 medical works thought to include the writings of Hippocrates himself as well as writings of his successors, but surprisingly, a discussion of hernias in not found in this body of work. It is possible that the manuscript was lost.[2]

Aulus Corneleuis Celsus provides us with a picture of the surgical art at the time of Christ. Celsus was probably not a physician but a literary man who summarized existing knowledge in scientific fields. His only surviving work is *De Re Medica Libri Octo* (Eight books on medicine). The last two books deal with surgery.[3] He discusses inguinal hernia anatomy and surgery and specifically mentions children: "And if in a young child intestine prolapses bandaging should be tried before the knife. For this a strip of linen is taken, to one end of which is stitched a ball of rags which is placed on the prolapse itself so as to push back the intestines: then the rest of the bandage is firmly tied all round; under this the intestines are forced inside and the tunics become aglutined together."[3]

The growth of Western medicine declined when the Roman Empire collapsed but began its slow revival at Salerno. William of Salicet (1210–1277) was one of the early surgeons of this period who helped elevate surgery. His *Cyrurgia* in 1275 was the first complete book on the subject in the Middle Ages. On hernias, he wrote: "...And if you were to be assured of this manner of opening, then permit the testicle to re-descend to its place, and do not dream in any fashion of extirpating it, as do some stupid and ignorant doctors who know nothing; but take the nerve (the spermatic cord) itself and the conduit through which the intestines descend ... and tie completely this conduit and nerve..."[5]

Operative surgery was shunned during this time partly due to the risks involved and the risk to the practitioner's reputation. Pierre Franco (1500–1561), who had little formal education and was apprenticed to either a barber or "cutter," published *Traite des Hernies* in Lyon in 1561. He described in great detail the technique for radical repair of hernia. Removal of the testicle was the usual procedure, but he devised a method that spared the testes for those patients who had one testis: "After having shown the manner and procedure of the cure of intestinal hernias by removing the sexual parts, we will now teach the procedure and manner of curing them without the waste of these parts." The operation involved excising and ligating the sac without sacrificing the cord structures.[6]

Ambroise Parè (1510–1590), one of the most celebrated surgeons of the Renaissance, was most noted for his military work but wrote on many subjects, including hernia. In his "Of the Cure of Ruptures" Parè wrote: "Because children are very subject to Ruptures, but those truly not fleshy or varicous, but watery, windy and especially of the Guts by reason of continual and painfull crying and coughing: Therefore in the first place we will treate of their cure." He goes on to describe a truss that he advocated: "...the chiefe of the cure consists in folded clothes, and Trusses, and ligatures artificially made, that the restored gut may be contained in its place, for which purpose he shall keepe child seated in his cradle for 30 or 40 dayes.... Truly I have healed many by the help of such remedies and have delivered them from the hands of Gelders, which are greedy of childrens testicles, by reason of the great gaine they receive from thence."[7] L. DeMause in *Foundations of Psychohistory* describes Parè's displeasure with "Gelders" greedy to get children's testicles for magical purposes.[8]

Parè's case reports and autopsy records give insight into this superb surgeon:

> Undescended Testis Mistaken for Hernia (MI, 418) At this point I want to advise the young surgeons that the testes are not yet descended into the scrotum. They are retained in the groin and make a painful tumor, and since it is considered an intestinal hernia, it is treated with astringent plasters,trusses and bandages to restrain it. This increases the pain and prevents descent of the testis.
>
> Not long ago I was called to such a case and after finding a single testis in the scrotum, the child not having been castrated, had the plaster and the truss he wore removed. I told the father to let the child run and jump to help the testis descend into its natural place, which it did little-by-little; without any complication.[9]

Caspar Stromayr, a German surgeon of the sixteenth century, wrote a manuscript, *Practia Copiosa*, in 1559 that was not published until 1925. It includes 186 illustrations dealing chiefly with hernia and to a lesser extent surgery of the eye. His operation for cure of hernia consisted of removal of the sac to the level of the internal ring together with the cord and testes using a groin approach. He was the first to differentiate indirect from direct hernias for which he spared the testes.[10]

At that time, barber surgeons removed both testes, a practice that may have led to the initial *castrati*, singers who were popular in church choirs and opera. Castrated young boys had voices that were ideal for soprano parts. If a boy had a good soprano voice, castration would ensure it remained so into adulthood. Once the news of the castrati spread, centers developed in many areas in Europe for this operation. Many boys, mainly poor, underwent castration with the hope of future fame and fortune. Sadly so, few reached such heights. The dominance of the castrati began to decline in the early 1800s. The last castrato in the Vatican was Alessandro Moreschi, who died in 1922 at the age of 64.[11]

The practice of orchiectomy for hernia repair ended in the late eighteenth century as surgeons such as Percival Pott (1714–1788) denounced the radical cure for hernia but would operate for strangulation. Pott described "congenital hernia," but this resulted in some controversy, since the observations had been taken from preparations made by John Hunter (1728–1793), renowned surgeon and anatomist.[12]

The post–Listerian age brought the repair of non-strangulated hernias to a test. The results were far from satisfactory, with most hernias recurring. Then came the work of Eduardo Bassini (1844–1924): "In order to achieve a radical cure (of inguinal hernia) it is absolutely essential to restore those conditions in the area of the hernial orifice which existed under normal conditions." He recommended physiologic reconstruction of the canal. His technique involved ligation and excision of the sac along with suturing the three layers, internal oblique, transverus abduminus muscle, and transversalis fascia, to the posterior edge of the inguinal ligament after splitting of the transversalis fascia. He initially presented his first 42 cases to the Italian Surgical Society in 1887.[13] His comprehensive article "The Treatment of Inguinal Hernias" was published in 1890 and described his experience with 262 cases. Eleven patients were under 5 years of age. Thirteen were 5 to 10 years of age. Twenty-four were 11 to 16 years of age. There were no deaths in the nonstrangulated cases. All but four patients were followed from 1 month to 4½ years. There were seven recurrences (2.7 percent).[14] No other technique had such good results. His technique was widely adopted and he became the creator of modern hernia surgery.

Dr. William T. Bull, one of New York's leading surgeons of the time, read a paper to the American Surgical Association in 1890 on hernia. He stated: "Of the cases in children, it may be said that they prove or disprove nothing; prompt recurrence in cases where the sac was not found, shows the importance of obliterating it by any method of cure as well as the uncertainty of simple closure of the pillars of the external ring with sutures."[15]

Drs. Bull and W. B. Coley in 1898 reported in "Observations upon the Operative Treatment of Hernias at the Hospital for Ruptured and Crippled" their experience over a ten year period. During the period 1889–1890 they operated on 19 cases of hernia in children, with a 50 percent recurrence rate. They then began using Bassini's method, with much improved results. From 1888 to 1898 they operated on a variety of hernias in 1,051 cases. Children under 14 years of age comprised 461 cases (16 prior to 1890). Bassini's method was employed in 371 children under the age of 14. There were three recurrences (0.75 percent). In the patients (children and adults) operated on since 1890, there were five deaths in 917 cases. One child, with a spinal cord disease, died of pneumonia, pericarditis and a wound infection. One 20-month-old infant died of shock secondary to an irreducible hernia containing cecum. Drs. Bull and Cole reported 19 hernias in children containing the cecum and/or appendix. In five children, they removed the appendix due to extensive adhesions. Seven children presented with strangulated hernias. Six were in children under two years of age.[16]

A. H. Ferguson in 1899 first suggested leaving the cord undisturbed during repair: "Tearing the cord out of its bed is without anatomic reason to recommend it, a physiologic act to suggest it, nor does it give brilliant surgical results to justify its continuance. Leave the cord alone, for it is the sacred pathway along which travel elements indispensable to the perpetuity of our race." The age of his patients ranged from 5 to 76 years.[17]

In a short time, P. Turner, A. MacLennan and R. H. Russell all stated that cure in children required simple removal of the sac.[18] Turner in "The Radical Cure of Inguinal Hernia in Children" in 1912 stated: "The essential point about an inguinal hernia in a child is the presence of a sac; there is no congenital weakness or deficiency of the abdominal wall." He felt a truss interfered with the development of abdominal wall musculature and was in fact harmful.[19]

MacLennan in 1922 reported on 1,038 hernia operations on 978 children in Glasgow, aged two weeks to 12 years, with eight deaths.[20] Four died due to "status lymphaticus," one with pneumonia, three from gastroenteritis. There were four, possibly five recurrences. All four children presented with strangulated hernias recovered. The appendix was removed on 15 occasions. MacLennan was the first to describe adrenal cortical rests in 1919. In this series he removed 14 adrenal cortical rests.[21]

Russell in 1925 described simple suture ligature of the freed sac. He stated the truss had fallen into complete disuse at the Melbourne Children's Hospital at that time.[22] Gertrude Herzfeld in her 1925 paper "The Radical Cure of Hernia in Infants and Young Children" reviewed 1,000 consecutive cases over a two year period of time.[23] She advocated outpatient surgery and claimed that the operation could be performed in three to five minutes. In 16 cases the appendix was present and 11 were removed. The ovary was present in the sac in 15 percent of cases (16/106). In 1 case the ovary was gangrenous and was removed. She felt that incarceration occurred rarely in children and usually in infants under 6 months of age. In her series 9 cases had been temporarily irreducible prior to operation. She also noted the presence of the bladder in the hernia sac in 7 cases and discussed abnormality in descent of the testicle in 32 cases. She had one mortality in a four-month infant who died on the operating table before the operation due to status lymphaticus. The vas deferens was cut and repaired in 1 case. One patient developed pneumonia. Herzfeld had one recurrence. She concluded that the operation might be safely performed at any age as long as the infant was doing well and advocated an outpatient approach.

Drs. William Ladd and Robert E. Gross in their 1941 text, *Abdominal Surgery of Infancy and Childhood*, discussed the use of a yarn truss for hernias in babies until herniorrhaphy could be more easily performed.[24] They did a modified Ferguson operation and felt there was some difficulty in operating on children younger than a year and a half or two years of age since the cord structures were delicate. There was also some concern about contamination of the wound by urine. They recommended a "Stiles" dressing, which consisted of a cradle from which the diaper was hung down between the legs absorbing the urine. The baby was restrained and kept on his back for a week in the hospital. Bed rest was recommended for the second week at home, after which walking was permitted. They operated on young infants if needed and repaired large hernias that were difficult to reduce regardless of age. If a child presented with an incarcerated hernia that could be reduced, they advocated waiting for two to three days until the edema related to the incarceration had resolved.

From 1915 to 1939, 4,133 inguinal herniorrhaphies were performed at the Boston Children's Hospital. The majority had been followed for at least one year. They knew of ten recurrences. They noted a slightly greater incidence of testicular atrophy than recurrences.

Dr. Willis J. Potts in "The Treatment of Inguinal Hernia in Infants and Children," published in 1950, stated that there was much misinformation concerning hernia repair in children, since most of the literature concerned adults.[25] Potts advocated simple removal of the sac and had only one recurrence in a series of six hundred hernias. There was one death in a four-pound six-week premature infant admitted in extremis with a strangulated hernia. Potts' patients were admitted the afternoon before surgery and discharged the day after. Children under five years of age had no restrictions. Older children were advised to refrain from "violent exercise."

J. W. Duckett published a similar series in 1952 describing a series of 380 herniorrhaphies during a six-year period.[26] He concluded that hernia repair should be done at whatever age diagnosis is made with few exceptions and suggested exploring the opposite side when there was even slight evidence of a contra-lateral hernia. There followed a continuing debate on the advisability of exploring the contra-lateral side if there was no sign of a hernia on the opposite side. In one of the darker episodes in the history of pediatric surgery, for a time some surgeons injected contrast material into the abdominal cavity in an attempt to diagnose a second hernia. Some, like R. E. Rothenberg and T. Barnett in 1955, concluded that bilateral exploration was justified.[27] Others decided that routine bilateral exploration was indicated in children under one year of age, but the issue was hotly debated with no conclusion. M. I. Rowe and H. W. Clatworthy in 1971 in 2,764 patients found a "significant" patent processus vaginalis on the contra-lateral side in 48 percent of patients.[28] The argument remained unsettled, because some surgeons were worried that complications would outweigh possibility of a second hernia developing at a later date.

The Section of Surgery on the American Academy of Pediatrics surveyed its members in 1993, looking at the practice of inguinal hernia repair in infants and young children.[29] 65 percent performed contra-lateral exploration in males if they were two years of age or younger. 80 percent use it in females up to four years of age. Laparoscopic evaluation of the contra-lateral internal ring was performed by only 6 percent of responders (40 percent use the open ipsilateral sac for introduction of the laparoscope).

G. W. Holcomb III advocated laparoscopy to examine the contra-lateral side when there was a known hernia on one side.[30] When he found a patent processus vaginalis, he repaired the opposite side. The argument continued as to whether a patent processus was significant.

P. Montupet and C. Esposito in 1999[31] and Schier in 2000[32] described their initial results with the laparoscopic repair of inguinal hernias. They then described their three-center experience with 933 laparosopic inguinal herniorrhaphies in 666 children.[33] The recurrence rate was 3.4 percent, with a follow-up on only two months to seven years, and four children had postoperative hydroceles. The authors blamed the high recurrence rate on an initial lack of experience with the instrumentation. Perhaps this is an instance when we should return to earlier techniques — such as those of Gertrude Herzfeld in the early part of the century.

CHAPTER 35

Atresias of the Jejunum, Ileum and Colon

RANDALL POWELL, M.D.

The term "atresia" derives from the Greek word *atrelos* which means "without opening or perforation," which in turn derives from the Greek *a* meaning "no" or "without" and the Greek *tresis* meaning "orifice." This definition is the commonly accepted term for this congenital anomaly, but throughout the recorded literature pertaining to the term "atresia" some liberties with the definition have been taken, even when the term has been defined in the body of the article.

Perhaps one of the best examples of this is represented by Charles Howes Evans in his collective review that was published in 1951.[1] For this paper he reviewed 1,498 cases of intestinal atresia as reported in 1,353 different articles, theses and textbooks, which represents a subset of over 4,100 original articles in 19 languages used for a larger study of problems resulting in "acute surgical condition of the abdomen" in the newborn and infant. All of the foreign-language articles were translated by either the Department of Literacy Research of the American College of Surgeons or the New York Academy of Medicine. After defining atresia in a footnote, Evans then proceeds to redefine the term to refer to a "subtotal or total atresia of the gastrointestinal tract, excluding the esophageal and rectoanal regions." This same freedom with the usage of the term "atresia" recurs throughout the recorded literature.

Evans reported another problem when attempting to review the incidence of the lesion and successful treatment. A number of the latter seem to have been published two or more times. An example is a duodenal atresia successfully treated by Weeks in 1916, which was reported by Porter and Carter in 1922 and then reported again in 1927 by Weeks and Delprat. Another example is an infant with ileal atresia treated by Carter in 1930 and reported in 1933. In 1937 Reisman reported the same case again in detail. In subsequent series these two examples were reported as four successfully treated patients.

Evans goes on to cite the difficulty in enumerating cases of atresia in Boston. In their textbook *Abdominal Surgery of Infancy and Childhood* published in 1941, Ladd and Gross list all cases located at the Children's Hospital. However, many of the cases were also either reported as case reports or series by a number of surgeons, including Quinland (1922), Loitman (1927), Thorndike (1927), Baty (1929), Ladd (1930, 1933, 1937), Neuhauser (1944) and Williams (1946).[2]

Historical Firsts

The first case of an atresia of the intestine was reported by J. N. Binninger in 1673 in a one-and-a-half-day old infant with an atresia of the colon.[3] In 1684 Goeller described an atresia of the terminal ileum in a female stillborn, one of triplets whose two siblings survived. The next case, reported by C. Horch in 1696, described a female infant who lived for 22 days with a lower ileal atresia with separation of the bowel.[4] The first report of an operative procedure was documented in N. I. Spriggs' extensive review published in 1910.[5] He refers to a report in an appendix titled "Other Operations, Enterostomies, Etc.," by Voison, in 1804.[6]

The first infant to be diagnosed correctly while still alive was reported by Abraham Jacoby in 1861.[7] The infant had four atresias in the lower jejunum and ileum. In this paper he stressed the salient features of the condition, one of which was the characteristics of the meconium. His observations on the absence of "epithelial cells" in the abnormal meconium pointed to an early-acquired atresia. These findings led S. Farber to describe a simple staining procedure to detect vernix epithelial cells in a meconium specimen.[8] In Ladd and Gross' *Abdominal Surgery of Infancy and Childhood* and Gross' *The Surgery of Infancy and Childhood* the test is described as follows: "A specimen of meconium is obtained, care being taken that it comes from the center of the stool, and is smeared on a glass slide. This is gently washed for about one minute with ether to extract the fat, is allowed to dry, and then is stained for one minute with Sterling's gentian violet. It is washed with running water and decolorized with acid alcohol. This decolorization removes the dye from the entire specimen except the cornified epithelial cells." The absence of such cells represents presumptive evidence of an intestinal or colonic atresia. If cells are seen the obstruction may be partial (stenosis or extrinsic pressure).[9]

History of Classifications

The first descriptions of intestinal atresia were mainly in the form of case reports such as Binninger (1673: colon), Goellar (1684: ileum) and Calder (1733: duodenum).[10] Following these single and dual case reports, series began to appear. J. F. Meckel was one of the first to review the literature in 1812.[11] In 1826, A. Schaefer is reported to have brought the subject up to date and was the first to classify the various types.[12] In 1877, E. Theremin reported the first planned study, observing two cases over 11 years at a hospital in Vienna and nine cases among 150,000 children in a St. Petersburg hospital.[13]

John Bland-Sutton reported three cases of ileal atresia, the first classification in the English literature, in 1889.[14] Two of his cases were stillborn infants in whom dissection demonstrated two "cul-de-sacs" side by side in one and a complete obstruction with separation of the ends in another. He also mentions a fibrous cord connection. He consulted on the third case and with a preoperative diagnosis he explored the abdomen, finding a blind-ending ileum approximately 18 inches from the ileocecal valve. The ends were separated by a gap of about one inch. He basically described five types of obstruction: (1) web obstruction with small orifice, (2) obstruction by a markedly narrow segment, (3) complete web obstruction, (4) complete obstruction with an impervious fibrous band, and (5) complete obstruction with two separate ends of the bowel. In his operative case he removed a portion of the dilated bowel and sutured the end of the bowel to the abdominal wound. Meconium and flatus passed and the infant took feedings. Six hours later the infant suddenly expired.

Spriggs reported 24 new cases of intestinal occlusion and also included 328 previously reported cases.[15] Of these five were duodenal obstructions, with three atresias and two stenoses. Of the cases involving the bowel distal to the duodenum table 1 depicts the site of the obstruction and the description of the obstruction. In a figure Spriggs had simple drawings

Table 1

Site	Web atresia	Atresia with cord	Atresia with defect	Atresia with coiled bowel	Multiple
Jejunum	0	0	0	1	3
Ileum*	3	4	2	1	2
Colon	3	0	1	0	0

*In the ileal group one was a stenosis and one was not described.

illustrating six different types of obstruction: (a) simple stenosis, (b) perforated diaphragm, (c) complete diaphragm with bowel wall continuity, (d) diaphragm with a short band connecting the bowel, (e) thread-like fibrous band along mesentery connecting the two ends of the bowel, and (f) gap between bowel that included mesentery. Spriggs further stated that types a, b and f were rare forms and of the others some type of band occurred three times as often as a simple diaphragm.

In 1966, J. J. Weitzman and R. S. Vanderhoof reported four cases of an unusual form of jejunal atresia with agenesis of the dorsal mesentery, which resulted in a "Christmas tree" deformity of the distal small intestine.[16] The term "Christmas tree" was suggested by Dr. Orvar Swenson, who trained Dr. Weitzman. The blood supply to the distal bowel was formed by a union of the right branch of the middle colic artery and the right colic artery, which supplied the cecum and then the distal small bowel in a retrograde manner resembling the trunk of a tree around which the bowel curled in a corkscrew fashion. The authors pointed out the precarious nature of this abnormal blood supply. In their discussion they referenced a case by Keith in 1910 in which there were similarities to their four cases. Weitzman and Vanderhoof postulated due to the absence of rotation anomalies in their cases that the event occurs after the tenth week. The coiling of the distal intestine occurs due to the rapid growth of the intestine, which outstrips the growth of the blood supply, resulting in the spiral coiling. They recommend great care and diligence in placing the bowel back in the abdomen to prevent kinking of the precarious blood supply.

A review by L. W. Martin and J. T. Zarella of 59 cases of jejunoileal atresia led to a proposed classification of four distinct groups based on associated disease, intra- and postoperative complications, subsequent management and prognosis.[17] They utilized four groupings: Type I: single atresia (diaphragm) with bowel continuity, Type II: single atresia with discontinuity of the bowel wall (may have thready fibrous tissue connection), Type III: multiple atresias, and Type IV: "apple peel" or "Christmas tree" deformity. In their study Type I patients had the best prognosis (11 of 13 survived). In Type II patients, when those with cystic fibrous were excluded, 17 of 18 survived (overall, 21 of 32 survived). Types III and IV had 29 percent and 57 percent survival, respectively.

The most recent classification system, described by J. L. Grosfeld and colleagues, utilized four types, with a subdivision of one of the types into two groups.[18] The system included: Type I: mucosal or web destruction, Type II: atretic ends connected by a fibrous cord, Type IIIa: atresia with ends separated by a V-shaped mesenteric defect, Type IIIb: "apple peel" or "Christmas tree" atresia, and Type IV: multiple atresias.

One of the earlier speculations on the etiology of atresias was proposed in 1812 by Meckel, who believed that the intestine developed in segments with atresia resulting from an arrest in development.[19]

In 1889, Bland-Sutton reported three cases of ileal atresia and in his discussion postulated that congenital obstructions occurred in areas of embryologic events, e.g., duodenum near the ampulla ileum and the area of the vitelline duct and the rectoanal junction.[20] In 1902, J. Tandler, from a study of human embryos, showed that the duodenum passes through a solid stage due to epithelial proliferation from the fifth to the eighth week of gestation.[21] Vacuoles develop and join to reconstitute the lumen. These findings were confirmed by others and Tandler's theory was widely adopted as the cause of atresias throughout the gastrointestinal tract. Other reports confirmed Tandler's findings in the duodenum, but F. P. Johnson demonstrated that this solid stage of development did not occur in the esophagus, stomach and other portions of the small intestine.[22]

In his extensive review in 1911, Spriggs expounded for 17 pages on possible causes of atresia.[23] He first mentions Meckel's theory but quickly rejects it. Then in order Spriggs discusses the pros and cons of Bland-Sutton's view regarding sites of embryologic events, the entrapment of a loop of bowel during abdominal wall closure, epithelial occlusion (Tandler), volvulus or "axial rotation," kinking of the bowel intussusception, strangulation via a mesenteric defect, inflammation, vascular anomalies, pressure of the head of the pancreas (duodenal atresia), mucosal inflammation and ulceration, hypertrophy of the valvulae commiventes, neoplasm, and other rare conditions such as mesenteric cyst, traction by a hernia, and omental bands. Spriggs then concluded the discussion with the following causes as the most likely to be responsible for the anomaly: developmental defects including snaring at the umbilicus, fetal accidents, e.g. intussusceptions, volvulus, kinks, and fetal diseases, e.g., peritonitis, and ulceration. In 1931, C. H. Webb and O. H. Vangensteen discuss many of the preceding causes and then state: "Perhaps no one of these factors will adequately account for all cases of intestinal atresia, but the failure of a portion of the intestine to acquire a normal lumen during its developmental period would seem the most plausible."[24]

Little changed as far as to the etiology of intestinal atresias until Louw and Barnard published their early work in 1955 after a review of the cases at Great Ormond Street suggested that interference with the blood supply to the fetal intestine was likely.[25] Observed features included anomalous vascular supply to the atretic portion, early necrosis of the proximal blind end, and postoperative atony and ileus. Also, in 1949, H. Laufman and colleagues demonstrated in dogs that isolated, devascularized and sterilized loops of bowel are converted into fibrous bands or entirely disappear.[26] Based on that study, Barnard performed ligation of the blood supply to the intestine in fetal canine pups. After many failures due to anesthesia, technical problems, fetal death, premature labor and cannibalism, two animals survived to term. Both had intestinal obstructions, one with a dilated proximal bowel with a short segment of necrotic bowel in the process of being absorbed. In the second, the proximal bowel ended blindly, with a fibrous cord connecting to the distal bowel and a V-shaped defect in the mesentery. Further canine experiments yielded the types of atresias as described by Bland-Sutton, depending on the method and extent of the vascular insult. The vascular theory has been studied and confirmed by studies in numerous models including fetal sheep, fetal canines, and chick embryos.[27]

It is not surprising, that after the work of Billroth and others with intestinal surgery attempts would be made to treat infants with intestinal atresia. In 1902, H. Braun reviewed 19 enterostomies for congenital atresias, but all patients died.[28] Spriggs in his extensive review published in 1911 found 82 patients who underwent various operations, mostly enterostomies, with no survivors.[29] There were also 12 infants undergoing anastomoses (3 duodenal, 5 small bowel to small bowel, and 4 small bowel to large bowel) and none survived. He discusses the recommendation by H. S. Clogg to abandon enterostomy due to the 100 percent mortality.[30] Clogg also suggested that distention of the bowel distal to the atresia with water pressure would improve the passage of succus after an anastomosis. Spriggs concludes his paper with a "few dogmatic rules": (1) demonstrate no obstruction within two inches of the anus; (2) spinal anesthesia if possible and avoid shock; (3) median laparotomy; (4) if obstruction is in the lower ileum or colon, dilate distal bowel and anastomose as quickly as possible; (5) duodenal obstruction above ampulla — gastro-enterostomy; (6) duodenal obstruction below ampulla: (a) stenosis with bile passage duodeno-enterostomy and (b) complete atresia with all distal bowel constricted close abdomen; (7) multiple atresias: (a) close proximity excluded/bypass and (b) widely spaced close abdomen, (8) infant in very poor condition: do enterostomy to see if child improves.

Paul Fockens (1876–1955), of Rotterdam, in 1911 published "Case History, — Congenital Atresia of the Bowel Healed by Surgery"[31] This was the first infant with an intestinal atresia to survive. The baby had been born on September 6, 1910, and was seen at the outpatient clinic of the Sophia Children's Hospital because of the failure to pass stool and the vomiting of all feedings. On examination there was no stool in the rectum, and the next day the baby had fecal vomiting and the abdomen was distended and tympanitic. Dr. Fockens diagnosed a low intestinal obstruction because of the visible dilated loops of intestine. He operated upon the baby under chloroform anaesthesia with the assistance of Dr. de Monchy, one of the founders of the Sophia hospital. There was an atresia at the junction of the lower and middle third of the ileum, with the two ends separated. In his paper and on inspection, there was no distal atresia. Fockens carried out a side-to-side anastomosis. On the first day after surgery the baby had a "smelly stool" and thereafter had normal stools. The baby was fed with 30 milliliters of mother's milk every three hours, despite vomiting during the first two days. At the age of five months, the baby was healthy, had normal stools and didn't vomit. Dr. Fockens' excellent paper discusses the various treatment options, such as the creation of an artificial anus, enterostomy with a later anastomosis and an immediate side-to-side

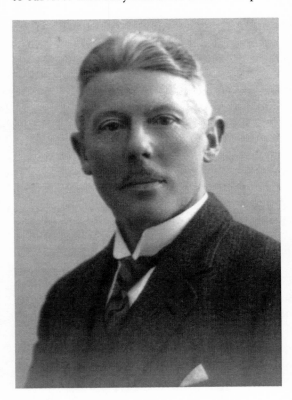

Paul Fockens was the first to successfully operate upon a baby with an intestinal atresia. At the time, Dr. Fockens had just finished his training and was substituting for the chief surgeon at the Sophia Children's Hospital in Rotterdam, the Netherlands (courtesy Paul Fockens, M.D., his grandson).

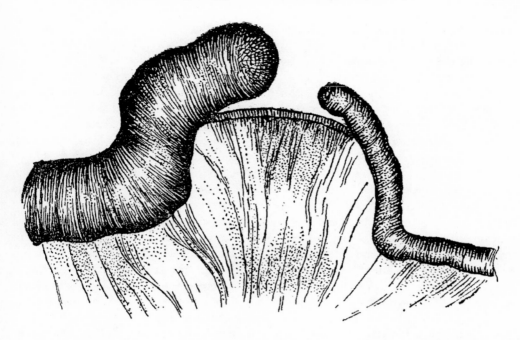

The hand-drawn diagram of Dr. Fockens' operative findings indicated the ileal atresia with separation of the two ends. This most likely represents an intrauterine vascular accident, such as a thrombosis of a small mesenteric vessel.

anastomosis. He thought that resection with an end-to-end anastomosis would be "unworkable." This remarkable paper ends: "Ein in dit sombere gebied maakt een zwaluw zoo geen zomer dan toch lente," which roughly translates as a swallow of summer has come into this bleak area. Paul Fockens' grandson, also named Paul, the professor of a gastroenterology and hepatology at the University of Amsterdam, provided the following information: Dr. Fockens graduated from the University of Groningen in 1903, did additional study in Vienna, then returned to Rotterdam for surgical training. He had just finished his surgical training and was 34 years old when he performed the first successful operation for an intestinal atresia. He was "on call" to the Sophia Children's Hospital because the Chief of Surgery, Dr. van Rossem was away. Dr. Fockens practiced surgery at the Jewish Hospital, Megon Hatsedek in Rotterdam until he retired in 1942.

In 1922, D. L. Davis and C. W. M. Poynter in a review of 401 cases and a report of one unsuccessful enterostomy recommended: (1) early diagnosis and operation, (2) procaine infiltration anesthesia, (3) adequate incision to visualize all bowel, and (4) enteroanastomosis (lateral or "atypical" end to end).[32] In 1931, Webb and Wangensteen reported 17 new cases (7 duodenal, 2 jejunal, 7 ileal and one colon) with unsuccessful operation in seven.[33] Based on their review of the literature they recommended an anastomotic procedure as best for chance of survival. Technically they recommended distal bowel distention and a single running Connell suture using a fine silk.

J. D. Martin, Jr., and D. C. Elkin reported two patients with ileal atresia treated initially with the ileostomy.[34] One succumbed 15 hours after the operation, but the other survived and a month later underwent a resection and lateral anastomosis. The authors stress the importance of the medical therapy, including 38 subcutaneous injections of Hartmann's solution, four blood transfusions and 5 percent glucose infusions. They recommend enteroanastomosis as the most desirable procedure, but the operative choice must be dependent on the individual situation.

J. H. Louw in the Moynihan Lecture to the Royal College of Surgeons in 1959 raised the problem of "post-operative obstruction" as a major cause of death in patients undergoing anastomosis.[35] He noted that the best results occurred in infants who had to have the bowel resected due to necrosis at the atretic ends. In 1952, Louw recommended resection of 10 to 15 centimeters of the proximal blind bowel and 2 to 3 centimeters of the distal blind end, with a subsequent reduction in mortality of 40 percent.[36] Experimental work by H. H. Nixon established that unresected dilated proximal bowel does not propulse well when luminal pressure is normal.[37] Nixon also noticed the improved course of infants with atresia who required resection of bowel due to ischemia (two patients in 1949). Another patient did not have ischemia and did not have bowel resected, which resulted in failure of the anastomosis to function, leading to death. The ward sister drew Nixon's attention to this by the fact that after feeding, the milk bolus could be felt to reach the right lower quadrant, where it seemed to churn without progression through the anastomosis. In a series of jejunoileal atresia patients from 1949 to 1955 Nixon reported 11 of 16 survivors in cases undergoing resection and anastomosis versus 5 of 17 in cases where simple anastomosis was performed.[38] C. D. Benson confirmed the efficacy of resection and anastomosis with a 70 percent survival in 14 patients.[39] Both Nixon and Benson utilized an end-to-end-side technique, but in 1971 Nixon recommended a tuck in the proximal bowel mesentery to prevent kinking due to the distal bowel mesentery being so much shorter.[40] In 1971, T. V. Santulli and W. A. Blanc reported a series of 76 patients with atresias, of which 59 were located in the jejunum, ileum, or colon.[41] They noted a distinct improvement in survival rates since 1948 and also noted a preference for enterostomy with delayed closure. They also recommended that a proximal enterostomy with the distal bowel anastomosed end-to-side to the proximal bowel with a catheter threaded through the enterostomy and across the anastomosis into the distal bowel. The enterostomy is left open for decompression and feedings instilled through the catheter. Then a Potts clamp is placed over the enterostomy to effectively close it and allow material to pass distally. Eventually the proximal stoma is closed under local anesthesia. Three of five cases were of the "apple peel" variety (Type IIIb) with prematurity. All five patients survived.

High jejunal atresias represent a particular problem. Nixon described

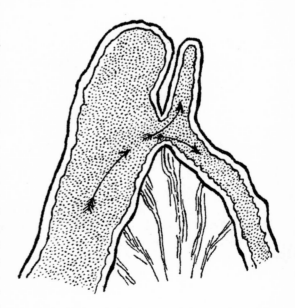

The successful side-to-side anastomosis performed by Dr. Fockens. This type of operation was commonly used until the 1960s when most surgeons adopted some form of end-to-end anastomosis. The disadvantage of the side-to-side anastomosis was the formation of a "blind loop" in the end of the bowel beyond the anastomosis.

resecting back to the duodenal flexure with a direct anastomosis, often with a gastrostomy and transanastomotic feeding tube.[42] In 1966, C. G. Thomas, Jr., reported a technique that involved a tapering jejunoplasty with a subsequent end-to-end or end-to-side anastomosis.[43] In a review of atresias reported in 1974, he reported six cases of proximal jejunal atresia that utilized the tapering, with all six surviving.

The advent of laparoscopy and the development of gastrointestinal anastomotic staplers led to the description of the use of endoscopic staplers for intestinal anastomosis in infants. In 1995, R. W. Powell reported the successful use of the endoscopic GIA in one patient with ileal atresia and three premature infants requiring closure of an ileostomy.[44] Due to limitations imposed by dilated intestine and a limited size of the peritoneal cavity the total laparoscopic approach to jejunoileal or colonic atresia has not been widely utilized.[45]

Perhaps the most significant contribution to the survival of infants with intestinal atresias has not been surgical technique but the development of total intravenous nutrition.

CHAPTER 36

Malrotation

RANDALL POWELL, M.D.

The difficult diagnostic and surgical challenges posed by children with defects in intestinal rotation and fixation require a knowledge of embryology and careful study of previous cases. The history of malrotation, as is true of most topics pertaining to pediatric surgery, originates in reports of unusual cases. Newbauer reported a case of a paraduodenal hernia in 1786.[1] This was followed by John Reid[2] in 1836 and James Y. Simpson[3] in 1839, both in Edinburgh, Scotland, who each described anomalies of intestinal rotation in human embryos. Numerous case reports of rotational anomalies followed but understanding was delayed until the embryologic process of the development of the gastrointestinal tract and the subsequent factors leading to the eventual position of the different portions of the intestinal tract were described.

The initial description of the rotation and fixation of the intestines was by Franklin P. Mall, professor of anatomy at Johns Hopkins University, in 1898.[4] Mall had studied with the German anatomist and embryologist Wilhelm His and utilized many of his human embryo specimens to aid in his description of intestinal development. Mall credits Meckel with the first description of the intestine moving into the umbilical cord in 1817 and describes the midgut loop as being horizontal to the long axis of the embryo's body with the blood supply from the omphalomesenteric artery, which becomes the superior mesenteric artery.[5] Mall then describes the developing coils of intestine with the upper loops moving toward the left side of the body. Due to the differential growth rates of the small and large intestine the small intestine is gradually turned from the right to left side of the body and as a result is rolled under the superior mesenteric artery (SMA). He then states that the return of the intestine occurs rapidly and no embryos have been seen that demonstrate the return. In a short paragraph titled "Marked Variations," Mall described one case of what is now recognized as malrotation.

The next advance in the embryology was when in 1915 J. Ernest Frazer and R. H. Robbins at the University of London and St. Mary's Hospital based their conclusions on microscopic examination and reconstruction of human embryos from the fourth week to the third month and dissection of embryos from the third month to birth. They divided the entire process into three stages: exit into cord to onset of return, return to cecum lying next to the dorsal abdominal wall, and from the end of the second stage to sometime after birth. In stage one a loop of intestine herniates into the umbilical cord with a proximal (right) and distal (left) limb, which occurs due to intestinal growth in a cavity too small to contain it. The proximal loop goes to the right because of rapid liver growth and the position of the left umbilical vein. The duodenal loop is shaped by the growth of the pancreatic head and the somewhat fixed aspect of the mesoduodenum distally. The proximal limb grows in length faster with the most proximal coil within the cord bending, and the duodenojejunal conjunction becomes apparent. During the second stage, rotation occurs. Frazer and Robbins describe the factors leading to the "sucked back" description given by Mall. The first is the decrease in the rate of liver growth along with an increased size of the abdominal cavity causing a relative decrease in intra-abdominal pressure. The second is the relative increase in amniotic fluid pressure. Frazer and Robbins then discuss the actual reduction of the bowel as an orderly but rapid event with the proximal limb reducing first in a coil by coil fashion, which occurs because of the larger size of the cecum and ascending colon. The coils enter below the right lobe of the liver, fill the lower abdomen and then push ventrally to the median septum. In the process the coils are forced to go below the distal limb and the mesenteric vessels. The colon then enters and lies on top of the coils and their mesentery with the cecum pointing to the right. In the third stage, extension and fixation of the colon occurs. With growth the cecum gradually progresses to the area of the right iliac crest. During this period the mesocolon extends itself as the colon grows and becomes fixed to the dorsal wall of the abdominal cavity. In their summary the authors point out the influence of the liver on the rotation and fixation of the gut.

Norman M. Dott, surgeon at the Royal Edinburgh Hospital for Sick Children, provided further enlightenment to the process in his 1923 paper.[7] Dott stated that understanding the process is critical to the surgeon for the following reasons: (1) to correctly diagnose the pathology, (2) because failure may lead to errors in the procedure, prolonged operation or abandonment of the operation, and (3) because errors of development may cause serious sequelae, e.g., volvulus. Dott basically confirms the work of Mall, Frazer and Robbins and emphasized the proximity of the duodenum and colon at the umbilical ring, the duodeno-colic isthmus. He also uses the terms "prearterial" and "postarterial" to describe the dorsal (right) and ventral (left) loops, respectively. The result of the second stage is a counterclockwise rotation about the axis of the superior mesenteric artery (SMA) of 270 degrees. This causes the duodenum to cross behind the SMA near its origin and the colon crossing anterior to the SMA. In the third stage, after growth and positioning of the cecum, the mesentery adheres to the posterior abdominal wall from above down, resulting in a broad-based mesentery. Dott further postulates that the departure from the process could occur with a widened umbilical ring and could result in all the bowel reducing together. He continues with a classification related to each stage. Stage I is seen in "extroversion of the cloaca." Stage II varies, but common to most is a narrow-based mesentery (persistent duodenocolic isthmus). Reverse rotation occurs very rarely, with a rotation of 90° clockwise with the colon passing posterior to the SMA and duodenum anterior to it. It usually presents as a transverse colon obstruction. The other form presents as a malrotation of the midgut in which both loops pass anterior to the SMA. Stage III abnormalities mainly relate to varying degrees of cecal position. Of the 45 cases Dott reviewed, 35 were discovered accidentally. He presented five cases: one elderly man with reverse rotation, three infants with acute obstruction due to volvulus, and a five-year-old male with a history of chronic abdominal pain and vomiting. All underwent operations, with only the five-year-old surviving. He was found to have a chronic volvulus, duodenal obstruction and his mesentery was narrowed to less than an inch in diameter. The surgeon, Rixford, reduced the volvulus in a counterclockwise fashion until the normal position was achieved. The child did well afterward, and in the words of the surgeon "he grew like the blossom stalk of an aloe, and is now a strapping, normal boy of 13."[8] Dott stressed that time was of the essence in the newborn, with the only hope being an early diagnosis and operation. Due to the findings in his two postmortem cases and the case of Rixford, Dott recommended reduction of the volvulus and then continuing the rotation to achieve normal positioning of the small bowel and colon. He suggested that fixing the cecum in the right lower quadrant might prevent recurrence.

In 1927, Dott reported a case of an eight-day-old female as the first newborn diagnosed from clinical observations and successfully treated by operation. He commented at the end of the report: "I regard this case with peculiar satisfaction, as it represents to me the outcome of former embryological and pathological researches in practical diagnosis and operative care."[9]

Two more papers with significant relevance to the embryology of these anomalies must be mentioned. Clarence E. Gardner, Jr. (Department of Surgery, Duke University School of Medicine), presented a thorough discussion of the process with superb colored illustrations.[10] He presented each stage of rotation and then described the anomalies associated with that stage as follows: First Stage: omphalocele, Second Stage: non-rotation, volvulus of the midgut, malrotation, internal hernia and reversed rotation, and Third Stage: subhepatic cecum, retrocecal appendix and mobile cecum. Cases with radiographs and anatomical illustrations are utilized to present the various anomalies. In 1954, William H. Snyder, Jr. (the lead editor of the first edition of the two-volume textbook *Pediatric Surgery*) and Lawrence Chaffin (Los Angeles Children's Hospital and the University of Southern California School of Medicine) presented the embryology in stages as far as the duodenojejunal loop and cecocolic loop rotations with a simple device.[11] The demonstration utilized a loop of rope attached at both ends to a board, with a wire extending at right angles from the board at the base of the loop. The top limb represented the duodenojejunal loop, the bottom represented the cecocolic loop and the wire the SMA. The loop is then rotated through a 270° counterclockwise rotation. As the rope rotates. the position of the two loops allows one to visualize the rotation process in the embryo. This illustration has been utilized in all six editions of the two-volume textbook *Pediatric Surgery* (1962–2006). The authors then present 40 cases from the Los Angeles Children's Hospital (from 1937 to 1952) which will be discussed later.

As one traces the history of malrotation and volvulus a number of generalities are realized: (1) the patients usually present with either an acute high gastrointestinal obstruction or chronic symptoms, which frequently have obstructive components, (2) patients may present at any age, and (3) a host of different surgical procedures have been described, although the basic procedure performed today was described by William E. Ladd in 1936.[12]

The early history of volvulus associated with rotational anomalies was well presented by Edward C. Brenner from New York in 1932.[13] In this paper he credits the first description of a volvulus due to malrotation by Kuljabzo-Koreski (1847) in a 22-year-old male who had experienced severe colic attacks since childhood. His last attack lasted five days before operation, and the patient succumbed that day. Postmortem examination revealed a four-complete-turn volvulus with gangrene. Brenner reported that in 1865 Valenta published a report of an infant who died from obstruction, but the postmortem was "somewhat confusing." In 1877, Theremin reported a male infant dying at 23 days of life without operation and autopsy revealed a 720° counterclockwise volvulus of small bowel, cecum and ascending colon. He credits Mohring with the first postoperative survival of a total volvulus in 1904, the patient being a 72-year-old female. Of the 30 cases described by Brenner, 25 were documented by operation or autopsy. Mortality following operation was 62 percent. He recommended urgent operation with detorsion and fixation of the cecum in the right lower quadrant of the abdomen.

George E. Waugh (London) in 1928 reported five patients, ages 6, 7, 10, 12, and 21, with more chronic courses.[14] He described chronic pain, which appeared in acute attacks, with vomiting being erratic in his patients. In four he described an "emptiness of the right iliac fossa" and asymmetric fullness on the left side in three and the episgastrium in one. As far as radiographic exams, he recommended the best method was to first give barium by mouth and when the small intestine is defined then perform a barium enema to obtain a view of colon position. All five patients had appendectomies and three also had lysis of mesenteric bands. Bowel positioning was not documented.

In 1933, Ladd reported ten cases of duodenal obstruction in children, six of which involved malrotation, and described the bands from the cecum to the lateral abdominal wall, which have come to bear his name.[15] In the six patients with malrotation, the cecum was placed to the left in two patients, to the right in two and not mentioned in two.

In 1934, Clarence E. Gardner, Jr., and Deryl Hart (Department of Surgery, Duke University School of Medicine) published 2 cases of their own and reviewed 103 cases from the literature.[16] Their two cases, ages two months and six years, respectively, had volvulus due to malrotation. After reduction of the volvulus the jejunum was moved to the left and the cecum placed in the right iliac fossa. Both survived and symptoms resolved. The two-month-old infant had a subsequent barium examination that showed the colon in a normal position. In ten pages done in table form the authors described 103 cases gathered from the literature organized under the headings: "Volvulus of the Entire Mesentery" (88 cases), "Reversed Rotation with Obstruction of the Colon by Torsion or Kinking" and "Duodenal Obstruction from Abnormal Intestinal Fixation." Of the 105 cases, 55 (52 percent) either were newborns or had had symptoms since several days of age. Sixty-two percent of the 97 in whom sex was reported were males. Complete mesenteric volvulus occurred in 88 patients (83 percent), and this represents the most common cause of bowel obstruction related to rotation anomalies. The rotation was clockwise in 56 (70 percent) of 79 cases where the direction was reported. Volvulus presenting as a duodenal obstruction occurred in 52 of the 75 cases (70 percent) where the description was adequate for this determination, with 32 cases being newborns. Roentgenograms with barium reveal obstruction usually of the third portion of the duodenum, but the characteristic finding in rotational anomalies is the presence of the entire duodenum on the right side of the abdomen, which to date represents the key radiographic finding in reaching the correct diagnosis. The authors state that operative treatment is the only hope for cure. They recommended adequate exposure, evisceration to clarify the anatomy, and detorsion of the volvulus with replacement of the viscera in their normal position as "the ideal operative procedure." They also advised fixation of the cecum and ascending colon in their normal position. In the entire series all 36 patients not undergoing operations succumbed while 36 of 69 operative cases survived (52 percent).

In 1936, Elmer G. Wakefield and Charles W. Mayo (Mayo Clinic, Rochester, Minnesota) reported 15 cases of intestinal obstruction with mesenteric bands associated with anomalies of intestinal rotation, with the youngest patient being 11 years of age. All had anomalies associated with the second stage of rotation.[17] Wakefield and Mayo pointed out the role of the duodenocolic isthmus. Operations performed included: division of bands only, division of bands with duodenojejunostomy, jejunojejunostomy, and gastrojejunostomy. Two patients had anomalies discovered during operations for other causes and two refused operation. In 1939, Drs. Rustin McIntosh and Edward J. Donovan (Babies' Hospital,

Department of Pediatrics and Surgery, Columbia University, New York) presented 20 patients, 16 less than one year of age and of these 15 less than one month of age.[18] Thirteen of the 20 had volvulus and presented as acute duodenal obstruction. The authors note an increased reliance on radiographic examinations and seemed to prefer the UGI. They also emphasized adequate and prompt preoperative preparation of the patients and the need to explore the duodenum to divide any obstructing bands as described by Ladd. They recommended fixation of the cecum and ascending colon in their proper position to perhaps lessen the chance of recurrence.

In his presentation to the New Hampshire Medical Society on May 26, 1936, Dr. Ladd described the technique he devised. Prior to the adoption of the Ladd operation, the mortality for volvulus at the Children's Hospital in Boston had been 100 percent and in the literature there had been only 15 survivors reported in 349 articles.[19] Dr. Ladd divided bands crossing over the duodenum from the cecum and separated the duodenocolic isthmus to place the cecum in the left upper quadrant of the abdomen. In the book titled *Abdominal Surgery in Infancy and Childhood* by Ladd and Gross, the procedure is described in more detail and the steps depicted in superb illustrations by Miss Etta Piotti.[20] In 1942, Dr. Owen H. Wangensteen (Chair, Department of Surgery, University of Minnesota) described an operation for non-rotation in which a volvulus if present is reduced, the small intestine is passed through a defect created in the transverse mesocolon, and the cecum and ascending colon are placed in their normal position.[21] Due to a kinking in the ascending colon the terminal ileum is divided and anastomosed to the ascending colon after the latter is unkinked. The small intestinal mesentery is then anchored by a "few well-placed sutures." The procedure places the intestine and colon in their normal positions. The necessity for the opening of the intestine probably limited this procedure's becoming popular in the face of the simplicity and aseptic nature of the procedure described by Ladd.

In the 1950s, as the procedure became widely accepted, there were numerous reports describing experience with the Ladd procedure for malrotation. Drs. William B. Keisewetter and John W. Smith reported the experience from the Children's Hospital of Pittsburgh from 1940 to 1957.[22] In a period of six years (1951 to 1957) they had 31 patients, and during the same period 81 patients were diagnosed as having malrotation by the Radiology Department. Operatively the authors stressed the importance of being able to follow the duodenum down into the upper jejunum to ensure no obstructions from volvulus, cecal bands, kinks or intrinsic bands or webs. Drs. Richard J. Andrassy and G. Hossein Mahour updated the Children's Hospital of Los Angeles experience and reported an increase in survival from 77 percent (1937–1951) to 96 percent (1951–1977).[23] They also described their technique for evaluating the duodenum for partial webs by passing a Foley catheter through the intestine from the stomach. Drs. Howard C. Filston and Donald R. Kirks reported the experience at Duke University from 1976 to 1980 and noted a significant increase in associated congenital anomalies[24] Of particular note was an association with duodenal and jejunal atresias. This represented one-half and one-third, respectively, of the total of such atresias during the same time period. In 1982, in a five-year review from the Children's Hospital of Philadelphia, Dr. Charles G. Howell and colleagues reported two main findings in their 50 patients: (1) volvulus was the main complication and (2) nutritional status at the time of operation was extremely poor in 70 percent of their patients.[25] In a mouse model they were able to demonstrate an increase in ischemic injury in malnourished rats related to the time length of ischemia. One of their recommendations was to perform UGI examinations in patients with failure to thrive.

Two series have placed emphasis on older children diagnosed with malrotation. Drs. Hugh V. Firor and Ezra Steiger from the Cleveland Clinic reported nine cases of rotational anomalies diagnosed after infancy (range 3–20 years, median 11.5 years). Eight of nine had chronic symptoms and two presented with acute volvulus and infarction.[26] The authors emphasize the "time bomb" nature of anomaly as related to the risk of volvulus and infarction. They recommend a Ladd procedure for patients with symptoms and also for asymptomatic patients whose rotation anomaly predisposes to volvulus. A review of 70 patients by Drs. David M. Powell, H. Biemann Othersen and C. D. Smith (Medical University of South Carolina, Charleston) led to the conclusion by the authors that all patients with a malrotation anomaly that carries a risk of volvulus should undergo a Ladd procedure.[27] In another review, Drs. A. Margarite Torres and Moritz M. Ziegler (Children's Hospital Medical Center, University of Cincinnati College of Medicine) reported 22 patients over an 18-month period.[28] Fifteen of the 22 presented with volvulus five, of which required bowel resection. Tables illustrated the present series and 16 others from the literature. Another table demonstrated the superior accuracy of the UGI for diagnosis, a study favored by numerous other authors. There are several reports that utilized both a UGI and BAE in non-acute patients.[29] Abdominal ultrasound can be utilized in the acute situation with the finding of a sonographic "whirlpool" pattern of the superior mesenteric vein and mesentery wrapping around the superior mesenteric artery.[30] This was seen in 15 of 18 patients with midgut volvulus.

Two areas of possible controversy remain to be addressed. The first is the fixation of the duodenum and cecum to the right lateral and left lateral abdominal walls, respectively. This was advocated by Dr. Alexander H. Bill, Jr., in two reports in the literature and in at least one textbook.[31] The reason for the fixation was to decrease the rate of recurrent volvulus. In a later report from Switzerland, Drs. U. G. Stauffer and P. Hermann found in a comparison of patients with and without fixation that there was no advantage in either group.[32] In a personal communication to Dr. Hugh Firor, Dr. Bill agreed that fixation was not necessary.[33] The other area of possible controversy involves the use of the laparoscopic approach for malrotation. At least three series report the safety and efficacy of the laparoscopic performance of a Ladd procedure.[34] There has been a report of a laparoscropic reduction of an acute volvulus in a neonate, although most authors do not recommend it because of the increased friability of ischemic bowel.[35]

CHAPTER 37

Coarctation of the Thoracic Aorta

JACK H. T. CHANG, M.D.,
AND JOHN BURRINGTON, M.D.

The earliest recorded report of narrowing of the thoracic aorta was by the Prussian anatomist Johann Friedrich Meckel, the Elder (1724–1774), patriarch of a most remarkable family of physicians. Meckel the Elder first described the sphenopalatine and submaxillary ganglions in his inaugural dissertation, *De Quinto Pari Nervorum*, 1748. In 1751 he became professor of anatomy, botany, and obstetrics at Berlin and taught midwifery at the Charité. His son, Philipp Friedrich Theodor Meckel (1756–1803), was professor of anatomy and surgery at Halle two years after delivering his dissertation on the internal ear, *De Labyrinthi Auria Contenti*, in 1777. He later turned to obstetrics and was highly honored in the court of the Czar. Philipp had two sons, August Albrecht (1790–1829) and Johann Friedrich, the Younger (1781–1833). August Albrecht became professor of anatomy and forensic medicine at Bern in 1821. Johann Friedrich, the Younger, was preeminent, becoming a noted pathologist and, before Mueller, the greatest comparative anatomist in Germany. He wrote treatises on pathologic anatomy (1812–1818), normal human anatomy (1815), and human abnormalities (1817–1826). His most significant contribution was his system of comparative anatomy (1821–1830) in which the doctrine of "ontogeny recapitulates phylogeny" was established. In addition, he translated Wolff's monograph on the development of the intestine and described the diverticulum of the small intestine, which bears his name.

The elder Meckel delivered his paper *Anatomical and Physiological Observations, Concerning Extraordinary Dilatation of the Heart, Which Came from the Fact that the Aortic Conduit Was Too Narrow*, before the Royal Academy of Sciences of Berlin in 1750. The paper was published 18 years later in the sixth volume of the *Memoirs of the Royal Academy*.

Meckel's report concerned an 18-year-old girl who had been "very choleric" from childhood. She suffered from palpatations of the heart, trembling of the limbs and amenorrhea. As her family was poor, her only treatment consisted of liquors, purges, emmenagogues (agents promoting menstrual discharge), and phlebotomies. Her symptoms progressed, and after a prolonged bedridden course she died in a state of "suffocation." The autopsy was as follows: "When I opened the thorax the ... heart ... occupied almost the whole left half of the small chest. As for the aorta [Fig. 1, G], it was so narrow that its diameter was smaller by half than that of the pulmonary artery, which it should have exceeded or at least equal in caliber."[1]

Meckel then discussed the hemodynamics of increased arterial resistance. His reasoning, naïve by modern physiology, reflected the concept of backward failure. The illustrations and measurements of the great vessels as they issued from the heart seemed to indicate that the process was one of hypoplasia of the aorta.

A subsequent case report was recorded by Giovanni Baptiste Morgagni in his classic, *De Sedibus et Causis Morborum per Anatomen Indagatis Libri Quinque,* published in 1761. The observation was made in October 1733 of a 33-year-old monk dying of "dropsy":

> In both the cavities of the thorax was a confiderable [the beginning and middle letter *s* was printed as a *f* as late as 1800] quantity of water. The lungs were contracted. The heart was not without polypous [clots] concretions; and the valves not without a bony portion. But on the internal furface of the great artery, from the fuperior branches quite to the emulgents [renal arteries], were beginnings of future offification. This artery, though in a body of tall ftature, was fcarcely thicker than a finger of a moderate size; and the other fanguiferous veffels, alfo, were narrow in the fame proportion.[2]

While this may certainly be another report of aortic hypoplasia, Morgagni has described the valvular and aortic atherosclerosis that is encountered in both adults and children.

The first undisputed description of a postductal coarctation of the aorta was made by M. Paris, *prosecteur de l'amphitheatre,* Hôtel-Dieu de Paris, in the *Journal de Chirurgie de Desault,* 1791. As with Meckel the Elder's case, the heart and vessels were injected by a compound of resin and tallow dyed by lampblack:

> Since the body was very thin, before the dissection it was possible to see distinctly, on the sides of the chest, the trunks and branches of the thoracic arteries, which were much thicker and more tortuous than the normal... The part of the aorta which is beyond the arch, between the ligamentum arteriosum and the first inferior intercostal, was so greatly narrowed that it had at most the thickness of a goosequill.... The part of the vessel which was above the constriction was slightly dilated, the distal part was of normal caliber...
>
> The carotids and their branches showed nothing unusual. The innominate artery, the first branch of the arch and also the subclavian which arise from it, were a third larger than normal. The left subclavian artery was half again as thick as the normal. The branches of the two subclavians had increased in the same proportion and described extensive and multiple zigzags.... The internal mammary arteries had a diameter of 2 lines (2.5 mm), the superior phrenic had a diameter of 1½ lines. The latter was very tortuous. The transverse cervicals were twice as thick as normal: all their posterior branches ran a long and sinuous course, and communicated with the posterior branches of the intercostals. The intercostals which arise from the subclavians had a diameter of 2 lines. The thoracic arteries, the common scapular, and the other principal branches which come from axillary arteries to branch out wholly or partly on the chest were as large again as the normal.
>
> The successive intercostal arteries which arose from the thoracic aorta below the narrowing were larger and larger the nearer one came to the constriction. The first and the second each had a diameter of 3 lines; the others diminished gradually and the last were almost normal. The anterior branches of these arteries were little enlarged but the posterior branches were so much and formed such intricate and closely approximated zigzags that they resembled the beads of a necklace placed one against another. Their communications with the transverse cervicals were large and very conspicuous.
>
> The branches of the abdominal aorta were unremarkable except for the inferior phrenic, which was abnormally thick and presented large communications with the superior phrenic; likewise the epigastric artery, which was as thick as the internal mammary with which it had a large number of very distinct anastomoses.
>
> From the circumstances which have just been described it is clear that in this woman the circulation worked in an extraordinary way. Instead of passing directly along the trunk of the

aorta, the blood went from the branches which originated above the narrowing, i.e. those from the subclavian and axillary arteries, into the branches which arose below the narrowing, such as the intercostals, the inferior phrenics, and the epigastrics, through the numerous communications which existed between these arteries, around the chest, and the anterior part of the abdomen.[3]

The skillfully described collateral circulation requires no further comment. Paris reported this case as rare but did not refer to any antecedent reports.

In 1827, August Albrecht Meckel reported in *Archives for Anatomy and Physiology* of a 35-year-old man who died from a ruptured right auricle after carrying a heavy load. At autopsy after dye injection, he described a postductal coarctation (fig. 2) with rib erosions from the tortuosity of the intercostal vessels as well as the extensive collateral circulation.

Diagnosis of coarctation of the aorta did not evolve until the mid-1800s. Although Auenbrugger's *Inventum Novum Ex Percussione Thoracis Humani* was published in 1761, the technique of percussion was not widely practiced. Laennec's *De l'Auscultation Mediate* provided the instrument for diagnosis at the beginning of the nineteenth century.

Legrand made the diagnosis of obstruction of the thoracic aorta in 1835 by observing the forcible pulsation in the carotids and periscapular pulsations of the collateral vessels. A. Mercier made a similar observation and at autopsy described the cause and coined the term "coarctation": "A part leur coarctation, les tissus qui forment ce rétrécissement paraissent à l'état sain. [Apart from their coarctation, the tissues that make up this narrowing appear to the healthy state.]"[5]

Oppolzer was credited with the first ante-mortem diagnosis of coarctation in a 38-year-old shoemaker in 1848. He described a murmur in the left interscapular space and attributed this to the stress of blood rushing through the greatly enlarged superior intercostal artery (intercostalis suprema). His diagnosis was later confirmed at autopsy.

In 1892, Potain from the Hôspital de la Charité called attention to the finding of hypertension in patients with coarctation. Woltman and Shelden emphasized the absence of aortic and femoral pulsations with this disease in 1920.

Pathologically, L. M. Bonnet, Chief of Clinical Medicine at the

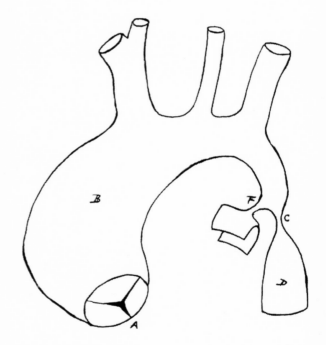

August Albrecht Meckel carried out an autopsy on a 35-year-old man who died while carrying a heavy load. The cause of death was rupture of the right auricle. A dye injection demonstrated this postductal coarctation of the thoracic aorta. The narrow portion is indicated by C and the closed ductus arteriosus is adjacent, at F. The ascending aorta, B is dilated and the aorta distal to the coarctation is smaller than normal (from A. A. Meckel's report in *Archives for Anatomy and Physiology* Vol. 2 [1837]: 345).

University of Lyon, reviewed his and other authors' experiences and introduced the classifications of "infantile" and "adult" types of coarctation. In the former, the stricture occurred proximal to the ductus arteriosus or ligamentum arteriosum; and in the latter, distal.[6]

In 1928, Maude E. Abbott, Curator of the Historical Medical Museum of McGill University, reviewed two hundred cases of coarctation of the aorta. She confirmed Bonnet's impression that the infantile type of coarctation was associated with a higher incidence of serious anomalies than the adult type:

> The contrast is well seen in the analysis of 212 cases of both types which I made in another connection. Among 82 of these which were in "infants under one year," 50 were complicated by "grave" or "major" anomalies, and 19 by "minor" ones, while in only 15 cases was the defect uncomplicated by any other anomaly. On the other hand in the 155 of these cases in which the coarctation was in subjects over one year ("adults"), there were only 13 cases complicating "grave" anomalies, against 57 in which "minor" anomalies were associated, and 86 in which the coarctation was the only defect. In these 13 cases complicated by other "grave" anomalies, the coarctation was either so slight as to be of no apparent importance...[7]

In the same year, L. Minor Blackford, Fellow in Medicine, the Mayo Clinic, reviewed the subject of coarctation and concluded: "The clinical diagnosis in such cases is of little or no actual importance, because coarctation of the infantile type is rapidly fatal, or, if of the adult type, hardly a factor in causing death."[8]

Interest in producing an animal model began in the early 1900s. Halsted unsuccessfully attempted to completely occlude the thoracic aorta of dogs with metal bands. Matas and Allen used placation of the aortic wall to produce occlusion but succeeded in only reducing flow. Finally, in 1942, J. C. Owings produced complete occlusion by using rubber bands in multiple-stage operations.

In 1944, Alfred Blalock and Edwards A. Parks, from the Johns Hopkins University and Hospital, reported an experimental technique for treating coarctation:

> The mediastinal pleural overlying the left subclavian artery was incised and the thoracic part of the subclavian was freed from adjacent structures. A bulldog clamp was placed on the subclavian artery at its most proximal part. The artery was then ligated about 5 cm. distal to this point and was divided just proximal to the ligature. The aorta immediately proximal and distal to the origin of the left subclavian artery was mobilized sufficiently to allow two rubber-shod clamps to be placed upon it. These clamps were placed about 6 cm. apart and the aorta was completely occluded by each of them. The aorta was then divided midway between the two rubber-shod clamps and each end was closed by two rows of very fine silk...
>
> A short transverse incision was made into the side of the distal aorta slightly beyond the point at which its end had been closed. The length of the incision was slightly greater than that of the diameter of the subclavian artery. It is important that this incision should be in a transverse direction because the wall of the aorta tears rather easily if the incision is a longitudinal direction. Furthermore, it is important not to try to clean the aorta of adventitia as is usually done in arterial anastomoses. An end-to-side anastomosis between the proximal end of the subclavian artery and the side of the aorta was then performed. As in all blood vessel anastomoses, the important point is that the intima should be approximated to intima by eversion.... The rubber-shod clamps were removed from the subclavian artery and the aorta.... A thrill was felt in the aorta distal to the anastomosis following the removal of the clamps.[9]

They performed 43 such procedures on dogs. Occlusion time varied from 40 to 65 minutes, only 10 of the dogs lived for any appreciable time: 33 died in an average of six days. The major postoperative complication was paralysis of the posterior portion of the animals.

Blalock suggested that the carotid artery may be a better vessel to use in man since it had no branches and the major source of collateral channeling, the subclavian artery, would be spared. Blalock concluded:

> Although this operation has not been attempted in man, it would appear that the enlarged collateral vessels which enter the aorta below the point of the stenosis in the patient with coarctation would make it difficult to obtain a dry field for the performance of the anastomosis. On the other hand, it would appear that the patient with a chronic partial occlusion of the aorta would tolerate a temporary complete occlusion better than the normal dog in which there has been no stimulus to the formation of collateral arterial pathways. In any case, the procedure, or a modification of it, should be considered only in those cases of coarctation in which the outlook is very grave since many patients with coarctation of the aorta have a fairly long life expectancy.[10]

The Blalock-Parks left-subclavian-artery-to-aorta bypass, successfully used by Clagett in 1949, is still occasionally used today in the surgical treatment of coarctation of the aorta.

The majority of coarctation is repaired by resection with an end-to-end anastomosis. This technique was developed independently by Clarence Crafoord, Surgeon in Chief of the Sabbatsberg Hospital, Stockholm and Robert E. Gross, then assistant professor of surgery at Harvard Medical School.

In experimental studies of pulmonary resection in dogs, circa 1935, Crafoord showed that circulation to all organs, except the brain, could be interrupted for as long as 20 to 25 minutes without ill effects. Also, during the repair of a persistent ductus arteriosus Crafoord noted that the aorta could be cross-clamped for as long as 27 minutes without distal organ damage.

After discussions with G. Nylin, Physician-in-Chief of the Heart Clinic, Crafoord performed two coarctation resections on October 19 and October 31, 1944:

> In both patients, there were powerful aortic pulsations to a two centimeter long stricture, but distally, the aorta was dilated and not moving. There were tortuos, dilated intercostal arteries and a fibrous remnant of the ductus arteriosus. Dr. Crafoord clamped the aorta and the intercostal vessels proximal and distal to the stricture, then resected the narrow area. He anastomosed the aorta with interrupted and running sutures.[11]

Both patients were doing well five months after operation, with satisfactory reduction of their pre-operative hypertensions.

In March of 1938, Robert E. Gross began experiments to find a surgical procedure for coarctation of the aorta. Clinically, he noted that the complications of aneurismal dilatation, dissecting aneurysm, aortic rupture, superimposed streptococcus infection, hypertension, cardiac failure, and cerebral hemorrhage greatly diminished the normal life expectancy of individuals with coarctation. Once he was joined by Charles A. Hufnagel, their experiments centered on two problems, the type of anastomosis and the complications of aortic occlusion. They attempted several types of anatomoses and decided upon a continuous mattress suture, which allowed for near-perfect hemostasis. As the dogs used for these experiments were fully grown, the inability of such an anastomosis to enlarge in a growing animal was not appreciated. Today, the majority of anastomoses are performed with a continuous running suture for the back wall and an interrupted anterior row allowing for growth potential.

Another salient observation by the authors was that the rapid removal of the aortic clams resulted in a greatly increased pulse rate as the heart attempted to compensate for the sudden increased vascular capacity. In one dog, death occurred "apparently to cardiac strain." Gross properly reasoned: "...that the momentary embarrassment occasioned by removal of the clamps could be greatly reduced if the clamps were taken off slowly in order to allow a gradual readjustment in the vascular system.[12] They confirmed Blalock and Parks' observations that a significant number of animals will sustain hindquarter paralysis after aortic occlusion. Interestingly, Gross and Hufnagel also took a number of animals and inflicted aortic occlusion while the dogs' backs were packed in ice and found the incidence of paraplegia reduced by nearly half. One must remember that W. G. Bigelow's classic paper on hypothermia and the body's oxygen requirement was not published until 1950 and the first successful atrial septal defect repair under hypothermia by F. J. Lewis was seven years in the future. Regarding the possibility of paraplegia in humans, the authors correctly concluded that "when aortic operations are performed in human subjects, there is little likelihood of neurologic complications from temporary aortic obstruction if there is am adequate collateral circulation, such as is uniformly found with coarctation of the aorta."[13]

As a footnote to the article, Gross reported on two cases of coarctation resection. The first, performed on June 28, 1945, on a six-year-old boy resulted in death when after completion of the anastomosis the aortic clamps were released suddenly, resulting in uncontrolled cardiac dilation and death. The second was performed on July 6, 1945, on a

> twelve-year-old girl for whom surgical therapy was undertaken because of marked hypertension. The systolic pressure was frequently recorded at 215, and at no examination was it below 190. No pulsations could be felt in the groins or legs, and no blood pressure readings could be obtained in the legs.... The aorta appeared to be completely blocked 1 cm. beyond the origin of the left subclavian artery. The aorta was doubly clamped, and the constricted area was excised. (Examination of the interior of the specimen showed no opening between the two ends.) The aorta was repaired by direct end-to-end anastomosis. The clamps were gradually [author's italics] released, a full ten minutes taken before opening them fully. There were no deleterious effects on the heart. The procedure was tolerated exceedingly well; the wound healed per primum. The patient was discharged from the hospital in a satisfactory condition on the nineteenth postoperative day. The systolic pressure in the arms had dropped to 140. Femoral pulsations could be readily felt, and the systolic pressure in the legs was 145.[14]

One must admire the courage and conviction of Robert E. Gross in performing the second procedure following the initial catastrophic failure. By 1948, Gross had reported on the successful use of human arterial grafts in the treatment of coarctation.

Not until the early 1950s was attention centered on neonates and infants with coarctation. Martin M. Calodney and Merl J. Carson from St. Louis reviewed 22 cases in this age group and showed that the diagnosis could be made with accuracy.[15] Besides the cardiac murmur, hypertension of the upper extremities was found in over 80 percent, while hypotension or absent blood pressure in the lower extremities was uniform. Due to a large persistent ductus arteriosus femoral pulsations were not always absent. Congestive heart failure was uniform and of grave prognosis unless immediately reversed by digitalis and diuretics. The authors advised early surgical repair but recognized that in 27 percent of their cases were accompanying severe congenital anomalies of the heart and great vessels. Only one of their cases underwent surgery. This 35-day-old male with a long juxta-ductal coarctation had the strictured segment replaced by a 21-millimeter-long arterial graft. Twenty minutes after the aortic clamps were removed, the infant arrested and died.[16] At autopsy, the anastomosis was intact, and one wonders if the aortic clamps were removed too rapidly and this infant met the same fate as Gross' first patient.

John W. Kirklin and his associates at the Mayo Clinic successfully operated upon a 10-week-old infant in 1952. This baby was in congestive heart failure secondary to a juxtaligamental coarctation. The stricture segment was resected and an end-to-end anastomosis performed with interrupted mattress sutures. Postoperatively, convalescence was uneventful and at 18 months of age the child was growing and developing normally.[17]

Today, resection of coarctation of the aorta is a fairly common procedure. The surgeon is well supported with correct anatomic information derived from echocardiography, magnetic resonance imaging and cardiac catheterization. The mortality of this procedure in the child above the age of one year is quite low. Mortality of the infant with this disease remains problematic secondary to associate cardiovascular anomalies. The pediatric cardiac surgeon may correct coarctation resection with primary anastomosis, patch aortoplasty, left subclavian flap angioplasty, or bypass graft repair. Concomitant cardiac surgical repair is performed with the aid of cardiac bypass. Recurrent stenosis after surgery may be treated with balloon angioplasty or reoperation.

Chapter Notes

Chapter 1

1. B. Webber and A. Vedder, *In the Kingdom of the Go-rillas: Fragile Species in a Dangerous Land* (New York, London: Simon and Schuster, 2001), 49.

2. S. Montgomery, *Walking with the Great Apes: Jane Goodall, Dian Fossey, Biruté Galdikas.* (Boston: Houghton-Mifflin, 1991), 7.

3. Dian Fossey, *Gorillas in the Mist* (Boston: Houghton-Mifflin, 1988), 75–76.

4. Murdoch Riley, *Maori Healing and Herbal* (Paraparaumu, New Zealand: Viking Sevenseas, fourth printing, 2010), 8.

5. H. N. Wardle, "Stone Implements of Surgery from San Miguel Island, California, *American Anthropologists*, New Series 15, no. 4 (October–December 1913): 656–659.

6. H. E. Sigerist, *History of Medicine*, vol. 1: *Primitive and Archaic Medicine* (New York, Oxford: Oxford University Press, 1951), 128; W. S. Lyon, *Encyclopedia of Native American Healing* (New York, London: W.W. Norton), 138.

7. D. Brothwell and A. T. Sandison, *Diseases in Antiquity* (Springfield, IL: Charles C. Thomas, 1967), 210 and 223–224.

8. V. Vogel, "American Indian Medicine," in *Civilization of the American Indian* series (Norman: University of Oklahoma Press, 1970), 1–11 and 183–184; Lyon, op. cit., 264.

9. Vogel, op. cit., 1–11.

10. A. Johnson, *Plants and the Blackfoot* (Lethbridge, Alberta: Lethbridge Historical Society, 1987), 51.

11. Vogel, op. cit., 175.

12. Johnson, op. cit., 15.

13. E. Stone, *Medicine Among the American Indians* (New York: Paul B. Hoeber, 1932), 78–87.

14. Vogel, op. cit., 224–226.

15. Personal communication, the Cheyenne Elders at Soaring Eagle, Hardin, Montana; Johnson, op. cit., 15.

16. B. Dulger, "A Short Report on Antibacterial Activity of Ten Lycoperdaceae," *Fitoterapia*, no. 76, published by Elsevier (2005): 352–354.

17. Vogel, op. cit., 215.

18. Leslie Spier, "Havasupai Ethnography," *Anthropological Papers of American Museum of Natural History* 29 (1928): 284–285.

19. N. B. Hunt, *Shamanism in North America* (Buffalo, NY: Firefly Books, 2003), 7–14.

20. Ibid., 58–59.

21. Ibid., 152–153.

22. Ibid., 175.

23. Lyon, op. cit., 233.

24. Sidney Greenfield, *Spirits with Scalpels* (Walnut Creek, CA: Left Coast Press, 2008).

25. Sigerist, op. cit., 128–130.

26. Hunt, op. cit., 100–102.

27. J. H. Cooper, *The Gros Ventre of Montana, Part II: Re-ligion and Ritual* (Washington, DC.: Catholic University of America Press, Anthropological Series #16, 1956), 351–356.

28. A. M. Bowers, *Mandan Social and Ceremonial Organization* (Chicago, IL.: University of Chicago Press, 1950), 177–178.

29. E. T. Deng, "Indian Tribes of the Upper Missouri," in *40th Annual Report of Bureau of American Ethnology* (1930), 422.

30. F. Densmore, "Teton Sioux Music," *Bureau of American Ethnology* Bulletin no. 61 (1916): 70.

31. Hunt, op. cit., 126.

32. Sigerist, op. cit., vol. I, illustration 3; Brothwell and Sandison, op. cit., 423–443, and Sigerist, op. cit., 527–528.

33. John Raffensperger, "Conjoined Twins of Polynesia," *Rapi Nui Journal: The Journal of Easter Island* 15, no. 2 (October 2001): 105–109.

34. C. Wells, *Bones, Bodies and Disease* (New York, Washington: Frederick A. Praeger, 1964), illustrations 5, 11, and 63.

35. C. B. Courville, M.D., and K. H. Abbott, M.D., "Cranial Injuries in Precolumbian Incas, with Comments on Their Mechanism, Effects and Lethality," *Bulletin of the Los Angeles Neurological Society* 7, number 5 (September 1942): 107–130.

36. Brothwell and Sandison, op. cit., 657.

37. Ibid., 666–667.

Chapter 2

1. John F. Nunn, *Ancient Egyptian Medicine* (Norman: University of Oklahoma Press, 1996), 24–41.

2. J. H. Breasted, *Edwin Smith Papyrus*, published in facsimile and hieroglyphic transliteration with translation and commentary, in two volumes (Chicago: University of Chicago Press, 1930).

3. H. E. Sigerist, *History of Medicine*, vol. 1:, *Primitive and Archaic Medicine* (New York, Oxford: Oxford University Press, 1951), 277–279.

4. Nunn, op. cit., 127.

5. Ibid., 165.

6. Ibid., 169–171.

7. R. Burger and T. Guthrie, "Why Circumcision," *Pediatrics* 54, no. 3 (September 1974): 362–364.

8. D. L. Gallaher, *Circumcision* (New York: Basic, 2000), 8.

9. I. Twersky, *A Maimonides Reader*, Library of Jewish Studies (Springfield, NJ: Behrman House, 1972), 99.

10. Ibid., 338.

11. D. Gairdner, "The Fate of the Foreskin, a Study of Circumcision," *British Medical Journal* (December 24, 1949): 1433–1437.

12. N. Sari, C. Buyukanal, and B. Zolficar, "Circumcision

Ceremonies at the Ottoman Palace," *Journal of Pediatric Surgery* 31, no. 7 (1996): 920–924.

13. J. Wright, "The Dawn of Surgery, the Ritual Mutilations of Primitive Magic and Circumcision," *New York Medical Journal and Medical Record* (January 17, 1923): 103–105.

14. E. T. Deng, "Indian Tribes of the Missouri," in the *48th Annual Report of the Bureau of American Ethnology* (1930), 427.

15. B. E. Gordon, *Medieval and Renaissance Medicine* (New York: Philosophical Library, 1959), 429–432.

16. L. M. Zimmerman and I. Veith, *Great Ideas in the History of Surgery,* second revised edition (New York: Dover, 1967), 68–71.

Chapter 3

1. Fred Rosner, translator and editor, *Julius Preuss' Biblical and Talmudic Medicine* (New York: Sanhedrin, 1978), 201.

2. Ibid., 129.

3. Ibid., 201.

4. Ibid., 215.

5. Ibid., 212.

Chapter 4

1. C. Muthu, *The Antiquity of Hindu Medicine and Civilization*, third edition (Boston: Milford House, 1931); G. N. Mukhopdhyay, *History of Indian Medicine*, in two volumes (Calcutta: Calcutta University Press, 1923–1929); P. V. Sharma, *History of Medicine in India* (Delhi: Indian National Academy of Science, 1992).

2. J. Marshall, *Mohenjo-Daro and the Indus Civilizations*, vol. 1 (Delhi: Indological Book House, 1973).

3. K. Kelly, "The History of Medicine — Early Civilizations: Prehistoric Times to 500 C.E.," *New York Facts on File* (2009): 51–69; R. C. Majumdar and A. D. Pusalker, eds., *The History and Culture of the Indian People*, vol. 1:, *The Vedic Age* (Bombay: Bharatiya Vidya Bhavan, 1951).

4. K. L. Bhishagratna, *The Sushruta Samhita*, an English translation based on original Sanskrit texts, in three volumes (New Delhi: Cosmo, 2006).

5. T. A. Wise, *Commentary on the Hindu System of Medicine* (London: Trubner, 1860); Anonymous, "Sushruta Samhita — the Compendium of Sushruta," *Lancet* 2 (1912): 1025–1026; M. Neuburger, "The Medicine of the Indians," in M. Neuburger (ed.), *History of Medicine*, vol. 1 (London: Oxford University Press, 1910), 43–60.

6. Kelly, op. cit., 51–69.

7. Bhishagratna, op. cit.

8. P. S. Chari, "Sushruta and Our Heritage," *Indian Journal of Plastic Surgery* 36 (2003): 4–13.

9. P. Johnston-Saint, "An Outline of the History of Medicine in India," *Indian Medical Record* 49 (1929): 289–299; V. K. Raju, "Sushruta of Ancient India," *Indian Journal of Ophthalmology* 51 (2003): 119–122; C. M. Tipton, "Sushruta of India, an Unrecognized Contributor to the History of Exercise Physiology," *Journal of Applied Physiology* 104 (2008): 1553–1556.

10. P. S. Sankaran and P. J. Deshpande, "Sushruta," in V. Raghvan (ed.), *Scientists* (Delhi: Publications Division of Government of India, 1990), 44–72.

11. P. J. Sarma, "Hindu Medicine and Its Antiquity," *Annals of Medical History* 3 (1931): 318–320.

12. Bhishagratna, op. cit.

13. "Dictionary of Spoken Sanskrit (Online)," accessed June 20, 2011, http://spokensanskrit.de.

14. Bhishagratna, op. cit., vol. 2, 57.

15. F. S. Hammett, "The Anatomical Knowledge of the Ancient Hindus," *Annals of Medical History* 1 (1929): 325–327.

16. Bhishagratna, op. cit.

17. Ibid.

18. G. Dwivedi and S. Dwivedi, "Sushruta — the Clinician — Teacher Par Excellence," *Indian Journal of Chest Diseases and Allied Sciences* 49 (2007): 243–244.

19. Bhishagratna, op. cit.

20. Ibid., vol. 2, 140.

21. Bhishagratna, op. cit.

22. J. E. Zimmerman, *Dictionary of Classical Mythology* (New York: Harper and Row, 1964).

23. Bhishagratna, op. cit.

24. Ibid., vol. 2, 29–30.

25. V. Raveenthiran, "Knowledge of Ancient Hindu Surgeons on Hirschsprung's Disease: Evidence from Sushruta Samhita of Circa 1200–600 BC," *Journal of Pediatric Surgery* 46, no. 11 (November 2011): 2204–2208.

26. Bhishagratna, op. cit., vol. 2, 333.

27. S. Das, "Sushruta of India: Pioneer in Vesicolithotomy," *Urology* 23 (1984): 317–319.

28. Bhishagratna, op. cit.; G. Mukhopadhyaya, *The Surgical Instruments of the Hindus, with a Comparative Study of the Surgical Instruments of Greek, Roman, Arab and the Modern European Surgeons*, vol. 1 (Calcutta: Calcutta University Press, 1913).

29. B. K. Killelea and M. S. Arkovitz, "Perforated Appendicitis Presenting as Appendicoumbilical Fistula," *Pediatric Surgery International* 22 (2006): 286–288.

Chapter 5

1. F. Li, *Zhang Zhong-jing's Academic Innovation*, Negative 2010 V1N1: 9–11; S. H. Wang, *Zhang Zhong-jing and H1N1*, Negative 2010 V1N1: 7–8.

2. S. H. Wang, *Hua Tuo, Military Doctor Career*, Negative 2010 V1N3: 13–15.

3. Y. P. Du, *Outstanding Achievements of Hua Tuo*, Negative 2010 V1N3: 15–16.

4. S. H. Wang, *Sun Si-Miao and Acupuncture*, Negative 2010 V1N2: 17–19; S. H. Wang, *Sun Si-Miao and Health Cultivation*, Negative 2010 V1N2:15–17.

5. C. C. Chang et al., "A Clinical Analysis of 1,474 Operations Under Acupuncural Anesthesia Among Children," *Chinese Medical Journal* 1 (1975): 369.

6. J. Z. Zhang, "Anal Fistula," in J. Z. Zhang, *Anorectal Diseases Among Children* (Beijing: International Academic Publisher, 1993), 235.

7. Y. X. She and E. C. Tong, *Textbook of Pediatric Surgery*, third edition (Beijing: Peoples Medical, 1995), 1.

8. J. Z. Zhang and L. Li, "Evolution of Surgical Pediatrics in China," *Journal of Pediatric Surgery*, supplement 1, vol. 38 (2003): 48–52.

Chapter 6

1. Homer, *The Iliad*, trans. Robert Fitzgerald (New York, Toronto, Sydney, Auckland: Anchor, Doubleday, 1974).

2. Ibid., 95.

3. Ibid., 277.

4. *Hippocrates*, vol. 2, trans. W. H. S. Jones (Cambridge, MA, London: Loeb Classic Library, Harvard University Press, 1923), 139.

5. *Hippocrates*, vol. 1, trans. W. H. S. Jones (Cambridge, MA: Harvard University Press, and London: William Heinemann, 1984), 29.

6. Plato, *The Collected Dialogues*, ed. Edith Hamilton and Huntington Cairns (Princeton, NJ: The Bollinger Series, LXXI, Princeton University Press, 1961), lines 309–311.

7. *Hippocrates*, vol. 4: *Heraclitus on the Universe*, trans. W. H. S. Jones (Cambridge, MA, London: Loeb Classic Library, Harvard University Press, 1923), 131–133.

8. *Hippocrates*, vol. 1, op. cit., 147–149.

9. Ibid., 277–279.

10. *Hippocrates*, vol. 7, ed. G. F. Goold (Cambridge, MA, London: Loeb Classical Library, Harvard University Press, 1994), 123.

11. Ibid., 359.

12. *Hippocrates*, vol. 2, op. cit., 19.

13. Ibid., 31.

14. *Hippocrates*, vol. 6, trans. Paul Potter (Cambridge, MA: Harvard University Press, and London: William Heinemann, 1988), 29–31.

15. Ibid., 31–51.

16. Ibid., 51–57.

17. *Hippocrates*, vol. 5, trans. Paul Potter (Cambridge, MA: Harvard University Press, and London: William Heinemann, 1988), 275.

18. *Hippocrates*, vol. 4, op. cit., 203.

19. *Hippocrates, Vol. III*, trans. Dr. E. T. Witherspoon (Cambridge, MA: Harvard University Press and London: William Heinemann, 1928), 41

20. *Hippocrates*, vol. 8, ed. and trans. Paul Potter (Cambridge, MA, London: Loeb Classic Library, Harvard University Press, 1995) 32.

21. *Hippocrates*, vol. 7, op. cit., 101.

22. Ibid., 167.

23. Ibid., 330.

24. Ibid., 95–173.

25. Ibid., 179.

26. Ibid., 225–231.

27. Ibid., 281–283.

28. Ibid., 319–331.

29. F. Douglas Stephens, DSO, FRCS, personal communication.

30. *Hippocrates*, vol. 7, op. cit., 347–351.

31. Ibid., 351–353.

32. *Hippocrates*, vol. 8, op. cit., 303–307.

33. Ibid., 315.

34. Ibid., 317; ibid., 35.

35. Ibid., 401–403.

36. *Hippocrates*, vol. 1, op. cit., 291–301.

37. Isaac A. Abt, M.D., and Arthur F. Abt, M.D., *Abt-Garrison History of Pediatrics* (Philadelphia, London: W.B. Saunders, 1965), 35 (quoted from *Plutarch's Lives*, A. H. Clough, sub voce "Lycurgus").

Chapter 7

1. Richard A. Leonardo, M.D., Ch.M., F.I.C.S., *A History of Surgery* (New York: Froben Press, 1943), 34–39; Robert Garland, *Daily Life of Ancient Greeks* (Westport, CT, London: Greenwood, 1998), 40–41.

2. Celsus, *De Medicina*, in three volumes, trans. W. G. Spencer, M.S., F.R.C.S. (Cambridge, MA: Harvard University Press, and London: William Heineman, 1938).

3. Celsus, *De Medicina*, vol. 2, op. cit., 49.

4. Ibid., 73.

5. Ibid., 81–115.

6. Ibid., 117–119.

7. Ibid., 139–141.

8. Don Brothwell and A. T. Sandison, *Diseases of Antiquity: A Survey of the Diseases and Injuries and Surgery of Early Populations* (Springfield, IL: Charles C. Thomas, 1967), 243.

9. Celsus, *De Medicina*, vol. 2, op. cit., 269–271.

10. Celsus, *De Medicina*, vol. 3, 307–309.

11. Celsus, *De Medicina*, vol. 2, op. cit., 373–377.

12. Ibid., 383.

13. C. Elgood, M.A., M.D., F.R.C.P., *A Medical History of Persia and the Eastern Caliphate* (Cambridge: University Press, 1951), 30.

14. Celsus, *De Medicina*, vol. 2, op. cit., 453.

15. T. N. K. Raju, M.D., D.C.H., chapter 27, "Soranus of Ephesus: Who Was He and What Did He Do?" *Neonatology on the Web.*

16. Soranus, *Gynecology*, book 2:, *Care of the Newborn*, trans. Owsei Temkin, M.D. (Baltimore, London: Johns Hopkins University Press, 1956), 79–127.

17. George F. Still, *The History of Pediatrics* (London: Dawson's of Pall Mall, 1965), 40–41.

18. Soranus, *Gynecology*, op. cit., 189–190 and 192–196.

19. Guido Majno, *The Healing Hand: Man and Wound in the Ancient World* (Cambridge, MA: Harvard University Press, 1970), 112–124 and 186–188.

20. "Galen," Wikipedia, http://en.wikipedia.org.

21. L. M. Zimmerman and I. Veith, *Great Ideas in the History of Surgery*, second revised edition (New York: Dover, 1867), 42–44.

22. R. Leonardo, *History of Surgery* (New York: Froben, 1943), 59–60.

23. John Scarborough, *Roman Medicine* (Ithaca, NY: Cornell University Press, 1969).

24. A. J. Brock, *Greek Medicine, Being Extracts Illustrative of Medical Writers from Hippocrates to Galen* (New York: J. M. Dent and Sons and E. P. Dutton, 1929), 130–246.

25. Still, op. cit., 46.

26. Galen, *On the Usefulness of the Parts of the Body*, trans. Margaret T. May (Ithaca, NY: Cornell University Press, 1967).

Chapter 8

1. A. Goldsworthy, *How Rome Fell* (New Haven, CT, New York: Yale University Press, 2009), 16–23.

2. J. Scarborough, *Roman Medicine* (Ithaca, NY: Cornell University Press, 1969).

3. N. Senn, "Pompeian Surgery and Surgical Instruments," *Medical News*, American Periodical Series Online (December 28, 1895): 26 and 67.

4. Scarborough, op. cit., 89–90.

5. G. F. Still, *The History of Pediatrics: The Progress of the Study of Diseases of Children to the End of the 18th Century* (London: Dawson's of Pall Mall, 1965), 40–42.

6. Sir William Osler, *The Evolution of Modern Medicine* (Classics in Medical Literature, from the collection of Yale University, the Harvey Cushing/John Hay Medical Library, 1921), 29–36.

7. C. Freeman, *The Closing of the Western Mind: The Rise of Faith and the Fall of Reason* (New York: Alfred A. Knopf, 2003), 233.

8. B. E. Gordon, *Medieval and Renaissance Medicine* (New York: Philosophical Library, 1959), 34–35.

9. J. J. Walsh, *Old Time Makers of Medicine: The Story of Students and Teachers of the Sciences Related to Medicine During the Middle Ages* (New York: Fordham University Press, 1911), 23–25.

10. D. Reisman, M.D., Sc.D., *The Story of Medicine in the Middle Ages* (New York: Paul B. Hoeber, Medical Book Department of Harper and Brothers, 1936), 23–24.

11. C. E. Bagwell, M.D., "'Respectful Surgeon,' Revenge of the Barber Surgeon," *Annals of Surgery* 241, no. 6 (June 2005): 874.

12. Gordon, op. cit., 73.

13. Ibid., 458–464.

14. Freeman, op. cit., 358.

15. Still, op. cit., 57–59.

16. R. A. Leonardo, *History of Surgery* (New York: Froben, 1943), 120–121.

Chapter 9

1. Dr. Mark Dickens, Cambridge University, .

2. G. F. Still, *The History of Pediatrics: The Progress of the Study of Diseases of Children Up to the End of the 18th Century* (London: Dawson's of Pall Mall, 1965), 48–50.

3. B. E. Gordon, *Medieval and Renaissance Medicine* (New York: Philosophical Library, 1959), 47–50.

4. Ibid., 60–65.

5. Still, op. cit., 50.

6. L. M. Zimmerman and I. Veith, *Great Ideas in the History of Surgery* (New York: Dover, 1867), 74–78.

7. A. O. Whipple, M.D., *The Role of the Nestorians and Muslims in the History of Medicine* (Princeton, NJ: Allen O. Whipple Surgical Society, printed by Princeton University Press, 1967).

8. Ibid., 11–12.

9. De Lacy O'Leary, D.D., *How Greek Science Passed to the Arabs* (London: Routledge and Kegan Paul, 1949), 184 (available at http://www.aina.org/books/hgsptta.htm).

10. C. Elgood, M.A., M.D., F.R.C.P., *A Medical History of Persia and the Eastern Caliphate* (Cambridge: University Press, 1951), 66–68.

11. E. G. Brown, *Arabian Medicine* (Cambridge: University Press, 1962), 23–32

12. Elgood, op. cit., 196–197.

13. Still, op. cit., 53–54.

14. Elgood, op. cit., 184–191.

15. Gordon, op. cit., 198–200.

16. M. S. Spink and G. L. Lewis, *Albucasis, on Surgery and Instruments* (Berkeley, Los Angeles: University of California Press, 1973).

17. Ibid., xi–xii.

18. Ibid., 50.

19. Ibid., 396–400.

20. Ibid., 558–650.

21. S. N. Cenk Buyukunal and N. Sari, "Serafeddin Sabuncuo lu, the Author of the Earliest Pediatric Surgical Atlas: Cerrahiye-I Ilhaniye," *Journal of Pediatric Surgery* 26 (1991): 1148–1151.

Chapter 10

1. B. E. Gordon, *Medieval and Renaissance Medicine* (New York: Philosophical Library, 1959), 313–320.

2. "Constantine the African," Wikipedia, ; Medieval Manuscripts of the National Library of Medicine (on the Internet).

3. "Gerard of Cremona," Wikipedia, http://en.wikipedia.org.

4. G. W. Corner, "Salernitan Surgery in the Twelfth Century," *British Journal of Surgery*, the Thomas Vicary Lecture delivered at the Royal College of Surgeons of England, December 10, 1936.

5. F. Heer, *The Medieval World: Europe, 1100–1350* (New York: A Mentor Book, New American Library, 1963), 242.

6. H. Graham, *The Story of Surgery* (New York: Doubleday, Doran, 1939), 127–133.

7. C. E. Bagwell, "'Respectful Image': Revenge of the Barber Surgeon," *Annals of Surgery* 241, no. 6 (June 2005): 876.

8. Ibid.

9. F. Cunha, "Hugo of Lucca and the School at Bologna," *American Journal of Surgery* 67, no. 1 (January 1940): 172–180.

10. *The Surgery of Theodoric*, vol. 1, books 1 and 2, trans. E. Campbell, M.D., and J. Colton, M.A. (New York: Appleton-Century-Croft, 1955); *The Surgery of Theodoric*, vol. 2, books 3 and 4, trans. E. Campbell, M.D., and J. Colton, M.A. (New York: Appleton-Century-Crofts, 1960).

11. L. M. Zimmerman and I. Veith, *Great Ideas in the History of Surgery*, second revised edition (New York: Dover, 1967), 124–129.

12. Ibid., 134–146.

13. Marie-Christine Pouchelle, *The Body and Surgery in the Middle Ages* (New Brunswick, NJ: Rutgers University Press, 1990), 15–18.

14. Zimmerman and Veith, op. cit., 138.

15. Pouchelle, op. cit., 119.

16. L. D. Rosenman, trans., *The Surgery of Jehan Yperman* (Xlibris, 2002), 1–27.

17. Ibid., 186.

18. "Guy de Chauliac," Wikipedia, .

19. Zimmerman and Veith, op. cit., 155–156.

20. Gordon, op. cit., 420.

21. L. D. Rosenman, M. D., trans., *The Major Surgery of Guy de Chauliac* (XLibris, 2007).

22. J. E. Pilcher, "Guy de Chauliac and Henri de Mondeville, a Surgical Retrospect," *Annals of Surgery* 21, no. 1 (1895): 84–102 and 92.

Chapter 11

1. "Anatomy," *Catholic Encyclopedia* (from the Internet), 3.

2. L. M. Zimmerman and I. Veith, *Great Ideas in the History of Surgery*, second revised edition (New York: Dover, 1967), 113–118.

3. D. Reisman, *The Story of Medicine in the Middle Ages* (New York: Paul B. Hoeber, Medical Book Division of Harper and Brothers, 1936), 202–231.

4. W. F. Richardson and J. B. Carman, trans., *Andreas Vesalius, on the Fabric of the Human Body*, vol. 1 (San Francisco: Norman, 1998).

5. Ibid., 382–383.

6. H. Cushing, *Andreas Vesalius* (New York: Schuman's, 1953), introduction, xxx.

7. Ibid., 158–159.

8. Richardson and Carman, op. cit., xi.

9. Ibid., 48.

10. Dr. Dan Garrison, Northwestern University, Evanston, Illinois, personal communication with the author.

11. W. F. Richardson and J. B. Carman, trans., *Andreas Vesalius, on the Fabric of the Human Body*, vol. 5 (Novato, CA: Norman, 2007), 65–66.

12. Ibid., 140.

13. H. Graham. *The Story of Surgery*. New York: Doubleday, Doran, 1939, 143.

Chapter 12

1. A. Paré, *The Workes of Ambrose Paréy, Translated Out of Latine and Compared with the French*, trans. Th. Johnson (London: Th. Cotes and R. Young, 1634).

2. P. Lewis, ed., *History of Medicine* (London: Chancellor, 2001), 89.

3. A. N. Williams, "'Labor Improbus Omnia Vincit': Ambroise Paré and Sixteenth Century Child Care," *Archives of Disease in Childhood*, no. 88 (2003): 985–989; A. N. Williams and J. Williams, "'Proper to the Duty of a Chirurgeon': Ambroise Paré and Sixteenth Century Paediatric Surgery," *Journal of the Royal Society of Medicine*, no. 97 (2004): 446–449.

4. G. Keynes, *The Apologie and Treatise of Ambroise Paré* (London: Falcon Educational, 1951), xi.

5. Ibid., xx.

6. A. Wear, *Knowledge & Practice in English Medicine, 1550–1680* (Cambridge: Cambridge University Press, 2000), 223.

7. Keynes, op. cit., 23.

8. Ibid., xx.

9. G. F. Still, *History of Pediatrics* (Oxford: 1932; reprinted 1996, College of Paediatrics and Child Health), 361–362.

10. Keynes, op. cit., 92.

11. Paré, *The Works of Ambrose Paréy*, op. cit., book 17: "Of the Cure That Is Rendered by Surgery," 664.

12. A. Paré, *Oeuvres Complètes (1585)*, vol. 3 (Genève: Facsimile Slatkine Reprints, 1970), 489.

13. Paré, *The Works of Ambroise Paréy*, op. cit., book 17: "Of Divers Preternaturall Affairs Whose Cure Is Performed by Surgery," 662.

14. J. Kiely Bridgens, "Current Management of Clubfoot (Congenital Talipes Equinovarus)," *British Medical Journal*, no. 340 (2010): 355.

15. D. Le Vay, *The History of Orthopaedics: An Account of the Study and Practice of Orthopaedics from the Earliest Times to the Modern Era* (London: Parthenon, 1990), p. 68, citing F. P. Verney, *The Memoirs of the Verney Family During the Civil War* (London: 1894).

16. Paré, *The Works of Ambrose Paréy*, op. cit., book 23: "Of the Meanes and Manner to Repaire or Supply the Natural or Accidental Defects or Wants to a Mans Body," 874.

17. Ibid.

18. A. H. Iason, *Hernia* (Philadelphia: Blackiston, 1941).

19. Paré, *The Works of Ambroise Paréy*, op. cit., book 25: "Of Monsters and Prodigies," 972.

20. L.M. Zimmerman and J. E. Zimmerman, "The History of Hernia Treatment," in I.M. Nyhus and R. E. Condon (eds.), *Hernia*, second edition (Philadelphia: J.B. Lippincott, 1978), 4.

21. Paré, *Oeuvres Complètes (1585)*, op. cit., vol. 111, 502.

22. W. B. Hanby, ed., *The Case Reports and Autopsy Records of Ambroise Paré*, translated from J. P. Malgaines, *Oeuvres Complètes d'Ambroise Paré, 1840* (Springfield, IL: Charles C. Thomas, 1960), 129.

23. Paré, *Oeuvres Complètes (1585)*, op. cit., vol. 111, 288.

24. Paré, *The Works of Ambroise Paréy*, op. cit., book 24: "Concerning the Generation of Man," 959–960.

25. Paré, *The Works of Ambroise Paréy*, op. cit., book 1: "An Introduction or Compendious Way to Chyrurgerie," 45; Wear, op. cit., 223.

26. Wear, op. cit., 223.

27. R. Viner, "Using the History of Paediatrics," *Health and History*, no. 1 (1999): 162–168.

Chapter 13

1. J. E. Pilcher, "Felix Wurtz and Pierre Franco — a Glimpse of the Sixteenth Century," *Annals of Surgery* 24 (October 1896): 505–535.

2. D. Seror, A. Szold, and S. Nissan, "Felix Wurtz, Surgeon and Pediatrician," *Journal of Pediatric Surgery* 26, no. 10 (October 1991): 1152–1155.

3. L. D. Rosenman, trans., *The Surgery of Pierre Franco, an English translation* (Xlibris, 2006).

4. Ibid., 269.

5. Ibid., 312–313.

6. Ibid., 380.

7. Ibid., 548.

8. A. F. Scharli, "Kinder mit Mibbildungen in der Renaissance (nach den Aufzeichnungen von Fabricius Hildanus, 1560–1634)," *Kinderchirurgie*, no. 39 (1984): 296–301.

9. P. P. Rickham, "The Dawn of Pediatric Surgery: Johannes Fatio (1649–1691), His Life, His Work and His Horrible End," *Progress in Pediatric Surgery*, vol. 20 (Heidelberg, Berlin: Springer-Verlag, 1986): 95–105.

10. E. J. O. Kompanjie, "The First Successful Separation of Conjoined Twins in 1689: Some Additions and Corrections," *Twin Research* 7, no. 6, 537–541.

11. A. M. C. Ribbink-Goslinga and J. C. Molenaar, "Pediatric Surgery, Past, Present and Future," *Bulletin de la Societé des Sciences Medicales du Grand-Duchie de Luxembourg, Chirurgie Pediatrique numero special* (1987): 20–30.

12. B. Haseker, "Mr. Job von Meekeren, 1611–1666, and Surgery of the Hand," *Plastic and Reconstructive Surgery* 82, issue 3 (September 1988): 539–546.

Chapter 14

1. L. M. Zimmerman and I. Veith, *Great Ideas in the History of Surgery*, second revised edition (New York: Dover, 1961), 230–238.

2. "William Harvey," Wikipedia, http://en.wikipedia.org.

3. William Harvey, *The Circulation of the Blood and Other Writings*, trans. Kenneth J. Franklin, D.M., F.R.S. (New York: Everyman's Library, Dutton, published in 1907, reissued in new translation 1967).

4. Ibid., 46–48.

5. Ibid., 161.

6. Giovanni Battista Morgagni, *The Seats and Causes of Disease, Investigated by Anatomy in Five Books*; trans. Benjamin Alexander, M.D. (New York: Published under the auspices of the Library of the New York Academy of Medicine by Hafner, 1960).

7. Morgagni, op. cit., book 1, 244–274.

8. Ibid., 313–315

9. Morgagni, op. cit., book 3, 154–163.

10. Ibid., 95–99.

11. Morgagni, op. cit., book 4, 204–211.

12. Morgagni, op. cit., book 3, 644–663 and 520.

13. Ibid., 750–770.

14. Ibid., 476–503.

Chapter 15

1. H. Ellis, "The Umbilical Hernia of Queen Caroline," *Contemporary Surgery* 17 (November 1980): 83–85.

2. Sir Zachary Cope, *William Cheseldon* (London: E. and S. Livingstone, 1953), 53.

3. Ibid., 7.

4. Ibid., 52.

5. Ibid., 15–16.

6. William Cheseldon, Surgeon to St. Thomas' Hospital in Southwark and F.R.S. London, *A Treatise on the High Operation for a Stone*, printed for John Osborn at the Oxford Arms in Lombard Street, 1723, in R. A. Leonardo, *History of Surgery* (New York: Froben, 1943), 207–208.

7. Cope, op. cit., 77–78.

8. Ibid., 85.

9. J. Dobson, "Percival Pott," *Annals of the Royal College of Surgeons, England* 50 (1972): 54–65.

10. L. M. Zimmerman and I. Veith, *Great Ideas in the History of Surgery*, second revised edition (New York: Dover, 1961), 324–337.

11. J. R. Brown and J. L. Thornton, "Percival Pott (1714–1788) and Chimney Sweepers' Cancer of the Scrotum," *British Journal of Industrial Medicine*, no. 1 (January 14, 1957): 68–70.

12. W. Moore, *The Knife Man: The Extraordinary Life and Times of John Hunter, Father of Modern Surgery* (New York: Broadway, 2005).

13. F. Beckman, "The Hernia Congenita, and an Account of the Controversy It Provoked Between William Hunter and Percival Pott," *Bulletin of the New York Academy of Medicine*, no. 22 (1946): 486–500.

14. Moore, op. cit., 102–108.

15. L. G. Stevenson, "The Stag of Richmond Park," *Bulletin of the History of Medicine*, no. 22 (1948): 467–475.

16. Moore, op. cit., 284–285.

17. Ibid., 286.

18. "Lord Byron's Lameness," *British Medical Journal* (March 31, 1923): 568–569.

19. P. M. Dunn, "George Armstrong, M.D. (1719–1789), and His Dispensary for the Infant Poor," *Archives of Disease in Childhood* (fetal, neonatal) 87 (2002): F288–F231.

20. "Nicolas Andry," Wikipedia, http://en.wikipedia.org.

21. N. Andry, *Orthopedia*, a facsimile reproduction of the

first edition in English, London 1743 (Philadelphia, Montreal: J. B. Lippincott, 1961).

22. Ibid., 101–122.

Chapter 16

1. G. F. Still, *The History of Pediatrics* (London: Davison of Pall Mall, 1965), 84–156.

2. S. X. Radbill, "A History of Children's Hospitals," *American Journal of Diseases of Children* 90 (1955): 411–416.

3. Ibid., 415.

4. T. E. C., Jr., M.D., "L'Hôpital des Enfants Malades, the World's First Children's Hospital Founded in Paris in 1802," *Pediatrics* 67, no. 5 (May 1981): 670.

5. Still, op. cit., 101.

6. Radbill, op. cit., 416.

7. L. Auenbrugger, *Inventum Novum ex Percussione Thoracis Humaniet Signo Abstruces Interni Pectoris Morbus Detendi, Vindobpmmae: Typis Joannis Thomae Trattner, 1761*, in L. A. Hochberg, *Thoracic Surgery Before the Twentieth Century* (New York, Washington, DC, Hollywood: Vantage, 1960), 630–641.

8. R. T. H. Laennec, *De l'Auscultation Mediate our Traite du Diagnostic des Maladies des Poumons et du Coeur* (Paris: J. A. Broson et J. S. Chaude, 1819), in Hochberg, op. cit., 641–655.

9. W. C. Roentgen, "On a New Kind of Rays," *Science New York*, no. 3 (February 14, 1896): 227–231.

10. E. P. Davis, "The Clinical Application of Roentgen Rays, the Study of the Infant's Body and of the Pregnant Womb by the Roentgen Rays," *American Journal of Medical Sciences*, no. 111 (1896): 262–270.

11. Hochberg, op. cit., 741.

12. "Humphrey Davy," Wikipedia, http://en.wikipedia.org/wiki/Humphrey_Davy.

13. R. A. Leonardo, *Lives of Master Surgeons* (New York: Froben, 1948), 444.

14. J. C. Warren, "Inhalation of Ethereal Vapor for the Prevention of Pain in Surgical Operations," *Boston Medical and Surgical Journal* 35 (1846): 375–379.

15. J. F. Fulton, *Harvey Cushing: A Biography* (Springfield, IL: Charles C. Thomas, 1946), 69–70.

16. Ibid., 93–94.

17. H. Graham, *The Story of Surgery* (New York: Doubleday, Doran, 1939), 324–329.

18. M. P. Guersant, *Surgical Diseases of Infants and Children*, trans. Richard J. Dunglison, M.D. (Philadelphia: Henry C. Lea, 1873).

19. A. A. Johnson, "Lectures on Surgery of Childhood, Delivered at the Hospital for Sick Children, *British Medical Journal* (January 7, 21, and 28, 1860): 1–4, 41–47, and 61–63.

20. J. G. Raffensperger, "A Review of the First Textbook of Pediatric Surgery in the English Language," *Journal of Pediatric Surgery* 4, no. 4 (August 1969): 403–405.

21. Ibid., 405.

22. J. G. Raffensperger, "John Cooper Forster and the First Textbook of Pediatric Surgery in the English Language," *Guy's Hospital Reports* 113, no. 2 (1964): 172–178

23. V. A. J. Swain, "Sketches of Surgical Cases Drawn from 1884–87 at the East London Hospital for Children, Shadwell," *Progress in Pediatric Surgery* 20 (1986): 265–280.

Chapter 17

1. R. J. Godlee, *Lord Lister*, third edition, revised (Oxford: Clarendon, 1924), 18.

2. Joseph Barron Lister, *Collected Papers of Joseph Barron Lister*, vols. 1 and 2 (Oxford: Clarendon Press, 1859; republished as a special edition [Birmingham AL: Classics of Medicine Library Division of Gryphon Editions, 1979]), vol. 2, 491.

3. Ibid., vol. 2, 516–517.

4. Godlee, op. cit., 29–34.

5. Ibid., 113–114.

6. Lister, op. cit., vol. 1, 69–84.

7. Ibid., vol. 2, 417–440.

8. Godlee, op. cit., 130.

9. Lister, op. cit., vol. 2, 1–2.

10. Godlee, op. cit., 187.

11. Lister, op. cit., vol. 2, 37–85.

12. Ibid., 253.

13. Ibid., 188 and 307.

14. Douglas Guthrie, *The Royal Edinburgh Hospital for Sick Children, 1860–1960* (Edinburgh, London: E. and S. Livingstone, 1960), 19.

15. Ely M. Liebow, *Dr. Joe Bell, Model for Sherlock Holmes* (Bowling Green, OH: Bowling Green University Popular Press, 1982), 12–13.

16. Joseph Bell, F.R.C.S. Edinburgh, *A Manual of Operations of Surgery for the Use of Senior Students, House Surgeons and Junior Practioners*, fifth edition (Edinburgh: Maclachan and Stewart, and London: Simpkin, Marshall, 1883).

17. F. H. Robarts, "The Origins of Paediatric Surgery in Edinburgh," *Journal of the Royal College of Surgeons of Edinburgh* 14 (November 1969): 307–308.

18. W. B. Bell, "A Brief Resumé of the Cases Treated in Mr. Joseph Bell's Ward in the Royal Hospital for Sick Children from November 9, 1894, to April 23, 1895," *Edinburgh Medical Journal* 41, part 1 (September 1885): 234.

19. Liebow, op. cit., 159–160, in Joseph Bell, *Notes on Surgery for Nurses*, sixth edition (New York: William Wood, 1906).

20. F. J. Jirka, *American Doctors of Destiny* (Chicago, IL: Normandie House, 1940), 69–81.

21. H. B. Otherson, M.D., "Ephraim McDowell, the Qualities of a Good Surgeon," *Annals of Surgery* 239, no. 5 (May 2004): 648.

22. L. A. Grey, "Lawson Tait, 1845–1899," from the Internet.

Chapter 18

1. "Claude Bernard," Wikipedia, http://en.wikipedia.org.

2. "Virchow," Wikipedia, http://en.wikipedia.org.

3. "Rokitansky," Wikipedia, http://en.wikipedia.org.

4. "Robert Koch," http://ocp.hul.harvard.edu/contagion/kock.html.

5. "Karl Landsteiner," Wikipedia, http://en.wikipedia.org.

6. "Tetanus," Wikipedia; "Edmond Nocard," Wikipedia, http://en.wikipedia.org.

7. S. Quinn, *Marie Curie: A Life* (New York, London, Toronto: Simon and Schuster, 1995), 158–159.

8. J. F. Fulton, *Harvey Cushing: A Biography* (Springfield, IL: Charles C. Thomas, 1946), 102.

9. J. G. Raffensperger, *The Old Lady on Harrison Street: Cook County Hospital, 1833–1995* (New York, Washington, DC: Peter Lang, 1997), 50.

10. J. G. Scannell, "Willy Meyer (1858–1932), Historical Perspective," *Journal of Thoracic and Cardiovascular Surgery* 111 (May 1996): 1112.

11. E. C. Burke, "Abraham Jacobi, M.D.: The Man and His Legacy," *Pediatrics* 101, no. 2 (February 1998): 309–312.

12. H. Clappesattle, *The Doctors Mayo* (Garden City, NY: Garden City Publishing, 1941), 241.

13. W. G. MacCallum, *William Stewart Halsted, Surgeon* (Baltimore: Johns Hopkins Press, 1930), 21–28.

14. Ibid., 160–176.

15. Fulton, op. cit., 161–201.

16. M. M. Ravitch, *A Century of Surgery, 1880–1980* (Philadelphia, Toronto: J. B. Lippincott, 1981), 238–398.

17. H. Cushing, *From a Surgeon's Journal, 1915–1918* (Boston: Little, Brown, 1936).

18. Ravitch, op. cit., 534–535.

19. Cushing, op. cit., 197.

Chapter 19

1. Edmund Owen, M.B., F.R.C.S., *The Surgical Diseases of Children* (London, Paris, Melbourne: Cassell, 1897).

2. E. F. Kermisson, *Précis de Chirurgie Infantile* (Paris: Masson, 1906).

3. D. F. T. Willard, *The Surgery of Childhood* (Philadelphia: J. B. Lippincott, 1910).

4. S. W. Kelley, *Surgical Diseases of Children: A Modern Treatise on Pediatric Surgery*, third revised edition (St. Louis: C.V. Mosby, 1929)

5. J. F. Fulton, *Harvey Cushing: A Biography* (Springfield, IL: Charles C. Thomas, 1946), 78.

6. V. Tosousy, "Salute to Pediatric Surgery in Czechoslovakia," *Journal of Pediatric Surgery* 3 (1968): 647–648.

7. R. Carachi and D. G. Young, "James Henderson Nicoll — 'Father of Day Surgery'— a History of Surgical Pediatrics," *World Scientific* (New Jersey, London, Singapore, 2009): 702–713.

8. F. H. Robarts, "The Origins of Paediatric Surgery in Edinburgh," *Journal of the Royal College of Surgeons of Edinburgh* 14 (November 1969): 299–315.

9. M. M. Ravitch, *A Century of Surgery, 1880–1980* (Philadelphia: J. B. Lippincott, 1981), 432.

10. Dr. Beiman Otherson, personal communication.

11. Gertrude Herzfeld, handwritten note to Dr. Otherson.

12. A. H. Bill, "William E. Ladd: Great Pioneer of North American Surgery," in *Historical Aspects of Pediatric Surgery, Progress in Pediatric Surgery* (Berlin, Heidelberg, New York, Tokyo: Springer-Verlag, 1986), 52–60.

13. D. A. Gillis, S. D. Lewis, and D. C. Little, "The Halifax Explosion and the Birth of a Surgical Specialty — Myth or Reality," *Journal of Pediatric Surgery* 45 (2010): 855–858 (see also letter to the editor, same issue, 1069, by A. Ein, S. Ein, and D. A. Gillis, now in the possession of Richard Ricketts, M.D., Atlanta, Georgia).

14. W. E. Ladd and R. E. Gross, *Abdominal Surgery of Infancy and Childhood* (Philadelphia: W. B. Saunders, 1941).

15. H. H. Hendren, "Introduction and Historical Overview: North American Perspective," in Mark Stringer, Keith Oldham, and Pierre Mouriquand, *Pediatric Surgery and Urology, Long Term Outcomes* (Cambridge: Cambridge University Press, 2006), 5.

16. J. G. Randolph, "History of the Section on Surgery, the American Academy of Pediatrics: The First 25 Years, 1948–1973," *Journal of Pediatric Surgery* 34, no. 5, supplement 1 (1999): 3–18.

17. R. Carrachi, D. G. Young, and C. Buyukunal, "A History of Surgical Pediatrics," *World Scientific* (New Jersey, London, Singapore, 2009): 525–528.

18. J. Crooks, "Denis Browne, Colleague," *Progress in Pediatric Surgery* 20 (1986): 60–66.

19. P. P. Rickham, "Denis Browne, Surgeon," *Progress in Pediatric Surgery* 20 (1986): 67–74.

20. J. L. Gamble, special article, "Early History of Fluid Replacement Therapy," *Pediatrics* 11 (1953): 554–567

21. Ravitch, Op. cit., 602–603.

22. J. L. Gamble and G. S. Ross, "Factors in the Dehydration Following Pyloric Obstruction," *Journal of Clinical Investigation* 1, no. 5 (1925): 402–423.

23. I. Evans et al., "Fluid and Electrolyte Requirements in Severe Burns," *American Journal of Surgery* 135 (1952): 804.

24. R. E. Gross and J. P. Hubbard, "Surgical Ligation of Patent Ductus Arteriosus," *Journal of the American Medical Association* 112 (1939): 112; C. Crafoord and G. Nylin, "Congenital Coarctation of the Aorta and Its Surgical Treatment," *Journal of Thoracic Surgery* 14 (1945): 347; H. Blalock and H. B. Taussig, "The Surgical Treatment of Malformations of the Heart in Which There Is Pulmonary Stenosis or Pulmonary Atresia," *Journal of the American Medical Association* 128 (1945): 189; W. J. Potts, S. Smith, and S. Gibson, "Anastomosis of the Aorta to the Pulmonary Artery for Certain Types

of Congenital Heart Disease," *Journal of the American Medical Association* 132 (1946): 627; R. C. Brock, "Pulmonary Valvotomy for Relief of Congenital Pulmonary Stenosis," *British Medical Journal* 1 (1948): 1121.

25. R. E. Gross, *The Surgery of Infancy and Childhood* (Philadelphia, London: W. B. Saunders, 1953)

26. Ibid.

27. M. Grob, M. Stockman, and M. Bettex, *Lehrbuch der Kinderchirurgie* (Stuttgart: Georg Thierm, 1957).

28. A. Oberniedermayr, *Lehrbuch der Chirurgie und Orthopadie des Kindesalters* (Berlin, Göttingen, Heidelberg: Springer, 1959).

29. W. J. Potts, *The Surgeon and the Child* (Philadelphia, London: W. B. Saunders, 1959).

30. C. E. Koop, "A Perspective on the Early Days of Pediatric Surgery," *Journal of Pediatric Surgery* 11 (July 1998): 553–560.

31. P. P. Rickham, *The Metabolic Response to Neonatal Surgery* (Cambridge, MA: Harvard University Press, 1957).

32. J. V. Aranda, N. Saheb, and I. Stern, "Arterial Oxygen Tension and Retinal Vasoconstriction in Newborn Infants," *American Journal of Diseases of Children* 122 (1971): 189.

33. A. B. Otherson, "Intubation Injuries of the Trachea in Children," *Annals of Surgery* 189, no. 5 (1979): 601.

34. Henry Rosenberg, M.D., and Jean K. Axelrod, B.A., http://www. anesthesia-analgesia.org.

35. Wikipedia.org/wiki/medical_ventilator

36. Ravitch, op. cit., 1046.

37. D. W. Wilmore and S. J. Dudrick, "Growth and Development of an Infant Receiving All Nutrients Exclusively by Vein," *Journal of the American Medical Association* 203 (1968): 860; S. J. Dudrick, D. B. Groff, and D. W. Wilmore, "Long-Term Venous Catheterization in Infants Surgery," *Gynecology and Obstetrics* 129 (1969): 805.

38. A. M. Waldman, "Medical Ethics and Hopelessly Ill Children," *Journal of Pediatrics Part II* 88 (1976): 890–892.

39. K. Moss, "The 'Baby Doe' Legislation, Its Rise and Fall," *Policy Studies Journal* 15, no. 4 (1987): 629–651.

40. M. Kasai et al., "Surgical Treatment of Biliary Atresia," *Journal of Pediatric Surgery* 3 (1968): 665.

41. M. Dunlop, *Bill Mustard, Surgical Pioneer* (Toronto: Fitzhenry and Whiteside, 1996).

42. S. L. Gans and G. Berci, "Advances in Endoscopy of Infants and Children," *Journal of Pediatric Surgery* 6 (1971): 199–223.

43. D. K. Gupta, A. R. Charles, and M. Srinivas, "Pediatric Surgery in India, a Specialty Comes of Age," *Pediatric Surgery International* 18 (2000): 649–652.

44. S. W. Bickler, J. Kyambi, and H. Rode, "Pediatric Surgery in Sub-Saharan Africa," *Pediatric Surgery International* 17 (2001): 442–447.

Chapter 20

1. R. E. Gross and J. P. Hubbard, "Surgical Ligation of a Patent Ductus Arteriosus. Report of First Successful Case," *Journal of the American Medical Association* 112 (1939): 729.

2. R. E. Gross, "Surgical Approach for Ligation of Patent Ductus Arteriosus," *New England Journal of Medicine* 220 (1939): 510.

3. A. Graybiel, J. W. Strieder, and N. H. Boyer, "An Attempt to Obliterate the Patent Ductus Arteriosus in a Patient with Subacute Bacterial Endocarditis," *American Heart Journal* 15 (1938): 621.

4. R. E. Gross, "Surgical Management of the Patent Ductus Arteriosus with Summary of Four Successfully Treated Cases," *Annals of Surgery* 110 (1939): 321.

5. J. C. Munro, "Ligation of the Ductus Arteriosus," *Annals of Surgery* 46 (1907): 335.

6. Jurgen Thorwald, *The Dismissal: The Incredible Story of the Last Years of Ferdinand Sauerbruch, One of the Great Surgeons of Our Time* (New York: Pantheon, 1961).

7. R. E. Gross, "Idiopathic Dilatation of Common Bile Duct in Children. Review of Literature and Report of the Two Cases," *Journal of Pediatrics* 3 (1933): 730

8. Gross and Hubbard, op. cit., 729.

9. W. E. Ladd and R. E. Gross, "Congenital Malformations of Anus and Rectum; Report of 162 Cases," *American Journal of Surgery* 23 (1934): 167; R. L. Patterson and R. E. Gross, "Adenocarcinoma of Stomach; Case Occurring in Man 27 Years of Age," *New England Journal of Medicine* 210 (1934): 1161; R. E. Zollinger and R. E. Gross, "Traumatic Subdural Hematoma; Explanation of Late Onset of Pressure Symptoms," *Journal of the American Medical Association* 103 (1934): 245; W. E. Ladd and R. E. Gross, "Intussusception in Infancy and Childhood; Report of 372 Cases," *Archives of Surgery* 29 (1934): 365; C. D. Branch and R. E. Gross, "Aberrant Pancreatic Tissue in Gastro-Intestinal Tract; Report of 24 Cases," *Archives of Surgery* 31 (1935): 200; R. E. Gross, "Congenital Anomalies of Gall-bladder; Review of 138 Cases, with Report of a Double Gallbladder," *Archives of Surgery* 33 (1936): 131; E. C. Cutler and R. E. Gross, "Surgical Treatment of Tumors of the Peripheral Nerves," *Annals of Surgery* 104 (1936): 436; E. C. Cutler and R. E. Gross, "Neurofibroma and Neurofibrosarcoma of Peripheral Nerves Unassociated with Rechlinghausen's Disease; a Report of 25 Cases," *Archives of Surgery* 33 (1936):733; E. C. Cutler and R. E. Gross, "Non Tuberculous Abscess of Lung; Etiology, Treatment and Results in 90 Cases," *Journal of Thoracic Surgery* 6 (1936): 125; R. E. Gross, "Recurring Myxomatous, Cutaneous Cysts of Fingers and Toes," *Surgery, Gynecology and Obstetrics* 65 (1937): 289 1937; W. E. Ladd and R. E. Gross, "Congenital Branchiogenic Anomalies; Report of 82 Cases," *American Journal of Surgery* 39 (1938): 234; R. E. Gross and W. W. Vaughan, " Plasma Cell Myeloma; Report of 2 Cases with Unusual Survivals of 6 and 10 Years," *Am J Roentgenol* 39 (1934): 344; R. E. Gross, "The Use of Vinyl Ether (Vinethene) in Infancy and Childhood; Report of 100 Cases, *New England Journal of Medicine* 220 (1939): 334.

10. W. E. Ladd and R. E. Gross, *Abdominal Surgery of Infancy and Childhood* (Philadelphia, London: W. B Saunders, 1941).

11. R. E. Gross, *The Surgery of Infancy and Childhood* (Philadelphia, London: W. B. Saunders, 1953).

12. R. E. Gross, *An Atlas of Children's Surgery* (Philadelphia, London, Toronto: W. B. Saunders, 1970).

13. R. E. Gross and C. A. Hufnagel, "Coarctation of the Aorta. Experimental Studies Regarding Its Surgical Correction," *New England Journal of Medicine* 233 (1945): 287.

14. C. Crafoord and G. Nylin, "Congenital Coarctation of the Aorta and Its Surgical Treatment," *Journal of Thoracic Surgery* 14 (1945): 347.

15. R. E. Gross, A. H. Bill, Jr., and E. C. Peirce II, "Methods of Preservation and Transplantation of Arterial Grafts," *Surgery, Gynecology and Obstetrics* 88 (1949): 689; R. E. Gross, "Treatment of Certain Coarctations by Homologous Grafts. A Report of Nineteen Cases," *Annals of Surgery* 134 (1951): 753.

16. R. E. Gross, "Surgical Relief for Tracheal Obstruction from a Vascular Ring," *New England Journal of Medicine* 233 (1945): 586; R. E. Gross and E. B. D. Neuhauser, "Compression of the Trachea or Esophagus by Vascular Anomalies; Surgical Therapy in 40 cases," *Pediatrics* 7 (1952): 69.

17. R. E. Gross and J. B. Blodgett, "Omphalocele (Umbilical Eventration) in the Newly Born," *Surgery, Gynecology and Obstetrics* 71 (1940): 520; S. R. Schuster, "A New Method for Surgical Treatment of Large Omphaloceles," *Surgery, Gynecology and Obstetrics* 125 (1967): 837.

18. R. E. Gross, "Congenital Hernia of the Diaphragm," *American Journal of Disease in Childhood* 71 (1946): 579; R. E. Gross and T. C. Chisholm, "Annular Pancreas Producing Duodenal Obstruction," *Annals of Surgery* 119 (1944): 759; R. E. Gross, E. B. D. Neuhauser, and L. A. Longino, "Thoracic Diverticula Which Originate from the Intestine," *Annals*

of Surgery 131 (1950): 363; R. E. Gross, H. W. Clatworthy, Jr., and I. A. Meeker, Jr:, "Sacrococcygeal Teratomas in Infants and Children: A Report of 40 Cases," *Surgery, Gynecology and Obstetrics* 92 (1951): 341.

19. R. E. Gross, E. Watkins, Jr., A. J. Pomeranz, and E. I. Goldsmith, "A Method for Surgical Closure of Interauricular Septal Defects," *Surgery, Gynecology and Obstetrics* 96 (1953): 1.

20. G. Wayne Miller, *King of Hearts* (New York: Times, 2000).

21. H. B. Taussig, "Tetrology of Fallot; Especially the Care of the Cyanotic Infant and Child," *Pediatrics* 1 (1948): 307.

22. W. J. Potts and S. Gibson, "Aortico–Pulmonary Anastomosis in Congenital Pulmonary Stenosis," *Journal of the American Medical Association* 137 (1948): 343.

23. R. Allen, "Presidential Address: The Evolution of Pediatric Surgery," *Journal of Pediatric Surgery* 15 (1980): 711.

Chapter 21

1. C. Mack, "A History of Hypertrophic Pyloric Stenosis and Its Treatment," *Bulletin of the History of Medicine* 12 (October 1942): 465–485, 595–615, and 666–689.

2. Mark Ravitch, "The Story of Pyloric Stenosis," *Surgery* 48, no. 6 (December 1960): 1117–1143.

3. H. Hirschsprung, "Falle von Angeborener Pylorustenose, Beobachtet bei Sauglingen," *Jahrb. D. Kindeh* 27 (1885): 61–68.

4. L. M. Zimmerman and I. Veith, *Great Ideas in the History of Surgery*, second revised edition (New York: Dover, 1967).

5. F. Schwyzer, "A Case of Congenital Hypertrophy and Stenosis of the Pylorus," *New York Medical Journal*, no. 64 (1896): 674.

6. C. Stern, "Uber Pylorus Stenose Beim Saugling nebst Bemerkungen uber deren Chirurgschen Benhandlung," *Deutsche Me. Wchnscr.* 24 (1898): 601.

7. S. J. Meltzer, "On Congenital Hypertrophic Stenosis of the Pylorus in Infants," *Medical Record of New York* 54 (August 1898): 253–259

8. Ravitch, op. cit., 1131; Mack, Op. cit., part 3, 603.

9. P. Loretta, "Divulsioni del Piloro e del Cardias," *Gazzete dii Ospedale Milano* 8 (1887): 803.

10. J. Nicoll, "Congenital Hypertrophic Stenosis of the Pylorus with an Account of a Case Successfully Treated by Operation," *British Medical Journal* 21 (1900): 571.

11. Mack, op. cit., part 2, 608.

12. C. Dent, "On Congenital Hypertrophic Stenosis of the Pylorus," *British Journal of Children's Disease*, no. 1 (1904): 16.

13. J. H. Nicoll, "Several Patients from a Further Series of Cases of Congenital Obstruction of the Pylorus Treated by Operation," *Glasgow Medico–Chirurgical Journal* 2, no. 65 (1906): 253.

14. H. Dufour and P. Fredet, "La Stenose Hypertrophique du Pylore chez le Nourrisson et Son Traitement Chirurgical," *Bulletin et Memoires, Société de Medecine de Paris* 24, no. 1221 (1907): 208–217.

15. G. Cerbonnet, "Pierre Fredet, 1870–1946. Dernier Président de la Société Nationale et Premier Président de l'Academie de Chirurgie," *Chirurgie [Memoires de l'Academie* 112, no. 1 (1986): 13–26.

16. Ibid., 24.

17. H. DuFour and P. Fredet, "La Stenose Hypertrophique du Pylore chez le Nourrisson et Son Traitment Chirurgical," *Revue de Chirurgie* 37 (1908): 208–253.

18. P. Fredet and L. Guillemot, "La Stenose du Pylore par Hypertrophic Musculaire chez les Nourrissons," *Annales de Gynecologie et d'Obstetrique* 67 (1910): 604–629.

19. P. Fredet and L. Guillemot, "La Stenose du Pylore par Hypertrophie Musculaire chez les Nourrissons," *Congres Nationale Periodique de Gynecologie, d'Obstetrique et de Pe-*

diatrie, Sixième Session, Toulouse, September 1910; *Memoires et Discussions* (Toulouse: J. Audebert, Imprimerie de Librairie Edouard Privat, 1912), 242–323.

20. P. Fredet and P. Pironneau, "La Stenose Hypertrophique du Pylore," *Bulletin et Memoires, Société Nationale de Chirurgie de Paris* 47 (1921): 1021.

21. P. Fredet, "La Cure de la Stenose Hypertrophique du Pylore chez les Nourrissons par la Pylorotomie — Extra Muqueuse,*" Journal de Chirurgie* 29, no. 4 (1927): 385–408.

22. Ibid.; P. Fredet et E. Lesne, "Stenose Hypertrophique du Pylore chez les Nourrissons: Resultat Anatomique de la Pylorotomie sur un Sujet Traite Gueri Depuis Trois Mois," *Bulletins et Memoires, Société de Chirurgie* 32 (July 11, 1928): 1050–1060.

23. W. Weber, "Ueber Einen Technische Neurerung be der Operation der Pylorus Stenoses des Sauglings," *Berlin Klinische Wehschr.* 47 (1910): 763.

24. C. Ramstedt, "Zur Operation der Angeborenen Pylorusstenose," *Medizin Klinische* 8 (1912): 1702.

25. Mack, op. cit., part 3, 676.

26. Ravitch, op. cit., 1140.

27. Mack, op. cit., part 3, 678.

28. Mack, op. cit., part 3, 679.

29. A. D. Bevan, "Congenital Pyloric Stenosis," *American Journal of Diseases of Children* 1, no. 2 (February 1911): 85–95.

30. D. Lewis and C. Grulee, "The Pylorus After Gastroenterostomy for Congenital Pyloric Stenosis," *Journal of the American Medical Association* 64 (January 30, 1915): 410–412.

31. H. M. Richter, "Congenital Pyloric Stenosis: A Study of Twenty-two Cases with Operation by the Author," *Journal of the American Medical Association* 62 (January 31, 1914): 353–356.

32. W. A. Downes, "Congenital Hypertrophic Pyloric Stenosis: Review of One Hundred and Seventy-five Cases in which the Fredet-Rammstedt Operation Was Performed," *Journal of the American Medical Association* 75 (June 24, 1920): 228–232.

33. W. E. Ladd, "Surgical Diseases of the Alimentary Tract in Infants," *New England Journal of Medicine* 215 (1936): 705–708.

34. Robert E. Gross, *The Surgery of Infancy and Childhood* (Philadelphia, London: W. B. Saunders, 1953), 143; W. J. Potts, *The Surgeon and the Child* (Philadelphia, London: W. B. Saunders, 1958), 57.

Chapter 22

1. A. F. Scharli, "Malformations of the Anus and Rectum and Their Treatment in Medical History," *Progress in Pediatric Surgery* 11 (1978): 141–172.

2. D. Fulbrook, "Medusa's Tails and Leonardo's Heads: Fantasies of Anal Creation in 19th-century Literature and Psychoanalytic Theory," UMI Dissertation Services, ProQuest, Michigan, 2003.

3. B. Rossiter, *Autopsy Reports on Connecticut Medical History,* 11–12 (1692).

4. W. Bodenhamer, *A Practical Treatise on the Etiology, Pathology and Treatment of the Congenital Malformations of the Rectum and Anus* (New York: S&S Wood, 1860), 41.

5. Scharli, op. cit., 148.

6. Ibid., 155.

7. Ibid., 156.

8. W. Wood and C. Kelsey, *Diseases, Injuries and Malformations of the Rectum and Anus* (London: 1857), 378.

9. Ibid. (The original reference can be found in *Emem. de l'Academy des Sciences,* vol. 10, page 36.)

10. G. Dodi and R. J. Spencer, *Outpatient Coloproctology* (1776).

11. Bodenhamer, op. cit.

12. H. Feidberg, "Recherches Clinique et Critiques sur l'Anus Artificialle," *Archives Generales de Medicine de Paris,* 1856.

13. J.-Z. Amussat, "Troisième Memoires sur la Possibilité d'Établire un Overture Artificialle sure le Colon Lombaire Gauche sans Ouvrier le Peritoine, chez les Enfants Imperforate," *Lu a l'Academie Royale des Sciences,* July 4, 1842.

14. W. W. Keen, *An American Text-book of Surgery for Practitioners and Students* (Philadelphia: W. B. Saunders, 1892), 37 and 1209.

15. A. Keith, M.D., "Malformations of Hind End of Body," *British Medical Journal,* December 1736.

16. Bodenhamer, op. cit., 55

17. R. P. Warren, F.R.C.S., "History of Excision of the Rectum," *Proceedings of the Royal Society of Medicine* 50 (1957): 599–600.

18. L. M. Corman, "Classic Articles in Colonic and Rectal Surgery," *Diseases of the Colon and Rectum* 27 (1984): 499–503; W. C. Hargrove, H. Gertner, and W. J. Fitts, "The Kraske Operation for Carcinoma of the Rectum," *Surgery, Gynecology and Obstetrics* 148 (1979): 931–933.

19. M. M. Ravitch, *A Century of Surgery, 1880–1980* (Philadelphia, London: J.B. Lippincott, 1981), 187.

20. R. Matas, "The Surgical Treatment of Congenital Ano-Rectal Imperforation Considered in the Light of Modern Operative Procedures," *Transactions of the American Surgical Association,* 1896, 453–553.

21. F. P. Johnson, "The Development of the Rectum in the Human Embryo," *American Journal of Anatomy* 16 (1914): 1; Sir A. Keith, "Malformations of the Hinder End of the Body," *British Medical Journal* 2 (1908): 1736.

22. O. H. Wangensteen and C. O. Rice, "Imperforate Anus: A Method of Determining the Surgical Approach," *Annals of Surgery* 92, no. 1 (1930): 77–81.

23. W. E. Ladd and R. E. Gross, *The Abdominal Surgery of Infancy and Childhood* (Philadelphia: W. B. Saunders, 1941), 166–187.

24. Ibid., 179–180.

25. J. E. Rhoads, R. L. Pipes, and J. P. Ranjale, "A Simultaneous Abdominal and Perineal Approach in Operations of Imperforate Anus with Atresia of the Rectum and Rectosigmoid," *Annals of Surgery* 127: 552.

26. J. E. Rhoads and C. E. Koop, "The Surgical Management of Imperforate Anus," *Surgical Clinics of North America* (1955): 1251–1257.

27. R. E. Gross, *The Surgery of Infancy and Childhood* (Philadelphia: W. B. Saunders, 1953), 359.

28. Ibid., 360–361.

29. W. J. Potts, *The Surgeon and the Child* (Philadelphia, London: W. B. Saunders, 1959), 202–213.

30. W. B. Kiesewetter, "Imperforate Anus: The Role and Results of the Sacro-Abdomino-Perineal Operation," *Annals of Surgery* 164 (1966): 655–661.

31. R. Carachi, D. G. Young, and C. Buykunal, "A History of Surgical Pediatrics," *World Scientific* (New Jersey, London, Singapore, Beijing, Shanghai, Hong Kong, Taipei, Chennai, 2009): 551–559.

32. S. Douglas, *Oral History Project*: F. Douglas Stephens, M.D., interviewed by John M. Hutson, M.D., May 30, 2007, in Melbourne, Australia (published by the American Academy of Pediatrics).

33. F. Douglas Stephens, "Congenital Imperforate Rectum, Recto-Urethral and Recto-Vaginal Fistulae," *Australia and New Zealand Journal of Surgery* 22, no. 3 (1953): 161–172.

34. F. Douglas Stephens, "Imperforate Anus," *Medical Journal of Australia* 46, no. 2 (1959): 803–805.

35. F. Douglas Stephens, *Photographic Album of Anorectal Anomalies and Sphincter Muscles* (Chicago, IL: Kascot, 1986).

36. Ibid., no. 35; F. Douglas Stephens and W. L. Donnellan, "'H-type' Urethroanal Fistula," *Journal of Pediatric Surgery* 12, no. 1 (1977): 95–102.

37. F. Douglas Stephens, "Wingspread Anomalies, Rarities, and Super Rarities of the Anorectum and Cloaca," *Birth Defects: Original Article Series* 24, no. 4 (1988): 581–585.

38. W. Hasse, "Associated Malformations with Anal and Rectal Atresia," *Progress in Pediatric Surgery* 9 (1976): 100.

39. F. Rehbein, "Imperforate Anus: Experiences with Abdomino-Perineal and Abdomino-Sacroperineal Pull-through Procedures," *Journal of Pediatric Surgery* 2 (1967): 99.

40. A. P. Peña and P. A. DeVries, "Posterior Sagittal Anorectoplasty: Important Technical Consideration and New Applications," *Journal of Pediatric Surgery* 17, no. 6 (1982): 796–811.

41. A. P. Peña, "Posterior Sagittal Anorectoplasty as a Secondary Operation for Fecal Incontinence Through Use of a Levator Sling," *Journal of Pediatric Surgery* 18 (1983): 762.

42. D. Nakayama et al., "Complications of Posterior Sagittal Anorectoplasty," *Journal of Pediatric Surgery* 21 (1986): 488.

43. A. P. Peña, "Posterior Sagittal Anorectoplasty: Results in the Management of 332 Cases of Anorectal Malformations," *Pediatric Surgery International* 3 (1988): 94–104; A. P. Peña et al., "The Effects of the Posterior Sagittal Approach on Rectal Function (Experimental Study), *Journal of Pediatric Surgery* 28, no. 6 (1993): 773–778;A. P. Peña, "Current Management of Anorectal Anomalies," *Surgical Clinics of North America* 72, no. 6 (December 1992): 1393–1416.

44. P. Mollard, J. Marechal, and M. DeBeaujeu, "Surgical Treatment of High Imperforate Anus with Definition of the Puborectalis by an Anterior Approach," *Journal of Pediatric Surgery* 13 (1978): 1499; J. Martin-Laberge et al., "The Anterior Perineal Approach for Pull-through Operations in High Imperforate Anus," *Journal of Pediatric Surgery* 18 (1983): 774.

45. K. E. Georgeson, T. H. Inge, and C. Albanese, "Laparoscopically Assisted Anorectal Pull-through for High Imperforate Anus — a New Technique," *Journal of Pediatric Surgery* 35 (June 2000): 927–933.

46. D. Kimura et al., "Laparoscopic Versus Open Abdomino-Perineal Rectoplasty for Infants with High Type Anorectal Malformation," *Journal of Pediatric Surgery* 45 (December 2010): 2390–2393.

47. F. Douglas Stephens and D. E. Smith, "Classification, Identification and Assessment of Surgical Treatment of Anorectal Anomalies," *Pediatric Surgery International* 1 (1986): 200.

48. L. Schnaufer et al., "Differential Sphincter Studies in the Diagnosis of Anorectal Disorders of Childhood," *Journal of Pediatric Surgery* 2, no. 6 (1967): 538–543.

49. H. Ikawa et al., "The Use of Computerized Tomography to Evaluate Anorectal Anomalies," *Journal of Pediatric Surgery* 20, no. 6 (1985): 640–644; H. P. Haber, S. W. Warmann, and J. Fuchs, "Transperineal Sonography of the Anal Sphincter Complex in Neonates and Infants: Differentiation of Anteriorly Displaced Anus from Low-type Imperforate Anus with Perineal Fistula," *Ultraschall Med* 29 (2008): 383–387; K. C. Pringle, Y. Sato, and R. T. Soper, "Magnetic Resonance Imaging as an Adjunct to Planning an Anorectal Pull-through," *Journal of Pediatric Surgery* 22, no. 6 (1987): 571–574.

50. E. J. Doolin et al., "Rectal Manometry, Computed Tomography and Functional Results of Anal Atresia Surgery," *Journal of Pediatric Surgery* 28, no. 2 (1993): 195–198.

51. J. A. Ditesheim and J. M. Templeton, Jr., "Short-term v. Long-term Quality of Life in Children Following Repair of High Imperforate Anus," *Journal of Pediatric Surgery* 22, no. 7 (1987): 581–587.

52. E. D. Smith, "The Bath Water Needs Changing, but Don't Throw Out the Baby: An Overview of Anorectal Anomalies," *Journal of Pediatric Surgery* 22, no. 4 (1987): 335–348.

53. R. Powel, J. Sherman and J. Raffensperger, "Megarectum: A Rare Complication of Imperforate Anus Repair and Its Surgical Correction by Endorectal Pull-through," *Journal of Pediatric Surgery* 17 (1982): 786; A. P. Peña and M. Behery, "Megasigmoid: A Source of Pseudo-incontinence in Children with Repaired Anorectal Malformations," *Journal of Pediatric Surgery* 28, no. 2 (1993): 199–203.

54. K. L. Pickrell et al., "Construction of a Rectal Sphincter and Restoration of Anal Continence by Transplanting the Gracilis Muscle," *Annals of Surgery* 135 (1952): 853.

55. J. Raffensperger, *Swenson's Pediatric Surgery*, fifth edition (East Norwalk, CT: Appleton and Lange, 1990), 617–619.

56. R. D. Madoff et al., "Standards for Anal Sphincter Replacement," *Diseases of the Colon and Rectum* 43, no. 2 (2000): 135–141.

57. M. Pescatori et al., "Transanal Electrostimulation for Fecal Incontinence: Clinical, Psychologic and Manometric Prospective Study," *Diseases of the Colon and Rectum* 34, no. 7: 540; O. Belyaev, C. Muller, and W. Uhl, "Neosphincter Surgery for Fecal Incontinence: A Critical and Unbiased Review of the Relevant Literature," *Surgery Today* 36 (2006): 295–303.

58. E. Arnbjornsson et al., *Z Kinderchir* 41 (1986): 101–103; V. Loening-Baucke, "Biofeedback Treatment for Chronic Constipation and Encopresis in Childhood: Long-term Outcome," *Pediatrics* 96, no. 1 (1995): 105–110.

59. A. Bischoff, M. A. Levitt, and A. Peña, "Bowel Management for the Treatment of Pediatric Fecal Incontinence," *Pediatric Surgery International* 25 (2009): 1027–1049.

60. P. S. Malone, P. G. Ransley, and E. M. Kiely, "Preliminary Report: The Antegrade Continence Enema," *Lancet* 336, no. 8725 (November 1990): 1217–1218.

Chapter 23

1. E. H. Strach, "Club-foot Through the Centuries," *Progress in Pediatric Surgery*, vol. 20, ed. P. P. Rickham (Berlin, Heidelberg: Springer-Verlag, 1986).

2. G. Elliot Smith and R. Dawson Warren, *Egyptian Mummies* (London: Allen and Unwin, 1924), 100.

3. Francis Adams, *The Genuine Works of Hippocrates Translated from the Greek*, vol. 1 (Sydenham Society, 1849).

4. "Galen," Internet Encyclopedia of Philosophy.

5. Paolo Santoni-Rugiu and Philip J. Sykes, *A History of Plastic Surgery* (Berlin, Heidelberg: Springer-Verlag, 2007).

6. H. S. Fang, "Footbinding in Chinese Women," *Canadian Journal of Surgery* 3 (1960): 195.

7. Joanne Snow-Smith, *Leonardo da Vinci: Ancient Medical Texts, History and Influence* (Seattle: University of Washington, 2004).

8. BBC History, "Andreas Vesalius 1514–1564," 2011.

9. Alain Dimeglio and Frederique Dimeglio, chapter 24 in Robert Hannon Fitzgerald, Herbert Kaufer, and Arthur L. Malkani, *Orthopaedics* (2002).

10. O. Bohne, "Orthopaedic Treatment of Clubfoot in the Sixteenth Century," *Z Krüppel Fürsorgei* 31: 104 11. F. Arcaeus, *De Curandis Vulneribus* (1658).

11. B. Barlow and T.V. Santulli, "Importance of Multiple Episodes of Hypoxia or Cold Stress on the Development of Enterocolitis in an Animal Model," *Surgery* 77, no. 5 (1975): 787–690.

12. Fabricius Hildanus, *Observationum et Curationum Medico-chirurgarum Centurae Sex. Lugduni* (1641).

13. N. Tulpius, *Observationes Medicae* (Amsterdam: 1685).

14. N. André, *Orthopaedia, or the Art of Preventing and Correcting Deformities in Children* (London: 1743).

15. J. A. Venel, *Memoires de la Société des Sciences Physiques de Lausanne*, vol. 2 (1789), 66 and 197.

16. August Brückner, *Uber die Natur, Ursachen und Behandlung der Einwarts Gekriimmten Füsse oder der Sogenannten Klumpfüsse* (Gotha: 1796).

17. E. M. Little, *Orthopaedics Before Stromeyer*, the Robert Jones birthday volume (Oxford: Oxford Medical Publications, 1928).

18. A. Scarpa, *A Memoir on the Congenital Club-foot of Children and the Mode of Correcting that Deformity* (Edinburgh: Constable, 1818).

19. J. M. Delpech, "Tenotomie du Tendon d'Achille," *Chirurgie Clinique Montpelier* 1 (1823): 184.

20. L. Stromeyer, "Contributions to Operative Orthopaedics, or Experiences with Subcutaneous Section of Shortened Muscles and Their Tendons," *Clinical Orthopedics* 97 (1973): 2–4.

21. L. A. Sayre, *Orthopedic Surgery* (New York: Appleton, 1885).

22. W. J. Little, *A Treatise on the Nature of Club-Foot and Analogous Distortions* (London: Jeffs, 1839).

23. http://www.museumofdisability.org/medicine_establishment.asp.

24. Ian A. Cameron, "Lister's Antiseptic Technique," *Canadian Family Physician* 54, no. 11 (November 2008): 1579–1580.

25. R. Baumgartner and W. Taillard, "Treatment of Congenital Club-foot at the Kinderspital Basel," *Annals of Paediatrics*, no. 200 (Basel, 1963): 363; A. M. Phelps, International Congress of Medical Science, Copenhagen, 1884.

26. J. C. McCauley, "Clubfoot," *Clinical Orthopedics* 44 (1966): 51.

27. J. R. Guerin, *Memoire sur l'Etiologie Generate de Pieds-bots Congenitaux* (Paris: 1838).

28. R. W. Parker and S. G. Shattock, "The Pathology and Etiology of Congenital Club-foot," *Transactions of the Pathologists' Society of London*, no. 35: 423.

29. E. M. Bick, *Source Book of Orthopedics* (Baltimore, MD: Williams and Wilkins, 1948).

30. Fritz Bessel-Hagen, *Die Pathologic und Therapie des Klumpfusses* (Heidelberg: 1889).

31. H. O. Thomas, "A New Wrench for Club-foot," *Provincial Medical Journal* 5 (1886): 286.

32. Gustave Flaubert, *Madame Bovary* (Harmandsworth: Penguin, 1950).

33. P. Gourineni and N. C. Carroll, "The Clubfoot Diagnosis and Treatment in Infancy," *Pediatric Orthopedic Problems, Foot and Ankle Clinics* 3, no. 4 (December 1998).

34. R. C. Elmslie, "The Principles of Treatment of Congenital Talipes Equinovarus," *Journal of Orthopedic Surgery* 2 (1920): 669.

35. D. Browne, "Talipes Equinovarus," *Lancet* 11 (1934): 969.

36. J. H. Kite, "The Treatment of Congenital Clubfeet," *Journal of the American Medical Association* 99 (1932): 1156.

37. I. Zadek and E. Barnett, "The Importance of the Ligaments of the Ankle in Correction of Congenital Clubfoot," *Journal of the American Medical Association* 69 (1917): 1057.

38. A. Codivilla, "Tendon Transplant in Orthopaedic Practice," *Clinical Orthopedics* 118 (1976): 2–6.

39. I. V. Ponseti, "Treatment of Congenital Clubfoot," *Journal of Bone and Joint Surgery* 74A (1992): 448–454.

40. V. J. Turco, "Resistant Congenital Clubfoot — One-stage Posteromedial Release with Internal Fixation: A Follow-up Note of a Fifteen-year Experience," *Journal of Bone and Joint Surgery* 61A (1979): 805.

41. J. L. Goldner, "Congenital Talipes Equinovarus: Fifteen Years of Surgical Treatment," *Current Practice in Orthopaedic Surgery* 4 (1969): 61–123.

42. D. W. McKay, "New Concept of and Approach to Clubfoot Treatment: Section I — Principles and Morbid Anatomy," *Journal of Pediatric Orthopedics* 2, no. 4 (1982): 347–356.

43. G. W. Simons, "The Diagnosis and Treatment of Deformity Combinations in Clubfeet," *Clinical Orthopaedics and Related Research*, no. 150 (1980): 229.

44. H. Bensahel et al., "Results of Physical Therapy for Idiopathic Clubfoot: A Long-Term Follow-up Study," *Journal of Pediatric Orthopedics* 10, no. 2 (1990): 189–192.

45. A. Dimeglio, F. Bonnet, P. Mazeau et al., "Orthopaedic Treatment and Passive Motion Machine: Consequences for the Surgical Treatment of Clubfoot," *Journal of Pediatric Orthopedics*, no. 5B (1996): 173.

46. N. C. Carroll, "Congenital Clubfoot: Pathoanatomy and Treatment," *American Academy of Orthopedic Surgeons*, Instructor Course Lecture No. 36 (1987): 117.

47. J. E. Herzenberg, N. C. Carroll, and M. R. Christoferson, "Clubfoot Analysis with Three-dimensional Computer Modeling," *Journal of Pediatric Orthopedics*, no. 8 (1988): 257.

48. N. C. Carroll, "Surgical Technique for Talipes Equinovarus," *Operative Technique in Orthopaedics* 3, no. 2 (1993): 1115.

49. Kenneth J. Noonan, M.D., and B. Stephens Richards, M.D., "Nonsurgical Management of Idiopathic Clubfoot," *Journal of the American Academy of Orthopedic Surgeons* 11, no. 6 (November/December 2003): 392–440.

Chapter 24

1. G. R. Williams, "Presidential Address: A History of Appendicitis," *Annals of Surgery* 197 (1983): 495–506.

2. J. A. Shepherd, "Acute Appendicitis: A Historical Survey," *Lancet* 2 (1954): 299–302; R. H. Meade, "The Evolution of Surgery for Appendicitis," *Surgery* 55 (1964): 741–752.

3. Shepherd, op. cit., 299–302.

4. Ibid.

5. Ibid.

6. Medical papers dedicated to Reginald Heber Fitz in honor of his sixty-fifth birthday, reprinted from *Boston Medical and Surgical Journal* 158, no. 19 (May 7, 1908).

7. J. Loveland, "Reginald Heber Fitz, the Exponent of Appendicitis," *Yale Journal of Biology and Medicine* 6 (1937): 509–520.

8. R. H. Fitz, "Perforating Inflammation of the Vermiform Appendix; with Special Reference to Its Early Diagnosis and Treatment," *The Transactions of the Association of American Physicians* (Philadelphia: Wm. J. Dornan, 1886).

9. W. W. Keen, "Reginald Heber Fitz, M.D., LL.D.: Dr. Fitz's Services to Surgery," *Boston Medical and Surgical Journal* 169 (1913): 893–895.

10. C. McBurney, "Experience with Early Operative Interference in Cases of Disease of the Vermiform Appendix," *New York Medical Journal* 50 (1889): 676–684.

11. J. F. Courtney, "The Celebrated Appendix of Edward VII," *Medical Times* 104 (1976): 176–181.

12. Fitz, op. cit.

13. McBurney, op. cit., 676–684.

14. J. B. Deaver, *Appendicitis*, third edition (Philadelphia: P. Blakiston's Son, 1905).

15. Ibid.

16. Ibid.

17. W. E. Ladd, "Immediate or Deferred Surgery for General Peritonitis Associated with Appendicitis in Children," *New England Journal of Medicine* 219 (1938): 329–333.

18. Ibid.

19. M. Z. Schwartz, D. Tapper, and R. I. Solenberger, "Management of Perforated Appendicitis in Children: The Controversy Continues," *Annals of Surgery* 197: 407–411.

20. R. E. Gross, *The Surgery of Infancy and Childhood* (Philadelphia: W.B. Saunders, 1953).

Chapter 25

1. A. Rossier and S. Sarrut, "Delplanque, l'Enterocolitis Ulcero-necrotique due Premature," *Annals of Pediatrics* 6 (1977): 1428–1436; A. Mizrahi et al., "Necrotizing Enterocolitis in Premature Infants," *Journal of Pediatrics* 66, no. 4 (1965): 697–706

2. J. C. Raffensperger, J. B. Condon, and J. Greengard, "Complications of Gastric and Duodenal Ulcers in Infancy and Childhood," *Surgery, Gynecology and Obstetrics* 123 (December 1966): 1269–1274; L. W. Martin and R. V. Perrin, "Neonatal Perforation of the Appendix in Association with Hirschsprung's Disease," *Annals of Surgery* 144 (November 1967): 799; R. T. Soper and J. M. Opitz, "Neonatal Pneu-

moperitoneum and Hirschsprung's Disease," *Surgery* 51 (April 1963): 527–533.

3. W. S. Keyting et al., "Pneumotosis Intestinalsis, a New Concept," *Radiology* 76 (May 1961): 733–741.

4. Utah State University Cooperative Extension, http://extension.usu.edu.

5. J. R. Lloyd, "Etiology of Gastrointestinal Perforations in the Newborn," *Journal of Pediatric Surgery* 4 (1969): 77.

6. R. J. Touloukian et al., "Surgical Experiences with Necrotizing Enterocolitis in the Infant," *Journal of Pediatric Surgery* 2, no. 5 (1967): 389–401; T. V. Santulli et al., "Acute Necrotizing Enterocolitis in Infancy: A Review of Sixty-Four Cases," *Pediatrics* 55, no. 3 (1975): 376–88; B. Barlow and T. V. Santulli, "Importance of Multiple Episodes of Hypoxia or Cold Stress on the Development of Enterocolitis in an Animal Model," *Surgery* 77, no. 5 (1975): 787–690; B. Barlow et al., "An Experimental Study of Acute Neonatal Enterocolitis: The Importance of Breast Milk," *Journal of Pediatric Surgery* 9, no. 5 (1974): 587–595.

7. R. R. Engel et al., "Origin of Mural Gas in Necrotizing Enterocolitis," *Pediatric Research* 7 (1973): 292.

8. A. M. Kosloske and J. R. Lilly, "Paracentesis and Lavage for Diagnosis of Intestinal Gangrene in Neonatal Necrotizing Enterocolitis," *Journal of Pediatric Surgery* 13 (1978): 315; R. R. Ricketts, "The Role of Paracentesis in the Management of Infants with Necrotizing Enterocolitis," *Annals of Surgery* 52 (1986): 61.

9. S. H. Ein, D. G. Marshall, and D. Girvan, "Peritoneal Drainage Under Local Anesthesia for Perforations in Necrotizing Enterocolitis," *Journal of Pediatric Surgery* 12 (1977): 963.

10. *Swenson's Pediatric Surgery* (Norwalk, CT: Appleton and Lange, 1990), 633–634.

11. R. L. Moss, M.D., R. R. Dimmit, M.D., M.S.P.H., and D. C. Barnhart, M.D., "Laparotomy Versus Peritoneal Drainage for Necrotizing Enterocolitis and Perforation," *New England Journal of Medicine* 354, no. 21 (May 25, 2006): 2225–2234.

12. C. M. Rees, MB, ChB. et al., "Peritoneal Drainage or Laparotomy for Neonatal Bowel Perforation? A Randomized Controlled Trial," *Annals of Surgery* 248, no. 1 (July 2008): 44–51.

13. M. A. Hull et al., "Surgery for Necrotizing Enterocolitis in the United States: Current Practice and Mortality," American Pediatric Surgical Associaiton meeting, May 16–19, 2010.

14. E. E. Zeigler and S. J. Carlson, "Early Nutrition of Very Low Birthweight Infants," *Journal of Fetal and Neonatal Medicine* 3 (March 2009): 191–197.

Chapter 26

1. N. A. Myers, "The History of Oesophageal Atresia and Tracheo-Oesophageal Fistula — 1670–1984," *Progress in Pediatric Surgery* 20 (1986): 106–157; K. W. Ashcraft and T. M. Holder, "The Story of Oesophageal Atresia and Tracheo-Esophageal Fistula," *Surgery* 65 (1969): 332–340.

2. T. M. Holder and K. W. Ashcraft, "Esophageal Atresia and Tracheo-Esophageal Fistula," in *Current Problems in Surgery* (Chicago, IL: Year Book Medical Publisher, 1965).

3. M. Martin, "Observateur des Sciences Medicales Marseille," *Exposé des Traveaux de la Société Royale de Medicine de Marseille*, no. 44 (1821), from Meyers, op. cit., 106–157; T. Mellor, "Malformations of the Oesophagus," *London Medical Gazette* 2 (1846): 542, from Meyers, op. cit.

4. T. P. Hill, "Congenital Malformation," *Boston Medical Surgical Journal* 21 (1840): 320, from Meyers, op. cit.

5. H. Hirschsprung, "Den Medfodte Tillerkning of Spiseroret [Congenital destruction of the esophagus] (4 Cases)," *Medico–Chirurgical Review* 30 (1861): 437.

6. M. Mackenzie, "Malformations of the Esophagus," *Archives of Laryngology* 1, no. 4 (December 1880): 301–315.

7. "Morell Mackenzie," Wikipedia, http://en.wikipedia.org.

8. L. A. Hochberg, *Thoracic Surgery Before the Twentieth Century* (New York: Vantage, 1960), 462–463.

9. C. Steele, M.D., F.R.C.S., "Case of Deficient Oesophagus," *Lancet*, October 20, 1888, 764.

10. Hochberg, op. cit., 474–475.

11. Isaac Abt and F. H. Garrison, *History of Pediatrics* (Philadelphia, London: W. B. Saunders, 1965), 99.

12. Joseph Barron Lister, *Collected Papers of Joseph Barron Lister*, vol. 1 (Oxford at the Clarendon Press; republished as a special edition, Birmingham, AL: Classics of Medicine Library Division of Gryphon Editions, 1979), 139–140.

13. J. O'Dwyer, "Oral Intubation for Diptheria," *Medical Record*, no. 32 (1887): 557.

14. M. Ravitch, *A Century of Surgery, 1880 to 1980: A History of the American Surgical Association* (Philadelphia, Toronto: J. B. Lippincott, 1981), 92–93.

15. R. Matas, "Intralaryngeal Insufflation for the Relief of Acute Surgical Pneumothorax, Its History and Methods with a Description of the Latest Devices for this Purpose," *Journal of the American Medical Association* 34 (1900): 1468–1473.

16. N. A. Gillespie, *Endotracheal Anesthesia* (Madison: University of Wisconsin Press, 1941), 8.

17. Ravitch, op. cit., 408–409.

18. C. A. Elsberg, "Anaesthesia by the Intratracheal Insufflation of Air and Ether, a Description of the Technic of the Method and of a Portable Apparatus for Use in Man," *Annals of Surgery* 53, no. 2 (February 1911): 161–168.

19. L. M. Zimmerman and I. Veith, *Great Ideas in the History of Surgery* (Baltimore, MD: Williams and Wilkins, 1961), 536–547.

20. J. Brenneman, "Congenital Atresia of the Esophagus, with Report of Three Cases," *American Journal of Diseases of Childhood* 5 (1913): 143–150; R. F. Zeit, "Congenital Atresia of the Esophagus with Esophago-Tracheal Fistula," *Journal of Medical Research* 26 (1912): 45–55; H. M. Richter, "Congenital Atresia of the Oesophagus; An Operation Designed for Its Cure. With a report of Two Cases Operated Upon by the Author," *Surgery, Gynecology and Obstetrics* (October 1913): 397–402.

21. H. M. Richter, "Pyloric Stenosis in Infancy, with a Study of Eleven Cases Personally Operated Upon," *Surgery, Gynecology and Obstetrics* (June 1911): 568–575.

22. H. M. Richter, "Positive Pressure Apparatus for Intrathoracic Operations. Preliminary Report," *Surgery, Gynecology and Obstetrics* (November 1908): 583–585.

23. F. Torek, "The First Successful Case of Resection of the Thoracic Portion of the Oesophagus for Carcinoma," *Surgery, Gynecology and Obstetrics* 16 (1913): 614–617.

24. H. M. Richter III, M.D., personal communication.

25. M. Gage and A. Ochsner, "The Surgical Treatment of Congenital Tracheo-Esophageal Fistula in the Newborn," *Annals of Surgery* 103, #5 (May 1936): 725–737.

26. T. H. Lanman, "Congenital Atresia of the Esophagus, a Study of Thirty-Two Cases," *Archives of Surgery* 41 (1940): 1060–1083.

27. N. L. Leven, M.D., "Congenital Atresia of the Esophagus with Tracheoesophageal Fistula, Report of Successful Extrapleural Ligation of Fistulous Communication and Cervical Esophagostomy," *Journal of Thoracic Surgery* 10 (1941): 648–657.

28. N. L. Leven, M.D. et al., "The Surgical Management of Congenital Atresia of the Esophagus and Tracheo-Esophageal Fistula," *Annals of Surgery* 136, no. 4 (October 1952): 701–717.

29. W. E. Ladd, "The Surgical Management of Esophageal Atresia and Tracheoesophageal Fistula," *New England Journal of Medicine* 230, no. 21 (May 25, 1944): 625–637.

30. C. Haight, M.D., and H. A. Tousley, "Congenital Atresia of the Esophagus with Tracheoesophageal Atresia. Extrapleural Ligation of the Fistula and End to End Anastomosis

of Esophageal Segments," *Surgery, Gynecology and Obstetrics* 73 (1943): 672–688.

31. C. Haight, M.D., "Total Removal of Left Lung for Bronchiectasis," *Surgery, Gynecology and Obstetrics* 58 (1934): 768.

32. P. B. Manning, M.D. et al., "Fifty Years' Experience with Esophageal Atresia and Tracheoesophageal Fistula, Beginning with Cameron Haight's First Operation in 1935," *Annals of Surgery* 204, no. 4 (October 1986): 446–451.

33. W. P. Longmire, "Congenital Atresia and Tracheo-Esophageal Fistula," *Archives of Surgery* 55 (1947): 330; R. Howard, "Oesophageal Atresia with Tracheoesophageal Fistula: Report of Six Cases with Two Successful Oesophageal Anastomoses," *Medical Journal of Australia*, no. 1 (1950): 401–404.

34. F. H. Franklin, "Congenital Atresia of the Esophagus, Two Cases Successfully Treated by Anastomosis," *Lancet* 2 (1947): 243.

35. W. E. Ladd, M.D., and O. Swenson, M.D., "Esophageal Atresia and Tracheo-Esophageal Fistula," *Annals of Surgery* 125, no. 1 (January 1947): 23–40.

36. R. E. Gross, *The Surgery of Infancy and Childhood* (Philadelphia, New York: W. B. Saunders, 1953), 75–101.

37. W. J. Potts, M.D., *The Surgeon and the Child* (Philadelphia, New York: W. B. Saunders, 1959), 51–61.

38. T. M. Holder, M.D., V. G. McDonald, M.D., and M. M. Wooley, M.D., "The Premature or Critically Ill Infant with Esophageal Atresia: Increased Survival with a Staged Approach," *Journal of Thoracic and Cardiovascular Surgery* 44, no. 3 (November 1962): 344–358.

39. T. M. Holder, M.D. et al., "Esophageal Atresia and Tracheoesophageal Fistula, a Survey of the Members of the Surgical Section of the American Academy of Pediatrics," *Pediatrics* 34, no. 4 (October 1964): 542–549.

40. D. J. Waterston, R. E. Bonham-Carter, and E. Aberdeen, "Oesophageal Atresia, Tracheo-Oesophageal Fistula: A Study of Survival in 218 Infants," *Lancet* 1 (1962): 819–822.

41. R. L. Replogle, "Esophageal Atresia: Plastic Sump Catheter for Drainage of the Proximal Pouch," *Surgery*, no. 54 (1963): 296–298.

42. D. E. Konkin et al., "Outcomes in Esophageal Atresia and Tracheo-Esophageal Fistula," *Journal of Pediatric Surgery*, no. 38 (2003): 1726–1729; T. M. Holder, M.D. et al., "Care of Infants with Esophageal Atresia, Tracheoesophageal Fistula, and Associated Anomalies," *Journal of Thoracic and Cardiovascular Surgery* 94, no. 6 (December 1987): 828–835; S. R. Choudhury et al., "Survival of Patients with Esophageal Atresia, Influence of Birthweight, Cardiac Anomalies and Late Respiratory Complications," *Journal of Pediatric Surgery* 34 (1999): 70–74; J. Oxford, D. T. Cass, and M. J. Glasson, "Advances in the Treatment of Oesophageal Atresia over Three Decades, the 1970s and the 1990s," *Pediatric Surgery International*, no. 20 (2004): 412–417.

43. A. K. Sharma et al., "Esophageal Atresia and Tracheo-Esophageal Fistula, a Review of 15 Years' Experience," *Pediatric Surgery International*, no. 16 (2000): 478–482.

44. R. Pieretti, B. Shandling, and C. A. Stephens, "Resistant Esophageal Stenosis with Reflux after Repair of Esophageal Atresia, a Therapeutic Approach," *Journal of Pediatric Surgery* 9 (1974): 355–357; K. W. Ashcraft, M.D. et al., "The Thal Fundoplication for Gastroesophageal Reflux," *Journal of Pediatric Surgery* 19 (1984): 480–483.

45. T. E. Lobe et al., "Thoracoscopic Repair of Esophageal Atresia in an Infant, a Surgical First," *Pediatric Endosurgery Innovation Techniques* 3 (1999): 141–148.

46. S. S. Rothenberg, "Thoracoscopic Repair of Tracheo-Esophageal Fistula in Newborns," *Journal of Pediatric Surgery* 37 (2002): 869–872; N. M. A. Bax and D. C. van der Zee, "Feasibility of Thoracoscopic Repair of Esophageal Atresia with Distal Fistula," *Journal of Pediatric Surgery* 37 (2002): 192–196.

47. G. W. Holcomb, M.D. et al., "Thoracoscopic Repair of Esophageal Atresia and Tracheo-Esophageal Fistula, a Multi-Institutional Analysis," *Annals of Surgery* 242, no. 3 (September 2005): 1–9.

48. G. A. MacKinlay, M.B., B.S, L.R.C.P., F.R.C.P.C.H., F.R.C.S. (ed.), "Esophageal Atresia Surgery in the 21st Century," *Seminars in Pediatric Surgery* 18 (2009): 20–22.

49. G. H. Humphries and J. M. Ferrer, "Management of Esophageal Atresia," *American Journal of Surgery*, no. 107 (1964): 406–411.

50. S. S. Yudin, M.D., F.A.C.S. (hon.), F.R.C.S. (hon.) Colonel, Red Army M.C., Moscow, U.S.S.R., "The Surgical Construction of 80 Cases of Artificial Esophagus," *Surgery, Gynecology and Obstetrics* 78, no. 6 (June 1944): 561–583.

51. J. H. Garlock, M.D. F.A.C.S., "The Re-Establishment of Esophagogastric Continuity Following Resection of Esophagus for Carcinoma of the Middle Third," *Surgery, Gynecology and Obstetrics* 78 (1944): 23–28.

52. J. S. Battersby, "Esophageal Replacement by Use of the Right Colon, a One-Stage Thoraco–Abdominal Procedure," *Surgical Forum*, no. 4 (1953): 279–284.

53. W. A. Dale and C. D. Sherman, "Late Reconstruction of Congenital Esophageal Atresia by Intrathoracic Colon Transplantation," *Journal of Thoracic Surgery* 29 (1953): 355; L. A. Longino, M. J. Wooley, and R. E. Gross, "Esophageal Replacement in Infants and Children with the Use of a Segment of Colon," *Journal of the American Medical Association* 171 (1959): 1187; D. J. Waterston, "Colonic Replacement of Esophagus (Intrathoracic)," *Surgical Clinics of North America* 44 (1964): 1441.

54. J. R. Raffensperger et al., "Intestinal Bypass of the Esophagus," *Journal of Pediatric Surgery* 31, no. 1 (1996): 38–47.

55. J. C. German and D. J. Waterston, "Colon Interposition for the Replacement of the Esophagus in Children," *Journal of Pediatric Surgery* 11 (1976): 227; M. Schiller, T. R. Frye, and E. T. Boles, "Evaluation of Colonic Replacement of the Esophagus in Children," *Journal of Pediatric Surgery* 6 (1971): 753.

56. R. Postlethwaite, "Colonic Interposition of Esophageal Replacement," *Surgery, Gynecology and Obstetrics* 156 (1983): 377; W. H. Hendren and W. G. Hendren, "Colon Interposition in Children," *Journal of Pediatric Surgery* 20 (1985): 829.

57. K. D. Anderson and J. G. Randolph, "Gastric Tube Interposition: A Satisfactory Alternative to the Colon for Esophageal Replacement in Children," *Annals of Thoracic Surgery* 6 (1978): 521; D. Viza, S. Ein, and B. Shandling, "Thirteen Years of Gastric Tubes," *Journal of Pediatric Surgery* 3 (1978): 638; J. G. Randolph, "The Gastric Tube for Esophageal Replacement in Children," *Pediatric Surgery International* 11 (1996): 221–223.

58. L. Spitz, E. Kiely, and T. Sparnon, "Gastric Transposition for Esophageal Replacement in Children," *Annals of Surgery* 206 (1987): 73; L. Spitz, "Gastric Transposition of Esophageal Replacement," *Pediatric Surgery International* 11 (1996): 218–220.

59. R. B. Hirschl, M.D. et al., "Gastric Transposition for Esophageal Replacement in Children, Experience with 41 Consecutive Cases with Special Emphasis on Esophageal Atresia," *Annals of Surgery* 236, no. 4 (2002): 531–541.

60. B. Ure et al., "Laparoscopically Assisted Gastric Pull-Up for Long Gap Esophageal Atresia," *Journal of Pediatric Surgery* 38, no. 11 (2003): 1661–1662; T. Nguyen et al., "Laparoscopic Transhiatal Gastric Transposition Preserving the Abdominal Esophagus for Long Gap Esophageal Atresia," *Journal of Pediatric Surgical Specialties*, no. 3 (2008): 32–33; R. M. Juza et al., "Laparoscopic-Assisted Transhiatal Gastric Transposition for Long Gap Esophageal Atresia in an Infant," *Journal of Pediatric Surgery* 45 (2010): 1534–1537.

61. D. K. Gupta et al., "Neonatal Gastric Pull Up: Reality or Myth?" *Pediatric Surgery International* 19 (2003): 100–103.

62. C. Petterson, "Experience in Esophageal Reconstruction," *Archives of Diseases of Surgery*, no. 37 (1962): 184–189.

63. J. F. R. Bentley, "Primary Colonic Substitution for Atresia of the Esophagus," *Surgery* 58 (1965): 731–736.

64. P. W. Johnston, "Elongation of the Upper Segment in Esophageal Atresia, Report of a Case," *Surgery* 58 (1965): 641–744.

65. G. H. Mahour, M. M. Wooley, and J. L. Gwin, "Elongation of the Upper Pouch and Delayed Anatomic Reconstruction in Esohageal Atresia," *Journal of Pediatric Surgery* 9 (1974): 373–383; B. H. Thomasson, "Congenital Esophageal Atresia: Mercury Bag Stretching of the Upper Pouch in a Patient without Tracheo-Esophageal Fistula," *Surgery* 71 (1972): 661–663; W. H. Hendren and J. R. Hale, "Esophageal Atresia Treated by Electromagnetic Bougienage and Subsequent Repair," *Journal of Pediatric Surgery* 11 (1976): 713–722.

66. A. Liviaditis, "Esophageal Atresia: A Method of Overcoming Large Segmental Gaps," *Z. Kindenchirurgie* 13 (1973): 298–306.

67. R. R. Ricketts, S. R. Luck, and J. G. Raffensperger, "Circular Myotomy for Primary Repair of Long Gap Esophageal Atresia," *Journal of Pediatric Surgery* 16, no. 3 (1981): 365–369.

68. J. E. Foker et al., "Development of a True Primary Repair for the Full Spectrum of Esophageal Atresia," *Annals of Surgery* 226 (1997): 533–543; D. C. van der Zee et al., "Thoracoscopic Elongation of the Esophagus in Long Gap Esophageal Atresia," *Journal of Pediatric Surgery* 42 (2007): 1785–1788.

69. L. Spitz et al., "Long Gap Esophageal Atresia," *Pediatric Surgery International* 11 (1996): 462–465.

70. V. Tommaselli et al., "Long-Term Evaluation of Esophageal Function in Patients Treated at Birth for Esophageal Atresia," *Pediatric Surgery International* 19 (2003): 40–43

71. G. S. Lipshutz et al., "A Strategy for Primary Reconstruction of Long Gap Esophageal Atresia Using Neonatal Colon Esophagoplasty: A Case Report," *Journal of Pediatric Surgery* 34, no. 1 (1999): 75–78.

72. C. T. Albanese, personal communication.

73. D. S. Lamb, "A Fatal Case of Congenital Tracheo-Esophageal Fistula," *Philadelphia Medical Times* 3 (1873): 705–707.

74. C. J. Imperatori, "Congenital Tracheo-Esophageal Fistula Without Atresia of the Esophagus," *Archives of Otolaryngology* 30 (1939): 352–359.

75. J. A. Helmsworth and C. V. Pryles, "Congenital Tracheo-Esophageal Fistula Without Esophageal Atresia," *Journal of Pediatrics* 38 (1951): 610–617; C. V. Pryles and A. Huros, "Congenital Tracheo-Esophageal Fistula Without Atresia: Report of a Case with Postmortem Findings," *New England Journal of Medicine* 253 (1955): 855–859.

76. D. A. Killen and H. B. Greennlee, "Transcervical Repair of an H-type Congenital Tracheo-Esophageal Fistula, Review of the Literature," *Annals of Surgery* 162 (1965): 145–150.

77. P. Bedard, D. P. Girvan, and B. Shandling, "Congenital H-type Tracheo-Esophageal Fistula," *Journal of Pediatric Surgery* 9 (1974): 666–668

78. S. L. Gans and R. O. Johnson, "Diagnosis and Surgical Management of H-Type Tracheo-Esophageal Fistula in Infants and Children," *Journal of Pediatric Surgery* 132 (1977): 233–236.

Chapter 27

1. A. Stewart et al., "Malignant Disease and Diagnostic Irradiation *in Utero*," *Lancet*, September 1, 1956, 447.

2. B. Thomasson and M. Ravitch, "Wilms' Tumor," *Urological Survey* 11 (1961): 83–100.

3. W. Osler, M.D. M.R.C.P.L., "Two Cases of Striated Myo-sarcoma of the Kidney," *Journal of Anatomy and Physiology* 14, no. 2 (1880): 229–233.

4. F. V. Birch-Hirschfeld, "Sarkomatose Drusengeschwulste der Niere im Kindesalter [Embryonales Adenosarcom]," *Beitrage zur Pathologischen Anatomie und zur Allgemeinen Pathologie* 24 (1898): 343–362.

5. M. Wilms, *Die Mischegeschwulste der Niere* (Leipzig: Verlag von Arthur Georgi, 1899).

6. "Max Wilms," Wikipedia, http://www.wikipedia.org.

7. E. Garceau, M.D., *Renal, Ureteral, Perirenal and Adrenal Tumors and Actinomycosis and Echinococcus of the Kidney* (New York, London: D. Appleton, 1909), 150–200.

8. I. E. Willetts, "Jessop and the Wilms' Tumor," *Journal of Pediatric Surgery* 38 (2004): 1496–1498.

9. Thomasson and Ravitch, op. cit., 87–89.

10. R. Park, M.D., "Successful Nephrectomy on a Patient of Twenty-three Months," *Transactions of the American Surgical Association* (1886), 259–262, and *Medical News* 48 (May 22, 1886): 567–569.

11. P. M. Rixey et al., "The Official Report of the Case of President McKinley," *Journal of the American Medical Association*. 37 (1901): 1029–1059

12. R. Abbe, "Sarcoma of the Kidney; Its Operative Treatment," *Annals of Surgery* 19 (1894): 58–69.

13. Thomasson and Ravitch, op. cit., 94.

14. A. Friedlander, "Sarcoma of the Kidney Treated by the Roentgen Ray," *American Journal of Diseases of Children* 12 (1915): 328–331.

15. W. E. Ladd and R. R. White, "Embryoma of the Kidney [Wilms' Tumor]," *Journal of the American Medical Association* 112 (1941): 1859–1863.

16. R. E. Gross, *The Surgery of Infancy and Childhood* (Philadelphia and London: W. B. Saunders, 1953), 662.

17. S. A. Waksman and H. B. Woodruff, "Bacteriostatic and Bacteriocidal Substances Produced by Soil Actinomycetes," *Proceedings of the Society of Experimental Biology* 45 (1941): 609–614.

18. W. J. Potts, *The Surgeon and the Child* (Philadelphia, London: W.B. Saunders, 1959), 243.

19. S. Farber et al., "Temporary Remissions in Acute Leukemia in Children Produced by Folic Antagonist 4-Aminopteroylglutamic Acid [Aminopterin]," *New England Journal of Medicine* 238 (1948): 787–793.

20. S. D. Farber et al., "Clinical Studies of Actinomycin-D with Special Reference to Wilms' Tumor in Children," *Annals of the New York Academy of Science* 89 (1960): 421–425.

21. M. M. Ravitch, *A Century of Surgery, 1880–1980: The History of the American Surgical Association* (Philadelphia, Toronto: J. B. Lippincott, 1981), 1252–1253.

22. G. J. D'Angio et al., "The Treatment of Wilms' Tumor: Results of the National Wilms' Tumor Study," *Cancer* 38 (1979): 633–646.

23. G. J. D'Angio et al., "The Treatment of Wilms' Tumor: Results of the Second National Wilms' Tumor Study," *Cancer* 47 (1981): 2302; N. Breslow et al., "Prognosis for Wilms' Tumor Patients with Metastatic Disease at Diagnosis; Results of the Second National Wilms' Tumor Study," *Journal of Clinical Oncology* 3 (1985): 521; G. J. D'Angio et al., "Results of the Third National Wilms' Tumor Study," *Cancer* 64 (1989): 349–360.

24. E. Weiner, "Bilateral Partial Nephrectomies for Large Bilateral Wilms' Tumors," *Journal of Pediatric Surgery* 11 (1976): 867; B. Wasiljew, A. Besser, and J. Raffensperger, "Treatment of Bilateral Wilms' Tumors, a Twenty-two Year Experience," *Journal of Pediatric Surgery* 17 (1982): 265.

25. R. Kubiak et al., "Renal Function and Outcome Following Salvage Surgery for Bilateral Wilms' Tumor," *Journal of Pediatric Surgery* 39, no. 11 (November 2004): 1667–1672.

26. T. E. Hamilton et al., "Bilateral Wilms' Tumor with Anaplasia, Lessons from the National Wilms' Tumor Study Group," *Journal of Pediatric Surgery* 41 (2006): 1641–1644.

27. D. A. Cozzi et al., "Nephron Sparing Surgery for Unilateral Primary Renal Tumors in Children," *Journal of Pediatric Surgery* 36, no. 2 (February 2001): 362–365.

28. P. E. Grundy et al., "Loss of Heterogyzosity for Chromosomes 16Q and 1p in Wilms Tumor Predicts Adverse Outcome," *Cancer Research* 54 (1994): 2331–2333.

29. M. L. Capra et al., "Wilms' Tumor, a Twenty-five Year Review of the Role of Pre-operative Chemotherapy," *Journal of Pediatric Surgery* 34, no. 4 (1999): 579–582.

30. S. Suita et al., "Clinical Characteristics and Outcome of Wilms' Tumors with a Favorable Histology in Japan, a Report from the Study Group for Pediatric Solid Malignant Tumors in the Kyushu Area, Japan," *Journal of Pediatric Surgery* 41 (2006): 1501–1505.

31. N. E. Breslow et al., "Second Malignant Neoplasms Following Treatment for Wilms' Tumors: A Report from the National Wilms' Tumor Study Group," *Journal of Clinical Oncology* 13 (1995): 1851–1859.

Chapter 28

1. "4th Century B.C.E.," in D. B. Guralnik (ed.), *Webster's New World Dictionary*, second college edition (Toronto: Nelson Foster and Scott, 1976), 797; L. S. Hamby, C. L. Fowler, and W. J. Pokorny, chapter 42: "Intussusception," in W. L. Donnellan (ed.), *Abdominal Surgery of Infancy and Childhood* (Austria: Harwood, 1996), 1–19.

2. J. G. Raffensperger, *The Acute Abdomen in Infancy and Childhood* (Philadelphia: J. B. Lippincott, 1970); M. M. Ravitch, *Intussusception in Infants and Children* (Springfield, IL: Charles C. Thomas, 1959); W. H. McAlister, "Intussusception: Even Hippocrates Did Not Standardize His Technique of Enema Reduction," *Radiology* 206 (1998): 595–598; G. Lloyd, *Hippocratic Writings*, fourth edition (London: Penguin, 1983).

3. J. G. Raffensperger, personal communication with Dr. Zhang, 2010.

4. M. D. Stringer and I. E. Willettz, "John Hunter, Frederick Treves and Intussusception," *Annals of the Royal College of Surgeons* 82 (2000): 18–23; O. Leichtenstern, "Intussusception, Invagination, und Darmein Schiebung," *Ziemssen's Cyclopaedia of the Practice of Medicine*, vol. 7 (1877), 610–624; C. F. Davis, A. J. McCabe, and P. A. M. Raine, "The Ins and Outs of Intussusception: History and Management over the Past Fifty Years," *Journal of Pediatric Surgery* 38 (2003): 60–64; J. Hunter, "An Introsusception," Transcript from the Society to Improve Medical and Surgical Knowledge Vol. 1 (1793): 103–118

5. Stringer and Willettz, op. cit.; Leichtenstern, op. cit.; Hunter, op. cit.

6. Davis, McCabe, and Raine, op. cit.

7. G. B. Morgagni, *The Seats and Causes of Diseases Investigated by Anatomy*, trans. B. Alexander (New York: Hafner, 1960), 154–163.

8. Ravitch, op. cit.; Stringer and Willettz, op. cit.; W. Dougall, "History of a Case of Ileus in Which a Considerable Portion of the Intestine Was Voided by Stool," *Medical Commentary* (London) 9 (1785): 278–281; J. Hull, "On Intussusception," *Medical and Physiological Journal* 7 (1802): 32–38; G. Langstaff, "Intussusception," *Edinburgh Medical and Chirurgical Journal* 3 (1807): 262–268.

9. Stringer and Willettz, op. cit.; Davis, McCabe, and Raine, op. cit.; Hunter, op. cit.; Hull, op. cit.

10. S. Mitchell, "Intussusception in Children," *Lancet* 904 (1836): 1837–1838; T. Spencer-Wells, "Intussusception of Caecum and Colon Replaced by Gastrostomy," *Transactions of the Pathological Society of London*, no. 26 (1863): 541–542.

11. Ravitch, op. cit.

12. Mitchell, op. cit.; Stringer and Willettz, op. cit.; Davis, McCabe, and Raine, op. cit.

13. H. Hachmann, "A Case of Intussusception," *Zeitschrift Ges Med* 14 (1840): 289–303.

14. D. Greig, "On Insufflation as a Remedy in Intussusception," *Edinburgh Medical Journal* 10 (1864): 306–315; V.

G. McDermott, "Childhood Intussusception and Approaches to Treatment: A Historical Review," *Pediatric Radiology* 24 (1994): 153–155.

15. Stringer and Willettz, op. cit.; Davis, McCabe, and Raine, op. cit.; D. G. Young, "Intussusception," in J. A. O'Neill, Jr. et al. (eds.), *Pediatric Surgery*, third edition (Chicago, IL: Year Book, 1998), 1185–1198; J. Hutchinson, "A Successful Case of Abdominal Section for Intussusception," *Proceedings of the Royal Medical and Chirurgical Society* 7 (1873): 195–198.

16. Ravitch, op. cit.

17. Stringer and Willettz, op. cit.; Davis, McCabe, and Raine, op. cit.; Hachmann, op. cit.; Spencer-Wells, op. cit.

18. Stringer and Willettz, op. cit.; Leichtenstern, op. cit.; Davis, McCabe, and Raine, op. cit.; S. Trombley, *Sir Frederick Treves, Surgeon and Extraordinary Edwardian* (London: Routledge, 1989); F. Treves, "Intussusception," in *Intestinal Obstruction: Its Varieties with their Pathology, Diagnosis and Treatment*, second edition (London: Cassell, 1899), 141–184; F. Treves, "The Treatment of Intussusception," *Proceedings of the Medical Society of London* 8 (1885): 83–94.

19. W. E. Forest, "Intussusception in Children," *American Journal of Obstetrics* 19 (1886): 673–697.

20. Ravitch, op. cit.

21. M. M. Ravitch and R. M. McCune, Jr., "Reduction of Intussusception by Hydrostatic Pressure: An Experimental Study," *Bulletin of Johns Hopkins Hospital* 82 (1948): 550–568.

22. Ravitch, op. cit.

23. Ibid.

24. M. M. Ravitch, "Intussusception," in K. J. Welch et al. (eds.), *Pediatric Surgery*, fourth edition (Chicago: Year Book, 1986), 868–882; Z. Cope, *Intussusception in the Early Diagnosis of the Acute Abdomen* (Oxford, England: Oxford University Press, 1948), 137–150; E. J. Berman and J. W. Kimble, "Barium Enema for Intussusception in Infants and Children," *Archives of Surgery* 92 (1966): 508–513.

25. Ravitch, *Intussusception in Infants and Children*, op. cit.; Davis, McCabe, and Raine, op. cit.; McDermott, op. cit.; S. H. Ein and A. Daneman, chapter 83: "Intussusception," in J. L. Grosfeld et al. (eds.), *Pediatric Surgery*, sixth edition (Philadelphia: Mosby, 2006), 1313–1341.

26. Ravitch, *Intussusception in Infants and Children*, p. cit.

27. Ibid.

28. Ibid.

29. Berman and Kimble, op. cit.

30. Davis, McCabe, and Raine, op. cit.; McDermott, op. cit.; Berman and Kimble, op. cit.; S. Monrad, "Acute Invagination of the Intestine in Small Children," *Archives of Disease in Childhood* 1 (1926): 323–338.

31. Ravitch, *Intussusception in Infants and Children*, op. cit.; Davis, McCabe, and Raine, op. cit.; Ein and Daneman, op. cit.; G. M. Retan, "Nonoperative Treatment of Intussusception," *American Journal of Disease in Childhood* 33 (1927): 765–770; J. Fraser, "Intussusception," in *Surgery of Childhood* (London: Edward Arnold, 1926), 839–850.

32. Ravitch, *Intussusception in Infants and Children*, op. cit.

33. Davis, McCabe, and Raine, op. cit.; Ravitch and McCune, op. cit.

34. Fraser, op. cit.; G. H. MacNab, "Intussusception," in E. R. Carling and J. P. Ross (eds.), *British Surgical Practice* (London: Butterworth, 1948), 160–168; Robert E. Gross, "Intussusception," in *The Surgery of Infancy and Childhood* (Philadelphia: W. B. Saunders, 1953), 281–300.

35. M. M. Ravitch and R. H. Morgan, "Reduction of Intussusception by Barium Enema," *Annals of Surgery* 135 (1952): 596–605; M. M. Ravitch, "Reduction of Intussusception by Barium Enema," *Surgery, Gynecology and Obstetrics* 99 (1954): 431–435; M. M. Ravitch, "Intussusception in Infancy and Childhood: An Analysis of 77 Cases Treated by Barium Enema," *New England Journal of Medicine* 259 (1958): 1058–1064.

36. Ravitch, "Intussusception," in *Pediatric Surgery*, op. cit.

37. R. B. Zachary, "Acute Intussusception in Children," *Archives of Disease in Childhood* 30 (1955): 32–36.

38. E. S. Fiorito and L. A. Recalde Cuestas, "Diagnosis and Treatment of Acute Intestinal Intussusception with Controlled Insufflation of Air," *Pediatrics* 24 (1959): 241–244; J. Z. Guo, X. Y. Ma, and Q. H. Zhou, "Results of Air Pressure Enema Reduction of Intussusception: 6,396 Cases in 13 Years," *Journal of Pediatric Surgery* 21 (1986): 1210–1213.

39. Davis, McCabe, and Raine, op. cit.

40. L. F. Burke and E. Clarke, "Ileo-colic Intussusception — a Case Report," *Journal of Clinical Ultrasound* 5 (1977): 346–347; A. Daneman et al., "Intussusception on Small Bowel Examination in Children," *American Journal of Roentgenology* 139 (1982): 299–304.

41. Davis, McCabe, and Raine, op. cit.

42. Guo, Ma, and Zhou, op. cit.

43. M. van der Laan et al., "The Role of Laparoscopy in the Management of Childhood Intussusception," *Surgical Endoscopy* 15 (2001): 373–376; S. A. Hay et al., "Idiopathic Intussusception: The Role of Laparoscopy," *Journal of Pediatric Surgery* 34 (1999): 577–578.

44. Ravitch, "Intussusception," in *Pediatric Surgery*, op. cit.; Ein and Daneman, op. cit.; A. Gorenstein et al., "Intussusception in Children: Reduction with Reported, Delayed Air Enema," *Radiology* 206 (1998): 721–724; J. Gonzales-Spinola et al., "Intussusception: The Accuracy of Ultrasound-guided Saline Enema and the Usefulness of a Delayed Attempt at Reduction," *Journal of Pediatric Surgery* 34 (1999): 1016–1020; A. D. Sandler et al., "Unsuccessful Air-enema Reduction of Intussusception: Is a Second Attempt Worthwhile?" *Pediatric Surgery International* 15 (1999): 214–216.

45. Davis, McCabe, and Raine, op. cit.

46. A. LeMasne et al., "Intussusception in Infants and Children: Feasibility of Ambulatory Management," *European Journal of Pediatrics* 158 (1999): 707–710.

47. L. R. Zanardi et al., "Intussusception Among Recipients of Rotavirus Vaccine: Reports to the Vaccine Adverse Event Reporting System," *Pediatrics* 107 (2001): E97; L. Simonsen et al., "Effect of Rotavirus Vaccination Programme on Trends in Admission of Infants to Hospital for Intussusception," *Lancet* 358 (2001): 1224–1229; E. A. Belongia et al., "Real-time Surveillance to Assess Risk of Intussusception and Other Adverse Events After Pentavalent, Bovine-derived Rotavirus Vaccine," *Pediatric Infectious Disease Journal* 29 (2010): 1–5; J. H. Tai et al., "Rotavirus Vaccination and Intussusception: Can We Decrease Temporally Associated Background Cases of Intussusception by Restricting the Vaccination Schedule?" *Pediatrics* 118 (2006): E258–264; M. M. Patel et al., "Intussusception and Rotavirus Vaccination: A Review of the Available Evidence," *Expert Review of Vaccines* 8 (2009): 1555–1564; P. Haber et al., "An Analysis of Rotavirus Vaccine Reports to the Vaccine Adverse Event Reporting System: More than Intussusception Alone?" *Pediatrics* 113 (2004): E353–359; H. G. Chang et al., "Intussusception, Rotavirus, Diarrhea, and Rotavirus Vaccine Use Among Children in New York State," *Pediatrics* 108 (2001): 54–60; E. J. Chang et al., "Lack of Association Between Rotavirus Infection and Intussusception: Implications for Use of Attenuated Rotavirus Vaccines," *Pediatric Infectious Disease Journal* 21 (2002): 97–102; A. Chouikha et al., "Rotavirus Infection and Intussusception in Tunisian Children: Implications for Use of Attenuated Rotavirus Vaccines," *Journal of Pediatric Surgery* 44 (2009): 2133–2138; R. Bahl et al., "Population-Based Incidence of Intussusception and a Case-control Study to Examine the Association of Intussusception with Natural Rotavirus Infection Among Indian Children," *Journal of Infectious Disease* 200 (2009): S277–281.

48. Ein and Daneman, pp. cit.

Chapter 29

1. P. T. Masiakos and S. H. Ein, "The History of Hirschsprung's Disease: Then and Now," *Seminar in Colon & Rectal Surgery* 17 (2006): 10–19.

2. W. K. Sieber, chapter 106: "Hirschsprung's Disease," in K. J. Welch, J. G. Randolph, M. M. Ravitch, J. A. O'Neill, Jr., and M. I. Rowe (eds.), *Pediatric Surgery*, fourth edition (Chicago, IL: Year Book, 1986), 995–1020.

3. E. Leenders and W. K. Sieber, "Congenital Megacolon Observation by Frederick Ruysch — 1691," *Journal of Pediatric Surgery* 5 (1970): 1–3.

4. R. Skaba, "Historic Milestones of Hirschsprung's Disease (Commemorating the 90th Anniversary of Professor Harald Hirschsprung's Death)," *Journal of Pediatric Surgery* 42 (2007): 249–251.

5. T. Ehrenpreis, *Hirschsprung's Disease* (Chicago, IL: Year Book, 1970), 13–25.

6. C. H. Parry, "Singular and Fatal Accumulation of Faeces," in C. H. Parry, *Collections from the Unpublished Medical Writings of the Late C. H. Parry*, vol. 2 (London: Underwoods, 1825), 380.

7. W. S. Haubrich, "Hirschsprung of Hirschsprung's Disease," *Gastroenterology* 127 (2004): 1299.

8. R. J. Touloukian, "Pediatric Surgery Between 1860 and 1900," *Journal of Pediatric Surgery* 30 (1995): 911–916.

9. Sieber, op. cit.

10. J. G. Raffensperger, "Hirschsprung's Disease: A Historical Review," *Bulletin de la Société des Sciences Medicales die Grand Duchy de Luxembourg* 124 (1987): 31–36.

11. H. Hirschsprung, "Dilatation Congénitale du Colon," in Grancher and Comby (eds.), *Traité des Maladies de l'Enfance*, second edition (Paris: 1904).

12. V. Jay, "Legacy of Harald Hirschsprung," *Pediatric and Developmental Pathology* 4 (2001): 203–204.

13. H. Hirschsprung, "Stuhlträgheit Neugeborener in Folge von Dilatation und Hypertrophie des Colons," *Jahrb Kinderh* 27 (1887): 1–7.

14. Raffensperger, op. cit.

15. W. Osler, "On Dilatation of the Colon in Young Children," *Archives of Pediatrics* 111 (1893): 59–62.

16. W. Osler, "Cases of Dilatation of the Colon in Young Children," *Johns Hopkins Hospital Bulletin*, no. 30 (1893): 41–43; H. Chaun, "Sir William Osler and Gastroenterology," *Canadian Journal of Gastroenterology* 24 (2010): 615–618.

17. G. Mya, "Due Osservazioni di Dilatazione ed Impertrofia Congenita del Colon," *Sperimentale* 48 (1894): 215–231; T. J. Walker and J. Griffiths, "Congenital Dilatation and Hypertrophy of Colon Fatal at Age of Eleven Years," *British Medical Journal* 2 (1893): 230–231; G. Genersich, "Ueber Angeborene Dilatation und Hypertrophie des Dickdarms," *JB Kinderhelik* 37 (1894): 91–100; L. Concetti, "Ueber einige Angeborene, bei Kindern die Habituelle Verstopfung, Hervorrufenden Missbildungen des Colon," *Archiv du Kinderhelik* 27 (1899): 319–353; A. Marfan, "De la Constipation des Nourrissons et en Particular de la Constipation d'Origine Congénitale," *Ren Mens Mal de Lent* 13 (1895): 153–157.

18. Marfan, op. cit., 153–157.

19. W. Lewitt, "Enlargement of the Left Colon," *Chicago Medical Journal* 24 (1897): 359–361.

20. F. Treves, "Idiopathic Dilatation of the Colon," *Lancet* 1 (1898): 276–279.

21. Ibid.

22. Ibid.

23. Johnson H. Daintree and D. H. Evans, "Hirschsprung's Disease," *Lancet* 1 (1957): 1147–1149.

24. W. M. Bayliss and E. H. Starling, "The Movements and Innervation of the Large Intestine," *Journal of Physiology* 26 (1900): 107–118.

25. M. Wilms, "Fall von Hirschsprunger Krankheit," *Münch Med Wschr* 42 (1905): 2061–2063; W. S. Fenwick,

"Hypertrophy and Dilatation of the Colon in Infancy," *British Medical Journal* 2 (1900): 564–567.

26. Wilms, op. cit.

27. Ibid.

28. Marfan, op. cit.; Skaba, op. cit.

29. K. Tittel, "Über eine Angeborener Mibbildung des Dickdarmes," *Wien Klinische Wochenschr.* 14 (1901): 903–907.

30. Hirschsprung, "Dilatation Congénitale du Colon," op. cit.

31. L. Kredel, "Über die Angeborener Dilatation und Hypertrophie des Dickdarmes," *Klinische Medizin* 53 (1904): 9–11.

32. J. Finney, "Congenital Idiopathic Dilatation of the Colon," *Surgery, Gynecology and Obstetrics* 6 (1908): 624–643.

33. H. P. Hawkins, "Remarks on Idiopathic Dilatation of the Colon," *British Medical Journal* 1 (1907): 477–483.

34. M. Wilms, "Dauerspasmus an Pylorus, Cardia, Sphincter der Blasé und des Mastdarmes," *Deutsche Zetschrift Chirurgie* 144 (1918): 68–71; E. Martin and V. G. Burden, "The Surgical Significance of the Rectosigmoid Sphincter," *Annals of Surgery* 86 (1927): 86–91.

35. R. B. Wade and N. D. Royle, "The Operative Treatment of Hirschsprung's Disease: A New Method with Explanation of Technique and Results of Operation," *Medical Journal of Australia* 1 (1927): 137–139; W. J. M. Scott and J. J. Morton, "Sympathetic Inhibition of Large Intestine in Hirschsprung's Disease," *Journal of Clinical Investigation* 9 (1930): 247–262.

36. A. W. Adson, "Hirschsprung's Disease, Indication for Treatment and Results Obtained by Sympathectomy," *Surgery* 22 (1947): 259–270.

37. V. P. Ross, "The Results of Sympathectomy," *British Journal of Surgery* 23 (1935): 433–443.

38. A. DallaValle, "Richirche isto Ogiche su di un Caso di Megacolon Congenito," *Pediatria* 8 (1920): 740–752.

39. H. E. Robertson and J. V. W. Kernohan, "The Myenteric Plexus in Congenital Megacolon," *Proceedings of Staff Meeting at the Mayo Clinic*, no. 13 (1938): 123–125.

40. W. A. D. Adamson and I. Aird, "Megacolon: Evidence in Favor of a Neurogenic Origin," *British Journal of Surgery* 20 (1932): 220–233.

41. K. S. Grimson, L. Vandergrift, and H. M. Datz, "Surgery in Obstinate Megacolon: One-Stage Resection and Ileosigmoidostomy," *Surgery, Gynecology and Obstetrics* 80 (1945): 164–173.

42. F. Whitehouse, J. A. Bargan, and C. F. Dixon, "Congenital Megacolon: Favourable End-Results of Treatment by Resection," *Gastroenterology* 1 (1943): 922–937.

43. T. Ehrenpreis, "Megacolon in the Newborn: A Clinical and Roentgenological Study with Special Regard to the Pathogenesis," *Acta Chirurgie Scandinavia* 94 (1946): 112–116.

44. Ibid.

45. O. Swenson, "Early History of the Therapy of Hirschsprung's Disease: Facts and Personal Observations over 50 Years," *Journal of Pediatric Surgery* 31 (1996): 1003–1008.

46. D. H. Teitelbaum et al., chapter 94: "Hirschsprung's Disease and Related Neuromuscular Disorders of the Intestine," in J. A. O'Neill, Jr., M. I. Rowe, J. L. Grosfeld, E. W. Fonkalsrud, and A. C. Coran (eds.), *Pediatric Surgery*, fifth edition (St. Louis: Mosby, 1998), 1381–1424.

47. O. Swenson and A. H. Bill, "Resection of Rectum and Rectosigmoid with Preservation of Sphincter for Benign Spastic Lesions Producing Megacolon," *Surgery* 214 (1948): 212–220.

48. O. Swenson and A. M. Holschneider, chapter 1: "Historical Review," in A. M. Holschneider and P. Puri (eds.), *Hirschsprung's Disease and Allied Disorders*, second edition (Amsterdam: Harwood, 2000), 3–7.

49. O. Swenson, "My Early Experience with Hirschsprung's Disease," *Journal of Pediatric Surgery* 24 (1989): 839–845.

50. Swenson and Bill, op. cit.

51. Raffensperger, op. cit.

52. W. W. Zuelzer and J. L. Wilson, "Functional Intestinal Obstruction on Congenital Neurogenic Basis in Infancy," *American Journal of Disease in Childhood* 75 (1948): 40–64.

53. O. Swenson, H. F. Rheinlander, and I. Diamond, "Hirschsprung's Disease: A New Concept of the Etiology, Operative Results in Thirty-Four Patients," *New England Journal of Medicine* 24 (1949): 551–556.

54. M. Bodian, F. D. Stephens, and B. L. H. Ward, "Hirschsprung's Disease and Idiopathic Megacolon," *Lancet* 1 (1949): 6–11.

55. R. B. Hiatt, "The Pathological Physiology of Congenital Megacolon," *Annals of Surgery* 133 (1951): 313–320.

56. D. State, "Surgical Treatment for Idiopathic Congenital Megacolon (Hirschsprung's Disease)," *Surgery, Gynecology and Obstetrics* 9 (1952): 201–212.

57. O. Swenson, J. H. Fisher, and H. E. MacMahon, "Rectal Biopsy as an Aid in the Diagnosis of Hirschsprung's Disease," *New England Journal of Medicine* 253 (1955): 632–635.

58. B. Duhamel, "Une Nouvelle Opération pour le Megacôlon Congénital: L'Abaissement Rétro-rectale et Transanale du Côlon, et son Application Possible au Traitment de Quelques Autres Malformatos," *Presse Médicale* 64 (1956): 2249–2250; B. Duhamel, "A New Operation for the Treatment of Hirschsprung's Disease," *Archives of Disease in Childhood* 35 (1960): 38–41; F. Rehbein, S. Von, and H. Zimmermann, "Result with Abdominal Resection in Hirschsprung's Disease," *Archives of Disease in Childhood* 35 (1960): 29–37; F. Soave, "Endorectal Pull-through: A Twenty-Year Experience," address by guest speaker to the American Pediatric Surgical Association in 1984," *Journal of Pediatric Surgery* 20 (1985): 568–571.

59. M. Grob, N. Genton, and V. von Tobel, "Experiences with Surgery of Congenital Megacolon and Suggestion of a New Surgical Technique," *Zentralb Chir* 84 (1959): 1781–1789.

60. R. Pagès, "Le Rôle du Sphincter Interne," *Annales de Chirurgie Infantile* 11 (1970): 145–149.

61. O. Swenson, "Partial Internal Sphincterectomy in the Treatment of Hirschsprung's Disease," *Annals of Surgery* 160 (1964): 540–550

62. M. Grob, "Intestinal Obstruction in the Newborn Infant," *Archives of Disease in Childhood* 35 (1960): 40–50.

63. R. T. Soper and F. E. Miller, "Modification of Duhamel Procedure: Elimination of Rectal Pouch and Colorectal Septum," *Journal of Pediatric Surgery* 3 (1968): 376–385.

64. Ibid.

65. F. Soave, "Hirschsprung's Disease: A New Surgical Technique," *Archives of Disease in Childhood* 39 (1964): 116–124; F. Soave, "A New Original Technique for Treatment of Hirschsprung's Disease," *Surgery* 56 (1964): 1007–1014.

66. S. J. Boley, "New Modification of the Surgical Treatment of Hirschsprung's Disease," *Surgery* 56 (1964): 1015–1017.

67. M. Kasai, H. Suzur, and K. Watanabe, "Rectal Myotomy with Colectomy: A New Radical Operation for Hirschsprung's Disease," *Journal of Pediatric Surgery* 6 (1971): 36–41.

68. Swenson, *Annals of Surgery*, op. cit.

69. M. Bodian, "Pathological Aids in the Diagnosis and Management of Hirschsprung's Disease," in S. C. Dyke, ed., *Recent Advances in Clinical Pathology*, series 3 (London: Churchill, 1960).

70. B. Shandling, "A New Technique in the Diagnosis of Hirschsprung's Disease," *Canadian Journal of Surgery* 4 (1961): 298–305.

71. W. O. Dobbins and A. H. Bill, Jr., "Diagnosis of Hirschsprung's Disease Excluded by Rectal Suction Biopsy," *New England Journal of Medicine* 272 (1965): 990–993.

72. L. Schnaufer et al., "Differential Sphincteric Studies

in the Diagnosis of Anorectal Disorders of Childhood," *Journal of Pediatric Surgery* 2 (1967): 538–543.

73. B. Shandling, personal communication, January 2011.

74. Ehrenpreis, op. cit.

75. S. Kleinhaus et al., "A Survey of the Members of the Surgical Section of the American Academy of Pediatrics, *Journal of Pediatric Surgery* 14 (1979): 588–597.

76. A. M. Holschneider, *Hirschsprung's Disease* (Stuttgart: Hippokrates, 1982).

77. W. Meier-Ruge, "Uberlein Erkrank Ungsbild des Colon mit Hirschsprung Symptomatik, *Verh Deutsche Ges Pathol* 55 (1971): 506–510

78. H. B. So et al., "Endorectal 'Pull-through' Without Preliminary Colostomy in Neonates with Hirschsprung's Disease," *Journal of Pediatric Surgery* 15 (1980): 470–471.

79. W. Webster, "Embryogenesis of the Enteric Ganglia in Normal Mice and in Mice That Develop Congenital Aganglionic Megacolon," *Journal of Embryology and Experimental Morphology* 30 (1973): 573–585.

80. D. Gaillard et al., "Colonic Nerve Network Demonstrated by Quinacrine," *Bulletin of the Association of Anatomists* 66 (1982): 63–70; C. Clavel et al., "Distribution of Fibronectin and Laminin During Development of the Human Myenteric Plexus and Hirschsprung Disease," *Gastroenterology and Clinical Biology* 12 (1988): 193–197.

81. G. Martucciello et al., "Immunohistochemical Localization of RET Protein in Hirschsprung's Disease," *Journal of Pediatric Surgery* 30 (1995): 433–436; M. S. Fewtrell et al., "Hirschsprung's Disease Associated with a Deletion of Chromosome 10 (q11.2q21.2) a Further Link with the Neurochrisopathies?" *Journal of Medical Genetics* 31 (1994): 325–327.

82. T. Kunieda et al., "A Mutation in Endothelin-B Receptor Gene Causes Myenteric Agangionosis and Coat Color Spotting in Rats," *DNA Research* 30 (1996): 101–105.

83. C. E. Gariepy et al., "Transgenic Expression of the Endothelin-B Receptor Prevents Congenital Intestinal Aganglionosis in a Rat Model of Hirschsprung Disease," *Journal of Clinical Investigation* 102 (1998): 1092–1101.

84. L. McCabe et al., "Overo Lethal White Foal Syndrome: Equine Model of Aganglionic Megacolon (Hirschsprung Disease)," *American Journal of Medical Genetics* 36 (1990): 336–340; G. C. Yang et al., "A Dinucleotide Mutation in the Endothelin-B Receptor Gene Is Associated with Lethal White Foal Syndrome (LWFS): A Horse Variant of Hirschsprung Disease," *Human Molecular Genetics* 7 (1998): 1047–1052.

85. L. De la Torre–Mondragon and J. A. Ortega-Selgado, "Transanal Endorectal Pull-through for Hirschsprung Disease," *Journal of Pediatric Surgery* 33 (1998): 1283–1286; J. C. Langer et al., "Transanal One-stage Soave Procedure for Infants with Hirschsprung Disease," *Journal of Pediatric Surgery* 34 (1999): 148–152.

86. J. C. Langer et al., "One-stage Transanal Soave Pull-through for Hirschsprung Disease: A Multicenter Experience with 141 Children," *Annals of Surgery* 238 (2003): 569–583.

87. K. E. Georgeson et al., "Primary Laparoscopic-assisted Endorectal Colon Pull-through for Hirschsprung's Disease: A New Gold Standard," *Annals of Surgery* 229 (1999): 678–683.

88. M. L. Proctor et al., "Correlation Between Radiographic Transition Zone and Level of Aganglionosis in Hirschsprung's Disease: Implications for Surgical Approach," *Journal of Pediatric Surgery* 38 (2003): 775–778.

89. C. J. Sauer, J. C. Langer, and P. W. Wales, "The Versatility of the Umbilical Incision in the Management of Hirschsprung's Disease," *Journal of Pediatric Surgery* 40 (2005): 385–389.

90. J. C. Hoehner, S. H. Ein, and B. Shandling, "Long-term Morbidity in Total Colonic Aganglionosis," *Journal of Pediatric Surgery* 33 (1998): 961–966.

91. R. Dasgupta and J. C. Langer, "Hirschsprung Disease," *Current Problems in Surgery* 41 (2004): 942–988; P.

Puri and T. Shinkai, "Pathogenesis of Hirschsprung's Disease and Its Variants: Recent Progress," *Seminars in Pediatric Surgery* 13 (2004): 18–24.

92. N. Wakamatsu et al., "Mutations in SIP1, Encoding Smad Interacting Protein-1, Cause a Form of Hirschsprung Disease," *Nature Genetics* 27 (2001): 369–370.

93. T. Iwashita et al., "Hirschsprung Disease Is Linked to Defects in Neural Crest Stem Cell Function," *Science* 301 (2003): 972–976.

Chapter 30

1. A. Paré, book 24, chapter 66, in *The Works of That Famous Chirugen* (London: Thomas Cotes and R. Young, 1634), 959.

2. G. B. Morgagni, book 3: *Of Diseases of the Belly*, letter XLVIII, article 53–54, in *The Seats and Causes of Diseases Investigated by Anatomy, in Five Books, Containing a Great Variety of Dissections, with Remarks*, trans. B. Alexander (London, 1769), 756–761.

3. Ibid.

4. Ibid.

5. Ibid.

6. W. Hey, "Case XXI," in *Practical Observations in Surgery, Illustrated with Cases* (London: L. Hansard, 1803), 226–232.

7. Ibid.

8. A. C. Robinson, "Case of Congenital Deformity," *Maryland Medical and Surgical Journal* 2 (1841): 162–165.

9. C. Visick, "An Umbilical Hernia in a Newly-Born Child," *Lancet* 1 (1873): 829.

10. W. Fear, "Congenital Extrusion of Abdominal Viscera: Return; Recovery," *British Medical Journal*, 1878, 518.

11. R. Z. Olshausen, "Zur Therapie der Nabelschnurhernien," *Archiv für Gynakologie*, no. 28 (1887): 443 (translated by Wolfgang Cerwinka, M.D.).

12. D. Power, "A Case of Congenital Umbilical Hernia," *Transactions of the Pathological Society of London* 39 (1888):108.

13. F. Ahlfeld, "Der Alkohol Als Desinficienz; (c) Der Alkohol Bei Der Behandlung Inoperabeler Bauchrüche," *Monatssohr Geburtsh Gynakologie* Vol. 10 (1899): 117–128 (translated by Wolfgang Cerwinka, M.D.).

14. T. S. Cullen, "Umbilical Hernia," in *Embryology, Anatomy, and Disease of the Umbilicus Together with Diseases of the Urachus* (Philadelphia, London: W. B. Saunders, 1916), 459–468.

15. Ibid.

16. E. J. Klopp, "Amniotic Hernia," *Annals of Surgery* 73 (1921): 462–463.

17. A. F. Herbert, "Hernia Funiculi Umbilicalis with Report of Three Cases," *American Journal of Obstetrics and Gynecology* 15 (1928): 86–88.

18. Ibid.

19. C. Williams, "Congenital Defects of the Abdominal Wall," *Surgical Clinics of North America* 10 (1930): 805–809.

20. R. E. Gross, "A New Method for Surgical Treatment of Large Omphaloceles," *Surgery* 24 (1948): 277–292.

21. N. M. Dott, "Clinical Record of Case of Exomphalos, Illustrating the Embryonic Type and Its Surgical Treatment," *Edinburgh Medical Journal* (1932): 105–108.

22. W. A. Niebuhr, C. A. Dresch, and F. W. Logan, "Hernia into the Umbilical Cord, Containing the Entire Liver and Gallbladder," *Journal of the American Medical Association* 103 (1934): 16–18; F. M. Dry, "Eventration," *Illinois Medical Journal*, 1934, 509–511; S. S. Peikoff, "Exomphalos," *Canadian Medical Journal* 52 (1945): 600–602; L. Rogers, "Exomphalos," *British Journal of Surgery* 29 (1941): 37–38; C. M. O'Leary and C. E. Clymer, "Umbilical Hernia," *American Journal of Surgery* 52 (1941): 38–43.

23. Rogers, op. cit.

24. O'Leary and Clymer, op. cit.

25. Gross, op. cit.

26. R. E. Gross, "Omphalocele (Umbilical Eventration)," in *The Surgery of Infancy and Childhood*, ed. R. E. Gross (Philadelphia, London: W. B. Saunders, 1953), 406–422.

27. R. H. Kahle, "Omphalocele: Analysis of Twenty-One Cases from Charity Hospital of Louisiana at New Orleans," *The American Surgeon* 17 (1951): 947.

28. A. A. Cunningham, "Exomphalos," *Archives of Disease in Childhood* 31 (1956): 144–151.

29. M. Grob, "Conservative Treatment of Exomphalos," *Archives of Disease in Childhood* 38 (1963): 148–150.

30. S. R. Schuster, "A New Method for the Staged Repair of Large Omphaloceles, *Surgery, Gynecology and Obstetrics* 125 (1967): 837–850.

31. Ibid.

32. R. C. Allen and E. L. Wrenn, "Silon as a Sac in the Treatment of Omphalocele and Gastroschisis," *Journal of Pediatric Surgery* 4 (1969): 3–8.

33. S. W. Beasley and P. G. Jones, "Use of Mercurochrome in the Management of the Large Exomphalos," *Australian Paediatric Journal* 22 (1986): 61–63; M. E. Mullins and Z. Horowitz, "Iatrogenic Neonatal Mercury Poisoning from Mercurochrome Treatment of a Large Omphalocele," *Clinical Pediatrics* 38 (1999): 111–112

34. S. H. Ein and B. Shandling, "A New Non-Operative Treatment of Large Omphaloceles with a Polymer Membrane," *Journal of Pediatric Surgery* 13 (1978): 255–257.

35. S. H. Kim, "Omphalocele," *Surgical Clinics of North America* 56 (1976): 361–371.

36. R. Foglia et al., "Management of Giant Omphalocele with Rapid Creation of Abdominal Domain," *Journal of Pediatric Surgery* 41 (2006): 704–709; O. M. Ramirez, E. Russ, and A. L. Dillon, "'Component Separation' Method for Closure of Abdominal Wall Defects: An Anatomical and Clinical Study," *Plastic and Reconstructive Surgery* 86 (1990): 519–526; F. C. Van Eijck et al., "Closure of Giant Omphalocele by Abdominal Wall Component Separation Technique in Infants," *Journal of Pediatric Surgery* 43 (2008): 246–250; M. S. Clifton et al., "Use of Tissue Expanders in the Repair of Complex Abdominal Wall Defects," *Journal of Pediatric Surgery* 46 (2011): 372–377.

37. M. D. Klein, "Congenital Defects of the Abdominal Wall," in J. L. Grosfeld, J. A. O'Neill, A. G. Coran et al., eds., *Pediatric Surgery*, sixth edition (Philadelphia: Mosby Elsevier, 2006), 1157–1171.

38. D. J. Thompson, "Obstructed Labour with Complicated Presentation and Exomphalos," *British Medical Journal* 2 (1944): 45.

39. J. R. Cantrell, J. A. Haller, and M. M. Ravitch, "A Syndrome of Congenital Defects Involving the Abdominal Wall, Sternum, Diaphragm, Pericardiaum, and Heart," *Surgery, Gynecology and Obstetrics* 107 (1958): 602–614.

40. A. Keith, "Three Demonstrations on Malformations of the Hind End of the Body," *British Medical Journal*, 1908, 1857–1861.

41. P. P. Rickham, "Vesico–Intestinal Fissure," *Archives of Disease in Childhood* 35 (1960): 97–102.

42. K. J. Welch, "Cloacal Exstrophy (Vesico–Intestinal Fissure)," in M. M. Ravitch and K. J. Welch, eds., *Pediatric Surgery* (Chicago, London: Year Book Medical, 1979), 802–808.

43. J. A. O'Neill, Jr., "Cloacal Exstrophy," in J. L. Grosfeld, J. A. O'Neill, A. G. Coran et al., eds., *Pediatric Surgery*, sixth edition (Philadelphia: Mosby Elsevier, 2006), 1859–1869.

44. D. P. Lund and W. H. Hendren, "Cloacal Exstrophy: A 25-Year Experience with 50 Cases," *Journal of Pediatric Surgery* 36 (2001): 68–75; R. R. Ricketts et al., "Modern Treatment of Cloacal Exstrophy," *Journal of Pediatric Surgery* 26 (1991): 444–450.

45. P. Bernstein, "Gastroschisis: A Rare Teratological Condition in the Newborn," *Archives of Pediatrics* 57 (1940): 505–513.

46. J. Calder, "XIV. Two Examples of Children Born with Preternatural Conformations of the Guts," in *Medical Essays*

and Observations (Edinburgh: T. and W. Ruddimans, 1733), 203–204.

47. Morgagni, op. cit.

48. Hey, op. cit.

49. E. N. Reed, "Infant Disemboweled at Birth — Appendectomy Successful," *Journal of the American Medical Association* 61 (1913): 199.

50. Bernstein, op. cit.

51. D. E. Watkins, "Gastroschisis, with Case Report," *Virginia Medical Monthly*, 1943, 42–44.

52. T. C. Moore and G. E. Stokes, "Gastroschisis. Report of Two Cases Treated by a Modification of the Gross Operation for Omphalocele," *Surgery* 33 (1953): 112–120.

53. Schuster, op. cit.; Allen and Wrenn, op. cit.

54. S. R. Luck et al., "Gastroschisis in 106 Consecutive Newborn Infants," *Surgery* 98 (1985): 677–683.

55. R. J. Izant,, Jr., F. Browen, and B. F. Rothman, "Current Embryology and Treatment of Gastroschisis and Omphalocele," *Archives of Surgery* 93 (1966): 49–53

56. D. W. Shermata and J.A. Haller, Jr., "A New Preformed Transparent Silo for the Management of Gastroschisis," *Journal of Pediatric Surgery* 10 (1975): 973–975.

57. J. D. Fischer et al., "Gastroschisis: A Simple Technique for Staged Silo Closure," *Journal of Pediatric Surgery* 30 (1995): 1169–1171.

58. R. K. Minkes et al., "Routine Insertion of a Silastic Spring-loaded Silo for Infants with Gastroschisis," *Journal of Pediatric Surgery* 35 (2000): 843–848; Y. Wu et al., "Primary Insertion of a Silastic Spring-loaded Silo for Gastroschisis," *The American Surgeon* 69 (2003): 1083–1086.

59. S. J. Dudrick, D. W. Wilmore, and H. M. Vars, "Long-term Total Parenteral Nutrition with Growth in Puppies and Positive Nitrogen Balance in Patients," *Surgical Forum* 18 (1967): 356–357.

60. S. J. Dudrick, oral history project interview, in *In Their Own Words* (American Academy of Pediatrics, History Center, 2008), 30–34.

61. D. W. Wilmore and S. J. Dudrick, "Growth and Development of an Infant Receiving All Nutrients Exclusively by Vein," *Journal of the American Medical Association* 203 (1968):140–144.

62. Dudrick, op. cit.

63. S. J. Dudrick, D. B. Groff, and D. W. Wilmore, "Long Term Venous Catheterization in Infants," *Surgery, Gynecology and Obstetrics* 129 (1969): 805–808.

64. D. W. Wilmore et al., "Total Parenteral Nutrition in Infants with Catastrophic Gastrointestinal Anomalies," *Journal of Pediatric Surgery* 4 (1969): 181–189.

65. G. L. Di Tanna, A. Rosano, and R. Mastroiacovo, "Prevalence of Gastroschisis at Birth: Retrospective Study," *British Medical Journal* 325 (2002): 389–390; M. D. Kilby, "The Incidence of Gastroschisis Is Increasing in the UK, Particularly Among Babies of Young Mothers," *British Medical Journal* 332 (2006): 250–251; M. Laughon et al., "Rising Birth Prevalence of Gastroschisis," *Journal of Perinatology* 23 (2003): 291–293.

66. R. W. Martin, "Screening for Fetal Abdominal Wall Defects," *Obstetrics and Gynecology Clinics of North America* 25 (1998): 517–526.

67. Kilby, op. cit.; Laughon et al., op. cit.; M. M. Werler, J. E. Sheehan, and A. V. Mitchell, "Maternal Medication Use and Risk of Gastroschisis and Small Intestinal Atresia," *American Journal of Epidemiology* 155 (2002): 26–31.

Chapter 31

1. M. S. Irish, B. A. Holm, and P. L. Glick, "Congenital Diaphragmatic Hernia: A Historical Review," *Clinics in Perinatology* 23, no. 4 (December 1996): 625–651.

2. Giovanni Battista Morgagni, *The Seats and Causes of*

Diseases, Investigated by Anatomy, in Five Books, trans. Benjamin Alexander, M.D. (New York: Hafner, 1960, published under the auspices of the Library of the New York Academy of Medicine), 204–212.

3. Ibid., 207 and 211.

4. Personal communication from Jay Wilson, Boston Children's Hospital, and Charles Stollar, Babies Hospital, New York. Dr. Stollar has the original manuscript: G. McCauley, "An Account of Visceral Herniation," *Philosophical Transactions of the Royal College of Physicians*, 1754, 625.

5. A. P. Cooper, *The Anatomy and Surgical Treatment of Abdominal Hernia,* second edition (London: Lea and Blanchard, 1844).

6. H. I. Bowditch, "A Peculiar Case of Diaphragmatic Hernia," *Buffalo Medical Journal and Monthly Review* 9 (1853): 1–39 and 65–94 (originally presented to the Boston Society for Medical Observation in 1847).

7. J. Felts, "Henry Ingersoll Bowditch and Oliver Wendell Holmes, Stethoscopist and Reformers," *Perspectives in Biology and Medicine* 45, no. 4 (Autumn 2002): 539–548.

8. S. Jarcho, "Henry I. Bowditch on Diaphragmatic Hernia, 1853," *American Journal of Cardiology*, August 12, 1963, 244–248.

9. D. Kachlik and P. Cech, "Vincenz Alexander Bochdalek, 1801–1883," *Journal of Medical Biography* 19 (2011): 38–43.

10. V. A. Bochdalek, "Einige Betrachtungen uber die Entstchung des Angeborenen Zwerchfellbruches. Als Beitrag zur Pathologischen Anatomie der Hernien," *Vierteljahrschrift die Practishe Heilkunde* 19 (1848): 89–97.

11. V. A. Bochdalek, "Von Prof. Praktische Bemerkungen uber Zwerchfellbruche nebst Beschreibung eines mit einer Frakture der Lendanwirbelsaule Komlizirten Falles," *Vierteljohrsschrift für die Praktische Heikunde* 24 (1867): 14–17.

12. J. O'Dwyer, "Operation for the Relief of Congenital Diaphragmatic Hernia," *Archives of Pediatrics* 9 (1889): 130–132.

13. M. M. Ravitch, *A Century of Surgery, 1880–1980* (Philadelphia, Toronto: J. B. Lippincott, 1981), 244.

14. J. B. Hume, "Congenital Diaphragmatic Hernia," *British Journal of Surgery* 10 (1922): 207–215 .

15. L. Heidenhain, "Geschicht eines Falles von Chronisher Inkarzeration des Magnes in einer Angeborenen Zwerchfellnernia, Welcher durch Laparotomie Geheiht Wurde mit Anschlressenden Bemerkungen über die Moglichkeit, das Cardiacrcinon der Peiserehre zu Reszeieren," *Deutsche Zetschrift für Chirurgie* 76 (1905): 394–403.

16. O. Aue, "Uber Angenborene Zwerchfellhernien," *Zentrablblatt für Chirurgie* 160 (1920): 14–35.

17. C. A. Hedblom, "Diaphragmatic Hernia," *Journal of the American Medical Association* 85, no. 13 (1925): 947–953.

18. H. M. Greenwald and M. Steiner, "Diaphragmatic Hernia in Infancy and in Childhood," *American Journal of Diseases of Childhood* 38 (1929): 361–392.

19. P. E. Truesdale, "Recurrent Hernia Through the Diaphragm," *Annals of Surgery* 79, no. 5 (May 1924): 751–757.

20. P. E. Truesdale, "Diaphragmatic Hernia in Children with a Report of Thirteen Operative Cases," *New England Journal of Medicine* 213, no. 24 (December 12, 1935): 1159–1172.

21. "Inverted Stomachs Declared Not Rare," *New York Times*, February 22, 1935.

22. "Operate to Right Stomach of Boy," *New York Times*, April 7, 1935.

23. H. Johnson and A. G. Bower, "Strangulated Diaphragmatic Hernia in an Infant," *California and Western Medicine* 36 (1932): 48–49.

24. K. A. Meyer, S. J. Hoffman, and J. K. Amtman, "Diaphragmatic Hernia in the Newborn, Review of the Literature and Report of a Case," *American Journal of Diseases of Children* 56 (1938): 600–607; E. M. Miller, A. H. Parmalee, and H.

N. Sanford, "Diaphragmatic Hernia in Infants, Report of Two Cases, *Archives of Surgery* 38, no. 6 (June 1939): 979–989.

25. W. E. Ladd and R. E. Gross, *Abdominal Surgery of Infancy and Childhood* (Philadelphia, London: W. B. Saunders, 1941), 333–348.

26. J. J. McNamara, A. J. Eraklis, and R. E. Gross, "Congenital Postero-Lateral Diaphragmatic Hernia in the Newborn," *Journal of Thoracic and Cardiobascular Surgery* 55 (1968): 55.

27. C. J. Cerilli, "Foramen of Bochdalek Hernia, a Review of the Experience at the Children's Hospital of Denver, Colorado," *Annals of Surgery* 159, no. 3 (March 1964): 385–389.

28. M. R. Harrison, R. Bjordal, and O. Knutrud, "Congenital Diaphragmatic Hernia: The Hidden Mortality," *Journal of Pediatric Surgery* 13 (1978): 337.

29. R. C. Raphaely and J. J. Downes, Jr., "Congenital Diaphragmatic Hernia: Prediction of Survival," *Journal of Pediatric Surgery* 8 (1973): 815.

30. A. W. Dibbin and E. S. Weiner, "Mortality from Neonatal Diaphragmatic Hernia," *Journal of Pediatric Surgery* 9 (1974): 653; W. M. Gersony et al., "The Hemodynamic Effects of IntrauterineHypoxia; an Experimental Model in Newborn Lambs," *Journal of Pediatrics* 89 (1976): 631; J. A. Haller et al., "Pulmonary and Ductal Hemodynamics in Studies of Simulated Diaphagmatic Hernia of Fetal and Newborn Lambs," *Journal of Pediatric Surgery* 11 (1976): 675.

31. D. S. Moodie et al., "Use of Tolazoline in Newborn Infants with Diaphragmatic Hernia and Severe Cardiopulmonary Disease," *Journal of Thoracic and Cardiovascular Surgery* 75 (1978): 725; R. J. Levy et al., "Persistent Pulmonary Hypertension in a Newborn with Congenital Diaphragmatic Hernia: Successful Management with Tolazoline," *Pediatrics* 60 (1977): 740.

32. J. German et al., "Management of Pulmonary Insufficiency in Diaphragmatic Hernia Using Extracorporeal Circulation with a Membrane Oxygenator [ECMO]," *Journal of Pediatric Surgery* 12 (1977): 905–912.

33. C. Stolar, P. Dillon, and C. Reyes, "Selective Use of ECMO in the Management of Congenital Diaphragmatic Hernia," *Journal of Pediatric Surgery* 23 (1988): 207; M. R. Langham et al., "ECMO Following Repair of Congenital Diaphragmatic Hernia," *Annals of Thoracic Surgery* 44 (1987): 247; B. J. Hardesty et al., "ECMO Successful Treatment of Persistent Fetal Circulation Following Repair of Diaphragmatic Hernia," *Journal of Thoracic and Cardiovascular Surgery* 81 (1981): 556.

34. M. V. Ravel et al., "Costs of Congenital Diaphragmatic Hernia Repair in the United States — Extracorporeal Membrane Oxygenation Foots the Bill," *Journal of Pediatric Surgery* 46 (2011): 617–624.

35. Y. S. Guner et al., "Outcome Analysis of Neonates with Congenital Diaphragmatic Hernia Treated with Venovenous vs. Venoarterial Extracorporeal Membrane Oxygenation," *Journal of Pediatric Surgery* 44 (2009): 1691–1701.

36. R. Carachik, D. G. Young, and C. Buyukunal, "History of Surgical Pediatrics," *World Scientific* (New Jersey, London, Singapore, 2009, citing Michael Harrison, M.D., chapter titled "Fetal Surgery"): 746–788

37. M. R. Harrison et al., "Correction of Congenital Diaphragmatic Hernia in Utero; Six Hard-earned Lessons," *Journal of Pediatric Surgery* 28 (1993): 1411–1417.

38. J. W. Difliore, D. O. Fauza, R. Slavin, C. A. Peters, J. C. Fackler, and J. M. Wilson, "Experimental Fetal Tracheal Ligation Reverses the Structural and Physiological Effects of Pulmonary Hypoplasia in Congenital Diaphragmatic Hernia, *Journal of Pediatric Surgery* 29 (1994): 248–257.

39. J. M. Laberge and H. Flageole, "Fetal Tracheal Occlusion for the Treatment of Congenital Diaphragmatic Hernia," *World Journal of Surgery* 31 (2007): 1577–1586.

40. C. S. Muratore and J. M. Wilson, "Congenital Diaphragmatic Hernia: Where Are We and Where Do We Go from Here?" *Seminars in Perinatology* 24, no. 6 (December 2000): 418–428.

41. H. Hedrick, "Management of Prenatally Diagnosed Congenital Diaphragmatic Hernia," *Seminars in Fetal and Neonatal Medicine* 15 (2010): 21–27.

42. D. M. Gourlay et al., "Beyond Feasibility: A Comparison of Newborns Undergoing Thoracoscopic and Open Repair of Congenital Diaphragmatic Hernias," *Journal of Pediatric Surgery* 44 (2009): 1702–1707.

43. W. J. Potts, *The Surgeon and the Child* (Philadelphia, London: W. B. Saunders, 1959), 66.

44. K. Al-Hathiol et al., "Perioperative Course of Pulmonary Hypertension with Congenital Diaphragmatic Hernia, Impact on Outcome," *Journal of Pediatric Surgery* 46 (2011): 625–629.

45. C. M. Burgos et al., "Gene Expression Analysis in Hypoplastic Lungs in the Nitrofen Model of Congenital Diaphragmatic Hernia," *Journal of Pediatric Surgery* 45 (2010): 1445–1454.

Chapter 32

1. G. Purnaropoules and K. Emmanuel, *Hippocrates: All His Works* (in Greek), vol. 1 (Athens: Martinos, 1967), 400–429.

2. W. G. Spencer, *Celsus' De Medicina*, vol. 1 (London: Heinemann, 1971), 364–369.

3. J. G. Lascaratos, I. G. Panourias, and D. E. Sakas, "Hydrocephalus According to Byzantine Writers," *Neurosurgery* 55 (2004): 214–221.

4. A. Vesalius, *De Humani Corporis Fabrica*, libri septem (Basel: 1555).

5. A. M. Brunori, R. Vagnozzi, and R. Giuffrè, "Antonio Pacchioni (1665–1726): Early Studies of the Dura Mater," *Journal of Neurosurgery* 78 (March 1993): 3.

6. B. Ljunggren and G. W. Bruyn (eds.), *The Nobel Prize in Medicine and the Karolinska Institute* (Basel: Karger, 2002).

7. W. E. Dandy, I. Blackfan, and D. Kenneth, "Internal Hydrocephalus, an Experimental, Clinical and Pathological Study," *American Journal of Diseases of Children* 8 (1914): 406.

8. E. J. O. Kompanje and E. J. Delwel, "The First Description of a Device for the Repeated External Ventricular Drainage in the Treatment of Congenital Hydrocephalus, Invented in 1744 by Claude-Nicolas Le Cat," *Pediatric Neurosurgery* 39 (2003): 10–13; C.-N. Le Cat, "A New Trocar for the Puncture in the Hydrocephalus and for Other Evacuations, Which Are Necessary to Be Made at Different Times," *Philosophical Transactions of the Royal Society of London* 157 (1751): 267–272.

9. J. A. Frederiks and P. J. Koehler, "The First Lumbar Puncture," *Journal of the History of Neuroscience* 6 (1997): 147–153.

10. W. W. Keen, "Tapping the Ventricles," *British Medical Journal*, no. 1574 (1891): 486; W. W. Keen, "Exploratory Trephining and Puncture of the Brain Almost to the Lateral Ventricle for Intracranial Pressure Supposed to be Due to an Abscess in the Temporo-Sphenoidal Lobe: Temporary Improvement, Death on the Fifth Day; Autopsy, Meningitis with Effusion into the Ventricles with a Description of a Proposed Operation to Tap and Drain the Ventricles as a Definite Surgical Procedure," *Medical News* 53 (1885): 603.

11. M. M. Ravitch, *A Century of Surgery, 1880–1980* (Philadelphia, Toronto: J. B. Lippincott, 1981), 131.

12. Ibid., 352 and 437.

13. J. Miculicz, "Beitrag zur Pathologie und Therapie des Hydrocephalus mit Grenzgeb," *Med Chir* 1 (1896): 264.

14. G. A. Sutherland and W. W. Cheyne "The Treatment of Hydrocephalus by Intra Cranial Drainage," *British Medical Journal* 2 (1898): 1155–1157.

15. R. H. Pudenz, "The Surgical Treatment of Hydrocephalus: An Historical Review," *Surgical Neurology* 15c (1981): 15–26.

16. E. Payr, "Drainage der Hirnventrikal Mittels Frei Transplantierter Blotgefabe Bremerkungen über Hydrocephalus," *Archiv der Klinische Chirurgie* 87 (1908): 801.

17. W. Kausch, "Die Behandlung des Hydrocephalus der Kleinen Kinder, *Archiv der Klinische Chirurgie* 87 (1908): 709–796.

18. C. Pendelton et al., "Harvey Cushing's Use of a Transplanted Human Vein to Treat Hydrocephalus in the Early 1900s," *Journal of Neurosurgery: Pediatrics* 5, no. 5 (2010): 423–427.

19. Ibid.; H. Cushing, "Surgery of the Head," in *Surgery, Its Principles and Practice*, third edition, ed. W. W Keen (Philadelphia: W. B. Saunders, 1908), 123–124.

20. W. E. Dandy, "The Diagnosis and Treatment of Hydrocephalus Due to Occlusions of the Foramina of Magendi and Lushka," *Surgery, Gynecology and Obstetrics* 32 (1921): 112.

21. W. E. Dandy, "Extirpation of the Chorid Plexus of the Lateral Ventricles in Communicating Hydrocephalus," *Annals of Surgery* 37 (1918): 569.

22. D. W. Matson, *Neurosurgery of Infancy and Childhood*, second edition (Springfield, IL: Charles C. Thomas, 1969), 224–258.

23. Ibid., 224.

24. A. Torkildsen, "A New Palliative Operation in Cases of Inoperable Occlusion of the Sylvian Aqueduct," *Acta Chirurgie Scandinavia* 82 (1939):117–124.

25. Matson, op. cit., 232–233.

26. B. Heile, "Uber Neue Operative Wege zur Druckentlastung bei Angeborenene Hydrocephalus (Uretero-Duraanastomosis)," *Zentrablblatt für Chirurgie* 52 (1925): 2229–2236; Matson, op. cit., 256.

27. Ibid., 247–250.

28. E. Ring-Mrozik and T. A. Angerpointer, "Historic Aspects of Hydrocephalus," *Progress in Pediatric Surgery* 20 (1986): 158–251.

29. G. R. Harsh III, "Peritoneal Shunt for Hydrocephalus, Utilizing the Fimbria of the Fallopian Tube for Entrance to the Peritoneal Cavity," *Journal of Neurosurgery* 11: 284–294.

30. F. E. Nulsen and E. B. Spitz, "Treatment of Hydrocephalus by Direct Shunt from Ventricle to Jugular Vein," *Surgery Forum*, no. 94 (1951): 399–403.

31. J. A. Bookvar, W. Loudon, and L. Sutton, "Development of the Spitz-Holter Valve in Philadelphia," *Journal of Neurosurgery* 95 (2001): 145–147.

32. R. H. Pudenz, "Experimental and Clinical Observations on the Shunting of Cerebrospinal Fluid into the Circulating System," in *Clinical Neurosurgery, Congress of Neurological Surgeons* (Baltimore, MD: Williams and Wilkins, 1958), 98–115.

33. A. J. Raimondi and W. Matsumoto, "A Simplified Technique for Performing the Ventriculo-Peritoneal Shunt: Technical Note," *Journal of Neurosurgery* 26 (1967): 357.

34. A. Reinprecht et al., "Medos Hakim Programmable Valve in the Treatment of Hydrocephalus," *Child's Nervous System* (1997); P. M. Black, R. Hakim, and N. O. Baily, "The Use of the Codman-Medos Hakim Programmable Valve in the Management of Patients with Hydrocephalus: Illustrative Cases," *Neurosurgery* 34 (1994): 1110–1113.

35. M. L. Walker, J. MacDonald, and L. C. Wright, "History of Ventriculoscopy: Where Do We Go from Here?" *Pediatric Neurosurgery* 18 (1992): 218–223.

36. W. E. Dandy, "The Operative Treatment of Communicating Hydrocephalus," *Annals of Surgery* 108 (1938): 194–202.

37. W. E. Dandy, "Diagnosis and Treatment of Strictures of the Aqueduct of Sylvius Causing Hydrocephalus," *Archives of Surgery* 51 (1945): 1–14.

38. J. E. Scarff, "Endoscopic Treatment of Hydrocephalus: Description of Aventriculoscope and Preliminary Report of Cases," *Archives of Neurology and Psychiatry* 35 (1935): 853–861.

39. M. P. Sayers and E. J. Kosnik, "Percutaneous Third

Ventriculostomy: Experience and Technique," *Child's Brain* 2 (1976): 24–30.

40. J. K. Vries, "An Endoscopic Technique for Third Ventriculostomy," *Surgical Neurology* 9 (1978): 165–168.

41. W. H. Bunch et al., *Modern Management of Myelomeningocele* (St. Louis: Warren H. Green, 1972).

42. J. T. Goodrich, "A Historical Review of the Surgical Treatment," in M. M. Ozek, G. Spinalli, and W. J. Maixner (eds.), *The Spina Bifida Management and Outcome* (Italy: Springer-Verlag, 2008).

43. J. B. Gool and J. D. Gool, *A Short History of Spina Bifida* (Manchester, England: Society for Research into Hydrocephalus and Spina Bifida, 1986); D. G. McLone, "Myelomeningocele," in *Youman's Jr. Edition of Neurological Surgery*, vol. 2, fourth edition (Philadelphia: W. B. Saunders, 1996), 843–860.

44. P. van Forest, "De Capitis et Cerebri Morbis ac Symptomatic," *Observationum Medicininalium*, book 3 (Leiden: Ex Officio Plantiniana Raphelemgii, 1587).

45. N. Tulp, *Observationum Medicarum*, book 3 (Amsterdam: Apud Ludovicum Elzevirum, 1641).

46. G. K. Smith, "The History of Spina Bifida, Hydrocephalus, Paraplegia, and Incontinence," *Pediatric Surgery International* 17 (2001): 424–432.

47. F. von Recklinghausen, "Untersuchungen über die Spina Bifida," *Virchows Archiv für Pathologische, Anatomie und Physiologie und für Klinische Medizin* 105 (1886): 243–330.

48. J. Morton, "Case of Spina Bifida Cured by Injection," *British Medical Journal* 1 (1872): 632–633.

49. J. Kinney, *Saga of a Surgeon: The Life of Daniel Brainard, M.D.* (Carbondale: Southern Illinois University School of Medicine, 1981), 98.

50. D. Brainard, "An Essay on the Treatment of Spina Bifida [Hydrorachitis] by Injections of Iodine," *Chicago Medical Journal* 2 (September 1859): 517–538.

51. C. Bayer, "The Surgical Treatment of Spina Bifida," in *The Retrospect of Practical Medicine and Surgery*, vols. 1–123, 1840–July 1901 (New York: W.A. Townsend, 1890).

52. A. A. Cohen-Gadol et al., "Cushing's Experience with the Surgical Treatment of Spinal Dysraphism," *Journal of Neurosurgery (Pediatrics 4)* 102 (2005): 441–444.

53. J. E. Moore, "Spina Bifida, with a Report of Three Hundred and Eighty-Five Cases Treated by Excision," *Surgery, Gynecology and Obstetrics* 1 (1905): 137–140.

54. J. H. Nicoll, "The Radical Cure of Spina Bifida, Observations of Certain Points in a Series of over Thirty Cases Treated by Open Operation," *British Medical Journal*, October 15, 1898, 1142–1146.

55. J. H. Nicoll, "Case of Hydrocephalus in Which Peritoneo-Menigeal Drainage Has Been Carried Out," *Glasgow Medical Journal* 63 (January–June 1905): 187–191.

56. F. D. Ingraham, *Spina Bifida and Cranium Bifidum* (Cambridge, MA: Harvard University Press, 1944).

57. P. Soare and A. J. Raimondi, "Intellectual and Perceptual Motor Characteristics of Treated Myelomeningocele Children," *American Journal of Diseases of Children* 131 (1977): 199–204.

58. D. G. McLone, D. Czyzeqski, and A. J. Raimondi, "The Effects of Complications on Intellectual Function in 173 Children with Myelomeningocele," in *Surgery of the Developing Nervous System* (New York: Grune and Stratton, 1982), 49–60.

59. J. Lorber, "Results of Treatment of Myelomeningocele: An Analysis of 524 Unselected Cases with Special References to Possible Selection for Treatment," *Developmental Medicine and Child Neurology* 13 (1971): 279.

60. D. G. McLone, "Treatment of Myelomeningocele and Arguments Against Selection," *Clinical Neurosurgery* 33 (1986): 359.

61. D. G. McClone and T. P. Naiditch, in H. J. Hoffman and F. Epstein (eds.), *Disorders of the Developing Nervous System, Diagnosis and Treatment* (Boston: Blackwell Scientific, 1986), 94–105.

62. T. P. Bruner, N. E. Tulipan, and W. O. Richards, "Endoscopic Coverage of Fetal Open Myelomeningocele *in Utero*," *American Journal of Obstetrics and Gynecology* 176, part 1 (June 1997): 256–257; N. Tulipan and J. P. Bruner, "Myelomeningocele Repair *in Utero*: A Report of Three Cases," *Pediatric Neurosurgery* 28 (1998): 177–180.

63. S. N. Adzick et al., "Successful Fetal Surgery for Spina Bifida," *Lancet* 352 (1998): 1675–1676; S. N. Adzick, "A Randomized Trial of Prenatal vs. Post-Natal Repair of Myelomeningocele," *New England Journal of Medicine* 364 (March 17, 2011): 993–1004.

Chapter 33

1. I. M. Rutkow, "Beaumont and St. Martin: A Blast from the Past," *Archives of Surgery* 133, no. 11 (November 1960): 1259.

2. W. Beaumont, *Experiments and Observations on the Gastric Juice and the Physiology of Digestion* (Edinburgh: Maclachlan and Stewart, 1838).

3. M. M. Ravitch, *A Century of Surgery, 1880–1980* (Philadelphia, Toronto: J. B. Lippincott, 1981), 45–46.

4. Ibid., 35.

5. Ibid., 80–81.

6. Nicholas Senn, M.D., Ph.D., *Experimental Surgery* (Chicago: W. T. Keener, 1889), 478–503.

7. Ravitch, op. cit., 103.

8. L. Schooler, "The Wounded from Santiago," pp. 99–106, in Jacob K. Berman (ed.), *The Western Surgical Association, 1891–1900* (Indianapolis: Hackett, 1976).

9. Giovanni Battista Morgagni, *The Seats and Causes of Disease*, book 4, letter 54, trans. Benjamin Alexander (London: 1769).

10. Ravitch, op. cit., 659–662.

11. Ibid., 730–732.

12. W. E. Ladd and R. R. Gross, *Abdominal Surgery of Infancy and Childhood* (Philadelphia, London: W. B. Saunders, 1941), 254–255.

13. R. E. Gross, *The Surgery of Infancy and Childhood* (Philadelphia, London: W. B. Saunders, 1953), 539 and 562–564.

14. C. H. Kempe, N. Silverman, and B. F. Steele, "The Battered Child Syndrome," *Journal of the American Medical Association* 181 (1962): 17.

15. P. Garnall et al., "Abdominal Injuries in the Battered Baby Syndrome," *Archives of Disease in Childhood* 47 (1972): 211; R. J. Touloukian, "Abdominal Visceral Injuries in Battered Children," *Pediatrics* 42 (1968): 642.

16. J. Haller, Jr., "Newer Concepts in Emergency Care of Children with Major Injuries," *Pediatrics* 52 (1973): 485; J. Haller, Jr. et al., "Use of a Trauma Registry in the Management of Children with Life-Threatening Injuries," *Journal of Pediatric Surgery* 11 (1976): 381.

17. D. E. Wesson, *Pediatric Trauma, Pathophysiology, Diagnosis and Treatment* (New York: Taylor and Francis, 2006), 34.

18. L. O. Persky and W. E. Forsythe, "Renal Trauma in Children," *Journal of the American Medical Association* 182 (November 17, 1962): 708–712; J. W. Chamberlain, "Minor Trauma with Major Injury," *Journal of Pediatric Surgery* 2 (October 1967): 455–457.

19. R. J. Touloukian, "Abdominal Trauma in Children," *Surgery, Gynecology and Obstetrics* 127 (September 1968): 561.

20. H. Levy, Jr. and L. H. Linder, "Major Abdominal Trauma in Children," *American Journal of Surgery* 122 (1970): 55.

21. H. King and H. B. Schumacker, "Splenic Studies: Increased Susceptibility to Infection After Splenectomy Performed in Infancy," *Annals of Surgery* 136 (1952): 239.

22. J. B. Belfauz et al., "Overwhelming Sepsis Following

Splenectomy for Trauma," *Journal of Pediatrics* 88 (1976): 458.

23. S. H. Ein et al., "Non-Operative Management of Traumatized Spleen in Children: How and Why," *Journal of Pediatric Surgery* 13 (1978): 117.

24. M. P. Karp et al., "The Role of Computerized Tomography in the Evaluation of Blunt Abdominal Trauma in Children," *Journal of Pediatric Surgery* 16 (1981): 316; R. Jeffrey, M. Federle, and R. Crass, "Computed Tomography of Pancreatic Trauma," *Radiology* 147 (1983): 491.

25. W. H. Hendren et al., "Traumatic Hemobilia: Non-Operative Management with Healing Documented by Angiography," *Annals of Surgery* 17 (1971): 991.

26. R. J. Touloukian, "Protocol for the Non-operative Treatment of Duodenal Hematoma in Children," *American Journal of Surgery* 145 (1983): 330.

27. D. J. Brenner, "Estimating Cancer Risks from Pediatric CT: Going from the Qualitative to the Quantitative," *Pediatric Radiology* 32 (2002): 228–233.

28. S. J. Fenton et al., "CT Scan and the Pediatric Trauma Patient — Are We Overdoing It," *Journal of Pediatric Surgery* 39 (2004): 1877–1881.

29. E. R. Scaife et al., "Use of Abdominal Sonography for Trauma at Pediatric and Adult Trauma Centers: A Survey," *Journal of Pediatric Surgery* 44 (2009): 1746–1749.

30. Wesson, op. cit., 5.

Chapter 34

1. L. M. Zimmerman and I. Veith, *Great Ideas in the History of Surgery* (New York: Dover, 1967.

2. Ibid; K. Haeger, *The Illustrated History of Surgery* (New York: Bell, 1988), 49.

3. Haeger, op. cit.

4. W. G. Spencer (ed.), *Celsus De Medicina* (Cambridge, MA: Harvard University Press, 1971).

5. Zimmerman and Veith, op. cit.

6. Ibid.

7. Ibid.

8. L. DeMause, Foundations of Psychohistory, 55, Institute for Psychohistory, New York.

9. W. B. Hamby, *The Case Reports and Autopsy Records of Ambroise Paré* (Springfield, IL: Charles C. Thomas, 1960), 21.

10. Simmerman and Veith, op. cit.

11. M. M. Melicow, "Castrati Singers and the Lost 'Cords,'" *Bulletin of the New York Academy of Medicine* 59 (1983): 744–764; J. M. Glass and N. A. Watkinn, "From NA. From Mutilation to Medication: The History of Orchidectomy," *British Journal of Urology* 80 (1997): 373 — 378; J. S. Jenkins, "The Voice of the Castrato," *Lancet* 351 (1998): 1877 —1880.

12. Zimmerman and Veith, op. cit.

13. Ibid.

14. E. Bassini, "Ueber die Behandlung des Leistenbruches," *Archiv für Klinische Chirurgie* 40 (1890): 429 — 476.

15. W. T. Bull and W. B. Coley, "Obervations upon the Operative Treatment of Hernia at the Hospital for Ruptured and Crippled," *Annals of Surgery* 28 (1898): 577–604.

16. Ibid.

17. A. H. Ferguson, "Oblique Inguinal Hernia-Typic Operation for Its Radical Cure," *Journal of the American Medical Association* 33 (1899): 6 —14.

18. P. Turner, "The Radical Cure of Inguinal Hernia in Children," *Proceedings of the Royal Society of Medicine* 5 (1912): 133–140; A. MacLennan, "The Radical Cure of Inguinal Hernia in Children, with Special Reference to the Embryonic Rests Found Associated with the Sacs," *British Journal of Surgery* 9 (1922): 445–448; R. H. Russell, "Inguinal Hernia and Operative Procedure," *Surgery, Gynecology and Obstetrics* 41 (1925): 605–609.

19. Turner, op. cit.

20. MacLennan, op. cit.

21. Ibid.

22. Russell, op. cit.

23. G. Herzfeld, "The Radical Cure of Hernia in Infants and Young Children," *Edinborough Medical Journal* 32 (1925): 281–290.

24. W. E. Ladd and R. E. Gross, *Abdominal Surgery of Infancy and Childhood* (Philadelphia: W. B. Saunders, 1941), 354–366.

25. W. J. Potts, W. L. Riker, and J. E. Lewis, "The Treatment of Inguinal Hernia in Infants and Children," *Annals of Surgery* 132 (1950): 566–574.

26. J. W. Duckett, "Treatment of Congenital Inguinal Hernia," *Annals of Surgery* 135 (1952): 879–884.

27. R. E. Rothenberg and T. Barnett, "Bilateral Herniotomy in Infants and Children," *Surgery* 37 (1955): 947–950.

28. M. I. Rowe and H. W. Clatworthy, *Surgical Clinics of North American* 51 (1971): 1371–1376.

29. E. S. Weiner, R. J. Touloukian, B. M. Rodgers, J. L. Grosfeld, E. L. Smith, M. M. Ziegler, A. G. Coran, "Hernia Survey of the Section of Surgery of the American Academy of Pediatrics, *Journal of Pediatric Surgery* 31 (1996): 1166–1169.

30. G. W. Holcomb III, J. W. Brock III, and W. M. Morgan III, "Laparoscopic Evaluation for a Contralateral Patent Processus Vaginalis," *Journal of Pediatric Surgery* 29 (1994): 970–977; G. W. Holcomb III, W. M Morgan III, and J. W. Brock III, "Laparoscopic Evaluation for Contralateral Processus Vaginalis: Part II," *Journal of Pediatric Surgery* 31 (1996): 1170–1173.

31. P. Montupet and C. Esposito, "Laparoscopic Treatment of Congenital Inguinal Hernia in Children, *Journal of Pediatric Surgery* 34 (1999): 420–423.

32. F. Schier, "Laparoscopic Surgery of Inguinal Hernias in Children: Initial Experience," *Journal of Pediatric Surgery* 35 (2000): 1331–1335.

33. F. Schier, P. Montupet, and C. Esposito, "Laparoscopic Inguinal Herniorraphy in Children; a Three-Center Experience with 933 Repairs, *Journal of Pediatric Surgery* 37 (2002): 395–397.

Chapter 35

1. C. H. Evans, "Atresias of the Gastrointestinal Tract," *Surgery, Gynecology and Obstetrics* 92 (1951): 1–8.

2. W. E. Ladd and R. E. Gross, *Abdominal Surgery of Infancy and Childhood* (Philadelphia: W. B. Saunders, 1941), 25–43.

3. J. N. Binninger, "Observationum et Curationum Medianalium, Centuriae Quinque," observ. 81, p. 22 (Montbelgardi: Hyppianis, 1673).

4. C. Horch, "C. De Puella cum Coalitu Intestini Ilei Nata, et per Viginti Duos dies Viventi," *Misc. Acad. Nat. Curios,* Francof 1694–1696, decuriae 3:1–4 and 188–189.

5. N. I. Spriggs, "Congenital Intestinal Occlusions: An Account of 24 Unpublished Cases with Remarks Based Thereon and Upon the Literature of the Subject, *Guy's Hospital Reports* 66 (1912): 143–218.

6. Voison, *Journ. Ger de Med et de Chir de la Soc de Med de Paris* 21 (1804): 353.

7. A. Jacobi, "Defective Development of the Intestine," *Am M Month NY* 16 (1861): 30–32.

8. S. Farber, "Congenital Atresia of the Alimentary Tract: Diagnosis by Microscopic Examination of Meconium," *Journal of the American Medical Association* 100 (1933): 1753–1754.

9. Ladd and Gross, op. cit.; R. E. Gross, "Congenital Atresia of the Intestine and Colon," in *The Surgery of Infancy and Childhood* (Philadelphia: W. B. Saunders, 1953), 150–166.

10. Binninger, op. cit.: J. Calder, "Two Examples of Chil-

dren Born with Preternatural Conformations of the Gut," *Med Essays and Obs. Soc, Edinb* 1 (1733): 203–206.

11. J. F. Meckel, *Handbuch der Pathologischen Anatomie*, vol. 6, 21–22, 179–180, and 493–507.

12. A. Schaefer, "Cas de Scission du Canal Intestinal en Plusieurs Portions, par Vice Primitif de Conformation," *J Compl du Dict d Sc Méd Paris* 24 (1926): 58–66.

13. E. Theremin, "Ueber Congenitale Occlusion des Dünndarms," *Deutsche Zeitschrift für Chirurgie* 8 (1877): 34–71.

14. J. Bland-Sutton, "Imperforate Ileum," *American Journal of Medical Science* 98 (1889): 457–462.

15. Spriggs, op. cit.

16. J. J. Weitzman and R. S. Vanderhoof, "Jejunal Atresia with Agenesis of the Dorsal Mesentery with "Christmas Tree" Deformity of the Small Intestine," *American Journal of Surgery* 111 (1966): 443–449.

17. L. W. Martin and J. T. Zerella, "Jejunoileal Atresia: A Proposed Classification," *Journal of Pediatric Surgery* 11 (1976): 399–403.

18. J. L. Grosfeld, V. N. Ballantine, and R. Shoemaker, "Operative Management of Intestinal Atresia and Stenosis Based on Pathologic Findings," *Journal of Pediatric Surgery* 14 (1979): 368–375.

19. Meckel, op. cit.

20. Bland-Sutton, op. cit.

21. J. Tandler, "Entwicklungsgeschichte des Menschlieben Duodenum in Früben Embryonal-studien," *Morphol Jahrb* 29 (1902): 187–216.

22. F. P. Johnson, "The Development of the Mucous Membrane of the Oesophagus, Stomach and Small Intestine in the Human Embryo," *American Journal of Anatomy* 10 (1910): 521–561.

23. Spriggs, op. cit.

24. C. H. Webb and O. H. Vangensteen, "Congenital Intestinal Atresia," *American Journal of the Diseases of Children* 41 (1931): 262–284.

25. J. H. Louw and C. N. Barnard, "Congenital Intestinal Atresia: Observations on Its Origin," *Lancet* 2 (1955): 1065–1067.

26. H. Laufman, W. B. Martin, H. Method, S. W. Tuell, and H. Harding, "Observations in Strangulation Obstruction: The Fate of Sterile Devascularized Intestine in the Peritoneal cavity," *Archives of Surgery* 59 (1949): 550–564.

27. J. S. Abrams, "Experimental Intestinal Atresia," *Surgery* 64 (1968): 185–191; Y. Koga, Y. Hayashida, K. Ikeda, K. Inokuchi, and N. Hashimoto, "Intestinal Atresia in Fetal Dogs Produced by Localized Ligation of Mesenteric Vessels," *Journal of Pediatric Surgery* 10 (1975): 949–953; R. J. Earlam, "A Study of the Aetiology of Congenital Stenosis of the Gut," *Annals of the Royal College of Surgeons, England* 51 (1972): 126–130; J. A. Tovar, M. Suñol, B. Lopez de Torre, C. Camarero, and J. Torrado, "Mucosal Morphology in Experimental Intestinal Atresia: Studies in the Chick Embryo," *Journal of Pediatric Surgery* 26 (1991): 184–189.

28. H. Braun, "Ueber den Angeberenen Verschluss des Dünndarms und Seine Operative Behandlung," *Beitz. Z Klin Zhir* 34 (1902): 993–1023.

29. Spriggs, op. cit.

30. H. S. Clogg, Congenital Intestinal Atresia," *Lancet* 2 (1904): 1770–1774.

31. P. Fockens, "Arts over Angeboren Atresia van den darm Met een Door Operate Genezem Geval," *Netherlands Tijdschrift vor Geneeskunde*, 1911, 1658–1655.

32. D. L. Davis and C. W. M. Poynter, "Congenital Occlusions of the Intestines," *Surgery, Gynecology and Obstetrics* 34 (1922): 35–41.

33. Webb and Vangensteen, op. cit.

34. J. D. Martin, Jr., and D. C. Elkin, "Congenital Atresia of the Colon," *Annals of Surgery* 105 (1937): 192–198.

35. J. H. Louw and C. N. Barnard, "Congenital Intestinal

Atresia: Observations on Its Origin," *Lancet* 2 (1955): 1065–1067.

36. J. H. Louw, "Congenital Intestinal Atresia and Stenosis in the Newborn," *S Afr J Clin Sci* 3 (1952): 109–129.

37. H. H. Nixon, "An Experimental Study of Propulsion in Isolated Small Intestine and Applications to Surgery in the Newborn," *Annals of the Royal College of Surgeons, England* 24 (1960): 105–124.

38. H. H. Nixon, "Intestinal Obstruction in the Newborn," *Archives of Disease in Childhood* 30 (1955): 13–22.

39. C. D. Benson, "Resection and Primary Anastomosis of the Jejunum and Ileum in the Newborn," *Annals of Surgery* 142 (1955): 478–485.

40. H. H. Nixon and R. Tawes, "Etiology and Treatment of Small Intestinal Atresia: Analysis of a Series of 127 Jejunoileal Atresias and Comparison with 62 Duodenal Atresias, *Surgery* 69 (1971): 41–51.

41. T. V. Santulli and W. A. Blanc, "Congenital Atresia of the Intestine: Pathogenesis and Treatment," *Annals of Surgery* 154 (1961): 939–948.

42. Nixon and Tawes, op. cit.

43. C. G. Thomas, Jr., "Jejunoplasty for the Correction of Jejuna Atresia, *Surgery, Gynecology and Obstetrics* 129 (1966): 545–546.

44. R. W. Powell, "Stapled Intestinal Anastomosis in Neonates and Infants: Use of the Endoscopic Intestinal Stapler, *Journal of Pediatric Surgery* 30 (1995): 195–197.

45. P. Aguayo and D. J. Ostlie, "Duodenal and Intestinal Atresia and Stenosis," in G. W. Holcomb III and J. P. Murphy, eds., *Ashcraft's Pediatric Surgery* (Philadelphia: Saunders-Elsevier, 2010), 400–415.

Chapter 36

1. G. Manson, "Anomalies of Intestinal Rotation and Mesenteric Fixation: Review of the Literature with Report of Nine Cases, *Journal of Pediatrics* 45 (1954): 214–233.

2. J. Reid, "Anatomical Observations," *Edinburgh Medical and Surgical Journal* 46 (1836): 70.

3. J. Y. Simpson, "On Foetal Peritonitis," *Edinburgh Medical and Surgical Journal* 52 (1839): 26.

4. F. P. Mall, "Development of the Human Intestine and Its Position in the Adult, *Bulletin of the Johns Hopkins Hospital* 9 (1898): 197–208.

5. J. E. Frazer and R. H. Robbins, "On the Factors Concerned in Causing Rotation of the Intestine in Man," *Journal of Anatomical Physiology* 50 (1915): 75–110.

6. N. M. Dott, "Anomalies of Intestinal Rotation: Their Embryology and Surgical Aspects with Report of 5 Cases," *British Journal of Surgery* 11 (1923): 251–286.

7. E. Rixford, "Failure of Primary Rotation of the Intestine (Left-Sided Colon) in Relation to Intestinal Obstruction," *Annals of Surgery* 72 (1920): 114–120.

8. N. M. Dott, "Volvulus Neonatorum," *British Medical Journal* 1 (1927): 230–231.

9. C. E. Gardner, Jr., "The Surgical Significance of Anomalies of Intestinal Rotation," *Annals of Surgery* 131 (1950): 879–896.

10. W. H. Snyder, Jr. and L. Chaffin, "Embryology and Pathology of the Intestinal Tract: Presentation of 40 Cases of Malrotation," *Annals of Surgery* 140 (1954): 368–379.

11. W. E. Ladd, "Surgical Diseases of the Alimentary Tract in Infants," *New England Journal of Medicine* 215 (1936): 705–708.

12. E. C. Brenner, "Total Volvulus," *American Journal of Surgery* 16 (1932): 34–44.

13. W. E. Ladd, "Congenital Obstruction of the Duodenum in Children," *New England Journal of Medicine* 206 (1933): 277–283.

14. G. E. Waugh, "Congenital Malformations of the Mesentery: A Clinical Entity," *British Journal of Surgery* 15 (1928): 438–449.

15. C. E. Gardner, Jr. and D. Hart, "Anomalies of Intestinal Rotation as a Cause of Intestinal Obstruction," *Archives of Surgery* 29 (1934): 942–981.

16. J. F. Meckel, "Blindengageschichte des Darmkanals der Sängeriere und Namentlich der Menschen," *Deutsche Archive I Physiol* 3 (1817): 1.

17. E. G. Wakefield and C. W. Mayo, "Intestinal Obstruction Produced by Mesenteric Bands in Association with Failure of Intestinal Rotation," *Archives of Surgery* 33 (1936): 47–67.

18. R. McIntosh and E. J. Donovan, "Disturbances of Rotation of the Intestinal Tract: Clinical Picture Based on Observations in 20 Cases," *American Journal of Disease in Childhood* 57:116–166, 1939.

19. W. E. Ladd, "Surgical Diseases of the Alimentary Tract in Infants," *New England Journal of Medicine* 215 (1936): 705–708.

20. W. E. Ladd and R. E. Gross, "Intestinal Obstruction Resulting from Malrotation of the Intestines and Colon," in W. E. Ladd and R. E. Gross, *Abdominal Surgery in Infancy and Childhood* (Philadelphia: W. B. Saunders, 1941), 53–70.

21. O. H. Wangensteen, "New Operative Techniques in the Management of Bowel Obstruction: (1) Aseptic Decompressive Suction Enterostomy (2) Aseptic Enterostomy for Removal of Obstructing Gallstone (3) Operative Correction of Non-rotation," *Surgery, Gynecology and Obstetrics* 75 (1942): 675–692.

22. W. B. Kiesewetter and J. W. Smith, "Malrotation of the Midgut in Infancy and Childhood," *Archives of Surgery* 77 (1958): 483–491.

23. R. J. Andrassy and G. H. Mahour, "Malrotation of the Midgut in Infants and Children," *Archives of Surgery* 116 (1981): 158–160.

24. H. C. Filston and D. R. Kirks, "Malrotation–the Ubiquitous Anomaly," *Journal of Pediatric Surgery* 16 (1981): 614–620.

25. C. G. Howell, F. Vozza , S. Shaw et al., "Malrotation, Malnutrition and Ischemic Bowel Disease," *Journal of Pediatric Surgery* 17 (1982): 469–473.

26. H. V. Firor and E. Steiger, "Morbidity of Rotational Abnormalities of the Gut Beyond Infancy," *Cleveland Clinic Quarterly* 50 (1983): 303–309.

27. D. M. Powell, H. B. Othersen, and C. D. Smith, "Malrotation of the Intestines in Children: The Effect of Age on Presentation and Therapy," *Journal of Pediatric Surgery* 24 (1989): 777–780.

28. A. M. Torres and M. M. Ziegler, "Malrotation of the Intestine," *World Journal of Surgery* 17 (1993): 326–331.

29. A. J. Simpson, J. C. Leonidas, I. H. Krasna, J. M. Becker, and K. M. Schneider, "Roentgen Diagnosis of Midgut Malrotation: Value of the Upper Gastrointestinal Radiographic Study," *Journal of Pediatric Surgery* 7 (1972): 243–252; E. L. Rubin and M. D. Liverp, "Radiological Aspects of Anomalies of Intestinal Rotation," *Lancet* 2 (1935): 1222–1226; W. L. Schey, J. S. Donaldson, and J. R. Sty, "Malrotation of Bowel: Variable Patterns with Different Surgical Considerations," *Journal of Pediatric Surgery* 28 (1993): 96–101.

30. J. P. Pracros, L. Sann, F. Genin et al., "Ultrasound Diagnosis of Midgut Volvulus: The 'Whirlpool' Sign," *Pediatric Radiology* 22 (1992):18–20.

31. A. H. Bill, Jr. and D. Grauman, "Rationale and Technic for Stabilization of the Mesentery in Cases of Non-Rotation of the Midgut," *Journal of Pediatric Surgery* 1 (1966): 127–

136; W. S. Brennom and A. H. Bill, "Prophylactic Fixation of the Intestine for Midgut Non-Rotation," *Surgery, Gynecology and Obstetrics* 138 (1974): 181–184.

32. U. G. Stauffer and P. Herrmann, "Comparison of Late Results in Patients with Corrected Intestinal Malrotation with and Without Fixation of the Mesentery," *Journal of Pediatric Surgery* 15 (1980): 9–12.

33. Firor and Steiger, op. cit.

34. M. V. Mazziotti, S. M. Strasberg, and J. C. Langer, "Intestinal Rotation Abnormalities Without Volvulus: The Role of Laparoscopy," *Journal of the American College of Surgeons* 185 (1997): 172–176; K. D. Bass, S. S. Rothenberg, and J. H. T. Chang, "Laparoscopic Ladd's Procedure in Infants with Malrotation," *Journal of Pediatric Surgery* 33 (1998): 279–281; N. M. A. Bax and D. C. van der Zee, "Laparoscopic Treatment of Intestinal Malrotation in Children," *Surg Endosc* 12 (1998): 1314–1316.

35. D. C. van der Zee and N. M. A. Bax, "Laparoscopic Repair of Acute Volvulus in a Neonate with Malrotation," *Surg Endosc* 9 (1995): 1123–1124.

Chapter 37

1. J. F. Meckel, "Anatomic and Physiological Observations, Concerning Extraordinary Dilation of the Heart, Which Came from the Fact That the Aortic Conduit Was Too Narrow," *Memoirs of the Royal Academy of Sciences,* Berlin, 1768.

2. G. B. Morgagni, *De Sedibus et Causis Morborum per Anatomen Indagatis Libri Quinque,* trans. B. Alexander (1766), book 3, letter 30, article 12.

3. M. Paris, "Retrécissement Considerable de l'Aorte Pectorale, Observé a l'Hôtel Dieu de Paris," *Journal de Chirurgie de Desalt* 2 (1791): 107.

4. A. A. Meckel, "Verschliessung der Aorta am Vierteu Brustwirbel," *Archiv für Anatomy und Physiology* (1827): 345.

5. A. Mercier, "Retrécissement avec oblitération presque complète de la portion thoracique de aorte," *Bulletins et Memoires de la Société Anatomique de Paris* 14 (1839): 153.

6. L. M. Bonnet, "Sur la lesion dite stenose congenitale de l'aorte dans la region de l'Isthme," *Rev. Med.* 23 (1903): 108.

7. M.E. Abbott, "Statistical Study and Historical Retrospect of 200 Recorded Cases, with Autopsy, of Stenosis or Obliteration of the Descending Arch," *Am. H. J.* 3 (1928): 92.

8. L.M. Blackford, "Coarctation of the Aorta," *Archives of Internal Medicine* 4 (1928): 702.

9. A. Blalock and E.A. Parks, "The Surgical Treatment of Experimental Coarctation (Atresia) of the Aorta," *Annals of Surgery* 119 (1944): 445.

10. C. Crafoord and G. Nylin, "Congenital Coarctation of the Aorta and its Surgical Treatment," *Journal of Thoracic Surgery* 14 (1945): 347.

11. R.E. Gross and C.A. Hufnagel, "Coarctati on of the Aorta: Experimental Studies Regarding its Surgical Correction," *New England Journal of Medicine* 233 (1945): 287.

12. M.M. Calodney and M.J. Carson, "Coarctation of the Aorta in Early Infancy," *Journal of Pediatrics* 37 (1950): 46.

13. J.W. Kirklin et al., "Surgical Treatment of Coarctation of the Aorta in a Ten Week Old Infant: Report of a Case," *Circulation* 6 (1952): 411.

Bibliography

Abbe, R. "Sarcoma of the Kidney; Its Operative Treatment." *Annals of Surgery* Vol. 19 (1894): 58–69.

Abbott, M.E. "Statistical Study and Historical Retrospect of 200 Recorded Cases, with Autopsy, of Stenosis or Obliteration of the Descending Arch." *Am. H. J.* 3 (1928): 92.

Abrams, J.S. "Experimental Intestinal Atresia." *Surgery* 64 (1968): 185–191.

Abt, Isaac A., M.D., and Arthur F. Abt, M.D. *Abt-Garrison History of Pediatrics* (Philadelphia, London: W. B. Saunders, 1965), 35 [quoted from Plutarch's *Lives*, A.H. Clough, sub voce "Lycurgus"].

Adams, Francis. *The Genuine Works of Hippocrates Translated from the Greek*, Volume 1 (Printed for the Sydenham Society, 1849). Galen Internet Encyclopedia of Philosophy.

Adamson, W.A.D., and I. Aird. "Megacolon: Evidence in Favor of a Neurogenic Origin." *British Journal of Surgery* Vol. 20 (1932): 220–233.

Adson, A.W. "Hirschsprung's Disease, Indication for Treatment and Results Obtained by Sympathectomy." *Surgery* Vol. 22 (1947): 259–270.

Adzick, S.N. "A Randomized Trial of Prenatal vs. Post-Natal Repair of Myelomeningocele." *New England Journal of Medicine* Vol. 364 (March 17, 2011): 993–1004.

Adzick, S.N. et. al. "Successful Fetal Surgery for Spina Bifida." *Lancet* Vol. 352 (2011): 1675–1676.

Aguayo, P., and D.J. Ostlie. "Duodenal and Intestinal Atresia and Stenosis." In *Ashcraft's Pediatric Surgery*, edited by G.W. Holcomb III and J.P. Murphy, 400–415. Philadelphia: Saunders-Elsevier, 2010.

Ahlfeld, F. "Der Alkohol Als Desinficienz; (c) Der Alkohol Bei Der Behandlung Inoperabeler Bauchrüche." *Monatssohr Geburtsh Gynakologie* Vol. 10 (1899): 117–128. [Translated by Wolfgang Cerwinka, M.D.].

Albanese, C.T. Personal communication.

Al-Hathiol, K., et al. "Perioperative Course of Pulmonary Hypertension with Congenital Diaphragmatic Hernia, Impact on Outcome." *Journal of Pediatric Surgery* Vol. 46 (2011): 625–629.

Allen, R. "Presidential Address: The Evolution of Pediatric Surgery." *Journal of Pediatric Surgery* 15 (1980): 711.

Allen, R.C., and E.L. Wrenn. "Silon as a Sac in the Treatment of Omphalocele and Gastroschisis." *Journal of Pediatric Surgery* Vol. 4 (1969): 3–8.

Amussat, J-Z. "Troisième memoires sur la possibilité d'établire un overture artificiale sure le colon lombaire gauche sans ouvrire le peritoine, chez les enfants imperforate." *Lu a l'Academie Royale des Sciences* (4 Juillet 1842).

Anderson, K.D., and J.G. Randolph. "Gastric Tube Interposition: A Satisfactory Alternative to the Colon for Esophageal Replacement in Children." *Annals of Thoracic Surgery* Vol. 6 (1978): 521.

Andrassy, R.J., and G.H. Mahour. "Malrotation of the Midgut in Infants and Children." *Arch Surg* 116 (1981):158–160.

Andry, N. *Orthopedia: A Facsimile Reproduction of the First Edition in English, London 1743*. Philadelphia, Montreal: J.B. Lippincott, 1961.

_____. *Orthopaedia, or the Art of Preventing and Correcting Deformities in Children*. London, 1743.

"Andry, Nicholas." Wikipedia, http://en.wikipedia.org.

Anonymous. "Sushruta Samhita — the Compendium of Sushruta." *Lancet* 2 (1912): 1025–1026.

Aranda, J. V., N. Saheb, and I. Stern, "Arterial Oxygen Tension and Retinal Vasoconstriction in Newborn Infants." *American Journal of Diseases of Children* 122 (1971): 189.

Arnbjornsson, E., U. Breland, C.M. Kullendorff, Okmian L Mikaelsson. *Z Kinderchir* 41 (1986): 101–103.

Ashcraft, K.W., M.D., et. al. "The Thal Fundoplication for Gastroesophageal Reflux." *Journal of Pediatric Surgery* Vol. 19 (1984): 480–483.

Ashcraft, K.W., and T.M. Holder. "The Story of Oesophageal Atresia and Tracheo-Esophageal Fistula." *Surgery* 65 (1969): 332–340.

Aue, O. "Uber Angenborene Zwerchfellhernien." *Zentralblatt für Chirurgie* Vol. 160 (1920): 14–35.

Auenbrugger, L. *Inventum Novum ex Percussione Thoracis Humaniet Signo Abstruces Interni Pectoris Morbus Detendi, Vindobpmmae: Typis Joannis Thomae Trattner*, 1761 [from *Thoracic Surgery Before the Twentieth Century*, L.A. Hochberg, pp. 630–641. New York, Washington, Hollywood: Vantage, 1960],

Bagwell, C.E., M.D., "'Respectful Surgeon,' Revenge of the Barber Surgeon." *Annals of Surgery* 241, no. 6 (June 2005): 874.

Bahl, R., et al. "Population-Based Incidence of Intussusception and a Case-Control Study to Examine the Association of Intussusception with Natural Rotavirus Infection Among Indian Children." *Journal of Infectious Disease* 200 (2009): S277–281.

Barlow, B., and T. V. Santulli. "Importance of Multiple Episodes of Hypoxia or Cold Stress on the Development of Enterocolitis in an Animal Model." *Surgery* 77, no. 5 (1975): 787–690.

Barlow, B., et al. "An Experimental Study of Acute

Neonatal Enterocolitis: The Importance of Breast Milk." *Journal of Pediatric Surgery* 9, no. 5 (1974): 587–595.

Bass, K.D., S.S. Rothenberg and J.H.T. Chang. "Laparoscopic Ladd's Procedure in Infants with Malrotation." *Journal of Pediatric Surgery* 33 (1998): 279–281.

Bassini, E. "Ueber die Behandlung des Leistenbruches." *Archive für Klinische Chirurgie* 40 (1890): 429–476.

Battersby, J.S. "Esophageal Replacement by Use of the Right Colon, a One-Stage Thoraco–Abdominal Procedure." *Surgical Forum*, no. 4 (1953): 279–284.

Baumgartner, R., and W. Taillard, "Treatment of Congenital Club-foot at the Kinderspital Basel." *Annals of Paediatrics*, no. 200 (Basel, 1963).

N.M.A. Bax and D.C. van der Zee. "Feasibility of Thoracoscopic Repair of Esophageal Atresia with Distal Fistula." *Journal of Pediatric Surgery* 37 (2002): 192–196.

_____. "Laparoscopic Treatment of Intestinal Malrotation in Children." *Surg Endosc* 12 (1998): 1314–1316.

Bayer, C. "The Surgical Treatment of Spina Bifida." In *The Retrospect of Practical Medicine and Surgery*, vols. 1–123, 1840–July 1901. New York: W.A. Townsend, 1890.

Bayliss, W.M., and E.H. Starling. "The Movements and Innervation of the Large Intestine." *Journal of Physiology* 26 (1900): 107–118.

BBC History. "Andreas Vesalius 1514–1564." 2011.

Beasley, S.W., and P.G. Jones. "Use of Mercurochrome in the Management of the Large Exomphalos." *Australian Paediatric Journal* 22 (1986): 61–63.

Beaumont, W. *Experiments and Observations on the Gastric Juice and the Physiology of Digestion*. Edinburgh: Maclachlan and Stewart, 1838.

Beckman, F. "The Hernia Congenita, and an Account of the Controversy it Provoked Between William Hunter and Percival Pott." *Bulletin of the New York Academy of Medicine* 22 (1946): 486–500.

Bedard, P., D.P. Girvan and B. Shandling. "Congenital H-Type Tracheo-Esophageal Fistula." *Journal of Pediatric Surgery* 9 (1974): 666–668.

Belfauz, J.B., et. al. "Overwhelming Sepsis Following Splenectomy for Trauma." *Journal of Pediatrics* 88 (1976): 458.

Bell, Joseph, F.R.C.S. *A Manual of Operations of Surgery for the Use of Senior Students, House Surgeons and Junior Practitioners*, 5th ed. Edinburgh: Maclachan and Stewart, and London: Simpkin, Marshall & Co., 1883.

Bell, W.B. "A Brief Resumé of the Cases Treated in Mr. Joseph Bell's Ward in the Royal Hospital for Sick Children from November 9, 1894, to April 23, 1895." *Edinburgh Medical Journal* 41, Part 1 (September 1885): 234.

Belongia, E.A., et. al. "Real-Time Surveillance to Assess Risk of Intussusception and Other Adverse Events after Pentavalent, Bovine-derived Rotavirus Vaccine." *Pediatric Infectious Disease Journal* 29 (2010): 1–5.

Belyaev, O., C. Muller and W. Uhl. "Neosphincter Surgery for Fecal Incontinence: A Critical and Unbiased Review of the Relevant Literature." *Surgery Today* 36 (2006): 295–303.

Bensahel, H., et. al. "Results of Physical Therapy for Idiopathic Clubfoot: A Long-Term Follow-Up Study." *Journal of Pediatric Orthopedics* 10, no. 2 (1990): 189–192.

Benson, C.D. "Resection and Primary Anastomosis of the Jejunum and Ileum in the Newborn." *Ann Surg* 142 (1955) :478–485.

Bentley, J.F.R. "Primary Colonic Substitution for Atresia of the Esophagus." *Surgery* 58 (1965): 731–736.

Berman, E.J., and J.W. Kimble. "Barium Enema for Intussusception in Infants and Children." *Archives of Surgery* 92 (1966): 508–513.

"Bernard, Claude." Wikipedia, http://en.wikipedia.org.

Bernstein, P. "Gastroschisis: A Rare Teratological Condition in the Newborn." *Archives of Pediatrics* 57 (1940): 505–513.

Bessel-Hagen, Fritz. *Die Pathologic und Therapie des Klumpfusses*. Heidelberg, 1889.

Bevan, A.D. "Congenital Pyloric Stenosis." *American Journal of Diseases of Children* vol. 1, no. 2 (February 1911): 85–95.

Bhishagratna, K.L. *The Sushruta Samhita: An English Translation Based on Original Sanskrit Texts*, in three volumes. New Delhi: Cosmo, 2006.

Bick, E.M. *Source Book of Orthopedics*. Baltimore, MD: Williams and Wilkins, 1948.

Bickler, S.W., J. Kyambi and H. Rode. "Pediatric Surgery in Sub-Saharan Africa." *Pediatric Surgery International* 17 (2001): 442–447.

Bill, A.H. "William E. Ladd: Great Pioneer of North American Surgery." In *Historical Aspects of Pediatric Surgery, Progress in Pediatric Surgery* (Berlin, Heidelberg, New York and Tokyo: Springer-Verlag, 1986), 52–60.

Bill, A.H., Jr., and D. Grauman. "Rationale and Technic for Stabilization of the Mesentery in Cases of Non-Rotation of the Midgut." *Journal of Pediatric Surgery* 1 (1966): 127–136.

Binninger, J.N. "Observationum et curationum medianalium, centuriae quinque." *Observ.* 81: 22. Montbelgardi: Hyppianis, 1673.

Birch-Hirschfeld, F.V. "Sarkomatose Drusengeschwulste der Niere im Kindesalter [Embryonales Adenosarcom]." *Beitrage zur Pathologischen Anatomie und zur Allgemeinen Pathologie* 24 (1898): 343–362.

Bischoff, A., M.A. Levitt and A. Pena. "Bowel Management for the Treatment of Pediatric Fecal Incontinence." *Pediatric Surgery International* 25 (2009): 1027–1049.

Black, P.M., R. Hakim and N.O. Baily. "The Use of the Codman-Medos Hakim Programmable Valve in the Management of Patients with Hydrocephalus: Illustrative Cases." *Neurosurgery* 34 (1994): 1110–1113.

Blackford, L.M. "Coarctation of the Aorta." *Arch. Int. Med* 4 (1928): 702.

Blalock, A., and E.A. Parks. "The Surgical Treatment of Experimental Coarctation (Atresia) of the Aorta." *Ann. Surg.* 119 (1944): 445.

Blalock, H., and H.B. Taussig. "The Surgical Treatment of Malformations of the Heart in Which There Is Pulmonary Stenosis or Pulmonary Atresia." *Journal of the American Medical Association* 128 (1945): 189.

Bland-Sutton, J. "Imperforate Ileum." *Am J Med Sci* 98 (1889): 457–462.

Bochdalek, V.A. "Einige Betrachtungen uber die Entstchung des Angeborenen Zwerchfellbruches. Als Beitrag zur Pathologischen Anatomie der Hernien." *Vierteljahrschrift die Practishe Heilkunde* 19 (1848): 89–97.

Bochdalek, Von, Prof. "Praktische Bemerkungen uber Zwerchfellbruche nebst Beschreibung eines mit einer Fraktur der Lendanwirbelsaule komlizirten Falles." *Vierteljohrsschrift für die Praktische Heikunde* 24 (1867): 14–17.

Bodenhamer, W. *A Practical Treatise on the Etiology,*

Pathology and Treatment of the Congenital Malformations of the Rectum and Anus. New York: S&S Wood, 1860, 41.

Bodian, M. "Pathological Aids in the Diagnosis and Management of Hirschsprung's Disease." In *Recent Advances in Clinical Pathology*, Series 3, edited by S.C. Dyke. London: Churchill, 1960.

_____, F.D. Stephens and B.L.H Ward. "Hirschsprung's Disease and Idiopathic Megacolon." *Lancet* 1 (1949): 6–11.

Bohne, O. "Orthopaedic Treatment of Clubfoot in the Sixteenth Century." *Z Krüppel Fürsorgei* 31: 104–11. [F. Arcaeus. *De Curandis Vulneribus.* 1658].

Boley, S.J. "New Modification of the Surgical Treatment of Hirschsprung's Disease." *Surgery* 56 (1964): 1015–1017.

Bonnet, L.M. "Sur la lesion dite stenose congenitale de l'aorte dans la region de l'isthme." *Rev. med.* 23 (1903): 108.

Bookvar, J.A., W. Loudon and L. Sutton. "Development of the Spitz-Holter Valve in Philadelphia." *Journal of Neurosurgery* 95 (2001): 145–147.

Bowditch, H.I. "A Peculiar Case of Diaphragmatic Hernia." *Buffalo Medical Journal and Monthly Review* 9 (1853): 1–39, 65–94 (originally presented to the Boston Society for Medical Observation in 1847).

Bowers, A.M. *Mandan Social and Ceremonial Organization.* Chicago, IL: University of Chicago Press, 1950, 177–178.

Brainard, D. "An Essay on the Treatment of Spina Bifida [Hydrorachitis] by Injections of Iodine." *Chicago Medical Journal* 2 (September 1859): 517–538.

Branch, C.D., R.E. Gross. "Aberrant Pancreatic Tissue in Gastro-Intestinal Tract; Report of 24 Cases." *Arch Surg* 31 (1935): 200.

Braun, H. "Ueber den angeberenen Verschluss des Dünndarms und seine operative Behandlung." *Beitz.z Klin Zhir* 34: (1902) 993–1023.

Breasted, J.H. *Edwin Smith Papyrus, Published in Facsimile and Hieroglyphic Transliteration with Translation and Commentary*, in two volumes. Chicago, IL: University of Chicago Press, 1930.

Brenneman, J. "Congenital Atresia of the Esophagus, with Report of Three Cases." *American Journal of Diseases of Childhood* 5 (1913): 143–150.

Brenner, D.J. "Estimating Cancer Risks from Pediatric CT: Going from the Qualitative to the Quantitative." *Pediatric Radiology* 32 (2002): 228–233.

Brenner, E.C. "Total volvulus." *Amer J Surg* 16 (1932): 34–44.

Brennom, W.S., and A.H. Bill. "Prophylactic Fixation of the Intestine for Midgut Non-Rotation." *Surgery, Gynecology and Obstetrics* 138 (1974): 181–184.

Breslow, N., et al. "Prognosis for Wilms' Tumor Patients with Metastatic Disease at Diagnosis; Results of the Second National Wilms' Tumor Study." *Journal of Clinical Oncology* 3 (1985): 521.

Breslow, N.E., et al. "Second Malignant Neoplasms Following Treatment for Wilms' Tumors: A Report from the National Wilms' Tumor Study Group." *Journal of Clinical Oncology* 13 (1995): 1851–1859.

Bridgens, J. Kiely. "Current Management of Clubfoot (Congenital Talipes Equinovarus)." *British Medical Journal* 340 (2010): 355

Brock, A.J. *Greek Medicine, Being Extracts Illustrative of Medical Writers from Hippocrates to Galen.* New York: J.M. Dent and Sons, E.P. Dutton, 1929, 130–246.

Brock, R.C. "Pulmonary Valvotomy for Relief of Congenital Pulmonary Stenosis." *British Medical Journal* 1 (1948): 1121.

Brothwell, D., and A.T. Sandison. *Diseases in Antiquity.* Springfield, IL: Charles C. Thomas, 1967, 210 and 223–224.

Brown, E.G. *Arabian Medicine.* Cambridge: Cambridge University Press, 1962, 23–32.

Brown, J.R., and J.L. Thornton. "Percival Pott (1714–1788) and Chimney Sweepers' Cancer of the Scrotum." *British Journal of Industrial Medicine* 1 (January 14, 1957): 68–70.

Browne, D. "Talipes Equinovarus." *Lancet* 11 (1934): 969.

Brückner, August. "Uber die Natur, Ursachen und Behandlung der Einwarts Gekriimmten Fiisse oder der Sogenannten Klumpfusse." Gotha, 1796.

Bruner, T.P., N.E. Tulipan and W.O. Richards. "Endoscopic Coverage of Fetal Open Myelomeningocele in Utero." *American Journal of Obstetrics and Gynecology* 176, Part 1 (June 1997): 256–257.

Brunori, R. Vagnozzi and R. Giuffrè. "Antonio Pacchioni (1665–1726): Early Studies of the Dura Mater." *Journal of Neurosurgery* 78 (March 1993): 3.

Bull, W.T., and W.B. Coley. "Observations Upon the Operative Treatment of Hernia at the Hospital for Ruptured and Crippled." *Annals of Surgery* 28 (1898): 577–604.

Bunch, W.H., et. al. *Modern Management of Myelomeningocele.* St. Louis: Warren H. Green, 1972.

Burger, R., and T. Guthrie. "Why Circumcision." *Pediatrics* 54, no. 3 (September 1974): 362–364.

Burgos, C.M., et. al. "Gene Expression Analysis in Hypoplastic Lungs in the Nitrofen Model of Congenital Diaphragmatic Hernia." *Journal of Pediatric Surgery* 45 (2010): 1445–1454.

Burke, E.C. "Abraham Jacobi, M.D.: The Man and His Legacy." *Pediatrics* Vol. 101, no. 2 (February 1998): 309–312.

Burke, L.F., and E. Clarke. "Ileo-Colic Intussusception: A Case Report." *Journal of Clinical Ultrasound* 5 (1977): 346–347.

Buyukunal, S.N.C., and N. Sari. "Serafeddin Sabuncuoglu, the Author of the Earliest Pediatric Surgical Atlas: Cerrahiye-I Ilhaniye." *Journal of Pediatric Surgery* 26 (1991): 1148–1151.

Calder, J. "XIV. Two Examples of Children Born with Preternatural Conformations of the Guts." In *Medical Essays and Observations.* Edinburgh: T. and W. Ruddimans, 1733, 203–204.

Calodney, M.M., and M.J. Carson. "Coarctation of the Aorta in Early Infancy." *Journal of Pediatrics* 37 (1950): 46.

Cameron, Ian A. "Lister's Antiseptic Technique." *Canadian Family Physician* 54, no. 11 (November 2008): 1579–1580.

Cantrell, J.R., J.A. Haller and M.M. Ravitch. "A Syndrome of Congenital Defects Involving the Abdominal Wall, Sternum, Diaphragm, Pericardiaum, and Heart." *Surgery, Gynecology and Obstetrics* 107 (1958): 602–614.

Capra, M.L., et al., "Wilms' Tumor, a Twenty-Five Year Review of the Role of Pre-Operative Chemotherapy." *Journal of Pediatric Surgery* Vol. 34, no. 4 (1999): 579–582.

Carachi, R., and D.G. Young. "James Henderson Nicoll—'Father of Day Surgery'—A History of Surgical Pediatrics." *World Scientific* (2009): 702–713.

_____, and C. Buyukunal. "A History of Surgical Pediatrics." *World Scientific* (2009): 525–528.

Carroll, N.C. "Congenital Clubfoot: Pathoanatomy and

Treatment." American Academy of Orthopedic Surgeons, Instructor Course Lecture no. 36 (1987): 117
_____. "Surgical Technique for Talipes Equinovarus." *Operative Technique in Orthopaedics* 3, no. 2 (1993): 1115.

Catholic Encyclopedia. Anatomy (from the Internet), 3.

Celsus. *De Medicina*, in three volumes, trans. W. G. Spencer, M.S., F.R.C.S. Cambridge, MA: Harvard University Press, and London: William Heineman; first printed 1938.

Cerbonnet, G. "Pierre Fredet, 1870–1946. Dernier Président de la Société Nationale et Premier Président de l'Academie de Chirurgie," *Chirurgie [Memoires de l'Academie]* 112, no. 1 (1986): 13–26.

Cerilli, C.J. "Foramen of Bochdalek Hernia: A Review of the Experience at the Children's Hospital of Denver Colorado." *Annals of Surgery* 159, no. 3 (March 1964): 385–389.

Chamberlain, J.W. "Minor Trauma with Major Injury." *Journal of Pediatric Surgery* 2 (October 1967): 455–457.

Chang, C.C., et. al. "A Clinical Analysis of 1,474 Operations under Acupunctural Anesthesia Among Children." *Chinese Medical Journal* New vol. 1 (1975): 369.

Chang, E.J., et al. "Lack of Association Between Rotavirus Infection and Intussusception: Implications for Use of Attenuated Rotavirus Vaccines." *Pediatric Infectious Disease Journal* 21 (2002): 97–102.

Chang, H.G., et al., "Intussusception, Rotavirus, Diarrhea, and Rotavirus Vaccine Use Among Children in New York State." *Pediatrics* 108 (2001): 54–60.

Chari, P.S. "Sushruta and Our Heritage." *Indian Journal of Plastic Surgery* 36 (2003): 4–13.

Chaun, H. "Sir William Osler and Gastroenterology." *Canadian Journal of Gastroenterology* 24 (2010): 615–618.

Cheseldon, William, Surgeon to St. Thomas' Hospital, in Southwark and F.R.S. London. *A Treatise on the High Operation for a Stone*, printed for John Osborn at the Oxford Arms in Lombard Street, 1723. [From R.A. Leonardo, *History of Surgery*. New York: Froben, 1943, 207–208].

Cheyenne Elders at Soaring Eagle, Hardin, Montana, personal communication.

Choudhury, S.R., et al. "Survival of Patients with Esophageal Atresia: Influence of Birthweight, Cardiac Anomalies and Late Respiratory Complications." *Journal of Pediatric Surgery* 34 (1999): 70–74.

Chouikha, A., et al. "Rotavirus Infection and Intussusception in Tunisian Children: Implications for Use of Attenuated Rotavirus Vaccines." *Journal of Pediatric Surgery* 44 (2009): 2133–2138.

Clappesattle, H. *The Doctors Mayo*. Garden City, NY: Garden City, 1941, 241.

Clavel, C., et. al. "Distribution of Fibronectin and Laminin During Development of the Human Myenteric Plexus and Hirschsprung Disease." *Gastroenterology and Clinical Biology* 12 (1988): 193–197.

Clifton, M.S., et al. "Use of Tissue Expanders in the Repair of Complex Abdominal Wall Defects." *Journal of Pediatric Surgery* 46 (2011): 372–377.

Clogg, H.S. "Congenital Intestinal Atresia." *Lancet* 2 (1904): 1770–1774.

Codivilla, A. "Tendon Transplant in Orthopaedic Practice." *Clinical Orthopedics* 118 (1976): 2–6.

Cohen-Gadol, A.A., et al. "Cushing's Experience with the Surgical Treatment of Spinal Dysraphism." *Journal of Neurosurgery* (Pediatrics 4) vol. 102 (2005): 441–444.

Collected Papers of Joseph Barron Lister, Volume I. Ox-

ford: Clarendon Press; republished as a special edition, Birmingham, AL: Classics of Medicine Library Division of Gryphon Editions, 1979, 139–140.

Collected Papers of Joseph Barron Lister, Volumes I and II. Oxford: Clarendon Press, 1859, republished as a special edition, Birmingham, AL: Classics of Medicine Library Division of Gryphon Editions, 1979, vol. II, 491.

Concetti, L. "Ueber einige Angeborene, bei Kindern die Habituelle Verstopfung, Hervorrufenden Missbildungen des Colon." *Archiv du Kinderhelik* 27 (1899): 319–353.

"Constantine the African." Wikipedia, http://en.wikipedia.org.

Cooper, A.P. *The Anatomy and Surgical Treatment of Abdominal Hernia*, 2d ed. London: Lea and Blanchard, 1844.

Cooper, J.H. *The Gros Ventre of Montana, Part II: Religion and Ritual*. Washington D.C.: Catholic University of America Press, Anthropological Series no. 16, 1956, 351–356.

Cope, Sir Zachary. *William Cheseldon*. London: E. and S. Livingstone, 1953, 53.

Cope, Z. *Intussusception in the Early Diagnosis of the Acute Abdomen*. Oxford, England: Oxford University Press, 1948, 137–150.

Corman, L.M. "Classic Articles in Colonic and Rectal Surgery." *Diseases, Colon and Rectum* 27 (1984): 499–503.

Corner, G.W. "Salernitan Surgery in the Twelfth Century." The British Journal of Surgery, the Thomas Vicary Lecture delivered at the Royal College of Surgeons of England, December 10, 1936.

Courtney, J.F. "The Celebrated Appendix of Edward VII." *Medical Times* 104 (1976):176–181.

Courville, C.B., M.D., and K.H. Abbott, M.D. "Cranial Injuries in Precolumbian Incas, with Comments on Their Mechanism, Effects and Lethality." *Bulletin of the Los Angeles Neurological Society* 7, no. 5 (September 1942): 107–130.

Cozzi, D.A., et al. "Nephron Sparing Surgery for Unilateral Primary Renal Tumors in Children." *Journal of Pediatric Surgery* 36, no. 2 (February 2001): 362–365.

Crafoord, C., and G. Nylin. "Congenital Coarctation of the Aorta and its Surgical Treatment." *Journal of Thoracic Surgery* 14 (1945): 347.

Crooks, J. "Denis Browne, Colleague." *Progress in Pediatric Surgery* 20 (1986): 60–66.

Cullen, T.S. "Umbilical Hernia." In *Embryology, Anatomy, and Disease of the Umbilicus Together with Diseases of the Urachus* (Philadelphia, London: W. B. Saunders, 1916), 459–468.

Cunha, F. "Hugo of Lucca and the School at Bologna." *American Journal of Surgery* 67, no. 1 (January 1940), 172–180.

Cunningham, A.A. "Exomphalos." *Archives of Disease in Childhood* 31 (1956): 144–151.

Cushing, H. *Andreas Vesalius*. New York: Schuman's, 1953, Introduction, p. xxx.

_____. *From a Surgeon's Journal, 1915–1918*. Boston: Little, Brown, 1936.

_____. "Surgery of the Head." In *Surgery, Its Principles and Practice*, 3d ed., edited by W.W Keen, 123–124. Philadelphia: W.B. Saunders Co., 1908.

Cutler, E.C., and R.E. Gross. "Neurofibroma and Neurofibrosarcoma of Peripheral Nerves Unassociated with Rechlinghausen's Disease; A Report of 25 Cases." *Archives of Surgery* 33 (1936): 733.

_____. "Non Tuberculous Abscess of Lung; Etiology, Treatment and Results in 90 Cases." *Journal of Thoracic Surgery* 6 (1936): 125.

_____. "Surgical Treatment of Tumors of the Peripheral Nerves." *Annals of Surgery* 104 (1936): 436.

D'Angio, G.J., et al., "Results of the Third National Wilms' Tumor Study." *Cancer* 64 (1989): 349–360.

_____. "The Treatment of Wilms' Tumor: Results of the National Wilms' Tumor Study." *Cancer* 38 (1979): 633–646.

_____. "The Treatment of Wilms' Tumor: Results of the Second National Wilms' Tumor Study." *Cancer* 47 (1981): 2302.

Daintree, J.H., and D.H. Evans. "Hirschsprung's Disease." *Lancet* 1 (1957): 1147–1149.

Dale, W.A., and C.D. Sherman. "Late Reconstruction of Congenital Esophageal Atresia by Intrathoracic Colon Transplantation." *Journal of Thoracic Surgery* 29 (1953): 355.

DallaValle, A. "Richirche isto Ogiche su di un Caso di Megacolon Congenito." *Pediatria* 8 (1920): 740–752.

Dandy, W.E. "The Diagnosis and Treatment of Hydrocephalus Due to Occlusions of the Foramina of Magendi and Lushka." *Surgery, Gynecology and Obstetrics* 32 (1921): 112.

_____. "Diagnosis and Treatment of Strictures of the Aqueduct of Sylvius Causing Hydrocephalus." *Archives of Surgery* 51 (1945): 1–14.

_____. "Extirpation of the Chorid Plexus of the Lateral Ventricles in Communicating Hydrocephalus." *Annals of Surgery* 37 (1918): 569.

_____. "The Operative Treatment of Communicating Hydrocephalus." *Annals of Surgery* 108 (1938): 194–202.

_____, I. Blackfan, and D. Kenneth, "Internal Hydrocephalus, an Experimental, Clinical and Pathological Study." *American Journal of Diseases of Children* 8 (1914): 406.

Daneman, A., et al. "Intussusception on Small Bowel Examination in Children." *American Journal of Roentgenology* 139 (1982): 299–304.

Das, S. "Sushruta of India: Pioneer in Vesicolithotomy." *Urology* 23 (1984): 317–319.

Dasgupta, R., and J.C. Langer. "Hirschsprung Disease." *Current Problems in Surgery* 41 (2004): 942–988.

Davis, C.F., A.J. McCabe, and P.A.M. Raine. "The Ins and Outs of Intussusception: History and Management over the Past Fifty Years." *Journal of Pediatric Surgery* 38 (2003): 60–64.

Davis, D.L., and C.W.M. Poynter. "Congenital Occlusions of the Intestines." *Surgery, Gynecology and Obstetrics* 34 (1922): 35–41.

Davis, E.P. "The Clinical Application of Roentgen Rays, the Study of the Infant's Body and of the Pregnant Womb by the Roentgen Rays." *American Journal of Medical Sciences* 111 (1896): 262–270.

"Davy, Humphrey." Wikipedia, http://en.wikipedia.org/wiki/Humphrey_Davy.

Deaver, J.B. *Appendicitis*, 3d ed. Philadelphia: P. Blakiston's Son, 1905.

De la Torre-Mondragon, L., and J.A. Ortega-Selgado. "Transanal Endorectal Pull-Through for Hirschsprung Disease." *Journal of Pediatric Surgery* 33 (1998): 1283–1286.

Delpech, J.M. "Tenotomie du Tendon d'Achille." *Chirurgie Clinique Montpelier* 1 (1823): 184.

DeMause L. "Foundations of Psychohistory." psychohistory.com, 55. [The Institute for Psychohistory, New York].

Deng, E.T. "Indian Tribes of the Missouri." 48th Annual Report of the Bureau of American Ethnology (1930): 427.

_____. "Indian Tribes of the Upper Missouri." In the 40th Annual Report of Bureau of American Ethnology (1930): 422.

Densmore, F. "Teton Sioux Music." *Bureau of American Ethnology Bulletin* 61 (1916): 70.

Dent, C. "On Congenital Hypertrophic Stenosis of the Pylorus." *British Journal of Children's Disease* 1 (1904): 16.

Dibbin, A.W., and E.S. Weiner. "Mortality from Neonatal Diaphragmatic Hernia." *Journal of Pediatric Surgery* 9 (1974): 653.

Dickens, Dr. Mark. Cambridge University.

Difliore, J.W., D.O. Fauza, R. Slavin, C.A. Peters, J.C. Fackler and J.M. Wilson. "Experimental Fetal Tracheal Ligation Reverses the Structural and Physiological Effects of Pulmonary Hypoplasia in Congenital Diaphragmatic Hernia." *Journal of Pediatric Surgery* 29 (1994): 248–257.

Dimeglio, A., F. Bonnet, P. Mazeau, et al. "Orthopaedic Treatment and Passive Motion Machine: Consequences for the Surgical Treatment of Clubfoot." *Journal of Pediatric Orthopedics* 5B (1996): 173.

Dimeglio Alain, and Frederique Dimeglio. Chapter 24, in *Orthopaedics*, by Robert Hannon Fitzgerald, Herbert Kaufer and Arthur L. Malkani. St. Louis: Mosby, 2002.

Di Tanna, G.L., A. Rosano, and R. Mastroiacovo. "Prevalence of Gastroschisis at Birth. Retrospective Study." *British Medical Journal* 325 (2002): 389–390.

Ditesheim, J.A., and J.M. Templeton, Jr. "Short-term V. Long-term Quality of Life in Children Following Repair of High Imperforate Anus." *Journal of Pediatric Surgery* 22, no. 7 (1987): 581–587.

Dobbins, W.O., and A.H. Bill, Jr. "Diagnosis of Hirschsprung's Disease Excluded by Rectal Suction Biopsy." *New England Journal of Medicine* 272 (1965): 990–993.

Dobson, J. "Percival Pott." *Annals of the Royal College of Surgeons, England* 50 (1972): 54–65.

Dodi, G., and R.J. Spencer. *Outpatient Coloproctology.* 1776.

Doolin, E.J., et al. "Rectal Manometry, Computed Tomography and Functional Results of Anal Atresia Surgery." *Journal of Pediatric Surgery* 28, no. 2 (1993): 195–198.

Dott, N.M. Anomalies of Intestinal Rotation: Their Embryology and Surgical Aspects with Report of 5 Cases." *Br J Surg* 11 (1923): 251–286.

_____. "Clinical Record of Case of Exomphalos, Illustrating the Embryonic Type and Its Surgical Treatment." *Edinburgh Medical Journal* (1932): 105–108.

_____. "Volvulus Neonatorum." *Br Med Jour* 1 (1927): 230–231.

Dougall, W. "History of a Case of Ileus in which a Considerable Portion of the Intestine was Voided by Stool." *Medical Commentary* (London) 9 (1785): 278–281.

Downes, W.A. "Congenital Hypertrophic Pyloric Stenosis: Review of One Hundred and Seventy-Five Cases in which the Fredet-Rammstedt Operation Was Performed." *Journal of the American Medical Association* 75 (June 24, 1920): 228–232.

Dry, F.M. "Eventration." *Illinois Medical Journal* (1934): 509–511.

Du, Y. "Outstanding Achievements of Hua Tuo." *Negative* 1, no. 3 (2010): 15–16.

Duckett, J.W. "Treatment of Congenital Inguinal Hernia." *Ann Surg* 135 (1952): 879 – 84.

Dudrick, S.J. Oral History Project Interview in *In Their Own Words*. American Academy of Pediatrics, History Center, 2008, 30–34.

Dudrick, S.J., D.B. Groff, and D.W. Wilmore. "Long Term Venous Catheterization in Infants." *Surgery, Gynecology and Obstetrics* 129 (1969): 805–808.

Dudrick, S.J., D.W. Wilmore, and H.M. Vars. "Long-Term Total Parenteral Nutrition with Growth in Puppies and Positive Nitrogen Balance in Patients." *Surgical Forum* 18 (1967): 356–357.

Dufour, H., and P. Fredet. "La Stenose Hypertrophique du Pylore Chez le Nourrisson et son Traitement Chirurgical." *Bulletin et Memoires, Société de Medecine De Paris* 24, no. 1221 (1907): 208–217.

_____. "La Stenose Hypertrophique du Pylore Chez le Nourrisson et son Traitment Chirurgical." *Revue de Chirurgie* 37 (1908): 208–253.

Duhamel, B. "A New Operation for the Treatment of Hirschsprung's Disease." *Archives of Disease in Childhood* 35 (1960): 38–41.

_____. "Une Nouvelle Opération pour le Megacôlon Congénital: l'Abaissement Rétro-rectale et Trans-anale du Côlon, et son Application Possible au Traitment de quelques autres Malformatos." *Presse Médicale* 64 (1956): 2249–2250.

Dulger, B. "A Short Report on Antibacterial Activity of Ten Lycoperdaceae." *Fitoterapia* 76 (2005): 352–354.

Dunlop, M. *Bill Mustard, Surgical Pioneer*. Toronto: Fitzhenry and Whiteside, 1996.

Dunn, P.M. "George Armstrong, M.D. (1719–1789) and his Dispensary for the Infant Poor." *Archives of Diseases of Childhood* (fetal, neonatal) 87 (2002): F288–F231.

Dwivedi, G., and S. Dwivedi. "Sushruta–the Clinician–Teacher Par Excellence." *Indian Journal of Chest Diseases and Allied Sciences* 49 (2007): 243–244.

Earlam, R.J. "A Study of the Aetiology of Congenital Stenosis of the Gut." *Ann Roy Coll Surg Engl* 51 (1972): 126–130.

Ehrenpreis, T. *Hirschsprung's Disease*. Chicago: Year Book, 1970, 13–25.

_____. "Megacolon in the Newborn: A Clinical and Roentgenological Study with Special Regard to the Pathogenesis." *Acta Chirugie Scandinavia* 94 (1946): 112–116.

Ein, S.H., and A. Daneman. "Chapter 83: Intussusception." In *Pediatric Surgery*, 6th ed., edited by J.L. Grosfeld, et al., , 1313–1341. Philadelphia: Mosby, 2006.

Ein, S.H., and B. Shandling. "A New Non-Operative Treatment of Large Omphaloceles with a Polymer Membrane." *Journal of Pediatric Surgery* 13 (1978): 255–257.

Ein, S.H., D.G. Marshall, and D. Girvan. "Peritoneal Drainage under Local Anesthesia for Perforations in Necrotizing Enterocolitis." *Journal of Pediatric Surgery* 12 (1977): 963.

Ein, S.H., et al. "Non-Operative Management of Traumatized Spleen in Children. How and Why." *Journal of Pediatric Surgery* 13 (1978): 117.

Elgood, C., M.A., M.D., F.R.C.P. *A Medical History of Persia and the Eastern Caliphate*. Cambridge: University Press, 1951, 30, 66–68.

Ellis, H. "The Umbilical Hernia of Queen Caroline." *Contemporary Surgery* 17 (November 1980): 83–85.

Elmslie, R.C. "The Principles of Treatment of Congenital Talipes Equinovarus." *Journal of Orthopedic Surgery* 2 (1920): 669.

Elsberg, C.A. "Anaesthesia by the Intratracheal Insufflation of Air and Ether, a Description of the Technic of

the Method and of a Portable Apparatus for Use in Man." *Annals of Surgery* 53, no. 2 (February 1911): 161–168.

Engel, R.R., et al., "Origin of Mural Gas in Necrotizing Enterocolitis." *Pediatric Research* 7 (1973): 292.

Evans, C.H. "Atresias of the Gastrointestinal Tract." *Surgery, Gynecology and Obstetrics* 92 (1951): 1–8.

Evans, E.I., et al. "Fluid and Electrolyte Requirements in Severe Burns." *American Journal of Surgery* 135 (1952): 804.

Fang, H.S. "Footbinding in Chinese Women." *Canadian Journal of Surgery* 3 (1960): 195.

Farber S. "Congenital Atresia of the Alimentary Tract: Diagnosis by Microscopic Examination of Meconium." *Journal of the American Medical Association* 100 (1933): 1753–54.

Farber, S.D., et al. "Clinical Studies of Actinomycin-D with Special Reference to Wilms' Tumor in Children." *Annals of the New York Academy of Science* 89 (1960): 421–425.

_____. "Temporary Remissions in Acute Leukemia in Children Produced by Folic Antagonist 4-Aminopteroylglutamic Acid [Aminopterin]." *New England Journal of Medicine* 238 (1948): 787–793.

Fear, W. "Congenital Extrusion of Abdominal Viscera: Return; Recovery." *British Medical Journal* (1878): 518.

Feidberg, H. "Recherches Clinique et Critiques sur l'Anus Artificialle." *Archives Generales de Medicine de Paris*, 1856.

Felts, J. "Henry Ingersoll Bowditch and Oliver Wendell Holmes, Stethoscopist and Reformers." *Perspectives in Biology and Medicine* 45, no. 4 (Autumn 2002): 539–548.

Fenton, S.J., et al. "CT Scan and the Pediatric Trauma Patient — Are We Overdoing It." *Journal of Pediatric Surgery* 39 (2004): 1877–1881.

Fenwick, W.S. "Hypertrophy and Dilatation of the Colon in Infancy." *British Medical Journal* 2 (1900): 564–567.

Ferguson, A.H. "Oblique Inguinal Hernia-Typic Operation for Its Radical Cure." *Journal of the American Medical Association* 33 (1899): 6–14.

Fewtrell, M.S., et al. "Hirschsprung's Disease Associated with a Deletion of Chromosome 10(q11.2q21.2) a Further Link with the Neurochrisopathies?" *Journal of Medical Genetics* 31 (1994): 325–327.

Filston, H.C., and D.R. Kirks. "Malrotation–the ubiquitous anomaly." *Journal of Pediatric Surgery* 16 (1981): 614–620.

Finney, J. "Congenital Idiopathic Dilatation of the Colon." *Surgery, Gynecology and Obstetrics* 6 (1908): 624–643.

Fiorito, E.S., and L.A. Recalde Cuestas. "Diagnosis and Treatment of Acute Intestinal Intussusception with Controlled Insufflation of Air." *Pediatrics* 24 (1959): 241–244.

Firor, H.V., and E. Steiger. "Morbidity of Rotational Abnormalities of the Gut Beyond Infancy." *Cleveland Clinic Quarterly* 50 (1983): 303–309.

Fischer, J.D., et al. "Gastroschisis: A Simple Technique for Staged Silo Closure." *Journal of Pediatric Surgery* 30 (1995): 1169–1171.

Fitz, R.H. *Perforating Inflammation of the Vermiform Appendix; with Special Reference to its Early Diagnosis and Treatment, Reprinted from the Transactions of the Association of American Physicians*. Philadelphia: Wm. J. Dornan, June 18, 1886.

Flaubert, Gustave. *Madame Bovary*. Harmondsworth: Penguin, 1950.

Fockens, P. "Arts Over Angeboren Atresia Van Den Darm, Met Een Door Operate Genezen Geval." *Netherlands Tijdschrift Voor Geneeskunde* (1911): 1658–1665.

Foglia, R., et al. "Management of Giant Omphalocele with Rapid Creation of Abdominal Domain." *Journal of Pediatric Surgery* 41 (2006): 704–709.

Foker, J.E., et al. "Development of a True Primary Repair for the Full Spectrum of Esophageal Atresia." *Annals of Surgery* 226 (1997): 533–543.

Forest, W.E. "Intussusception in Children." *American Journal of Obstetrics* 19 (1886): 673–697.

Fossey, Dian. *Gorillas in the Mist.* Boston: Houghton-Mifflin, 1988, 75–76.

Franklin, F.H. "Congenital Atresia of the Esophagus, Two Cases Successfully Treated by Anastomosis." *Lancet* 2 (1947): 243.

Fraser, J. "Intussusception." In *Surgery of Childhood.* London: Edward Arnold, 1926, 839–850.

Frazer, J.E., and R.H. Robbins. "On the Factors Concerned in Causing Rotation of the Intestine in Man." *J Anat Physiol* 50 (1915): 75–110.

Frederiks, J.A., and Koehler, P.J. "The First Lumbar Puncture." *Journal of the History of Neuroscience* 6 (1997): 147–153.

Fredet, P. "La Cure de la Stenose Hypertrophique du Pylore Chez les Nourrissons par la Pylorotomie — Extra Muqueuse." *Journal de Chirurgie* 29, no. 4 (1927): 385–408.

Fredet, P., and L. Guillemot. "La Stenose du Pylore par Hypertrophic Musculaire Chez les Nourrissons." *Annales de Gynecologie et d'Obstetrique* 67 (1910): 604–629.

_____. "La Stenose du Pylore par Hypertrophie Musculaire Chez les Nourrissons." Congres Nationale Periodique de Gynecologie, d'Obstetrique et de Pediatrie, Sixième Session, Toulouse, Septembre 1910; *Memoires et Discussions.* Toulouse: J. Audebert, Imprimerie de Librairie Edouard Privat, 1912, 242–323.

Fredet, P., and E. Lesne. "Stenose Hypertrophique du Pylore Chez les Nourrissons: Resultat Anatomique de la Pylorotomie sur un Sujet Traite Gueri Depuis Trois Mois." *Bulletins et Memoires, Société de Chirurgie* 32 (July 11, 1928): 1050–1060.

Fredet, P., and P. Pironneau. "La Stenose Hypertrophique du Pylore." *Bulletin et Memoires, Société Nationale de Chirurgie de Paris* 47 (1921): 1021.

Freeman, C. *The Closing of the Western Mind, The Rise of Faith and the Fall of Reason.* New York: Alfred A. Knopf, 2003, 233.

Friedlander, A. "Sarcoma of the Kidney Treated by the Roentgen Ray." *American Journal of Diseases of Children* 12 (1915): 328–331.

Fulbrook, D. "Medusa's Tails and Leonardo's Heads: Fantasies of Anal Creation in 19th-Century Literature and Psychoanalytic Theory." UMI Dissertation Services, ProQuest, Michigan, 2003.

Fulton, J.F. *Harvey Cushing: A Biography.* Springfield, IL: Charles C. Thomas, 1946, 69–70.

Gage, M., and Ochsner, A. "The Surgical Treatment of Congenital Tracheo-Esophageal Fistula in the Newborn." *Annals of Surgery* 103, no. 5 (May 1936): 725–737.

Gaillard, D., et al. "Colonic Nerve Network Demonstrated by Quinacrine." *Bulletin of the Association of Anatomists* 66 (1982): 63–70.

Gairdner, D. "The Fate of the Foreskin, a Study of Circumcision." *British Medical Journal* (December 24, 1949): 1433–1437.

"Galen." Wikipedia, http://en.wikipedia.org.

_____. *On the Usefulness of the Parts of the Body,* trans. Margaret T. May. Ithaca, NY: Cornell University Press, 1967.

Gallaher, D.L. *Circumcision.* New York: Basic, 2000, 8.

Gamble, J.L. "Early History of Fluid Replacement Therapy." *Pediatrics* Vol. 11 (1953): 554–567.

_____, and S.G. Ross. "Factors in the Dehydration Following Pyloric Obstruction." *Journal of Clinical Investigation* 1, no. 5 (1925): 402–423.

Gans, S.L., and G. Berci. "Advances in Endoscopy of Infants and Children." *Journal of Pediatric Surgery* 6 (1971): 199–223.

_____, and R.O. Johnson. "Diagnosis and Surgical Management of H-Type Tracheo-esophageal Fistula in Infants and Children." *Journal of Pediatric Surgery* 132 (1977): 233–236.

Garceau, E., M.D. *Renal, Ureteral, Perirenal and Adrenal Tumors and Actinomycosis and Echinococcus of the Kidney.* New York, London: D. Appleton, 1909, 150–200.

Gardner, C.E., Jr. "The Surgical Significance of Anomalies of Intestinal Rotation." *Annals of Surgery* 131 (1950): 879–896.

_____, and D. Hart. "Anomalies of Intestinal Rotation as a Cause of Intestinal Obstruction." *Archives of Surgery* 29 (1934): 942–981.

Gariepy, C.E., et al. "Transgenic Expression of the Endothelin-B Receptor Prevents Congenital Intestinal Aganglionosis in a Rat Model of Hirschsprung Disease." *Journal of Clinical Investigation* 102 (1998): 1092–1101.

Garland, Robert. *Daily Life of Ancient Greeks.* Westport, CT, and London: Greenwood, 1998, 40–41.

Garlock, J.H., M.D., F.A.C.S. "The Re-Establishment of Esophagogastric Continuity Following Resection of Esophagus for Carcinoma of the Middle Third." *Surgery, Gynecology and Obstetrics* 78 (1944): 23–28.

Garnall, P., et al. "Abdominal Injuries in the Battered Baby Syndrome." *Archives of Diseases of Children* Vol. 47 (1972): 211.

Garrison, Dan, Dr. Northwestern University, Evanston, Illinois. Personal communication.

Genersich, G. "Ueber Angeborene Dilatation und Hypertrophie des Dickdarms." *JB Kinderhelik* Vol. 37 (1894): 91–100.

Georgeson, K.E., T.H. Inge, and C. Albanese. "Laparoscopically Assisted Anorectal Pull-Through for High Imperforate Anus — A New Technique." *Journal of Pediatric Surgery* 35 (June 2000): 927–933.

_____, et al. "Primary Laparoscopic-Assisted Endorectal Colon Pull-Through for Hirschsprung's Disease: A New Gold Standard." *Annals of Surgery* 229 (1999): 678–683.

"Gerard of Cremona." Wikipedia, http://en.wikipedia.org.

German, J., et al. "Management of Pulmonary Insufficiency in Diaphragmatic Hernia Using Extracorporeal Circulation with a Membrane Oxygenator [ECMO]." *Journal of Pediatric Surgery* 12 (1977): 905–912.

German, J.C., and D.J. Waterston. "Colon Interposition for the Replacement of the Esophagus in Children." *Journal of Pediatric Surgery* 11 (1976): 227.

Gersony, W.M., et al. "The Hemodynamic Effects of Intrauterine Hypoxia: An Experimental Model in Newborn Lambs." *Journal of Pediatrics* 89 (1976): 631.

Gillespie, N.A. *Endotracheal Anesthesia.* Madison, WI: University of Wisconsin Press, 1941, 8.

Gillis, D.A., S.D. Lewis, and D.C. Little. "The Halifax

Explosion and the Birth of a Surgical Specialty — Myth or Reality." *Journal of Pediatric Surgery* Vol. 45 (2010): 855–858 [see also letter to the editor, same issue, p. 1069, A. Ein, S. Ein and D. A. Gillis. The letter is in the possession of Richard Rickets, M.D., Atlanta, GA.]

Glass, J.M., and N.A. Watkinn. "From Mutilation to Medication: The History of Orchidectomy." *British Journal of Urology* (80) 1997: 373 – 378.

Godlee, R.J. *Lord Lister*, 3d ed., rev. Oxford: Clarendon Press, 1924, 18.

Goldner, J.L. "Congenital Talipes Equinovarus: Fifteen Years of Surgical Treatment." *Current Practice in Orthopaedic Surgery* Vol. 4 (1969): 61–123.

Goldsworthy, A. *How Rome Fell*. New Haven, CT, and New York: Yale University Press, 2009, 16–23.

Gonzales-Spinola, J., et al. "Intussusception: The Accuracy of Ultrasound-Guided Saline Enema and the Usefulness of a Delayed Attempt at Reduction." *Journal of Pediatric Surgery* 34 (1999): 1016–1020.

Goodrich, J.T. "A Historical Review of the Surgical Treatment." In *The Spina Bifida Management and Outcome*, edited by M.M. Ozek, G. Spinalli and W.J. Maixner. Milan, Italy: Springer-Verlag, 2008.

Gool, J.B., and J.D. Gool. *A Short History of Spina Bifida*. Manchester, England: Society for Research into Hydrocephalus and Spina Bifida, 1986.

Gordon, B.E. *Medieval and Renaissance Medicine*. New York: Philosophical Library, 1959, 34–35, 429–432.

Gorenstein, A., et al. "Intussusception in Children: Reduction with Reported, Delayed Air Enema." *Radiology* 206 (1998): 721–724.

Gourineni, P., and N.C. Carroll. "The Clubfoot Diagnosis and Treatment in Infancy." *Pediatric Orthopedic Problems, Foot and Ankle Clinics* 3, no. 4 (December 1998).

Gourlay, D.M., et al. "Beyond Feasibility: A Comparison of Newborns Undergoing Thoracoscopic and Open Repair of Congenital Diaphragmatic Hernias." *Journal of Pediatric Surgery* 44 (2009): 1702–1707.

Graham, H. *The Story of Surgery*. New York: Doubleday, Doran, 1939, 127–133.

Graybiel, A., J.W. Strieder, and N.H. Boyer. "An Attempt to Obliterate the Patent Ductus Arteriosus in a Patient with Subacute Bacterial Endocarditis." *American Heart Journal* 15 (1938): 621.

Greenfield, S. *Spirits with Scalpels*. Walnut Creek, CA: Left Coast, 2008.

Greenwald, H.M., and M. Steiner. "Diaphragmatic Hernia in Infancy and in Childhood." *The American Journal of Diseases of Childhood* 38 (1929): 361–392.

Greig, D. "On Insufflation as a Remedy in Intussusception." *Edinburgh Medical Journal* 10 (1864): 306–315.

Grimson, K.S., L. Vandergrift, and H.M. Datz. "Surgery in Obstinate Megacolon: One-Stage Resection and Ileosigmoidostomy." *Surgery, Gynecology and Obstetrics* 80 (1945): 164–173.

Grob, M. "Conservative Treatment of Exomphalos." *Archives of Disease in Childhood* 38 (1963): 148–150.

_____. "Intestinal Obstruction in the Newborn Infant," *Archives of Disease in Childhood* 35 (1960): 40–50.

Grob, M., N. Genton, and V. von Tobel. "Experiences with Surgery of Congenital Megacolon and Suggestion of a New Surgical Technique." *Zentralb Chir* 84 (1959): 1781–1789.

Grob, M., M. Stockman, and M. Bettex. *Lehrbuch der Kinderchirurgie*. Stuttgart: Georg Thierm, 1957.

Grosfeld, J.L., V.N. Ballantine, and R. Shoemaker. "Operative Management of Intestinal Atresia and Stenosis

Based on Pathologic Findings." *Journal of Pediatric Surgery* 14 (1979): 368–375.

Gross, R.E. *An Atlas of Children's Surgery*. Philadelphia, London, Toronto: W.B. Saunders, 1970.

_____. "Congenital Anomalies of Gall-Bladder; Review of 138 Cases, with Report of a Double Gallbladder." *Archives of Surgery* 33 (1936): 131.

_____. "Congenital Hernia of the Diaphragm." *Am J Dis Child* 71 (1946): 579.

_____. "Idiopathic Dilatation of Common Bile Duct in Children: Review of Literature and Report of the Two Cases." *Journal of Pediatrics* 3 (1933): 730.

_____. "A New Method for Surgical Treatment of Large Omphaloceles." *Surgery* 24 (1948): 277–292.

_____. "Recurring Myxomatous, Cutaneous Cysts of Fingers and Toes." *Surgery, Gynecology, Obstetrics* 65 (1937): 289.

_____. *The Surgery of Infancy and Childhood*. Philadelphia, London: W.B. Saunders, 1953.

_____. "Surgical Approach for Ligation of Patent Ductus Arteriosus." *New England Journal of Medicine*, 220 (1939): 510.

_____. "Surgical Management of the Patent Ductus Arteriosus with Summary of Four Successfully Treated Cases." *Annals of Surgery* 110 (1939): 321.

_____. "Surgical Relief for Tracheal Obstruction from a Vascular Ring." *New England Journal of Medicine* 233 (1945): 586.

_____. "Treatment of Certain Coarctations by Homologous Grafts: A Report of Nineteen Cases." *Annals of Surgery* 134:753, 1951.

_____. "The Use of Vinyl Ether (Vinethene) in Infancy and Childhood: Report of 100 Cases." *New England Journal of Medicine* 220 (1939): 334.

Gross, R.E., and C.A. Hufnagel. "Coarctation of the Aorta: Experimental Studies Regarding its Surgical Correction." *New England Journal of Medicine* 233 (1945): 287.

Gross, R.E., and E.B.D. Neuhauser. "Compression of the Trachea or Esophagus by Vascular Anomalies: Surgical Therapy in 40 Cases." *Pediatrics* 7 (1952): 69.

Gross, R.E., and J.B. Blodgett. "Omphalocele (Umbilical Eventration) in the Newly Born." *Surgery, Gynecology, Obstetrics* 71 (1940): 520.

Gross, R.E., and J.P. Hubbard. "Surgical Ligation of Patent Ductus Arteriosus." *Journal of the American Medical Association* 112 (1939): 729.

Gross, R.E., and T.C. Chisholm. "Annular Pancreas Producing Duodenal Obstruction." *Annals of Surgery* 119 (1944): 759.

Gross, R.E., and W.W. Vaughan. "Plasma Cell Myeloma: Report of 2 Cases with Unusual Survivals of 6 and 10 Years." *Am J Roentgenol* 39 (1934): 344.

Gross, R.E., A.H. Bill, Jr., and E.C. Peirce II. "Methods of Preservation and Transplantation of Arterial Grafts." *Surgery, Gynecology, Obstetrics* 88 (1949): 689.

Gross, R.E., E. Watkins, Jr., A.J. Pomeranz and E.I. Goldsmith. "A Method for Surgical Closure of Interauricular Septal Defects." *Surgery, Gynecology, Obstetrics* 96 (1953): 1.

Gross, R.E., E.B.D. Neuhauser and L.A. Longino. "Thoracic Diverticula Which Originate from the Intestine." *Annals of Surgery* 131 (1950): 363.

Gross, R.E., H.W. Clatworthy, Jr., and I.A. Meeker, Jr. "Sacrococcygeal Teratomas in Infants and Children: A Report of 40 Cases." *Surgery, Gynecology, Obstetrics* 92 (1951): 341.

Grundy, P.E., et al. "Loss of Heterogyzosity for Chromosomes 16Q and 1p in Wilms Tumor Predicts Adverse Outcome." *Cancer Research* 54 (1994): 2331–2333.

Guerin, J. R. "Memoire sur l'Etiologie Generate de Piedsbots." *Congenitaux*. Paris, 1838.

Guersant, M.P. *Surgical Diseases of Infants and Children*, trans. Richard J. Dunglison, M.D. Philadelphia: Henry C. Lea, 1873.

Guner, Y.S., et al. "Outcome Analysis of Neonates with Congenital Diaphragmatic Hernia Treated with Venovenous Vs. Venoarterial Extracorporeal Membrane Oxygenation." *Journal of Pediatric Surgery* 44 (2009): 1691–1701.

Guo, J.Z., X.Y. Ma, and Q.H. Zhou. "Results of Air Pressure Enema Reduction of Intussusception: 6,396 Cases in 13 Years." *Journal of Pediatric Surgery* 21 (1986): 1210–1213.

Gupta, D.K., A.R. Charles, and M. Srinivas. "Pediatric Surgery in India, a Specialty Comes of Age." *Pediatric Surgery International* 18 (2000): 649–652.

Gupta, D.K., et al. "Neonatal Gastric Pull Up: Reality or Myth?" *Pediatric Surgery International* 19 (2003): 100–103.

Guthrie, Douglas. *The Royal Edinburgh Hospital for Sick Children, 1860–1960*. Edinburgh and London: E. and S. Livingstone, 1960, 19.

"Guy de Chauliac." Wikipedia, http://en.wikipedia.org.

Haber, H.P., S.W. Warmann, and J. Fuchs. "Transperineal Sonography of the Anal Sphincter Complex in Neonates and Infants: Differentiation of Anteriorly Displaced Anus from Low-Type Imperforate Anus with Perineal Fistula." *Ultraschall Med* 29 (2008): 383–387.

Haber, P., et al. "An Analysis of Rotavirus Vaccine Reports to the Vaccine Adverse Event Reporting System: More than Intussusception Alone?" *Pediatrics* 113 (2004): E353–359.

Hachmann, H. "A Case of Intussusception." *Zeitschrift Ges Med* 14 (1840): 289–303.

Haeger K. *The Illustrated History of Surgery*. New York: Bell, 1988: 49.

Haight, C., M.D. "Total Removal of Left Lung for Bronchiectasis." *Surgery, Gynecology and Obstetrics* 58 (1934): 768.

Haight, C., M.D., and H.A. Tousley. "Congenital Atresia of the Esophagus with Tracheoesophageal Atresia: Extrapleural Ligation of the Fistula and End to End Anastomosis of Esophageal Segments." *Surgery, Gynecology and Obstetrics* 73 (1943): 672–688.

Haller, J.A., Jr., "Newer Concepts in Emergency Care of Children with Major Injuries." *Pediatrics* 52 (1973): 485.

Haller, J.A., et al. "Pulmonary and Ductal Hemodynamics in Studies of Simulated Diaphagmatic Hernia of Fetal and Newborn Lambs." *Journal of Pediatric Surgery* 11 (1976): 675.

_____. "Use of a Trauma Registry in the Management of Children with Life-Threatening Injuries." *Journal of Pediatric Surgery* 11 (1976): 381.

Hamby, L.S., C.L. Fowler, and W.J. Pokorny. "Intussusception." Chapter 42 in *Abdominal Surgery of Infancy and Childhood*, edited by W. L. Donnellan, 1–19. Austria: Harwood, 1996.

Hamilton, T.E., et al. "Bilateral Wilms' Tumor with Anaplasia, Lessons from the National Wilms' Tumor Study Group." *Journal of Pediatric Surgery* 41 (2006): 1641–1644.

Hammett, F.S. "The Anatomical Knowledge of the Ancient Hindus." *Annals of Medical History* 1 (1929): 325–327.

Hanby, W.B., ed. *The Case Reports and Autopsy Records of Ambroise Paré*, translated from J. P. Malgaines, Oeuvres Complètes d'Ambroise Paré, 1840. Springfield, IL: Charles C. Thomas, 1960, 129.

Hardesty, B.J., et al. "ECMO Successful Treatment of Persistent Fetal Circulation Following Repair of Diaphragmatic Hernia." *Journal of Thoracic and Cardiovascular Surgery* 81 (1981): 556.

Hargrove, W.C., H. Gertner and W.J. Fitts. "The Kraske Operation for Carcinoma of the Rectum." *Surgery, Gynecology and Obstetrics* 148 (1979): 931–933.

Harrison, M.R., R. Bjordal, and O. Knutrud. "Congenital Diaphragmatic Hernia: The Hidden Mortality." *Journal of Pediatric Surgery* 13 (1978): 337.

Harrison, M.R., et al. "Correction of Congenital Diaphragmatic Hernia in Utero: Six Hard-earned Lessons." *Journal of Pediatric Surgery* 28 (1993): 1411–1417.

Harsh, G.R., III. "Peritoneal Shunt for Hydrocephalus, Utilizing the Fimbria of the Fallopian Tube for Entrance to the Peritoneal Cavity." *Journal of Neurosurgery* 11 (1954): 284–294.

"Harvey, William." Wikipedia, http://en.wikipedia.org.

Harvey, William. *The Circulation of the Blood and Other Writings*, trans. Kenneth J. Franklin, D.M., F.R.S. New York: Everyman's Library, Dutton, 1907, reissued in new translation, 1967.

Haseker, B. "Mr. Job von Meekeren, 1611–1666, and Surgery of the Hand." *Plastic and Reconstructive Surgery* 82, no. 3 (September 1988): 539–546.

Hasse, W. "Associated Malformations with Anal and Rectal Atresia." *Progress in Pediatric Surgery* 9 (1976): 100.

Haubrich, W.S. "Hirschsprung of Hirschsprung's Disease." *Gastroenterology* 127 (2004): 1299.

Hawkins, H.P. "Remarks on Idiopathic Dilatation of the Colon." *British Medical Journal* 1 (1907): 477–483.

Hay, S.A. et al. "Idiopathic Intussusception: The Role of Laparoscopy." *Journal of Pediatric Surgery* 34 (1999): 577–578.

Heldbom, C.A. "Diaphragmatic Hernia." *Journal of the American Medical Association* 85, no. 13 (1925): 947–953.

Hedrick, H. "Management of Prenatally Diagnosed Congenital Diaphragmatic Hernia." *Seminars in Fetal and Neonatal Medicine* 15 (2010): 21–27.

Heer, F. *The Medieval World: Europe, 1100–1350*. New York: Mentor/New American Library, 1963, 242.

Heidenhain, L. "Geschicht eines Falles von Chronisher Inkarzeration des Magnes in einer Angeborenen Zwerchfellnernia, welcher durch Laparotemie Geheiht wurde mit Anschlressenden Bemerkungen uber die Moglichkeit, das Cardiacrcinon der Peiserehre zu Resezieren." *Deutsche Zetschrift für Chirurgie* 76 (1905): 394–403.

Heile, B. "Uber Neue Operative Wege zur Druckentlastung bei Angeborenene Hydrocephalus (Uretero-Duraanastomosis)." *Zentralblatt für Chirurgie* 52 (1925): 2229–2236.

Helmsworth, J.A., and C.V. Pryles. "Congenital Tracheo-Esophageal Fistula without Esophageal Atresia." *Journal of Pediatrics* 38 (1951): 610–617.

Hendren, W.H. "Introduction and Historical Overview: North American Perspective." In *Pediatric Surgery and Urology: Long Term Outcomes* by Mark Stringer, Keith Oldham and Pierre Mouriquand, 5. Cambridge: Cambridge University Press, 2006.

Hendren, W.H., and J.R. Hale. "Esophageal Atresia Treated by Electromagnetic Bougienage and Subsequent Repair." *Journal of Pediatric Surgery* 11 (1976): 713–722.

Hendren, W.H., and W.G. Hendren. "Colon Interposition in Children." *Journal of Pediatric Surgery* 20 (1985): 829.

Hendren, W.H., et al. "Traumatic Hemobilia: Non-Operative Management with Healing Documented by Angiography." *Annals of Surgery* 17 (1971): 991.

Herbert, A.F. "Hernia Funiculi Umbilicalis with Report of Three Cases." *American Journal of Obstetrics and Gynecology* 15 (1928): 86–88.

Herzenberg, J.E., N.C. Carroll, and M.R. Christoferson. "Clubfoot Analysis with Three-Dimensional Computer Modeling." *Journal of Pediatric Orthopedics* 8 (1988): 257.

Herzfeld, G. "The Radical Cure of Hernia in Infants and Young Children." *Edinburgh Medical Journal* 32 (1925): 281–90.

Herzfeld, Gertrude. Handwritten note to Dr. Otherson.

Hey, W. "Case XXI." In *Practical Observations in Surgery, Illustrated with Cases*, 226–232. London: L. Hansard, printer, 1803.

Hiatt, R.B. "The Pathological Physiology of Congenital Megacolon." *Annals of Surgery* 133 (1951): 313–320.

Hildanus. *Hildanus Observationum et Curationum Medico-chirurgarum Centurae Sex*. Lugduni, 1641.

Hill, T.P. "Congenital Malformation." *Boston Medical Surgical Journal* 21 (1840): 320.

Hippocrates, Vol. I, trans. W.H.S. Jones. Cambridge, MA: Harvard University Press, and London: William Heinemann, 1984, 29.

Hippocrates, Vol. II, trans. W.H.S. Jones. Cambridge, MA, and London: Loeb Classic Library, Harvard University Press, 1923, 139.

Hippocrates, Vol. III, trans. Dr. E.T. Witherspoon. Cambridge, MA: Harvard University Press, and London: William Heinemann, 1928, 41.

Hippocrates, Vol. IV: Heraclitus on the Universe, trans. W.H.S. Jones. Cambridge, MA, and London: Loeb Classic Library, Harvard University Press, 1923, 131–133.

Hippocrates, Vol. V, trans. Paul Potter. Cambridge, MA: Harvard University Press, and London: William Heinemann, 1988, 275.

Hippocrates, Vol. VI, trans. Paul Potter. Cambridge, MA: Harvard University Press, and London: William Heinemann, 1988, 29–31.

Hippocrates, Vol. VII, G.F. Goold, ed. Cambridge, MA, and London: Loeb Classical Library, Harvard University Press, 1994, 123.

Hippocrates, Vol. VIII, ed. and trans. by Paul Potter. Cambridge, MA, and London: Loeb Classical Library, Harvard University Press, 1995, 32.

Hirschl, R.B., M.D., et al. "Gastric Transposition for Esophageal Replacement in Children: Experience with 41 Consecutive Cases with Special Emphasis on Esophageal Atresia." *Annals of Surgery* 236, no. 4 (2002): 531–541.

Hirschprung, H. "Den Medfodte Tillerkning of Spiseroret (4 Cases) [Congenital Destruction of the Esophagus]." *Medico–Chirurgical Review* 30 (1861): 437.

_____. "Dilatation congénitale du colon," in Grancher and Comby, eds., Traité Des Maladies de l'Enfance, second edition (Paris, 1904)

_____. "Falle Von Angeborener Pylorustenose, Beobachtet bei Sauglingen." *Jahrb. D. Kindeh* 27 (1885): 61–68.

_____. "Stuhlträgheit Neugeborener in Folge von Dilatation und Hypertrophie des Colons." *Jahrb Kinderh* 27 (1887): 1–7.

Hochberg, L.A. *Thoracic Surgery Before the Twentieth Century*. New York: Vantage, 1960, 462–463.

Hoehner, J.C., S.H. Ein, and B. Shandling. "Long-Term Morbidity in Total Colonic Aganglionosis." *Journal of Pediatric Surgery* 33 (1998): 961–966.

Holcomb, G.W., III, J.W. Brock III, and W.M. Morgan III. "Laparoscopic Evaluation for a Contralateral Patent Processus Vaginalis." *Journal of Pediatric Surgery* 29 (1994): 970–77.

_____. "Laparoscopic Evaluation for Contralateral Processus Vaginalis: Part II." *Journal of Pediatric Surgery* 31 (1996): 1170–73.

Holcomb, G.W., M.D., et al. "Thoracoscopic Repair of Esophageal Atresia and Tracheo-esophageal Fistula: A Multi-Institutional Analysis." *Annals of Surgery* 242, no. 3 (September 2005): 1–9.

Holder, T.M., and K.W. Ashcraft. "Esophageal Atresia and Tracheo-Esophageal Fistula." In *Current Problems in Surgery*. Chicago, IL: Year Book Medical, August 1966.

Holder, T.M., M.D., V.G. McDonald, M.D., and M.M. Wooley, M.D. "The Premature or Critically Ill Infant with Esophageal Atresia: Increased Survival with a Staged Approach." *Journal of Thoracic and Cardiovascular Surgery* 44, no. 3 (November 1962): 344–358.

Holder, T.M., M.D., et al. "Care of Infants with Esophageal Atresia, Tracheoesophageal Fistula, and Associated Anomalies." *The Journal of Thoracic and Cardiovascular Surgery* 94, no. 6 (December 1987): 828–835.

_____. "Esophageal Atresia and Tracheoesophageal Fistula: A Survey of the Members of the Surgical Section of the American Academy of Pediatrics." *Pediatrics* 34, no. 4 (October 1964): 542–549.

Holschneider, A.M. *Hirschsprung's Disease*. Stuttgart: Hippokrates, 1982.

Homer. *The Iliad*, trans. Robert Fitzgerald. New York, Toronto, Sydney, Auckland: Anchor/Doubleday, 1974.

Horch, C. "De puella cum coalitu intestini ilei nata, et per viginti duos dies viventi." Misc Acad. nat.curios. Francof 1694–1696, decuriae 3:1–4 188–189.

Howard, R. "Oesophageal Atresia with Tracheoesophageal Fistula: Report of Six Cases with Two Successful Oesophageal Anastomoses." *Medical Journal of Australia* 1 (1950): 401–404.

Howell, C.G., F. Vozza, and S. Shaw, et al. "Malrotation, Malnutrition and Ischemic Bowel Disease." *Journal of Pediatric Surgery* 17 (1982): 469–473.

Hull, J. "On Intussusception." *Medical and Physiological Journal* VII (1802): 32–38.

Hull, M.A., et al. "Surgery for Necrotizing Enterocolitis in the United States: Current Practice and Mortality." APSA meeting, May 16–19, 2010.

Hume, J.B. "Congenital Diaphragmatic Hernia." *British Journal of Surgery* 10 (1922): 207–215.

Humphries, G.H., and J.M. Ferrer. "Management of Esophageal Atresia." *American Journal of Surgery* 107 (1964): 406–411.

Hunt, N.B. *Shamanism in North America*. Buffalo, NY: Firefly, 2003, 7–14.

Hunter, J. "An Introsusception." *Transcript from the Society to Improve Medical and Surgical Knowledge*, vol. 1 (1793), 103–118.

Hutchinson, J. "A Successful Case of Abdominal Section for Intussusception." *Proceedings of the Royal Medical and Chirurgical Society* 7 (1873): 195–198.

Iason, A.H. *Hernia*. Philadelphia: Blackiston, 1941.

Ikawa, H., J. Yokoyama, T. Sanbonmatsu, et al. "The Use

of Computerized Tomography to Evaluate Anorectal Anomalies." *Journal of Pediatrics Surgery* 20, no. 6 (1985): 640–644.

Imperatori, C.J. "Congenital Tracheo-Esophageal Fistula without Atresia of the Esophagus." *Archives of Otolaryngology* 30 (1939): 352–359.

Ingraham, F.D. *Spina Bifida and Cranium Bifidum.* Cambridge, MA: Harvard University Press, 1944.

Irish, M.S., B.A. Holm, and P.L. Glick. "Congenital Diaphragmatic Hernia: A Historical Review." *Clinics in Perinatology* 23, no. 4 (December 1996): 625–651.

Iwashita, T., et al. "Hirschsprung Disease is Linked to Defects in Neural Crest Stem Cell Function." *Science* 301 (2003): 972–976.

Izant, R.J., Jr., F. Browen, and B.F. Rothman. "Current Embryology and Treatment of Gastroschisis and Omphalocele." *Archives of Surgery* 93 (1966): 49–53.

Jacobi A. "Defective Development of the Intestine." *Am M Month NY* (1861) 16: 30–32.

Jarcho, S. "Henry I. Bowditch on Diaphragmatic Hernia, 1853." *American Journal of Cardiology* (August 12, 1963): 244–248.

Jay, V. "Legacy of Harald Hirschsprung." *Pediatric and Developmental Pathology* 4 (2001): 203–204.

Jeffrey, R., M. Federle, and R. Crass. "Computed Tomography of Pancreatic Trauma." *Radiology* 147 (1983): 491.

Jenkins, J.S. "The Voice of the Castrato." *Lancet* 351 (1998): 1877 –1880.

Jirka, F.J. *American Doctors of Destiny.* Chicago, IL: Normandie House, 1940, 69–81.

Johnson, A. *Plants and the Blackfoot.* Lethbridge, Alberta: Lethbridge Historical Society, Historical Society of Alberta, 1987, 51.

Johnson, A.A. "Lectures on Surgery of Childhood, Delivered at the Hospital for Sick Children." *British Medical Journal* (January 7, 21 and 28, 1860): 1–4, 41–47, 61–63.

Johnson, F.P. "The Development of the Mucous Membrane of the Oesophagus, Stomach and Small Intestine in the Human Embryo." *Am J Anat* 10 (1910): 521–561.

_____. "The Development of the Rectum in the Human Embryo." *American Journal of Anatomy* 16 (1914): 1.

Johnson, H., and A.G. Bower. "Strangulated Diaphragmatic Hernia in an Infant." *California and Western Medicine* 36 (1932): 48–49.

Johnston, P.W. "Elongation of the Upper Segment in Esophageal Atresia, Report of a Case." *Surgery* 58 (1965): 641–744.

Johnston-Saint, P. "An Outline of the History of Medicine in India." *Indian Medical Record* 49 (1929): 289–299.

Juza, R.M., et al. "Laparoscopic-Assisted Transhiatal Gastric Transposition for Long Gap Esophageal Atresia in an Infant." *Journal of Pediatric Surgery* 45 (2010): 1534–1537.

Kachlik, D., and Cech, P. "Vincenz Alexander Bochdalek, 1801–1883." *Journal of Medical Biography* 19 (2011): 38–43.

Kahle, R.H. "Omphalocele: Analysis of Twenty-One Cases from Charity Hospital of Louisiana at New Orleans." *The American Surgeon* 17 (1951): 947.

Karp, M.P., et al. "The Role of Computerized Tomography in the Evaluation of Blunt Abdominal Trauma in Children." *Journal of Pediatric Surgery* 16 (1981): 316.

Kasai, M., H. Suzur, and K. Watanabe. "Rectal Myotomy with Colectomy: A New Radical Operation for Hirschsprung's Disease." *Journal of Pediatric Surgery* 6 (1971): 36–41.

Kasai, M., et al. "Surgical Treatment of Biliary Atresia." *Journal of Pediatric Surgery* 3 (1968): 665.

Kausch, W. "Die Behandlung des Hydrocephalus der Kleinen Kinder." *Archiv der Klinische Chirurgie* 87 (1908): 709–796.

Keen, W.W. *An American Text-Book of Surgery for Practitioners and Students.* Philadelphia: W.B. Saunders Co., 1892), 37, 1209.

_____. "Exploratory Trephining and Puncture of the Brain Almost to the Lateral Ventricle for Intracranial Pressure Supposed to be Due to an Abscess in the Temporo-Sphenoidal Lobe: Temporary Improvement, Death on the Fifth Day; Autopsy, Meningitis with Effusion into the Ventricles with a Description of a Proposed Operation to Tap and Drain the Ventricles as a Definite Surgical Procedure." *Medical News* 53 (1885): 603.

_____. "Reginald Heber Fitz, M.D., LL.D.: Dr. Fitz's Services to Surgery." *Boston Medical and Surgical Journal* 169 (1913): 893–895.

_____. "Tapping the Ventricles." *British Medical Journal* 1, no. 1574 (1891): 486.

Keith, A. "Three Demonstrations on Malformations of the Hind End of the Body." *British Medical Journal* (1908): 1857–1861.

Keith, Sir A. "Malformations of the Hinder End of the Body." *British Medical Journal* 2 (1908): 1736.

Kelley, S.W. *Surgical Diseases of Children: A Modern Treatise on Pediatric Surgery*, 3d rev. ed. St. Louis: C.V. Mosby, 1929.

Kelly, K. "The History of Medicine — Early Civilizations: Prehistoric Times to 500 C.E." New York: Facts on File (2009): 51–69.

Kempe, C.H., N. Silverman, and B.F. Steele. "The Battered Child Syndrome." *Journal of the American Medical Association* 181 (1962): 17.

Kermisson, E.F. *Précis de Chirurgie Infantile.* Paris: Masson, 1906.

Keynes, G. *The Apologie and Treatise of Ambroise Paré.* London: Falcon Educational, 1951, xi.

Keyting, W.S., et al. "Pneumotosis Intestinalis, a New Concept." *Radiology* 76 (May 1961): 733–741.

Kiesewetter, W.B. "Imperforate Anus: The Role and Results of the Sacro-Abdomino-perineal Operation." *Annals of Surgery* 164 (1966): 655–61.

Kiesewetter, W.B., and J.W. Smith. "Malrotation of the Midgut in Infancy and Childhood." *Archives of Surgery* 77 (1958): 483–491.

Kilby, M.D. "The Incidence of Gastroschisis Is Increasing in the UK, Particularly Among Babies of Young Mothers." *British Medical Journal* 332 (2006): 250–251.

Killelea, B.K., and M.S. Arkovitz. "Perforated Appendicitis Presenting as Appendicoumbilical Fistula." *Pediatric Surgery International* 22 (2006): 286–288.

Killen, D.A., and H.B. Greennlee. "Transcervical Repair of an H-Type Congenital Tracheo-Esophageal Fistula, Review of the Literature." *Annals of Surgery* 162 (1965): 145–150.

Kim, S.H. "Omphalocele." *Surgical Clinics of North America* 56 (1976): 361–371.

Kimura, D., N. Iwai, Y. Sasaki, et al. "Laparascopic Versus Open Abdominoperineal Rectoplacty for Infants with High Type Anorectal Malformation." *Journal of Pediatric Surgery* 45 (December 2010): 2390–2393.

King, H., and H.B. Schumacker. "Splenic Studies, Increased Susceptibility to Infection after Splenectomy Performed in Infancy." *Annals of Surgery* 136 (1952): 239.

Kinney, J. *Saga of a Surgeon: The Life of Daniel Brainard,*

M.D. Carbondale, IL: Southern Illinois University School of Medicine, 1981, 98.

Kirklin, J.W., et al. "Surgical Treatment of Coarctation of the Aorta in a Ten Week Old Infant: Report of a Case." *Circulation* 6 (1952): 411.

Kite, J.H. "The Treatment of Congenital Clubfeet." *Journal of the American Medical Association* 99 (1932): 1156.

Klein, M.D. "Congenital Defects of the Abdominal Wall." In *Pediatric Surgery*, 6th ed., edited by J.L. Grosfeld, J.A. O'Neill, A.G. Coran, et al., 1157–1171. Philadelphia: Mosby Elsevier, 2006.

Kleinhaus, S., et al. "A Survey of the Members of the Surgical Section of the American Academy of Pediatrics." *Journal of Pediatric Surgery* 14 (1979): 588–597.

Klopp, E.J. "Amniotic Hernia." *Annals of Surgery* 73 (1921): 462–463.

Koga, Y., Y. Hayashida, K. Ikeda, K. Inokuchi, and N. Hashimoto. "Intestinal Atresia in Fetal Dogs Produced by Localized Ligation of Mesenteric Vessels." *Journal of Pediatric Surgery* 10 (1975): 949–953.

Kompanjie, E.J.O. "The First Successful Separation of Conjoined Twins in 1689: Some Additions and Corrections." *Twin Research* 7, no. 6: 537–541.

Kompanje, E.J.O., and E.J. Delwel. "The First Description of a Device for the Repeated External Ventricular Drainage in the Treatment of Congenital Hydrocephalus, Invented in 1744 by Claude-Nicolas Le Cat." *Pediatric Neurosurgery* 39 (2003): 10–13.

Konkin, D.E., et al. "Outcomes in Esophageal Atresia and Tracheo-Esophageal Fistula." *Journal of Pediatric Surgery* 38 (2003): 1726–1729.

Koop, C.E. "A Perspective on the Early Days of Pediatric Surgery." *Journal of Pediatric Surgery* 11 (July 1998): 553–560.

Kosloske, A.M., and J.R. Lilly. "Paracentesis and Lavage for Diagnosis of Intestinal Gangrene in Neonatal Necrotizing Enterocolitis." *Journal of Pediatric Surgery* 13 (1978): 315.

Kredel, L. "Über die Angeborener Dilatation und Hypertrophie des Dickdarmes." *Klinische Medizin* 53 (1904): 9–11.

Kubiak, R., et al. "Renal Function and Outcome Following Salvage Surgery for Bilateral Wilms' Tumor." *Journal of Pediatric Surgery* 39, no. 11 (November 2004): 1667–1672.

Kunieda, T., et al. "A Mutation in Endothelin-B Receptor Gene Causes Myenteric Agangionosis and Coat Color Spotting in Rats." *DNA Research* 30 (1996): 101–105.

Laberge, J.M., and H. Flageole. "Fetal Tracheal Occlusion for the Treatment of Congenital Diaphragmatic Hernia." *World Journal of Surgery* 31 (2007): 1577–1586.

Ladd, W.E. "Congenital Obstruction of the Duodenum in Children." *New England Journal of Medicine* 206 (1933): 277–283.

_____. "Immediate or Deferred Surgery for General Peritonitis Associated with Appendicitis in Children." *New England Journal of Medicine* 219 (1938): 329–333.

_____. "Surgical Diseases of the Alimentary Tract in Infants." *New England Journal of Medicine* 215 (1936): 705–708.

_____. "The Surgical Management of Esophageal Atresia and Tracheoesophageal Fistula." *New England Journal of Medicine* 230, no. 21 (May 25, 1944): 625–637.

Ladd, W.E., and Gross, R.E. *Abdominal Surgery of Infancy and Childhood.* Philadelphia: W. B. Saunders, 1941.

_____. *Congenital Atresia of Intestine and Colon in Abdominal Surgery of Infancy and Childhood.* Philadelphia: W.B. Saunders, 1941, 25–43.

_____. "Congenital Branchiogenic Anomalies: Report of 82 Cases." *American Journal of Surgery* 39 (1938): 234.

_____. "Congenital Malformations of Anus and Rectum: Report of 162 Cases." *American Journal of Surgery* 23 (1934): 167.

_____. "Intestinal Obstruction Resulting from Malrotation of the Intestines and Colon." In *Abdominal Surgery in Infancy and Childhood*, W.E. Ladd and R.E. Gross, 53–70. Philadelphia: WB Saunders, 1941.

_____. "Intussusception in Infancy and Childhood: Report of 372 Cases." *Archives of Surgery* 29 (1934): 365.

Ladd, W.E., M.D., and O. Swenson, M.D. "Esophageal Atresia and Tracheo-Esophageal Fistula." *Annals of Surgery* 125, no. 1 (January 1947): 23–40.

Ladd, W.E., and R.R. White. "Embryoma of the Kidney [Wilms' Tumor]." *Journal of the American Medical Association* 112 (1941): 1859–1863.

Laennec, R.T.H. *De l'Auscultation Mediate our Traite du Diagnostic des Maladies des Poumons et du Coeur.* Paris: J.A. Broson et J.S. Chaude, 1819 [from Hochberg, *Thoracic Surgery Before the Twentieth Century*, 641–655].

Lamb, D.S. "A Fatal Case of Congenital Tracheo-Esophageal Fistula." *Philadelphia Medical Times* 3 (1873): 705–707.

"Landsteiner, K." Wikipedia, http://en.wikipedia.org.

Langer, J.C., et al. "One-Stage Transanal Soave Pull-Through for Hirschsprung Disease: A Multicenter Experience with 141 Children." *Annals of Surgery* 238 (2003): 569–583.

_____. "Transanal One-Stage Soave Procedure for Infants with Hirschsprung Disease." *Journal of Pediatric Surgery* 34 (1999): 148–152.

Langham, M.R., et al. "ECMO Following Repair of Congenital Diaphragmatic Hernia." *Annals of Thoracic Surgery* 44 (1987): 247.

Langstaff, G. "Intussusception." *Edinburgh Medical and Chirurgical Journal* 3 (1807): 262–268.

Lanman, T.H. "Congenital Atresia of the Esophagus, a Study of Thirty-Two Cases." *Archives of Surgery* 41 (1940): 1060–1083.

Lascaratos, J.G., I.G. Panourias, and D.E. Sakas. "Hydrocephalus According to Byzantine Writers." *Neurosurgery* 55 (2004): 214–221.

Laufman, H., W.B. Martin, H. Method, S.W. Tuell, and H. Harding. "Observations in Strangulation Obstruction: The Fate of Sterile Devascularized Intestine in the Peritoneal Cavity." *Archives of Surgery* 59 (1949): 550–564.

Laughon, M., et al. "Rising Birth Prevalence of Gastroschisis." *Journal of Perinatology* 23 (2003): 291–293.

Le Cat, C.N. "A New Trocar for the Puncture in the Hydrocephalus and for Other Evacuations, which are Necessary to be Made at Different Times." *Philosophical Transactions of the Royal Society of London* 157 (1751): 267–272.

Leenders, E., and W.K. Sieber. "Congenital Megacolon Observation by Frederick Ruysch —1691." *Journal of Pediatric Surgery* 5 (1970): 1–3.

Leichtenstern, O. "Intussusception, Invagination, und Darmein Schiebung." *Ziemssen's Cyclopaedia of the Practice of Medicine* 7 (1877): 610–624.

LeMasne, A., et al. "Intussusception in Infants and Children: Feasibility of Ambulatory Management." *European Journal of Pediatrics* 158 (1999): 707–710.

Leonardo, R.A., M.D., Ch.M., F.I.C.S. *A History of Surgery.* New York: Froben, 1943, 34–39.

Le Vay, D. *The History of Orthopaedics: An Account of the*

Study and Practice of Orthopaedics from the Earliest Times to the Modern Era. London: Parthenon, 1990, p. 68 [citing F.P. Verney, *The Memoirs of the Verney Family During the Civil War*, London, 1894].

Leven, N.L., M.D., "Congenital Atresia of the Esophagus with Tracheoesophageal Fistula, Report of Successful Extrapleural Ligation of Fistulous Communication and Cervical Esophagostomy." *Journal of Thoracic Surgery* 10 (1941): 648–657.

_____, et al. "The Surgical Management of Congenital Atresia of the Esophagus and Tracheo-Esophageal Fistula." *Annals of Surgery* 136, no. 4 (October 1952): 701–717.

Levy, H., Jr., and L.H. Linder. "Major Abdominal Trauma in Children." *American Journal of Surgery* 122 (1970): 55.

Levy, R.J., et al. "Persistent Pulmonary Hypertension in a Newborn with Congenital Diaphragmatic Hernia: Successful Management with Tolazoline." *Pediatrics* 60 (1977): 740.

Lewis, D., and C. Grulee. "The Pylorus After Gastroenterostomy for Congenital Pyloric Stenosis." *Journal of the American Medical Association* 64 (January 30, 1915): 410–412.

Lewis, P. ed. *History of Medicine.* London: Chancellor, 2001, 89.

Lewitt, W. "Enlargement of the Left Colon." *Chicago Medical Journal* 24 (1897): 359–361.

Li, F. "Zhang Zhong-Jing's Academic Innovation." *Negative* 1, no. 1 (2010): 9–11.

Liebow, E.M. *Dr. Joe Bell, Model for Sherlock Holmes* (Bowling Green, OH: Bowling Green University Popular Press, 1982), 12–13.

Lipshutz, G.S., et al. "A Strategy for Primary Reconstruction of Long Gap Esophageal Atresia Using Neonatal Colon Esophagoplasty: A Case Report." *Journal of Pediatric Surgery* 34, no. 1 (1999): 75–78.

Little, E.M. *Orthopaedics Before Stromeyer: The Robert Jones Birthday Volume.* Oxford: Oxford Medical, 1928.

Little, W.J. *A Treatise on the Nature of Club-Foot and Analogous Distortions.* London: Jeffs, 1839.

Liviaditis, A. "Esophageal Atresia: A Method of Overcoming Large Segmental Gaps." *Z. Kindenchirurgie* 13 (1973): 298–306.

Ljunggren, B., and G.W. Bruyn, eds. *The Nobel Prize in Medicine and the Karolinska Institute.* Basel: Karger, 2002.

Lloyd, G. *Hippocratic Writings*, 4th ed. London: Penguin, 1983.

Lloyd, J.R. "Etiology of Gastrointestinal Perforations in the Newborn." *Journal of Pediatric Surgery* 4 (1969): 77.

Lobe, T.E., et al. "Thoracoscopic Repair of Esophageal Atresia in an Infant, a Surgical First." *Pediatric Endosurgery Innovation Techniques* 3 (1999): 141–148.

Loening-Baucke, V. "Biofeedback Treatment for Chronic Constipation and Encopresis in Childhood: Long-term Outcome." *Pediatrics* 96, no. 1 (1995): 105–110.

Longino, L.A., W.J. Wooley, and R.E. Gross. "Esophageal Replacement in Infants and Children with the Use of a Segment of Colon." *Journal of the American Medical Association* 171 (1959): 1187.

Longmire, W.P. "Congenital Atresia and Tracheo-Esophageal Fistula." *Archives of Surgery* 55 (1947): 330.

Lorber, J. "Results of Treatment of Myelomeningocele: An Analysis of 524 Unselected Cases with Special References to Possible Selection for Treatment." *Developmental Medicine and Child Neurology* 13 (1971): 279.

Loretta, P. "Divulsioni del Piloro e del Cardias." *Gazzete Di Ospedale Milano* 8 (1887): 803.

Louw, J.H. "Congenital Intestinal Atresia and Stenosis in the Newborn." *S Afr J Clin Sci* 3 (1952): 109–129.

_____. "Congenital Intestinal Atresia and Stenosis in the Newborn: Observations on its Pathogenesis and Treatment." *Annals Royal College Surgeons England* 25 (1959): 209–234.

_____, and Barnard, C.N. "Congenital Intestinal Atresia: Observations on its Origin." *Lancet* 2 (1955): 1065–1067.

Loveland, J. "Reginald Heber Fitz, the Exponent of Appendicitis." *Yale Journal of Biology and Medicine* 6 (1937): 509–520.

Luck, S.R., et al. "Gastroschisis in 106 Consecutive Newborn Infants." *Surgery* 98 (1985): 677–683.

Lund, D.P., and W.H. Hendren. "Cloacal Exstrophy: A 25-Year Experience with 50 Cases." *Journal of Pediatric Surgery* 36 (2001): 68–75.

Lynn, H.B., and E.E. Espinas. "Intestinal Atresia: An Attempt to Relate Location to Embryologic Processes." *Archives of Surgery* 79 (1959): 357–361.

Lyon, W.S. *Encyclopedia of Native American Healing.* New York, London: W.W. Norton, 138.

MacCallum, W.G. *William Stewart Halsted, Surgeon.* Baltimore: The Johns Hopkins Press, 1930, 21–28.

Mack, C. "A History of Hypertrophic Pyloric Stenosis and Its Treatment." *Bulletin of the History of Medicine* 12 (October 1942): 465–485, 595–615, 666–689.

"Mackenzie, M." Wikipedia, http://en.wikipedia.org.

_____. "Malformations of the Esophagus." *Archives of Laryngology* 1, no. 4 (December 1880): 301–315.

MacKinlay, G.A., M.B., B.S, L.R.C.P., F.R.C.P.C.H., F.R.C.S., ed. "Esophageal Atresia Surgery in the 21st Century." *Seminars in Pediatric Surgery* 18 (2009): 20–22.

MacLennan, A. "The Radical Cure of Inguinal Hernia in Children, with Special Reference to the Embryological Rests found Associated with the Sacs." *British Journal of Surgery* 9 (1922): 445–448.

MacNab, G.H. "Intussusception." In *British Surgical Practice*, edited by E.R. Carling and J.P. Ross, 160–168. London: Butterworth, 1948.

Madoff, R.D., et al. "Standards for Anal Sphincter Replacement." *Diseases of the Colon and Rectum* 43, no. 2 (2000): 135–141.

Mahour, G.H., M.M. Wooley and J.L. Gwin. "Elongation of the Upper Pouch and Delayed Anatomic Reconstruction in Esohageal Atresia." *Journal of Pediatric Surgery* 9 (1974): 373–383.

Majno, Guido. *The Healing Hand: Man and Wound in the Ancient World.* Cambridge, MA: Harvard University Press, 1970, 112–124 and 186–188.

Majumdar R.C., and A.D. Pusalker, eds. *The History and Culture of the Indian People, Volume 1: The Vedic Age.* Bombay: Bharatiya Vidya Bhavan, 1951.

Mall, F.P. "Development of the Human Intestine and its Position in the Adult." *Bull Johns Hopkins Hosp* 9 (1898): 197–208.

Malone, P.S., P.G. Ransley and E.M. Kiely. "Preliminary Report: The Antegrade Continence Enema." *Lancet* 336, no. 8725 (November 1990): 1217–1218.

Manning, P.B., M.D., et al. "Fifty Years' Experience with Esophageal Atresia and Tracheoesophageal Fistula, Beginning with Cameron Haight's First Operation in 1935." *Annals of Surgery* 204, no. 4 (October 1986): 446–451.

Manson G. "Anomalies of Intestinal Rotation and Mesenteric Fixation: Review of the Literature with Report of Nine Cases." *Journal of Pediatrics* 45 (1954): 214–233.

Marfan, A. "De la Constipation des Nourrissons et en Particular de la Constipation d'Origine Congénitale." *Ren Mens Mal De Lent* 13 (1895): 153–157.

Marshall, J. *Mohenjo-Daro and the Indus Civilizations*, Vol. I. Delhi: Indological Book House, 1973.

Martin, E., and V. Burden. "The Surgical Significance of the Rectosigmoid Sphincter." *Annals of Surgery* Vol. 86 (1927): 86–91.

Martin, J.D., Jr., and D.C. Elkin. "Congenital Atresia of the Colon." *Annals of Surgery* 105 (1937): 192–198.

Martin, L.W., and J.T. Zerella. "Jejunoileal Atresia: A Proposed Classification." *Journal of Pediatric Surgery* 11 (1976): 399–403.

Martin, L.W., and R.V. Perrin. "Neonatal Perforation of the Appendix in Association with Hirschprung's Disease." *Annals of Surgery* 144 (November 1967): 799.

Martin, M. "Observateur des Sciences Medicales Marseille." *Exposé des Traveaux de la Société Royale de Medicine de Marseille* 44 (1821) [from N.A. Meyers, "The History of Oesophageal Atresia and Tracheo-Oesophageal Fistula, 1670–1984." *Progress in Pediatric Surgery* 20 (1986): 106–157].

Martin, R.W. "Screening for Fetal Abdominal Wall Defects." *Obstetrics and Gynecology Clinics of North America* 25 (1998): 517–526.

Martin-Laberge, J., O. Bose, S. Yazbeck, et al. "The Anterior Perineal Approach for Pullthrough Operations in High Imperforate Anus." *Journal of Pediatric Surgery* 18 (1983): 774.

Martin-Laberge, J., et al. "The Anterior Perineal Approach for Pull-Through Operations in High Imperforate Anus." *Journal of Pediatric Surgery* 18 (1983): 774.

Martucciello, G., et al. "Immunohistochemical Localization of RET Protein in Hirschsprung's Disease." *Journal of Pediatric Surgery* 30 (1995): 433–436.

Masiakos, P.T., and S.H. Ein. "The History of Hirschsprung's Disease: Then and Now." *Seminar in Colon and Rectal Surgery* 17 (2006): 10–19.

Matas, R. "Intralaryngeal Insufflation for the Relief of Acute Surgical Pneumothorax: Its History and Methods with a Description of the Latest Devices for this Purpose." *Journal of the American Medical Association* 34 (1900): 1468–1473.

_____. "The Surgical Treatment of Congenital Anal Rectal Imperforation Considered in the Light of Modern Operative Procedures." *Transactions of the American Surgical Association* (1896): 453–553.

Matson, D.W. *Neurosurgery of Infancy and Childhood*, 2d ed. (Springfield, IL: Charles C. Thomas, 1969, 224–258.

Mazziotti, M.V., S.M. Strasberg, and J.C. Langer. Intestinal Rotation Abnormalities without Volvulus: The Role of Laparoscopy." *J Am Coll Surg* 185 (1997): 172–176.

McAlister, W.H. "Intussusception: Even Hippocrates Did Not Standardize His Technique of Enema Reduction." *Radiology* 206 (1998): 595–598.

McBurney, C. "Experience with Early Operative Interference in Cases of Disease of the Vermiform Appendix." *New York Medical Journal* 50 (1889): 676–684.

McCabe, L., et al. "Overo Lethal White Foal Syndrome: Equine Model of Aganglionic Megacolon (Hirschsprung Disease)." *American Journal of Medical Genetics* 36 (1990): 336–340.

McCauley, J.C. "Clubfoot." *Clinical Orthopedics* 44 (1966): 51.

McClone, D.G., et al, eds. *Disorders of the Developing Nervous System, Diagnosis and Treatment*. Boston: Blackwell Scientific, 1986, 94–105.

McDermott, V.G. "Childhood Intussusception and Approaches to Treatment: A Historical Review." *Pediatric Radiology* 24 (1994): 153–155.

McIntosh, R., and E.J. Donovan. "Disturbances of Rotation of the Intestinal Tract: Clinical Picture Based on Observations in 20 Cases." *Am J Dis Child* 57 (1939): 116–166.

McKay, D.W. "New Concept of and Approach to Clubfoot Treatment: Section I — Principles and Morbid Anatomy." *Journal of Pediatric Orthopedics* 2, no. 4 (1982): 347–56.

McLone, D.G. "Myelomeningocele." In *Neurological Surgery*, vol. 2, 4th ed., by Julian R. Youmans, 843–860. Philadelphia: W.B. Saunders.

_____. "Treatment of Myelomeningocele and Arguments Against Selection." *Clinical Neurosurgery* 33 (1986): 359.

_____, D. Czyzeqski, and A.J. Raimondi. "The Effects of Complications on Intellectual Function in 173 Children with Myelomeningocele." In *Surgery of the Developing Nervous System*, 49–60. New York: Grune and Stratton, 1982.

McNamara, J.J., A.J. Eraklis, and R.E. Gross. "Congenital Postero-Lateral Diaphragmatic Hernia in the Newborn." *Journal of Thoracic and Cardiovascular Surgery* 55 (1968): 55.

Meade, R.H. "The Evolution of Surgery for Appendicitis." *Surgery* 55 (1964): 741–752.

Meckel, A.A. "Verschliessung der Aorta am vierteu Brustwirbel." *Archiv. f. Anat. u Physiol.* (1827): 345.

Meckel, J.F. "Anatomic and Physiological Observations, Concerning Extraordinary Dilation of the Heart, Which Came from the fact that the Aortic Conduit Was Too Narrow." *Memoirs of the Royal Academy of Sciences*, Berlin, 1768.

_____. "Blindengagageschichte des darmkanals der sängeriere und namentlich der menschen." *Deutsche Arch 1 Physiol* 3 (1817): 1.

_____. *Handbuch der Pathologischen Anatomie* VI, 1812, 21–22, 179–180, 493–507.

Medical papers dedicated to Reginald Heber Fitz in honor of his 65th birthday; reprinted from *Boston Medical and Surgical Journal* 158, no. 19 (May 7, 1908).

Medieval Manuscripts of the National Library of Medicine. http://www.nlm.nih.gov/.

Meier-Ruge, W. "Uberlein Erkrank Ungsbild des Colon mit Hirschsprung Symptomatik." *Verh Deutsche Ges Pathol* 55 (1971): 506–510, 91.

Melicow, M.M. "Castrati Singers and the Lost 'Cords.'" *Bull NY Acad Med* (1983) 59: 744–764.

Mellor, S.T. "Malformations of the Oesophagus." *London Medical Gazette* 2 (1846): 542.

Meltzer, S.J. "On Congenital Hypertrophic Stenosis of the Pylorus in Infants." *Medical Record of New York* 54 (August 1898): 253–259.

Mercier, A. "Retrécissement avec oblitération presque complète de la portion thoracique de aorte." *Bulletins et memoires de la societe anatomique de Paris* 14 (1839): 153.

Meyer, K.A., S.J. Hoffman, and J.K. Amtman. "Diaphragmatic Hernia in the Newborn, Review of the Literature and Report of a Case." *American Journal of Diseases of Children* 56 (1938): 600–607.

Miculicz, J. "Beitrag zur Pathologie und Therapie des Hydrocephalus mitt Grenzgeb," *Med Chir.* Vol. 1 (1896): 264.

Miller, E.M., A.H. Parmalee, and H.N. Sanford. "Diaphragmatic Hernia in Infants, Report of Two Cases. *Archives of Surgery* 38, no. 6 (June 1939): 979–989.

Miller, Wayne G. *King of Hearts*. New York: Times Books, 2000.

Minkes, R.K., et al. "Routine Insertion of a Silastic Spring-Loaded Silo for Infants with Gastroschisis." *Journal of Pediatric Surgery* 35 (2000): 843–848.

Mitchell, S. "Intussusception in Children." *Lancet* 904 (1836): 1837–1838.

Mizrahi, A., et al. "Necrotizing Enterocolitis in Premature Infants." *Journal of Pediatrics* 66 no. 4 (1965): 697–706.

Mollard, P., J. Marechal and M. DeBeaujeu. "Surgical Treatment of High Imperforate Anus with Definition of the Puborectalis by an Anterior Approach." *Journal of Pediatric Surgery* 13 (1978): 1499.

Monrad, S. "Acute Invagination of the Intestine in Small Children." *Archives of Disease in Childhood* 1 (1926): 323–338.

Montgomery, S. *Walking with the Great Apes: Jane Goodall, Dian Fossey, Biruté Galdikas*. Boston: Houghton-Mifflin, 7.

Montupet, P., and C. Esposito. "Laparoscopic Treatment of Congenital Inguinal Hernia in Children." *Journal of Pediatric Surgery* 34 (1999): 420–23.

Moody, D.S., et al. "Use of Tolazoline in Newborn Infants with Diaphragmatic Hernia and Severe Cardiopulmonary Disease." *Journal of Thoracic and Cardiovascular Surgery* 75 (1978): 725.

Moore, J.E. "Spina Bifida, with a Report of Three Hundred and Eighty-five Cases Treated by Excision." *Surgery, Gynecology and Obstetrics* 1 (1905): 137–140.

Moore, T.C., and G.E. Stokes. "Gastroschisis: Report of Two Cases Treated by a Modification of the Gross Operation for Omphalocele." *Surgery* 33 (1953): 112–120.

Moore, W. *The Knife Man: The Extraordinary Life and Times of John Hunter, Father of Modern Surgery*. New York: Broadway, 2005.

Morgagni, G.B. Book III, Of Diseases of the Belly; Letter XLVIII, Article 53–54. In *The Seats and Causes of Diseases Investigated by Anatomy, in Five Books, Containing a Great Variety of Dissections, with Remarks*, trans. B. Alexander. London, 1769, 756–761.

_____. *De Sedibus et Causis Morborum per Anatomen Indagatis Libri Quinque*, trans. B. Alexander. Book III, Letter XXX, Article 12. 1761.

_____. *The Seats and Causes of Diseases Investigated by Anatomy*, trans. B. Alexander. New York: Hafner, 1960, 154–163.

Morgagni, Giovanni Battiste. *The Seats and Causes of Disease, Investigated by Anatomy, in Five Books*, trans. Benjamin Alexander, M.D. New York: Library of the New York Academy of Medicine/Hafner, 1960.

Morton, J. "Case of Spina Bifida Cured by Injection." *British Medical Journal* 1 (1872): 632–633.

Moss, K. "The 'Baby Doe' Legislation, Its Rise and Fall." *Policy Studies Journal* 15 no. 4 (1987): 629–651.

Moss, R.L., M.D., RR. Dimmit, M.D., M.S.P.H., and D.C. Barnhart, M.D. "Laparotomy Versus Peritoneal Drainage for Necrotizing Enterocolitis and Perforation." *New England Journal of Medicine* 354, no. 21 (May 25, 2006): 2225–2234.

Mukhopadhyaya, G. *The Surgical Instruments of the Hindus, with a Comparative Study of the Surgical Instruments of Greek, Roman, Arab and the Modern European Surgeons*, vol. 1. Calcutta: Calcutta University Press, 1913.

Mukhopdhyay, G.N. *History of Indian Medicine*, in two volumes. Calcutta: Calcutta University Press, 1923–29.

Mullins, M.E., and Z. Horowitz. "Iatrogenic Neonatal Mercury Poisoning from Mercurochrome Treatment of a Large Omphalocele." *Clinical Pediatrics* 38 (1999) 111–112.

Munro, J.C. "Ligation of the Ductus Arteriosus." *Annals of Surgery* 46 (1907): 335.

Muratore, C.S., and J.M. Wilson. "Congenital Diaphragmatic Hernia: Where Are We and Where Do We Go From Here?" *Seminars in Perinatology* 24, no. 6 (December 2000): 418–428.

Museum of Disability. http://www.museumofdisability.org/medicine_establishment.asp.

Muthu, C. *The Antiquity of Hindu Medicine and Civilization*, 3d ed. Boston: Milford House, 1931.

Mya, G. "Due Osservazioni di Dilatazione ed Impertrofia Congenita del Colon." *Sperimentale* 48 (1894): 215–231.

Myers, N.A. "The History of Oesophageal Atresia and Tracheo-Oesophageal Fistula, 1670–1984." *Progress in Pediatric Surgery* 20 (1986): 106–157.

Nakayama, D., J. Templeton, and M. Zeigler, et al. "Complications of Posterior Sagittal Anorectoplasty." *Journal of Pediatric Surgery* 21 (1986): 488.

Neuburger, M. "The Medicine of the Indians." In *History of Medicine*, vol. 1, edited by M. Neuburger, 43–60. London: Oxford University Press.

Nguyen, T., et al. "Laparoscopic Transhiatal Gastric Transposition Preserving the Abdominal Esophagus for Long Gap Esophageal Atresia." *Journal of Pediatric Surgical Specialties* 3 (2008): 32–33.

Nicoll, J. "Congenital Hypertrophic Stenosis of the Pylorus with an Account of a Case Successfully Treated by Operation." *British Medical Journal* 21 (1900): 571.

_____. "Several Patients from a Further Series of Cases of Congenital Obstruction of the Pylorus Treated by Operation." *Glasgow Medico–Chirurgical Journal* 2, no. 65 (1906): 253.

Nicoll, J.H. "Case of Hydrocephalus in Which Peritoneo-Menigeal Drainage has been Carried Out." *Glasgow Medical Journal* 63 (January-June 1905): 187–191.

_____. "The Radical Cure of Spina Bifida, Observations of Certain Points in a Series of over Thirty Cases Treated by Open Operation." *British Medical Journal* (October 15, 1898): 1142–1146.

Niebuhr, W.A., C.A. Dresch, and F.W. Logan. "Hernia into the Umbilical Cord, Containing the Entire Liver and Gallbladder." *Journal of the American Medical Association* 103 (1934): 16–18.

Nixon, H.H. "An Experimental Study of Propulsion in Isolated Small Intestine and Applications to Surgery in the Newborn." *Ann Roy Coll Surg Engl* 24 (1960): 105–124.

_____. "Intestinal Obstruction in the Newborn." *Arch Dis Child* 30 (1955): 13–22.

_____, and R. Tawes. "Etiolocty and Treatment of Small Intestinal Atresia: Analysis of a Series of 127 Jejunoileal Atresias and Comparison with 62 Duodenal Atresias." *Surgery* 69 (1971): 41–51.

"Nocard, E." Wikipedia, http://en.wikipedia.org.

Noonan, K.J., M.D., and B.S. Richards, M.D. "Nonsurgical Management of Idiopathic Clubfoot." *Journal of the American Academy of Orthopedic Surgeons* 11, no. 6 (November/December 2003): 392–40.

Nulsen, F.E., and E.B. Spitz. "Treatment of Hydrocephalus by Direct Shunt from Ventricle to Jugular Vein." *Surgery Forum* 94 (1951): 399–403.

Nunn, J.F. *Ancient Egyptian Medicine*. Norman: University of Oklahoma Press, 1996, 24–41.

Oberniedermayr, A. *Lehrbuch der Chirurgie und Orthopadie des Kindesalters*. Berlin, Göttingen, Heidelberg: Springer, 1959.

O'Dwyer, J. "Operation for the Relief of Congenital Diaphragmatic Hernia." *Archives of Pediatrics* 9 (1889): 130–132.

_____. "Oral Intubation for Diptheria." *Medical Record* 32 (1887): 557.

O'Leary, C.M., and C.E. Clymer. "Umbilical Hernia." *American Journal of Surgery* 52 (1941): 38–43.

O'Leary, De Lacy, D.D. *How Greek Science Passed to the Arabs*. London: Routledge and Kegan Paul, 1949, 184 [available at http://www.aina.org/books/hgsptta.htm].

Olshausen, R.Z. "Zur Therapie der Nabelschnurhernien." *Archiv für Gynakologie* 28 (1887): 443 [translated by Wolfgang Cerwinka, M.D.].

O'Neill, J.A., Jr., "Cloacal Exstrophy." In *Pediatric Surgery*, 6th ed., edited by J.L. Grosfeld, J.A. O'Neill, A.G. Coran, et al., 1859–1869. Philadelphia: Mosby Elsevier, 2006.

"Oral History Project: F. Douglas Stephens, M.D." Interviewed by John M. Hutson, M.D., May 30, 2007, in Melbourne, Australia. American Academy of Pediatrics.

Osler, Sir William. *The Evolution of Modern Medicine*. New Haven, CT: Yale University Press, 1921, 29–35.

Osler, W. "Cases of Dilatation of the Colon in Young Children." *Johns Hopkins Hospital Bulletin* 30 (1893): 41–43.

_____. "On Dilatation of the Colon in Young Children." *Archives of Pediatrics* 111 (1893): 59–62.

Osler, W., M.D., M.R.C.P.L. "Two Cases of Striated Myo-Sarcoma of the Kidney." *Journal of Anatomy and Physiology* 14, no. 2 (1880): 229–233.

Otherson, A.B. "Intubation Injuries of the Trachea in Children." *Annals of Surgery* 189, no. 5 (1979): 601.

Otherson, H.B., M.D. "Ephraim McDowell, the Qualities of a Good Surgeon." *Annals of Surgery* 239, no. 5 (May 2004): 648.

Owen, E., M.B., F.R.C.S. *The Surgical Diseases of Children*. London, Paris and Melbourne: Cassell and Company, Limited, 1897.

Oxford, J., D.T. Cass, and M.J. Glasson. "Advances in the Treatment of Oesophageal Atresia over Three Decades, the 1970s and the 1990s." *Pediatric Surgery International* 20 (2004): 412–417.

Pagès, R. "Le Rôle du Sphincter Interne." *Annales de Chirurgie Infantile* 11 (1970): 145–149.

Paré, A. Book 1, *An Introduction or Compendious Way to Chyrurgerie*. London, 1634, 45

_____. Book 23, *Of the Meanes and Manner to Repaire or Supply the Natural or Accidental Defects or Wants to a Mans Body*. London, 1634, 874.

_____. Book 24, Chapter 66, in *The Works of that Famous Chirugen*. London: Thomas Cotes and R. Young, 1634, 959.

_____. Book 25, Of Monsters and Prodigies (London, 1634), 972

_____. "Of Divers Preternaturall Affairs Whose Cure is Performed by Surgery." In Book 17. London: 1634, 662

_____. "Of the Cure that is Rendered by Surgery." In Book 17. London: 1634, 664

_____. *Oeuvres Complètes*, 1585, vol. 111. Genève: Facsimile Slatkine Reprints, 1970, 489

_____. *The Workes of Ambrose Paréy, Translated Out of Latine and Compared with the French*, trans. Th. Johnson. London: Th. Cotes and R. Young, 1634.

Paris, M. "Retrécissement considerable de l'aorte pectorale, observé a l'Hôtel Dieu de Paris." *J. Chir. de Desalt* 2 (1791): 107.

Park, R., M.D. "Successful Nephrectomy on a Patient of Twenty-Three Months." *Transactions of the American Surgical Association* (1886): 259–262, and *Medical News* 48 (May 22, 1886): 567–569.

Parker, R.W., and S.G. Shattock. "The Pathology and Etiology of Congenital Club-Foot." *Transactions of the Pathologists' Society of London* 35: 423

Parry, C.H. "Singular and Fatal Accumulation of Faeces." In *Collections from the Unpublished Medical Writings of the Late C.H. Parry*, vol. 2, edited by C. H. Parry, 380. London: Underwoods, 1825.

Patel, M.M., et al. "Intussusception and Rotavirus Vaccination: A Review of the Available Evidence." *Expert Review of Vaccines* 8 (2009): 1555–1564.

Patterson, R.L., and R.E. Gross. "Adenocarcinoma of Stomach: Case Occurring in Man 27 Years of Age." *New England Journal of Medicine* 210 (1934): 1161.

Payr, E. "Drainage der Hirnventrikal Mittels Frei Transplantierter Blotgefabe Bremerkungen uber Hydrocephalus." *Archiv der Klinische Chirurgie* 87 (1908): 801.

Peikoff, S.S. "Exomphalos." *Canadian Medical Journal* 52 (1945): 600–602.

Peña, A., D. Amroch, C. Baeza, L. Csury and G. Rodriguez. "The Effects of the Posterior Sagittal Approach on Rectal Function (Experimental Study)." *Journal of Pediatric Surgery* 28, no. 6 (1993): 773–778.

Peña, A.P. "Current Management of Anorectal Anomalies." *Surgical Clinics of North America* 72, no. 6 (December 1992): 1393–1416.

_____. "Posterior Sagittal Anorectoplasty as a Secondary Operation for Fecal Incontinence Through Use of a Levator Sling." *Journal of Pediatric Surgery*18 (1983): 762.

_____. "Posterior Sagittal Anorectoplasty: Results in the Management of 332 Cases of Anorectal Malformation. *Pediatric Surgery International* 3 (1988): 94–104.

Peña, A.P., and M. Behery. "Megasigmoid: A Source of Pseudo-Incontinence in Children with Repaired Anorectal Malformations." *Journal of Pediatric Surgery* 28 no. 2 (1993): 199–203.

Peña, A.P., and P.A. Devries. "Posterior Sagittal Anorectoplasty: Important Technical Consideration and New Applications." *Journal of Pediatric Surgery* 17, no. 6 (1982): 796–811.

Pendelton, C., et al. "Harvey Cushing's Use of a Transplanted Human Vein to Treat Hydrocephalus in the Early 1900s." *Journal of Neurosurgery: Pediatrics* 5, no. 5 (2010): 423–427.

Persky, L.O., and W.E. Forsythe. "Renal Trauma in Children." *Journal of the American Medical Association* 182 (November 17, 1962): 708–712.

Pescatori, M., et al. "Transanal Electrostimulation for Fecal Incontinence: Clinical, Psychologic and Manometric Prospective Study." *Diseases of the Colon and Rectum* 34, no. 7: 540.

Petterson, C. "Experience in Esophageal Reconstruction." *Archives, Diseases of Surgery* 37 (1962): 184–189.

Phelps, A.M. *International Congress of Medical Science*. Copenhagen, 1884.

Pickrell, K.L., T.R. Bradbent, W. Masters, et al. "Construction of a Rectal Sphincter and Restoration of Anal Continence by Transplanting the Gracilis Muscle." *Annals of Surgery* 135, (1952): 853.

Pieretti, R., B. Shandling, and C.A. Stephens. "Resistant

Esophageal Stenosis with Reflux after Repair of Esophageal Atresia, a Therapeutic Approach." *Journal of Pediatric Surgery* 9 (1974): 355–357.

Pilcher, J.E. "Felix Wurtz and Pierre Franco — A Glimpse of the Sixteenth Century," *Annals of Surgery* 24 (October 1896): 505–535.

_____. "Guy de Chauliac and Henri de Mondeville, a Surgical Retrospect." *Annals of Surgery* 21, no. 1 (1895): 84–102.

Plato. *The Collected Dialogues.* Edith Hamilton and Huntington Cairns, eds. Bollinger Series, LXXI. Princeton, NJ: Princeton University Press, 1961, lines 309–311.

Ponseti, I.V. "Treatment of Congenital Clubfoot." *Journal of Bone and Joint Surgery* 74A (1992): 448–454.

Postlethwaite, R. "Colonic Interposition of Esophageal Replacement." *Surgery, Gynecology and Obstetrics* 156 (1983): 377.

Potts, W.J. *The Surgeon and the Child.* Philadelphia, London: W.B. Saunders, 1959.

Potts W.J., and S. Gibson. "Aortico–Pulmonary Anastomosis in Congenital Pulmonary Stenosis." *Journal of the American Medical Association* 137 (1948): 343.

Potts, W.J., S. Smith and S. Gibson, S. "Anastomosis of the Aorta to the Pulmonary Artery for Certain Types of Congenital Heart Disease." *Journal of the American Medical Association* 132 (1946): 627.

Potts, W.J., W.L. Riker and J.E. Lewis. "The Treatment of Inguinal Hernia in Infants and Children." *Annals of Surgery* 132 (1950): 566–74.

Pouchelle, Marie-Christine. *The Body and Surgery in the Middle Ages.* New Brunswick, NJ: Rutgers University Press, 1990, 15–18.

Powel, R., J. Sherman, and J. Raffensperger. "Megarectum: A Rare Complication of Imperforate Anus Repair and Its Surgical Correction by Endorectal Pull-Through." *Journal of Pediatric Surgery* 17 (1982): 786.

Powell, D.M., H.B. Othersen and C.D. Smith. "Malrotation of the Intestines in Children: The Effect of Age on Presentation and Therapy." *Journal of Pediatric Surgery* 24 (1989) :777–780.

Powell, R.W. "Stapled Intestinal Anastomosis in Neonates and Infants: Use of the Endoscopic Intestinal Stapler." *Journal of Pediatric Surgery* 30 (1995): 195–197.

Power, D. "A Case of Congenital Umbilical Hernia." *Transactions of the Pathological Society of London* XXXIX (1888): 108.

Pracros, J.P., L. Sann, F. Genin, et al. "Ultrasound Diagnosis of Midgut Volvulus: The 'Whirlpool' Sign." *Pediatr Radiol* 22 (1992): 18–20.

Pringle, K.C., Y. Sato, and R.T. Soper. "Magnetic Resonance Imaging as an Adjunct to Planning an Anorectal Pull-Through." *Journal of Pediatric Surgery* 22 no. 6 (1987): 571–574.

Proctor, M.L., et al. "Correlation Between Radiographic Transition Zone and Level of Aganglionosis in Hirschsprung's Disease: Implications for Surgical Approach." *Journal of Pediatric Surgery* 38 (2003): 775–778.

Pryles, C.V., and A. Huros. "Congenital Tracheo-Esophageal Fistula without Atresia: Report of a Case with Postmortem Findings." *New England Journal of Medicine* 253 (1955): 855–859.

Pudenz, R.H. "Experimental and Clinical Observations on the Shunting of Cerebrospinal Fluid into the Circulating System." In *Clinical Neurosurgery, Congress of Neurological Surgeons,* 98–115. Baltimore: Williams and Wilkins, 1958.

_____. "The Surgical Treatment of Hydrocephalus: An Historical Review." *Surgical Neurology* 15c (1981): 15–26.

Puri, P., and T. Shinkai, "Pathogenesis of Hirschsprung's Disease and its Variants: Recent Progress." *Seminars in Pediatric Surgery* 13 (2004): 18–24.

Purnaropoules, G., and K. Emmanuel. *Hippocrates: All His Works (in Greek),* vol. 1. Athens: Martinos, 1967, 400–429.

Quinn, S. *Marie Curie: A Life.* New York, London and Toronto: Simon and Schuster, 1995, 158–159.

Radbill, S.X. "A History of Children's Hospitals." *American Journal of Diseases of Children* 90 (1955): 411–416.

Raffensperger, J. *Swenson's Pediatric Surgery,* 5th ed. East Norwalk, CT: Appleton and Lange, 1990, 617–619, 633–634.

_____. "Conjoined Twins of Polynesia." *Rapi Nui Journal, The Journal of Easter Island* 15, no. 2 (October 2001): 105–109.

Raffensperger, J.G. *The Acute Abdomen in Infancy and Childhood.* Philadelphia: J.B. Lippincott, 1970.

_____. "Hirschsprung's Disease: A Historical Review." *Bulletin de la Société des Sciences Medicales die Grand Duchy de Luxembourg* 124 (1987): 31–36.

_____. "John Cooper Forster and the First Textbook of Pediatric Surgery in the English Language." *Guy's Hospital Reports* 113, no. 2 (1964): 172–178.

_____. *The Old Lady on Harrison Street: Cook County Hospital, 1833–1995.* New York and Washington, D.C.: Peter Lang, 1997, 50.

_____. "A Review of the First Textbook of Pediatric Surgery in the English Language." *Journal of Pediatric Surgery* 4, no. 4 (August 1969): 403–405.

Raffensperger, J.G., J.B. Condon and J. Greengard. "Complications of Gastric and Duodenal Ulcers in Infancy and Childhood." *Surgery, Gynecology and Obstetrics* 123 (December 1966): 1269–1274.

Raffensperger, J.G., et al. "Intestinal Bypass of the Esophagus." *Journal of Pediatric Surgery* 31 no. 1 (1996): 38–47.

Raimondi, A.J., and W. Matsumoto. "A Simplified Technique for Performing the Ventriculo-Peritoneal Shunt: Technical Note." *Journal of Neurosurgery* 26 (1967): 357.

Raju, T.N.K., M.D., D.C.H. "Soranus of Ephesus: Who Was He and What Did He Do?" Neonatology on the Web, http://www.neonatology.org/.

Raju, V.K. "Sushruta of Ancient India." *Indian Journal of Ophthalmology* 51 (2003): 119–122.

Ramirez, O.M., E. Russ and A.L. Dillon. "'Component Separation' Method for Closure of Abdominal Wall Defects: An Anatomical and Clinical Study." *Plastic and Reconstructive Surgery* 86 (1990): 519–526.

Ramstedt, C. "Zur Operation der Angeborenen Pylorusstenose." *Medizin Klinische* 8 (1912): 1702.

Randolph, J.G. "The Gastric Tube for Esophageal Replacement in Children." *Pediatric Surgery International* 11 (1996): 221–223.

_____. "History of the Section on Surgery, the American Academy of Pediatrics: The First 25 Years, 1948–1973." *Journal of Pediatric Surgery* 34, no. 5, Supplement 1 (1999): 3–18.

Raphaely, R.C., and J.J. Downes, Jr. "Congenital Diaphragmatic Hernia: Prediction of Survival." *Journal of Pediatric Surgery* 8 (1973): 815.

Raveenthiran, V. "Knowledge of Ancient Hindu Surgeons on Hirschsprung's Disease: Evidence from Sushruta Samhita of 1200–600 BC" *Journal of Pediatric Surgery* 46, no. 11 (November 2011): 2204–2208.

Ravel, M.V., et al. "Costs of Congenital Diaphragmatic Hernia Repair in the United States — Extracorporeal Membrane Oxygenation Foots the Bill." *Journal of Pediatric Surgery* 46 (2011): 617–624.

Ravitch, M.M. *A Century of Surgery, 1880–1980.* Philadelphia and Toronto: J.B. Lippincott, 1981), 238–398.

_____. "Intussusception." In *Pediatric Surgery*, 4th ed., edited by K.J. Welch, et al., 868–882. Chicago: Year Book, 1986.

_____. "Intussusception in Infancy and Childhood: An Analysis of 77 Cases Treated by Barium Enema." *New England Journal of Medicine* 259 (1958): 1058–1064.

_____. *Intussusception in Infants and Children.* Springfield, IL: Charles C. Thomas, 1959.

_____. "Reduction of Intussusception by Barium Enema." *Surgery, Gynecology and Obstetrics* 99 (1954): 431–435.

Ravitch, M.M., and R.H. Morgan. "Reduction of Intussusception by Barium Enema." *Annals of Surgery* 135 (1952): 596–605.

Ravitch, M.M., and R.M. McCune, Jr. "Reduction of Intussusception by Hydrostatic Pressure: An Experimental Study." *Bulletin of Johns Hopkins Hospital* 82 (1948): 550–568.

Ravitch, Mark. "The Story of Pyloric Stenosis." *Surgery* 48, no. 6 (December 1960): 1117–1143.

Reed, E.N. "Infant Disemboweled at Birth — Appendectomy Successful." *Journal of the American Medical Association* 61 (1913): 199.

Rees, C.M., MB, ChB., et al. "Peritoneal Drainage or Laparotomy for Neonatal Bowel Perforation? A Randomized Controlled Trial." *Annals of Surgery* 248, no. 1 (July 2008): 44–51.

Rehbein, F. "Imperforate Anus: Experiences with Abdomino-Perineal and Abdomino-Sacroperineal Pull-Through Procedures." *Journal of Pediatric Surgery* 2 (1967): 99.

_____, S. Von, and H. Zimmermann. "Result with Abdominal Resection in Hirschsprung's Disease." *Archives of Disease in Childhood* 35 (1960): 29–37.

Reid, J. "Anatomical Observations." *Edinburgh M and S J* 46 (1836): 70.

Reinprecht, A., et al. "Medos Hakim Programmable Valve in the Treatment of Hydrocephalus." *Child's Nervous System* (1997).

Reisman, D., M.D., Sc.D. *The Story of Medicine in the Middle Ages.* New York: Paul B. Hoeber/ Harper and Brothers, 1936, 23–24.

Replogle, R.L. "Esophageal Atresia: Plastic Sump Catheter for Drainage of the Proximal Pouch." *Surgery* 54 (1963): 296–298.

Retan, G.M. "Nonoperative Treatment of Intussusception." *American Journal of Disease in Childhood* 33 (1927): 765–770.

Rhoads, J.E., and C.E. Koop. "The Surgical Management of Imperforate Anus." *Surgical Clinics of North America* (1955): 1251–1257.

_____, R.L. Pipes and J.P. Ranjale. "A Simultaneous Abdominal and Perineal Approach in Operations of Imperforate Anus with Atresia of the Rectum and Rectosigmoid." *Annals of Surgery* 127: 552.

Ribbink-Goslinga, A.M.C., and J.C. Molenaar. "Pediatric Surgery, Past, Present and Future." *Bulletin de la Societé des Sciences Medicales du Grand-Duchie de Luxembourg, Chirurgie Pediatrique Numero Special* (1987): 20–30.

Richardson, W.F., and J.B. Carman, trans. *Andreas Vesalius: On the Fabric of the Human Body*, vol. I. San Francisco: Norman, 1998.

_____. *Andreas Vesalius: On the Fabric of the Human Body*, vol. V. Novato, CA: Norman, 2007, 65–66.

Richter, H.M. "Congenital Atresia of the Oesophagus: An Operation Designed for Its Cure. With a Report of Two Cases Operated Upon by the Author." *Surgery, Gynecology and Obstetrics* (October 1913): 397–402.

_____. "Congenital Pyloric Stenosis: A Study of Twenty-Two Cases with Operation by the Author." *Journal of the American Medical Association* 62 (January 31, 1914): 353–356.

_____. "Positive Pressure Apparatus for Intrathoracic Operations: Preliminary Report.," *Surgery, Gynecology and Obstetrics* (November 1908): 583–585.

_____. "Pyloric Stenosis in Infancy, with a Study of Eleven Cases Personally Operated Upon." *Surgery, Gynecology and Obstetrics* (June 1911): 568–575.

Richter, H. M., III, M.D. Personal communication.

Ricketts, R.R. "The Role of Paracentesis in the Management of Infants with Necrotizing Enterocolitis." *Annals of Surgery* 52 (1986): 61.

Ricketts, R.R., S.R. Luck, and J.G. Raffensperger. "Circular Myotomy for Primary Repair of Long Gap Esophageal Atresia." *Journal of Pediatric Surgery* 16, no. 3 (1981): 365–369.

Ricketts, R.R., et al. "Modern Treatment of Cloacal Exstrophy." *Journal of Pediatric Surgery* 26 (1991): 444–450.

Rickham, P.P. "The Dawn of Pediatric Surgery: Johannes Fatio (1649–1691), His Life, His Work and His Horrible End." *Progress in Pediatric Surgery* 20 (1986): 95–105.

_____. "Denis Browne, Surgeon." in *Progress in Pediatric Surgery* 20 (1986): 67–74.

_____. *The Metabolic Response to Neonatal Surgery.* Cambridge, MA: Harvard University Press, 1957.

_____. "Vesico-Intestinal Fissure." *Archives of Disease in Childhood* 35 (1960): 97–102.

Riley, Murdoch. *Maori Healing and Herbal.* Paraparaumu, New Zealand: Viking Sevenseas, 2010, 8.

Ring-Mrozik, E., and T.A. Angerpointer. "Historic Aspects of Hydrocephalus." *Progress in Pediatric Surgery* 20 (1986): 158–251.

Rixey, P.M., et al. "The Official Report of the Case of President McKinley."

Rixford E. "Failure of Primary Rotation of the Intestine (Left-Sided Colon) in Relation to Intestinal Obstruction." *Annals of Surgery* 72 (1920): 114–120.

Robarts, F.H. "The Origins of Paediatric Surgery in Edinburgh." *Journal of the Royal College of Surgeons of Edinburgh* 14 (November 1969): 307–308.

Robertson, H.E., and J.V.W Kernohan. "The Myenteric Plexus in Congenital Megacolon." *Proceedings of Staff Meeting at the Mayo Clinic* 13 (1938): 123–125.

Robinson, A.C. "Case of Congenital Deformity." *Maryland Medical and Surgical Journal* 2 (1841): 162–165.

Roentgen, W.C. "On a New Kind of Rays." *Science New York* 3 (February 14, 1896): 227–231.

Rogers, L. "Exomphalos." *British Journal of Surgery* 29 (1941): 37–38.

"Rokitansky." Wikipedia, http://en.wikipedia.org.

Rosenberg, H., M. D., and Jean Axelrod, K.B.A. http://www.anesthesia-analgesia.org.

Rosenman, L.D., M.D. *The Surgery of Jehan Yperman.* Xlibris, 2002, 1–27.

_____. trans. *The Major Surgery of Guy de Chauliac.* Xlibris, 2007.

Rosenman, L.D. *The Surgery of Pierre Franco, an English translation.* Xlibris, 2006.

Rosner, Fred. Trans. and ed. *Julius Preuss' Biblical and Talmudic Medicine.* New York: Sanhedrin, 1978, 201.

Ross, V.P. "The Results of Sympathectomy." *British Journal of Surgery* 23 (1935): 433–443.

Rossier, R., and S. Sarrut. "Delplanque, l'Enterocolitis Ulcero-necrotique due Premature." *Annals of Pediatrics* 6 (1977): 1428–1436.

Rossiter, B. *Autopsy Reports on Connecticut Medical History,* 11–12. 1692.

Rothenberg, R.E., and T. Barnett. "Bilateral Herniotomy in Infants and Children." *Surgery* 37 (1955): 947 – 50.

Rothenberg, S.S. "Thoracoscopic Repair of Tracheo-Esophageal Fistula in Newborns." *Journal of Pediatric Surgery* 37 (2002): 869–872.

Rowe, M.I., and H.W. Clatworthy. "The Other Side of the Pediatric Inguinal Hernia." *Surgical Clinics of North America* 51 (1971): 1371–76.

Rubin, E.L., and M.D. Liverp. "Radiological Aspects of Anomalies of Intestinal Rotation." *Lancet* 2 (1935): 1222–1226.

Russell, R.H. "Inguinal Hernia and Operative Procedure." *Surgery, Gynecology, Obstetrics* 41 (1925): 605 – 9.

Rutkow, I.M. "Beaumont and St. Martin: A Blast from the Past." *Archives of Surgery* 133, no. 11 (November 1960): 1259.

Sandler, A.D., et al. "Unsuccessful Air-Enema Reduction of Intussusception: Is a Second Attempt Worthwhile?" *Pediatric Surgery International* 15 (1999): 214–216.

Sankaran, P.S., and P.J. Deshpande. "Sushruta." In *Scientists,* edited by V. Raghvan, 44–72. Delhi: Publications Division of Government of India, 1990.

Santoni-Rugiu, Paolo, and Phillip J. Sykes. *A History of Plastic Surgery.* Berlin, Heidelberg: Springer-Verlag, 2007.

Santuli, T.V., and W.A. Blanc. "Congenital Atresia of the Intestine: Pathogenesis and Treatment." *Annals of Surgery* 154 (1961): 939–948.

Santulli, T.V., et al. "Acute Necrotizing Enterocolitis in Infancy: A Review of Sixty-Four Cases." *Pediatrics* 55, no. 3 (1975): 376–88.

Sari, N., C. Buyukanal and B. Zolficar. "Circumcision Ceremonies at the Ottoman Palace." *Journal of Pediatric Surgery* 31, no. 7 (1996): 920–924.

Sarma, P.J. "Hindu Medicine and Its Antiquity." *Annals of Medical History* 3 (1931): 318–320.

Sauer, C.J., J.C. Langer and P.W. Wales. "The Versatility of the Umbilical Incision in the Management of Hirschsprung's Disease." *Journal of Pediatric Surgery* 40 (2005): 385–389.

Sayers, M.P., and E.J. Kosnik. "Percutaneous Third Ventriculostomy: Experience and Technique." *Child's Brain* 2 (1976): 24–30.

Sayre, L.A. *Orthopedic Surgery.* New York: Appleton, 1885.

Scaife, E.R., et al. "Use of Abdominal Sonography for Trauma at Pediatric and Adult Trauma Centers: A Survey." *Journal of Pediatric Surgery* 44 (2009): 1746–1749.

Scannell, J.G. "Willy Meyer (1858–1932), Historical Perspective." *Journal of Thoracic and Cardiovascular Surgery* 111 (May 1996): 1112.

Scarborough, John. *Roman Medicine.* Ithaca, NY: Cornell University Press, 1969.

Scarff, J.E. "Endoscopic Treatment of Hydrocephalus: Description of Aventriculoscope and Preliminary Report of Cases." *Archives of Neurology and Psychiatry* 35 (1935): 853–861.

Scarpa, A. *A Memoir on the Congenital Club-foot of Children and the Mode of Correcting that Deformity.* Edinburgh: Constable, 1818.

Schaefer A. "Cas de scission du canal intestinal en plusieurs portions, par vice primitif de conformation." *J Compl du dict d sc méd Paris* 24 (1926): 58–66.

Scharli, A.F. "Kinder Mid Mibbildungen in der Renaissance (nach den Aufzeichnungen von Fabricius Hildanus, 1560–1634)." *Kinderchirurgie* 39 (1984): 296–301.

_____. "Malformations of the Anus and Rectum and Their Treatment in Medical History." *Progress in Pediatric Surgery* 11 (1978) 141–172.

Schey, W.L., J.S. Donaldson and J.R. Sty. Malrotation of Bowel: Variable Patterns with Different Surgical Considerations." *Journal of Pediatric Surgery* 28 (1993): 96–101.

Schier F. "Laparoscopic Surgery of Inguinal Hernias in Children: Initial Experience." *Journal of Pediatric Surgery* 35 (2000): 1331– 35.

_____, P. Montupet, and C. Esposito. Laparoscopic Inguinal Herniorraphy in Children: A Three-Center Experience with 933 Repairs." *Journal of Pediatric Surgery* 37 (2002): 395 – 97.

Schiller, M., T.R. Frye and E.T. Boles. "Evaluation of Colonic Replacement of the Esophagus in Children." *Journal of Pediatric Surgery* 6 (1971): 753.

Schnaufer, L., J.L. Talbert and A. Haller, et al. "Differential Sphincter Studies in the Diagnosis of Ano-Rectal Disorders of Childhood." *Journal of Pediatric Surgery* 2, no. 6 (1967): 538–543.

Schooler, L. "The Wounded from Santiago." In *The Western Surgical Association, 1891–1900,* edited by Jacob K. Berman, 99–106. Indianapolis: Hackett, 1976.

Schuster, S.R. "A New Method for the Staged Repair of Large Omphaloceles." *Surgery, Gynecology, Obstetrics* 125 (1967): 837–850.

Schwartz, M.Z., D. Tapper and R.I. Solenberger. "Management of Perforated Appendicitis in Children: The Controversy Continues." *Annals of Surgery* 197: 407–411.

Schwyzer, F. "A Case of Congenital Hypertrophy and Stenosis of the Pylorus." *New York Medical Journal* 64 (1896): 674.

Scott, W.J.M., and J.J. and Morton. "Sympathetic Inhibition of Large Intestine in Hirschsprung's Disease." *Journal of Clinical Investigation* 9 (1930): 247–262.

Senn, N. "Pompeian Surgery and Surgical Instruments." *Medical News, American Periodical Series Online* (December 28, 1895): 26, 67.

Senn, N., M.D., Ph.D. *Experimental Surgery.* Chicago: W.T. Keener, 1889, 478–503.

Seror, D., A. Szold and S. Nissan. "Felix Wurtz, Surgeon and Pediatrician." *Journal of Pediatric Surgery* 26, no. 10 (October 1991): 1152–55.

Shalkow, J., J.A. Quiros and N.A. Shorter. "Small Intestinal Atresia and Stenosis." Web MD Professional, 8 March 2010. Accessed 9 November 2010, http://emedicine.medscape.com/article/939258-overview.

Shandling, B. "A New Technique in the Diagnosis of Hirschsprung's Disease." *Canadian Journal of Surgery* 4 (1961): 298–305.

Sharma, A.K., et al., "Esophageal Atresia and Tracheo-Esophageal Fistula, a Review of 15 Years' Experience." *Pediatric Surgery International* 16 (2000): 478–482.

Sharma, P.V. *History of Medicine in India.* Delhi: Indian National Academy of Science, 1992.

She, Y.X., and E.C. Tong. *Textbook of Pediatric Surgery,* 3d ed. Beijing: Peoples Medical, 1995, 1.

Shepherd, J.A. "Acute Appendicitis: A Historical Survey." *Lancet* 2 (1954): 299–302.

Shermata, D.W., and J.A. Haller, Jr. "A New Preformed Transparent Silo for the Management of Gastroschisis." *Journal of Pediatric Surgery* 10 (1975): 973–975.

Sieber, W.K. "Hirschsprung's Disease." Chapter 106 in *Pediatric Surgery*, 4th ed., edited by K.J. Welch, J.G. Randolph, M.M. Ravitch, J.A. O'Neill, Jr. and M.I. Rowe, 995–1020. Chicago: Year Book, 1986.

Sigerist, H.E. *History of Medicine: Primitive and Archaic Medicine*, vol. 1. New York, Oxford: Oxford University Press, 1951, 128.

Simons, G.W. "The Diagnosis and Treatment of Deformity Combinations in Clubfeet." *Clinical Orthopaedics and Related Research* 150 (1980): 229.

Simonsen, L., et al. "Effect of Rotavirus Vaccination Programme on Trends in Admission of Infants to Hospital for Intussusception." *Lancet* 358 (2001): 1224–1229.

Simpson, A.J., J.C. Leonidas, I.H. Krasna, J.M. Becker and K.M. Schneider. "Roentgen Diagnosis of Midgut Malrotation: Value of the Upper Gastrointestinal Radiographic Study." *Journal of Pediatric Surgery* 7 (1972): 243–252.

Simpson, J.Y. "On Foetal Peritonitis." *Edinburgh M and S J* 52 (1839): 26.

Skaba, R. "Historic Milestones of Hirschsprung's Disease (Commemorating the 90th Anniversary of Professor Harald Hirschsprung's Death)." *Journal of Pediatric Surgery* 42 (2007): 249–251.

Smith, E.D. "The Bath Water Needs Changing, but Don't Throw Out the Baby: An Overview of Anorectal Anomalies." *Journal of Pediatric Surgery* 22 no. 4 (1987): 335–348.

Smith, G. Elliot, and R. Dawson Warren. *Egyptian Mummies.* London: Allen and Unwin, 1924, 100.

Smith, G.K. "The History of Spina Bifida, Hydrocephalus, Paraplegia, and Incontinence." *Pediatric Surgery International* 17 (2001): 424–432.

Snow-Smith, Joanne. *Leonardo da Vinci: Ancient Medical Texts, History and Influence.* Seattle: University of Washington, 2004.

Snyder, W.H., Jr., and L. Chaffin. "Embryology and Pathology of the Intestinal Tract: Presentation of 40 Cases of Malrotation." *Annals of Surgery* 140 (1954): 368–379.

So, H.B., et al. "Endorectal 'Pull-through' without Preliminary Colostomy in Neonates with Hirschsprung's Disease," *Journal of Pediatric Surgery* Vol. 15 (1980): 470–471.

Soare, P., and A.J. Raimondi. "Intellectual and Perceptual Motor Characteristics of Treated Myelomeningocele Children." *American Journal of Diseases of Children* 131 (1977): 199–204.

Soave, F. "Endorectal Pull-Through: A Twenty-Year Experience," address by guest speaker to the American Pediatric Surgical Association in 1984. *Journal of Pediatric Surgery* 20 (1985): 568–571.

_____. "Hirschsprung's Disease: A New Surgical Technique." *Archives of Disease in Childhood* 39 (1964): 116–124.

_____. "A New Original Technique for Treatment of Hirschsprung's Disease." *Surgery* 56 (1964): 1007–1014.

Soper, R.T., and F.E. Miller. "Modification of Duhamel Procedure: Elimination of Rectal Pouch and Colorectal Septum." *Journal of Pediatric Surgery* 3 (1968): 376–385.

Soper, R.T., and J.M. Opitz. "Neonatal Pneumoperitoneum and Hirschsprung's Disease." *Surgery* 51 (April 1963): 527–533.

Soranus. *Gynecology, Book II, Care of the Newborn*, trans. Owsei Temkin, M.D. Baltimore, London: Johns Hopkins University Press, 1956, 79–127.

Spencer, W.G. *Celsus De Medicina*, vol. 1. London: Heinemann, 1971, 364–369.

_____, ed. *Celsus De Medicina.* Cambridge: Harvard University Press, 1971.

Spencer-Wells, T. "Intussusception of Caecum and Colon Replaced by Gastrostomy." *Transactions of the Pathological Society of London* 26 (1863): 541–542.

Spier, L. "Havasupai Ethnography." *Anthropological Papers of American Museum of Natural History*, Vol. 29 (1928): 284–85.

Spink, M.S., and G.L. Lewis. *Albucasis: On Surgery and Instruments.* Berkeley, Los Angeles: University of California Press, 1973.

Spitz, L. "Gastric Transposition of Esophageal Replacement." *Pediatric Surgery International* 11 (1996): 218–220.

Spitz, L., L. Kiely, and T. Sparnon. "Gastric Transposition for Esophageal Replacement in Children." *Annals of Surgery* 206 (1987): 73.

Spitz, L., et al. "Long Gap Esophageal Atresia." *Pediatric Surgery International* 11 (1996): 462–465.

Spriggs, N.I. "Congenital Intestinal Occlusions: An Account of 24 Unpublished Cases with Remarks Based Thereon and Upon the Literature of the Subject." *Guys Hosp Rep Lond* 66 (1912): 143–218.

State, D. "Surgical Treatment for Idiopathic Congenital Megacolon (Hirschsprung's Disease)." *Surgery, Gynecology and Obstetrics* 9 (1952): 201–212.

Stauffer, U.G., and P. Herrmann. "Comparison of Late Results in Patients with Corrected Intestinal Malrotation with and without Fixation of the Mesentery." *Journal of Pediatric Surgery* 15 (1980): 9–12.

Steele, C., M.D., F.R.C.S. "Case of Deficient Oesophagus." *Lancet* (October 20, 1888): 764.

Stephens, F. Douglas "Congenital Imperforate Rectum, Recto-Urethral and Recto-Vaginal Fistulae." *Australia and New Zealand Journal of Surgery* 22, no. 3 (1953): 161–172.

_____. "Imperforate Anus." *Medical Journal of Australia* 46, no. 2 (1959): 803–805.

_____. *Photographic Album of Anorectal Anomalies and Sphincter Muscles.* Chicago: Kascot, 1986.

_____. "Wingspread Anomalies, Rarities, and Super Rarities of the Anorectum and Cloaca." *Birth Defects: Original Article Series* 24, no. 4 (1988): 581–585.

Stephens, F. Douglas, and W. Donnellan. "'H-Type' Urethroanal Fistula." *Journal of Pediatric Surgery* 12, no. 1 (1977): 95–102.

Stephens, F.D., and D.E. Smith. "Classification, Identification and Assessment of Surgical Treatment of Anorectal Anomalies." *Pediatric Surgery International* 1 (1986): 200.

Stephens, Douglas S. Interviewed by John M. Hutson, M.D., May 30, 2007, Melbourne, Australia. "Oral History Project," published by the American Academy of Pediatrics.

Stern, C. "Uber Pylorus Stenose Beim Saugling nebst Bemerkungen uber deren Chirurgschen Benhandlung." *Deutsche Me. Wchnscr.* 24 (1898): 601.

Stevens, F.D., DSO, FRCS. Personal communication.

Stevenson, L.G. "The Stag of Richmond Park." *Bulletin of the History of Medicine* 22 (1948): 467–475.

Stewart, A., et al. "Malignant Disease and Diagnostic Irradiation in Utero," *Lancet* (September 1, 1956): 447.

Still, G.F. *The History of Pediatrics.* London: Dawson's of Pall Mall, 1965, 40–41.

Stolar, C., P. Dillon and C. Reyes. "Selective Use of ECMO in the Management of Congenital Diaphragmatic Hernia." *Journal of Pediatric Surgery* 23 (1988): 207.

Stone, E. *Medicine Among the American Indians.* New York: Paul B. Hoeber, 1932, 78–87.

Strach, E.H. "Club-Foot Through the Centuries." *Progress in Pediatric Surgery* 20 (1986).

Stringer, M.D., and I.E. Willettz. "John Hunter, Frederick Treves and Intussusception." *Annals of the Royal College of Surgeons* 82 (2000): 18–23.

Stromeyer, L. "Contributions to Operative Orthopaedics, or Experiences with Subcutaneous Section of Shortened Muscles and their Tendons." *Clinical Orthopedics* 97 (1973): 2–4.

Suita, S., et al. "Clinical Characteristics and Outcome of Wilms' Tumors with a Favorable Histology in Japan: A Report from the Study Group for Pediatric Solid Malignant Tumors in the Kyushu Area, Japan." *Journal of Pediatric Surgery* 41 (2006): 1501–1505.

The Surgery of Theodoric, vol. I, Books I and II, trans. E. Campbell, M.D., and J. Colton, M.A. New York: Appleton-Century-Croft, 1955.

The Surgery of Theodoric, vol. II, Books III and IV, trans. E. Campbell, M.D., and J. Colton, M.A. New York: Appleton-Century-Crofts, 1960.

Sutherland, G.A., and W.W. Cheyne. "The Treatment of Hydrocephalus by Intra Cranial Drainage." *British Medical Journal* 2 (1898): 1155–1157.

Swain, V.A.J. "Sketches of Surgical Cases Drawn from 1884–87 at the East London Hospital for Children, Shadwell." *Progress in Pediatric Surgery* 20 (1986): 265–280.

Swenson, O. "Early History of the Therapy of Hirschsprung's Disease: Facts and Personal Observations over 50 Years." *Journal of Pediatric Surgery* 31 (1996): 1003–1008.

_____. "My Early Experience with Hirschsprung's Disease." *Journal of Pediatric Surgery* 24 (1989): 839–845.

_____. "Partial Internal Sphincterectomy in the Treatment of Hirschsprung's Disease." *Annals of Surgery* 160 (1964): 540–550.

Swenson, O., and A.H. Bill. "Resection of Rectum and Rectosigmoid with Preservation of Sphincter for Benign Spastic Lesions Producing Megacolon." *Surgery* 214 (1948): 212–220.

Swenson, O., and A.M. Holschneider. "Historical Review." Chapter 1 in *Hirschsprung's Disease and Allied Disorders,* 2d ed., edited by A.M. Holschneider and P. Puri, 3–7. Amsterdam: Harwood, 2000.

Swenson, O., H.F. Rheinlander and I. Diamond. "Hirschsprung's Disease: A New Concept of the Etiology, Operative Results in Thirty-Four Patients." *New England Journal of Medicine* Vol. 24 (1949): 551–556.

Swenson, O., J.H. Fisher and H.E. MacMahon. "Rectal Biopsy as an Aid in the Diagnosis of Hirschsprung's Disease." *New England Journal of Medicine* 253 (1955): 632–635.

T.E.C., Jr., M.D. "L'Hôpital des Enfants Malades, the World's First Children's Hospital Founded in Paris in 1802." *Pediatrics* 67, no. 5 (May 1981): 670.

Tai, J.H., et al. "Rotavirus Vaccination and Intussusception: Can We Decrease Temporally Associated Background Cases of Intussusception by Restricting the Vaccination Schedule?" *Pediatrics* 118 (2006): E258–264.

Tandler J. "Entwicklungsgeschichte des menschlieben Duodenum in früben Embryonal-studien." *Morphol Jahrb* 29 (1902): 187–216.

Taussig, H.B. "Tetrology of Fallot: Especially the Care of the Cyanotic Infant and Child." *Pediatrics* 1 (1948): 307.

Teitelbaum, D.H., et al. "Hirschsprung's Disease and Related Neuromuscular Disorders of the Intestine." Chapter 94 in *Pediatric Surgery,* 5th ed., edited by J.A. O'Neill, Jr., M.I. Rowe, J.L. Grosfeld, E.W. Fonkalsrud and A.C. Coran, 1381–1424. St. Louis: Mosby, 1998.

"Tetanus." Wikipedia, http://en.wikipedia.org.

Theremin E. "Ueber congenitale occlusion des dünndarms." *Deutsche Ztschr f. Chir* 8 (1877): 34–71.

Thomas, C.G., Jr. "Jejunoplasty for the Correction of Jejuna Atresia." *Surgery, Gynecology, Obstetrics* 129 (1966): 545–546.

_____, and J.M. Carter. "Small Intestinal Atresia: The Critical Role of a Functioning Anastomosis." *Annals of Surgery* 179 (1974): 663–370.

Thomas, H.O. "A New Wrench for Club-Foot." *Provincial Medical Journal* 5 (1886): 286.

Thomasson, B., and M. Ravitch. "Wilms' Tumor." *Urological Survey* 11 (1961): 83–100.

Thomasson, B.H. "Congenital Esophageal Atresia: Mercury Bag Stretching of the Upper Pouch in a Patient without Tracheo-Esophageal Fistula." *Surgery* 71 (1972): 661–663.

Thompson, D.J. "Obstructed Labour with Complicated Presentation and Exomphalos." *British Medical Journal* 2 (1944): 45.

Thorwald, Jurgen. *The Dismissal: The Incredible Story of the Last Years of Ferninand Saurbruch, One of the Great Surgeons of Our Time.* New York: Pantheon, 1961.

Tipton, C.M. "Sushruta of India, an Unrecognized Contributor to the History of Exercise Physiology." *Journal of Applied Physiology* 104 (2008): 1553–1556.

Tittel, K. "Über eine Angeborener Mibbildung des Dickdarmes." *Wien Klinische Wochenschr.* 14 (1901): 903–907.

Tomaselli, V., et al. "Long Term Evaluation of Esophageal Function in Patients Treated at Birth for Esophageal Atresia." *Pediatric Surgery International* 19 (2003): 40–43.

Torek, F. "The First Successful Case of Resection of the Thoracic Portion of the Oesophagus for Carcinoma." *Surgery, Gynecology, Obstetrics* 16 (1913): 614–617.

Torkildsen, A. "A New Palliative Operation in Cases of Inoperable Occlusion of the Sylvian Aqueduct." *Acta Chirurtgie Scandinavia* 82 (1939): 117–124.

Torres, A.M., and M.M. Ziegler. "Malrotation of the Intestine." *World J Surg* 17 (1993): 326–331.

Tosousy, V. "Salute to Pediatric Surgery in Czechoslovakia." *Journal of Pediatric Surgery* 3 (1968): 647–648.

Touloukian, R.J. "Abdominal Trauma in Children." *Surgery, Gynecology, Obstetrics* 127 (September 1968): 561.

_____. "Abdominal Visceral Injuries in Battered Children." *Pediatrics* 42 (1968): 642.

_____. "Pediatric Surgery Between 1860 and 1900." *Journal of Pediatric Surgery* 30 (1995): 911–916.

_____. "Protocol for the Non-Operative Treatment of Duodenal Hematoma in Children." *American Journal of Surgery* 145 (1983): 330.

_____, et al. "Surgical Experiences with Necrotizing Enterocolitis in the Infant." *Journal of Pediatric Surgery* 2, no. 5 (1967): 389–401.

Tovar, J.A., M. Suñol, B. Lopez de Torre, C. Camarero and J. Torrado. "Mucosal Morphology in Experimental Intestinal Atresia: Studies in the Chick Embryo." *Journal of Pediatric Surgery* 26 (1991): 184–189.

Treves, F. "Idiopathic Dilatation of the Colon." *Lancet* 1 (1898): 276–279.

_____. "Intussusception." In *Intestinal Obstruction: Its Varieties with their Pathology, Diagnosis and Treatment*, 2d ed. London: Cassell, 1899, 141–184.

_____. "The Treatment of Intussusception." *Proceedings of the Medical Society of London* 8 (1885): 83–94.

Trombley, S. *Sir Frederick Treves, Surgeon and Extraordinary Edwardian*. London: Routledge, 1989.

Truesdale, P.E. "Diaphragmatic Hernia in Children with a Report of Thirteen Operative Cases." *New England Journal of Medicine* 213, no. 24 (December 12, 1935): 1159–1172.

_____. "Recurrent Hernia through the Diaphragm." *Annals of Surgery* 79, no. 5 (May 1924): 751–757.

Tulipan, N., and J.P. Bruner. "Myelomeningocele Repair in Utero: A Report of Three Cases." *Pediatric Neurosurgery* 28 (1998): 177–180.

Tulp, N. *Observationum Medicarum, Libri III*. Amsterdam: Apud Ludovicum Elzevirum, 1641.

Tulpius, N. *Observationes Medicae*. Amsterdam, 1685.

Turco, V.J. "Resistant Congenital Clubfoot — One-Stage Posteromedial Release with Internal Fixation: A Follow-Up Note of a Fifteen-Year Experience." *Journal of Bone and Joint Surgery* 61A (1979): 805.

Turner P. "The Radical Cure of Inguinal Hernia in Children." *Proceedings of the Royal Society of Medicine* 5 (1912): 133 –140.

Twersky, I. *A Maimonides Reader*. Library of Jewish Studies. Springfield, NJ: Behrman House, 1972, 99.

Ure, B., et al. "Laparoscopically Assisted Gastric Pull-Up for Long Gap Esophageal Atresia." *Journal of Pediatric Surgery* 38, no. 11 (2003): 1661–2.

Utah State University Cooperative Extension. http://extension.usu.edu.

van der Laan, M., et al. "The Role of Laparoscopy in the Management of Childhood Intussusception." *Surgical Endoscopy* 15 (2001): 373–376.

van der Zee, D.C., and N.M.A. Bax. "Laparoscopic Repair of Acute Volvulus in a Neonate with Malrotation." *Surg Endosc* 9 (1995): 1123–1124.

van der Zee, D.C., et al. "Thoracoscopic Elongation of the Esophagus in Long Gap Esophageal Atresia." *Journal of Pediatric Surgery* 42 (2007): 1785–1788.

Van Eijck, F.C., et al. "Closure of Giant Omphalocele by Abdominal Wall Component Separation Technique in Infants." *Journal of Pediatric Surgery* 43 (2008): 246–250.

van Forest, P. "De Capitis et Cerebri Morbis ac Symptomatic." *Observationum Medicininalium*, Libri III. Leiden: Ex Officio Plantiniana Raphelemgii, 1587.

Venel, J.A. *Memoires de la Société des Sciences Physiques de Lausanne*, vol. 2. 1789, 66, 197.

Vesalius, A. *De Humani Corporis Fabrica, Libri Septem*. Basel, 1555, 5.

Viner, R. "Using the History of Paediatrics." *Health and History* 1 (1999): 162–168.

"Virchow." Wikipedia, http://en.wikipedia.org.

Visick, C. "An Umbilical Hernia in a Newly Born Child." *Lancet* 1 (1873): 829.

Viza, D., S. Ein and B. Shandling. "Thirteen Years of Gastric Tubes." *Journal of Pediatric Surgery* 3 (1978): 638.

Vogel, V. "American Indian Medicine." In *Civilization of the American Indian* series. Norman: University of Oklahoma Press, 1970, 1–11 and 183–184.

Voison. *Journ. Ger de Med et de Chir de la Soc de Med de Paris* xxi (1804) : 353.

von Recklinghausen, F. "Untersuchungen uber die Spina Bifida." *Virchows Archiv für Pathologische, Anatomie und Physiologie und für Klinische Medizin* 105 (1886): 243–330.

Vries, J.K. "An Endoscopic Technique for Third Ventriculostomy." *Surgical Neurology* 9 (1978): 165–168.

Wade, R.B., and Royle, N.D. "The Operative Treatment of Hirschsprung's Disease: A New Method with Explanation of Technique and Results of Operation." *Medical Journal of Australia* 1 (1927): 137–139.

Wakamatsu, N., et al. "Mutations in SIP1, Encoding Smad Interacting Protein-1, Cause a Form of Hirschsprung Disease." *Nature Genetics* 27 (2001): 369–370.

Wakefield, E.G., and C.W. Mayo. "Intestinal Obstruction Produced by Mesenteric Bands in Association with Failure of Intestinal Rotation." *Archives of Surgery* 33 (1936): 47–67.

Waksman, S.A., and H.B. Woodruff. "Bacteriostatic and Bacteriocidal Substances Produced by Soil Actinomycetes." *Proceedings of the Society of Experimental Biology* 45 (1941): 609–614.

Waldman, A.M. "Medical Ethics and Hopelessly Ill Children," Part II. *Journal of Pediatrics* 88 (1976): 890–892.

Walker, M.L., J. MacDonald and L.C. Wright. "History of Ventriculoscopy: Where Do We Go from Here?" *Pediatric Neurosurgery* 18 (1992): 218–223.

Walker, T.J., and J. Griffiths. "Congenital Dilatation and Hypertrophy of Colon Fatal at Age of Eleven Years." *British Medical Journal* 2 (1893): 230–231.

Walsh, J.J. *Old Time Makers of Medicine: The Story of Students and Teachers of the Sciences Related to Medicine During the Middle Ages*. New York: Fordham University Press, 1911, 23–25.

Wang, S.H. "Hua Tuo, Military Doctor Career." *Negative* 1, no. 3 (2010): 13–15.

_____. "Sun Si-Miao and Acupuncture." *Negative* 1, no. 2 (2010): 17–19.

_____. "Sun Si-Miao and Health Cultivation." *Negative* 1, no. 2 (2010): 15–17.

_____. "Zhang Zhong-jing and H1N1." *Negative* 1, no. 1 (2010): 7–8.

Wangensteen, O.H. "New Operative Techniques in the Management of Bowel Obstruction: (1) Aseptic Decompressive Suction Enterostomy (2) Aseptic Enterostomy for Removal of Obstructing Gallstone (3) Operative Correction of Non-Rotation." *Surgery, Gynecology, Obstetrics* 75 (1942): 675–692.

_____, and C.O. Rice. "Imperforate Anus; A Method of Determining the Surgical Approach." *Annals of Surgery* 92, no. 1 (1930): 77–81.

Wardle, H.N. "Stone Implements of Surgery from San Miguel Island, California." *American Anthropologists, New Series* 15, no. 4 (October-December 1913): 656–659.

Warren, J.C. "Inhalation of Ethereal Vapor for the Prevention of Pain in Surgical Operations." *Boston Medical and Surgical Journal* 35 (1846): 375–379.

Warren, R.P., F.R.C.S. "History of Excision of the Rectum." *Proceedings of the Royal Society of Medicine* 50 (1957): 599–600.

Wasiljew, B., A. Besser and J. Raffensperger. "Treatment of Bilateral Wilms' Tumors, a Twenty-Two Year Experience." *Journal of Pediatric Surgery* 17 (1982): 265.

Waterston, D.J. "Colonic Replacement of Esophagus (Intrathoracic)." *Surgical Clinics of North America* 44 (1964): 1441.

_____, R.E. Bonham-Carter and E. Aberdeen. "Oesophageal Atresia, Tracheo-Oesophageal Fistula: A Study of Survival in 218 Infants." *Lancet* 1 (1962): 819–822.

Watkins, D.E. "Gastroschisis, with Case Report." *Virginia Medical Monthly* (1943): 42–44.

Waugh, G.E. "Congenital Malformations of the Mesentery: A Clinical Entity." *Brit J Surg* 15 (1928): 438–449.

Wear, A. *Knowledge and Practice in English Medicine, 1550–1680.* Cambridge: Cambridge University Press, 2000, 223.

Webb, C.H., and O.H. Vangensteen. "Congenital Intestinal Atresia." *Am J Dis Child* 41 (1931): 262–284.

Webber, B., and A. Vedder. *In the Kingdom of the Gorillas: Fragile Species in a Dangerous Land.* New York, London: Simon and Schuster, 2001, 49.

Weber, W. "Ueber Einen Technische Neurerung be der Operation der Pylorus Stenoses des Sauglings." *Berlin Klinische Wehschr.* 47 (1910): 763.

Webster, W. "Embryogenesis of the Enteric Ganglia in Normal Mice and in Mice that Develop Congenital Aganglionic Megacolon." *Journal of Embryology and Experimental Morphology* 30 (1973): 573–585.

Weiner, E. "Bilateral Partial Nephrectomies for Large Bilateral Wilms' Tumors." *Journal of Pediatric Surgery* 11 (1976): 867.

Weiner, E.S., R.J. Touloukian, B.M. Rodgers, J.L. Grosfeld, E.S.I. Smith, M.M. Ziegler and A.G. Coran. "Hernia Survey of the Section of Surgery of the American Academy of Pediatrics." *Journal of Pediatric Surgery* 31 (1996): 1166 — 69.

Weitzman, J.J., and R.S. Vanderhoof. "Jejunal Atresia with Agenesis of the Dorsal Mesentery with 'Christmas Tree' Deformity of the Small Intestine." *American Journal of Surgery* 111 (1966): 443–449.

Welch, K.J. "Cloacal Exstrophy (Vesico-Intestinal Fissure)." In *Pediatric Surgery*, edited by M.M. Ravitch and K.J. Welch, 802–808. Chicago, London: Year Book Medical, 1979,

Wells, C. *Bones, Bodies and Disease.* New York, Washington: Frederick A. Praeger, 1964, Illustrations 5, 11 and 63.

Werler, M.M., J.E. Sheehan, and A.V. Mitchell. "Maternal Medication Use and Risk of Gastroschisis and Small Intestinal Atresia." *American Journal of Epidemiology* 155 (2002): 26–31.

Wesson, D.E. *Pediatric Trauma: Pathophysiology, Diagnosis and Treatment.* New York: Taylor and Francis, 2006, 34.

Whipple, A.O., M.D. *The Role of the Nestorians and Muslims in the History of Medicine.* Princeton, NJ: Allen O. Whipple Surgical Society/Princeton University Press, 1967.

Whitehouse, F., J.A. Bargan and C.F. Dixon. "Congenital Megacolon: Favourable End-Results of Treatment by Resection." *Gastroenterology* 1 (1943): 922–937.

Wilms, M. "Fall von Hirschsprunger Krankheit." *Münch Med Wschr* 42 (1905): 2061–2063.

Willard, D.F.T. *The Surgery of Childhood.* Philadelphia: J.B. Lippincott, 1910.

Willetts, I.E. "Jessop and the Wilms' Tumor." *Journal of Pediatric Surgery* 38 (2004): 1496–1498.

Williams, A.N. "Labor Improbus Omnia Vincit": Ambrose Paré and Sixteenth Century Child Care." *Archives of Disease in Childhood* 88 (2003): 985–989.

_____, and J. Williams. "Proper to the Duty of a Chirurgeon": Ambroise Paré and Sixteenth Century Paediatric Surgery." *Journal of the Royal Society of Medicine* 97 (2004): 446–449.

Williams, C. "Congenital Defects of the Abdominal Wall." *Surgical Clinics of North America* 10 (1930): 805–809.

Williams, G.R. "Presidential Address: A History of Appendicitis." *Annals of Surgery* 197 (1983): 495–506.

Wilmore, D.W., and S.J. Dudrick. "Growth and Development of an Infant Receiving All Nutrients Exclusively by Vein." *Journal of the American Medical Association* 203 (1968): 140–144.

Wilmore, D.W., et al. "Total Parenteral Nutrition in Infants with Catastrophic Gastrointestinal Anomalies." *Journal of Pediatric Surgery* 4 (1969): 181–189.

Wilms, M. "Dauerspasmus an Pylorus, Cardia, Sphincter der Blasé und des Mastdarmes." *Deutsche Zetschrift Chirurgie* 144 (1918): 68–71.

_____. *Die Mischegeschwulste der Niere.* Leipzig: Verlag von Arthur Georgi, 1899.

"Wilms, Max." Wikipedia, http://www.wikipedia.org.

Wilson, Jay, Boston Children's Hospital, and Charles Stollar, Babies Hospital, New York. Personal communication. Dr. Stollar has the original manuscript: G. McCauley, "An Account of Visceral Herniation." *Philosophical Transactions of the Royal College of Physicians* (1754): 625.

Wise, T.A. *Commentary on the Hindu System of Medicine.* London: Trubner, 1860.

Wood, W., and C. Kelsey. *Diseases, Injuries and Malformations of the Rectum and Anus.* London, 1857, 378 [the reference can be found in *Emem. de l'Academy des Sciences*, vol. 10, page 36].

Wright, J. "The Dawn of Surgery, the Ritual Mutilations of Primitive Magic and Circumcision." *New York Medical Journal and Medical Record* (January 17, 1923): 103–105.

Wu, Y., et al. "Primary Insertion of a Silastic Spring-Loaded Silo for Gastroschisis." *The American Surgeon* 69 (2003): 1083–1086.

Yang, G.C., et al. "A Dinucleotide Mutation in the Endothelin-B Receptor Gene Is Associated with Lethal White Foal Syndrome (LWFS): A Horse Variant of Hirschsprung Disease." *Human Molecular Genetics* 7 (1998): 1047–1052.

Young, D.G. "Intussusception." In *Pediatric Surgery*, 3d ed., edited by J.A. O'Neill, Jr., et al., 1185–1198. Chicago: Year Book, 1998.

Yudin, S.S., M.D., F.A.C.S. (hon.), F.R.C.S. (hon.) Colonel, Red Army M.C., Moscow, U.S.S.R. "The Surgical Construction of 80 Cases of Artificial Esophagus." *Surgery, Gynecology and Obstetrics* 78, no. 6 (June 1944): 561–583.

Zachary, R. B. "Acute Intussusception in Children." *Archives of Disease in Childhood* 30 (1955): 32–36.

Zadek, I., and E. Barnett. "The Importance of the Ligaments of the Ankle in Correction of Congenital Clubfoot." *Journal of the American Medical Association* 69 (1917): 1057.

Zanardi, L.R., et al. "Intussusception Among Recipients of Rotavirus Vaccine: Reports to the Vaccine Adverse Event Reporting System." *Pediatrics* 107 (2001): E97.

Zeigler, E.E., and S.J. Carlson. "Early Nutrition of Very Low Birthweight Infants." *Journal of Fetal and Neonatal Medicine* 3 (March 2009): 191–197.

Zeit, R.F. "Congenital Atresia of the Esophagus with Esophago-Tracheal Fistula." *Journal of Medical Research* 26 (1912): 45–55.

Zhang, J-z. "Anal Fistula." In *Anorectal Diseases Among Children*, J-z. Zhang, 235. Beijing: International Academic, 1993.

_____. Personal communication with John G. Raffensperger, 2010.

_____, and Li, L. "Evolution of Surgical Pediatrics in

China." *Journal of Pediatric Surgery* Supplement 1, vol. 38 (2003): 48–52.

Zimmerman, J.E. *Dictionary of Classical Mythology.* New York: Harper and Row, 1964.

Zimmerman, L.M., and I. Veith. *Great Ideas in the History of Surgery,* 2d rev. ed. New York: Dover, 1967, 68–71.

Zimmerman, L.M., and J.E. Zimmerman. "The History of Hernia Treatment." In *Hernia,* 2d ed. edited by I.M. Nyhus and R. E. Condon, 4. Philadelphia: J. B. Lippincott, 1978.

Zollinger, R.E., and R.E. Gross. "Traumatic Subdural Hematoma: Explanation of Late Onset of Pressure Symptoms." *Journal of the American Medical Association* 103 (1934): 245.

Zuelzer, W.W., and J.L. Wilson. "Functional Intestinal Obstruction on Congenital Neurogenic Basis in Infancy." *American Journal of Disease in Childhood* 75 (1948): 40–64.

About the Contributors

John **Burrington**, M.D., has been chief of pediatric surgery at the Denver Children's Hospital and professor of surgery at the University of Colorado and later was the chief of pediatric surgery at the University of Chicago. He is now involved with the El Paso County Medical Society in promoting public health.

Norris **Carroll**, M.D., formerly chief of orthopedic surgery at the Children's Memorial Hospital in Chicago, is an emeritus professor of orthopedic surgery at Northwestern University. He is noted for his work on children with clubfoot and the orthopedic problems associated with spina bifida.

Jack H. T. **Chang**, M.D., formerly chair of the department of surgery at the Denver Children's Hospital and then an associate professor of pediatric surgery at the Texas Health Sciences Center in Dallas, then became director of pediatric surgery, Presbyterian/St. Luke's Medical Center in Denver. He is the pediatric liaison for the Rocky Mountain Hospital for Children in Denver and the author of *Timelines in Pediatric Surgery*.

Catherine M. **Cosentino**, M.D., trained for pediatric surgery at Children's Memorial Hospital in Chicago. She is the senior pediatric surgeon in her home city in Arizona.

Stephen **Dolgin**, M.D., formerly chief of pediatric surgery at Mt. Sinai Hospital and Medical School and surgeon in chief at the Schneider Children's Hospital on Long Island, is a professor of surgery at the Hofstra NS-LTD Medical School.

Edward **Doolin**, M.D., practices general pediatric and fetal surgery at the Philadelphia Children's Hospital. He has carried out research on such varied problems as intestinal atresia and the culture of human cells for reconstructing the trachea.

Arlene **Ein**, R.N., has been since its inception the meeting coordinator of the Canadian Association of Paediatric Surgeons. She and her husband Sigmund H. Ein extensively researched the history of pediatric surgery in Canada and in 2009 published the *History of Pediatric Surgery in Canada* with *The History of the Canadian Association of Paediatric Surgeons: The First 40 years.*

Sigmund H. **Ein**, M.D., former president of the Canadian Association of Pediatric Surgeons 1991–1993, is an associate professor of the Adjunct Clinical Faculty of the University of Toronto and an Honorary Staff Surgeon at the Hospital for Sick Children, Toronto. He retired in 2004, and he and his wife Arlene live in Oshawa, Canada. He continues to write and reviews manuscripts for the *Journal of Pediatric Surgery*. He is also on the courtesy surgical staff at Lakeridge Health, Oshawa, and has been honored by an annual Simpson-Ein lecture at the Toronto Children's Hospital.

Praveen **Goyal**, M.D., MRCPCH, is a consultant pediatrician for the child health unit for the Oxford Radcliffe Hospital of the National Health Trust. He is especially interested in pediatric neuro-disability, children in public care and adopted children. With Dr. Andrew Williams he has published on the pediatric surgical work of Ambrois Paré in the *Journal of Pediatric Surgery*.

W. Hardy **Hendren**, M.D., established the department of pediatric surgery at Massachusetts General Hospital and then was the chief of surgery at Boston Children's Hospital from 1982 until

1998. In 1985, he was appointed the first Distinguished Robert E. Gross Professor of Surgery at Harvard. The American Urological Association gave him an award for his efforts in reconstructing complex uro-genital malformations in children. He travels worldwide to see former patients, is on the staff of the Boston Children's Hospital and is an honorary surgeon at the Massachusetts General Hospital.

Juda **Jona**, M.D., practiced pediatric surgery in Milwaukee, Wisconsin, and then became the chief of pediatric surgery at the Evanston Hospital in Evanston, Illinois. He was also an attending pediatric surgeon at the Children's Memorial Hospital. In 2005, the March of Dimes gave Dr. Jona the Health Leadership Award for his work with children with birth defects. He is the senior pediatric surgeon at Sparrow Hospital and clinical professor of surgery at Michigan State University, Lansing.

Randall **Powell**, M.D., a former staff surgeon at the Naval Hospital in San Diego and later a professor of surgery and pediatric surgeon at the University of South Alabama in Mobile, in 2009 became an emeritus professor at the university. He has written on colon atresia and trauma in children and has an abiding interest in teaching residents and medical students.

John G. **Raffensperger**, M.D., was director of pediatric surgery at the Cook County Children's Hospital and in 1970 went to Children's Memorial Hospital in Chicago, where he eventually became the surgeon in chief. After retiring, he spent short terms doing surgery in Haiti and St. Lucia, then returned to work at the Cook County and Children's Hospital before finally retiring with his wife, Susan Luck, also a pediatric surgeon, to Sanibel, an island off the west coast of Florida.

V. **Raveenthiran**, M.D., was born in a small town in southern India. He and his brother both suffered with congenital bilateral talipes equinovarus, a form of clubfoot. The resulting treatment, which included extensive hospitalization and exposure to surgeons, kindled his interest in medicine. He is an honorary fellow of the Royal College of Surgeons, Glasgow, and a professor of pediatric surgery at the SRM University of Chennai. His interests range from laparoscopic surgery to the treatment of the many common injuries and surgical diseases seen in India.

Richard **Ricketts**, M.D., is chief of pediatric surgery at Emory University in Atlanta, Georgia. His clinical work and teaching skills led in 1996 to the establishment of a training program in pediatric surgery at Emory. He was the chairman of the Surgical Section of the American Academy of Pediatrics from 2007 to 2008.

John **Ruge**, M.D., is the medical director of the Midwest Children's Brain Tumor Center and an attending pediatric neurosurgeon at the Advocate Lutheran Children's Hospital in Park Ridge, Illinois. He has developed techniques for using ultrasound to guide the insertion of tubes to shunt spinal fluid into the brain and for neuro-endoscopy and is on the faculty of the Rush Medical Center, Chicago.

Andrew **Williams**, M.D., is a consultant community pediatrician and the curator of archives at the Northhampton General Hospital in the United Kingdom, where he specializes in pediatric neuro-disability. He is also a medical historian with a special interest in child health from the sixteenth to the nineteenth centuries. A Fellow of the Royal Historical Society, he is a past president of the British Society for the History of Paediatrics and Child Health.

Jin-zhe **Zhang**, M.D., was appointed in 1950 to establish the first surgical unit in the department of pediatrics of the Peking University Hospital. In 1955, he went to the 750-bed Beijing Children's Hospital as chief of surgery. There he started training programs for pediatric surgeons and almost single-handedly brought Western surgical methods to China. In 2000 the British Association of Pediatric Surgeons awarded him the Denis Brown Gold Medal.

Index

337